Microsurgery in Periodontal and Implant Dentistry

Hsun-Liang (Albert) Chan
Diego Velasquez-Plata
Editors

Microsurgery in Periodontal and Implant Dentistry

Concepts and Applications

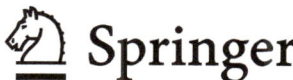 Springer

Editors
Hsun-Liang (Albert) Chan
School of Dentistry
University of Michigan
Ann Arbor, MI, USA

Diego Velasquez-Plata
School of Dentistry
University of Michigan
Ann Abor, MI, USA

ISBN 978-3-030-96873-1   ISBN 978-3-030-96874-8   (eBook)
https://doi.org/10.1007/978-3-030-96874-8

This Springer imprint is published by the registered company Springer Nature Switzerland AG
The registered company address is: Gewerbestrasse 11, 6330 Cham, Switzerland

For my family Chu-chun (June) Hsiao and Claire Chan, who gave full support and understanding while I was away for assembling this impactful book!

For my mentor Dr. Velasquez, who invited me to this exciting journey, guided me through the learning curve, and showed me what can be accomplished with the operating microscope!

For Dr. Wen-Xiang Zhang, who spent countless hours of practicing microsuturing with me and inspired me to think outside the box.

For Ms. Kay Demonge, who gives endless support and resources for us to provide microsurgery training courses and the warm friendship!

For my mentor Dr. Hom-Lay Wang, who showed me what endurance and perseverance mean and gave me full freedom to pursue microsurgery learning and education!

Hsun-Liang (Albert) Chan

Soli Deo Gloria.

To my wife Jeanine, for her love and support.

To Kieran, Braden, Fiona, and Rafe, my inspiration and joy.

Diego Velásquez-Plata

Foreword

Microsurgery has catapulted the entire field of minimally invasive surgery to new heights by operating with less damage to the body than conventional surgical procedures. Furthermore, minimally invasive surgery is typically associated with less pain, a shorter postoperative recovery, and fewer complications compared to traditional techniques. Microsurgery has truly become a "game changer" to advance all fields of medicine and dentistry. Clinicians can now deliver highly precise and exquisite operations with improved visualization and more idealized assessment of the soft and hard tissues. In this text, *Microsurgery in Periodontal and Implant Dentistry: Concepts and Applications*, Drs. Chan and Velásquez-Plata thoughtfully deliver a landmark textbook on the subject encompassing all aspects of these techniques focused on periodontal and dental implant surgical operations. The book not only provides outstanding technical information but also shows corresponding high-quality illustrations and video links for readers. It is an informative book on the evolving field of oral and periodontal surgery. This comprehensive textbook will be of great value to both early stage clinicians and expert practitioners alike to be informed on the state-of-the-art in microsurgery to advance patient care and clinical outcomes.

The opening chapter by the book's editors provides an illuminating historical perspective on the transition from traditional surgical procedures to microsurgery in both medicine and dentistry. This chapter underscores the tremendous advancements that have been made in optics and instrumentation to allow the delivery of exquisite surgical operations. The subsequent chapter on *wound healing in microsurgical procedures* (Burkhardt) provides the oral tissue repair perspective on the strong rationale on why microsurgery, how it can optimize clinical care, and promote greater wound stability above conventional macroscopic techniques. This is the direction that all fields of medicine are headed and for those in periodontology and implant dentistry. It is incumbent on practitioners to implement forms of microsurgical techniques into their practices to optimize clinical outcomes. The next three chapters on fundamentals of the *operating microscope* (Marron-Tarrazzi), *design requirements of the microsurgical instruments* (Burkhardt), and *suturing techniques* (Velásquez-Plata and Cross) focus on critical elements required with surgical microscopes corresponding surgical instrumentation and suturing materials. The microscopes and instrumentation go hand in hand in the proper preparation and implementation of microsurgical techniques. These chapters provide excellent overviews on the technical details and corresponding information on the major enhancements in the microscopy, instrumentation, and suturing biomaterials that make minimally invasive surgical operations a clinical reality. These major technical achievements highlight clinical improvements in intraoral soft tissue wound closure and stability with microsurgery and how these approaches are superior to traditional procedures that usually exhibit suboptimal incision placements and suturing.

The *practical considerations of incorporating microsurgery into the daily workflow* of clinical practice is pragmatically displayed by Dr. Velásquez-Plata. This chapter demonstrates to practitioners on how a busy practice setting delivering complex clinical care can be efficiently organized. This section highlights all aspects from infection control to ergonomic recommendations in working clinically with a surgical microscope setup in the clinical care environment.

The second half of the book carefully applies the concepts of microsurgery and minimally invasive intraoral surgical techniques to clinical periodontology, oral surgery, and implant dentistry. These chapters not only provide overviews on *microscope-assisted periodontal and peri-implant surgery* (Duran) by traditional incisions with microsurgical blades, but also the use of *laser ablation techniques for soft tissue plasty procedures to address intraoral pigmentation (Aoki, Mizutani, and Mikami)*. The successive chapters on *periodontal regenerative procedures* (Cortellini and Velásquez-Plata) demonstrate the ability to use minimally invasive techniques for reconstructive procedures, with and without biomaterials to rebuild lost periodontal support. *Pre-prosthetic procedures* (Nakata) combining periodontal and prosthodontic aspects are well highlighted for optimizing esthetic and functional outcomes in complex restorative cases.

The final four chapters provide a comprehensive overview on microsurgical techniques that prepare the patient for dental implant reconstructive procedures for oral rehabilitation. These chapters include *microscope-assisted ridge augmentation* (Llamosa), *sinus floor augmentation* (Sirinirund, Testori, Scaini, Velásquez-Plata, and Chan), *immediate implant placement* (Tibbetts, Pearson, and Cross), and the *peri-implant complication management* (Gomez-Meda and Esquivel). These sections provide the technical details for improved minimally invasive clinical approaches through microsurgery.

I am confident that you will greatly profit by this book in your improved understanding and clinical application of microsurgery for the successful delivery of oral and periodontal procedures. Drs. Chan and Velásquez-Plata have illuminated our clinical community with this text on the "new standard" of quality oral, periodontal, and implant microsurgical therapy to benefit our patients. Please Enjoy!

William V. Giannobile, DDS, MS, DMedSc
Dean and Professor
Department of Oral Medicine
Infection, and Immunity
Harvard School of Dental Medicine
Member of the Faculty of Medicine
Harvard Medical School
Boston, MA, USA

A Tribute to Dennis A. Shanelec, DDS:
The Father of Periodontal Microsurgery

Dennis Shanelec and I became friends as members of the twelve-person Periodontal Practice Development Network Study Club in 1985. It was a unique group of talented clinicians brought together initially to develop and strengthen overall practice management documentation techniques and evolved to include treatment planning and clinical treatment techniques. Membership restrictions required no overlapping practice areas, resulting in complete openness and sharing of propriety office information, and clinical techniques, so that it was a continuum of our periodontal education.

While the entire group of members became much more than casual friends, Dennis and I quickly bonded into an extraordinary friendship that lasted 34 years. We were both interested in expanding and sharing our mutual knowledge and understanding of periodontal anatomy, physiology, disease and its treatments. Early on I recognized that Dr. Shanelec was one of the most forward thinking, talented, and detail-oriented teachers that I had ever known and was a microsurgeon with the highest level of knowledge of periodontal anatomy and physiology who was willing to share his knowledge and microsurgical techniques and applications with those who wanted to become better therapists. I particularly admired the treatment results achieved with autogenous soft tissue grafts and root coverage. Even for experienced surgeons, those outcomes were difficult to consistently achieve. Dr. Shanelec shared autogenous soft tissue graft techniques, emphasizing precise right-angle incisions in preparing the graft recipient sites and precise suturing techniques using microsurgical instruments and much smaller suture needles and sutures than were normally used at the time. After detailed discussions at study club meetings, and personal visits to his Santa Barbara office in the late 1980s and early 1990s, I realized the critical importance of enhanced vision offered by microsurgery and the significantly improved outcomes that could be achieved compared to those using macrosurgery. I strongly urged Dr. Shanelec to publish some of his microsurgical material and results. He agreed to do so, but only if I coauthored the material with him. Over the years, we published over 15 papers in referred journals and textbooks.

The application of enhanced vision to all periodontal plastic surgery, diagnoses, and initial nonsurgical therapy as well as other periodontal surgical procedures became obvious. In discussing the consistently excellent results Dr. Shanelec achieved with microsurgical approaches to periodontal plastic surgical procedures and dental implant placements, I was led, in 1990, to purchase a set of 4.5× loupes and a surgical microscope. The enhanced visual acuity offered by the surgical microscope and microsurgical techniques readily surpassed the visual as well as the dexterity limits of what periodontal macrosurgery can routinely achieve.

Being in the officer chain of the American Academy of Periodontology and looking for new annual meeting material, I convinced Dr. Shanelec to give the first continuing education course on Periodontal Microsurgery at the 1992 AAP Annual Meeting in Orlando. He agreed only on the condition that I would present with him. As a result, Dr. Shanelec presented the results from several years of his experience with microsurgery. I presented what he had taught me over the previous three years. Dr. Shanelec and I presented a second program entitled "The Status of Periodontal Microsurgery" at the 1993 AAP Annual Scientific meeting, and in 1994 both a lecture and hands-on course entitled, "Periodontal Microsurgery in Private Practice," were given in June to the Washington State Society of Periodontists. At the 1996 AAP Annual Scientific Meeting in New Orleans, a special video session entitled "A Morning with the Masters" was given, with two of the three presenters being Drs. Shanelec and Tibbetts. Dr. Shanelec presented a video on a microsurgical connective tissue graft technique, and Dr. Tibbetts presented a video on a microsurgical technique for a posterior sextant of osseous surgery. The courses were well received and the AAP considered having us provide hands-on microsurgery courses in the various districts, but that was not ultimately feasible.

In 1993, using his personal resources Dr. Shanelec planned, built, and equipped the Shanelec Microsurgical Training Institute in Santa Barbara, California. He developed a curriculum and began to teach and share his knowledge and skills in periodontal microsurgery with all those who were eager and motivated to become better, more highly skilled periodontal microsurgeons. Dr. Shanelec developed microsurgical instruments, training models, suture platforms, and many other things to teach microsurgical incisions and suturing techniques at the MTI, he taught over 600 dentists, and he lectured extensively both nationally and internationally.

In 2006 Drs. Shanelec and Tibbetts founded the Dentorati Microsurgical Study Club. Both served as mentors to this seven-member group of Periodontists who had already been using surgical microscopes in their own private practices. Dr. Shanelec allowed the group to utilize the Microsurgical Training Institute for meetings, with the goal of members sharing experiences, and working to improve microsurgical procedures.

Dr. Shanelec developed the Simplified Microsurgical Implant Lifelike Esthetics (SMILE) Technique for the extraction and immediate replacement of teeth in the anterior esthetic zone. He treated over 600 cases with a long-term success rate of over 98% on very complex cases. His technique is described in detail in Chapter 13 of this textbook.

Dr. Dennis A. Shanelec was an incredibly unique visionary and truly a brilliant thinker and creative problem solver. His personal commitment to practicing and teaching periodontal and implant microsurgery has transformed what is now possible for our patients. He is definitely the "Father of Periodontal Microsurgery." For his contributions to the profession, Dr. Shanelec was awarded the American

Academy of Periodontology Master Clinician Award in 2010. His passing in 2019 was a significant loss to his wife, his friends and colleagues, the field of dentistry and Periodontology in particular!

Leonard S. Tibbetts, DDS, JMSD

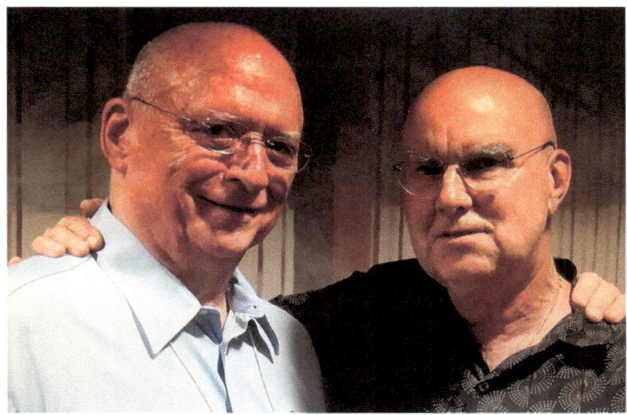

Dr. Leonard Tibbetts (left) and Dr. Dennis Shanelec (right)

Acknowledgments

Once it became clear that the operating microscope was to become an essential part of our clinical practice and for education, countless hours were dedicated towards learning about this technology and its application in periodontics and implant dentistry. The primary sources of information were scattered throughout the digital world in the form of articles, books, and videos, mainly found in the scientific libraries of the medical microsurgical specialties. The same thirst of knowledge drove us to seek hands-on training opportunities to enhance our skills and continue learning about this discipline and its applications. These learning experiences allowed us to interact with world-renowned opinion leaders in the field of microsurgery in periodontics and implant dentistry.

Over the years, it became apparent that there was a void in the literature when it came down to having a primary source of information that would guide and help both the novice and the more experienced microsurgeon in the quest of exploring the full potential that the operating microscope has to offer in the field of periodontics and implant dentistry. Writing a textbook about this topic had been an idea that we had been toying around with until one day in May of 2020 the opportunity to write a book to fill such a void manifested itself unambiguously, and the rest is history. We started inviting mentors, friends, and colleagues who have been instrumental in the development and promulgation of the benefits of implementing the operating microscope in the clinical periodontal and dental implant practice. We were very fortunate to find positive and supporting answers to collaborate in this project from the members of this "dream team" in this discipline.

The editors would like to express their most sincere appreciation to those individuals who have dedicated countless hours of hard work sharing their knowledge and expertise making this book a tangible reality. Dr. William Giannobile, Dean of Harvard School of Dental Medicine, Boston, Massachusetts, has been very kind to write the foreword of this book. Dr. Giannobile had been an advocate of the incorporation of microsurgery training while he served as Chairman of the Department of Periodontics and Oral Medicine (POM) at the University of Michigan. Dr. Leonard Tibbetts from Arlington, Texas, has written a heartfelt eulogy on his friend and colleague, Dr. Dennis Shanelec, the father of microsurgery in periodontics and dental implants. Dr. Rino Burkhardt from Zurich, Switzerland, has contributed to two chapters related to wound healing and instrument design for microsurgical applications. Dr. Irene Marron Tarrazi from Miami, Florida, shared her knowledge in the fundamentals of the operating microscope. Dr. David Cross from Springfield, Illinois, coauthored a chapter on the science and art of microsuturing. Dr. Juan Carlos Duran from Santiago, Chile, developed a chapter regarding microscope-assisted periodontal and peri-implant plastic surgery. Drs. Akira Aoki, Koji Mizutani, and Risako Mikami from Tokyo, Japan, put together a chapter illustrating the combination of the operating microscope and lasers for ablation of intraoral pigmentations. Dr. Pierpaolo Cortellini from Florence, Italy, participated by sharing his game changing experience dealing with minimally invasive procedures in microscope-assisted periodontal regenerative therapy. Dr. Kotaro Nakata, from Kyoto, Japan, has elaborated material dealing with microscope-assisted pre-prosthetic surgery. Dr. Lizette Llamosa, from Monterrey, Mexico, crafted a chapter illustrating the application of the microscope in ridge augmentation procedures and site preparation for implant placement. Dr. Benyapha Sirinirund from Ann Arbor, Michigan, in collaboration with Dr. Tiziano Testori from Cuomo, Italy, and Dr. Riccardo Scaini from Melzo, Italy, has assembled a chapter focused on the incorporation of the operating microscope in sinus augmentation procedures. Dr. Bryan Pearson from Lafayette, Louisiana, together with Drs. Leonard Tibbetts and David Cross has coauthored a chapter describing the SMILE technique introduced by the late Dr. Shanelec utilized for immediate implant placement in the anterior area. Last, but not least, Dr. Ramon Gomez-Meda from Leon, Spain, and Dr. Jonathan Esquivel from New Orleans, Louisiana, worked together in a chapter showcasing the management of implant complications assisted by the operating microscope.

Acknowledgments are also expressed to the editorial expertise from Ms. Allison Wolf, Ms. Smitha Diveshan, Mr. Vishal Anand and Mr. Dhanapal Palanisamy at Springer for their support and expertise guiding us throughout the process associated with the assembling of all this information in such manner that a textbook can be finally produced for the educational advantage of those interested in the fascinating world of microsurgery applied into periodontics and implant dentistry.

With most sincere gratitude to all,

Dr. Hsun-Liang (Albert) Chan, Dr. Diego Velásquez-Plata

Contents

Introduction to Microsurgery

Hsun-Liang (Albert) Chan and Diego Velasquez-Plata

Contents

Abstract

The operating microscope (OM) was first adopted by otorhinolaryngology professionals for performing surgeries in the early twentieth century. Soon after, it was used by other medical specialties, for example, ophthalmologists, vascular surgeons, reconstructive and plastic surgeons, etc. It was not until the late 1990s when incorporation of OM training in the accreditation standards for advanced specialty education programs in endodontics took place in the USA. The main advantages of using the OM over surgical loupes are unprecedented and adjustable magnification, and confocal illumination, among others. The use of OM for

H.-L. (A.) Chan (✉)
Periodontics Graduate Program, University of Michigan School of Dentistry,
Ann Arbor, MI, USA

D. Velasquez-Plata
Private Practice, Fenton, Michigan, USA

Adjunct Clinical Assistant Professor Periodontics and Oral Medicine Department,
The University of Michigan School of Dentistry, Ann Arbor, MI, USA

© The Author(s), under exclusive license to Springer Nature Switzerland AG 2022
H.-L. (A.) Chan, D. Velasquez-Plata (eds.), *Microsurgery in Periodontal and Implant Dentistry*, https://doi.org/10.1007/978-3-030-96874-8_1

1

performing periodontal and implant surgeries is on a rise. Its uses are justified by improved wound healing at tissue and clinical levels, as documented in the literature. Moving forward, more high-quality studies are encouraged to support the use of OM. A systematic and strategic approach should be developed among interested stakeholders to explore the full capacity of OM for elevating patient care quality and to create innovative learning modules and simulators for improving microsurgical education.

Keywords

Microsurgery · Minimally invasive surgical procedures · Periodontics Dental implant

1 Introduction

Curiosity has kindled humanity's passion for knowledge and understanding by harnessing realities and deciphering codes that explain the mysteries of its tangible existence. The world continually poses challenges that entice the intellect to interpret its secret language and unmask hidden truths that help us formulate axioms that define our own understanding of being. Unraveling our physical reality has been a fundamental task in the lives of researchers, entrepreneurs, and science leaders following the same common objective: to understand the how and the why of the mechanisms that make up the universe we live in. Whether elevating our gaze at the stars or looking down at the soil, we have been using visual aids to empower the naked eye in its quest for seeing beyond its inherent physiological limitations.

Understanding the world that surrounds us became a necessity to many. Simple lenses crafted with primitive tools opened a door hundreds of years ago that was not to be closed. According to Bradbury, the first individual credited with utilizing a convex lens to magnify an object's image was Ibn al Haitham (962–1038) [1]. It would take hundreds of years for the lens making industry to figure out how to eliminate chromatic aberrations, become proficient in lens polishing, and assembling mechanical contraptions that would facilitate the operation of magnifying tools for industrial and medical applications.

It is hard not to take for granted today's advances in technology that allows clinical operators to incorporate magnifying tools in their daily activities for use as extensions of their own body when providing patient care. In the field of microsurgery, dentistry has greatly benefited from trials and errors, discoveries, and challenges faced by medical colleagues. While otolaryngologists were at the tip of the spear and are credited with the first incursions utilizing an OM, techniques and armamentarium have been refined by an orchestrated collection of efforts by physicians applying microsurgical principles into their respective fields.

The specialty of endodontics embraced the OM as an essential part of their curriculum and mode of practice. The adoption by other dental specialties has advanced at a slow and steady pace. In the fields of periodontics and implant dentistry magnification has been acknowledged as advantageous for the delivery of care. The incorporation of the OM provides significant advantages that benefit patient care and operator well-being simultaneously. This textbook is a unique collaborative effort that brings together experts in the field of microsurgery from different geographical locations. The main goal of all the authors is to compile practical information that will help both novice and advanced clinician alike, to begin, improve, and master the utilization of the OM and microsurgical principles and philosophies with the ultimate goal of enhancing patient care and mental and physical well-being to those willing to challenge themselves to grow by adopting this discipline.

Within the pages of this textbook, the reader will be exposed to key information related to this topic; from wound healing principles, to understanding the mechanisms that regulate the OM and the armamentarium needed by the operator to execute its craft; from recommendations on incorporation of microsurgery to the daily clinical flow to rationale behind microscope-assisted care delivery in periodontal and peri-implant plastic surgery, periodontal regenerative therapy, pre-prosthetic applications, ridge augmentation related procedures, including maxillary antral augmentations and ending with immediate implant therapy and handling surgical and prosthetic complications in implant dentistry.

After studying this book and its supporting visual material, the reader will be able to embrace the rationale behind the incorporation of the OM in periodontics and implant dentistry and will be able to answer the question at the core of this endeavor: why bother working with an OM in periodontics and dental implant dentistry? The primary answer is simple: to see what needs to be done, so the hand can be told what to do. Once this is accomplished, the rest will follow: more delicate tissue manipulation and more accurate surface modifications via precise instrumentation will translate into less trauma, passive tissue approximation, clot stability, enhanced vascularization, thus increasing the predictability in successful clinical outcomes that depend on attention to regal minutia.

Welcome this book and its contents as a tool to help conquer a self-imposed challenge; an intellectual and psychomotor challenge that will help grow and explore the potential of your mind and your skills in a field that is waiting to be discovered and mastered.

2   History of Operating Microscope in Medicine

Names of opticians, scientists, textile and wine merchants like those of Zacharias and Hans Janssen, Galileo Galilei, Giovanni Faber, Anton von Leeuwenhoek, Robert Hook, and Jackson Lister are intimately associated with the assembling of the first microscopes, crafting chromatic-aberration free lenses and scoring numerous discoveries of micro-organisms and cells for the first time in the history of humankind. This craft would be elevated to a science by the work of Carl Zeiss and Ernst Abbé in Jena, Germany, who applied mathematical formulas to allow for a predictable and standardized lens making enterprise [2].

Sweden became the epicenter of microsurgical therapy in 1922 when an otolaryngologist, Carl-Olof Nylén reported his experience with a monocular OM he had designed to perform ear operations [3]. Like most innovations, the OM was not embraced immediately as the go to magnification tool to perform otic surgical procedures; contemporary key opinion leaders were still using surgical loupes with limited magnification. There was a lengthy hiatus until the OM became an indispensable tool in the operating room. In ophthalmology, Perritt reported in 1946, the use of a stationary microscope with an accessory illumination source to perform a superficial keratectomy [4, 5]. In 1954, H. Littmann published an article describing a binocular OM that allowed working at different magnification levels without having to exchange objective lenses or ocular pieces [6]. In vascular surgery, the next logical step to elevate the refinement of treatment execution was the incorporation of the OM as demonstrated by Jacobson and Suarez in 1960 [7, 8]. The advancements achieved on microvascular anastomosis opened the door to neurosurgeons, reconstructive surgeons (plastic, hand, and orthopedic surgeons), gastroenterologists, trauma specialists, urologists, and gynecologists to perform procedures that were not feasible before, thus enhancing the predictability of outcomes to levels not seen previously [9–13]. The following years witnessed a constant improvement on microscope design and versatility geared toward facilitating maneuverability, documentation, and performance. The addition of foot controls to operate zooming and mobility mechanisms, access ports to incorporate photographic and video cameras, dual binoculars for additional operators or assistant personnel, suspension arm features with locking breaks to provide positional stability to the supporting structures, optical filters, different source types of coaxial illumination, the addition of stereoscopic 3D vision and integrated laser applications are some of the most common additions that have made this technology a must have in the operating theater.

The adoption of the OM propelled the design of surgical armamentarium that could support the visual and psychomotor demands inherent to work being performed at high magnification levels. Reduced operating visual fields combined with a vertical plane of vision demand the utilization of instruments that do not interfere with the eye-to-target visual path. Therefore, most instruments that were used for conventional, macro-surgical procedures were adapted by reducing their size, incorporating specially designed finish features in active instrument sections, increasing the handle length, decreasing weight to maximize operational efficiency by reducing hand fatigue, and refining the cross-sectional profile and surface topography of the handle to facilitate execution of delicate digital movements in the presence of equally delicate tissue structures. In order to avoid coaxial light reflection by shiny and highly polished instrument surfaces, extrinsic finish coatings and treatments that mitigate luminous eye-fatigue sources for the operator have been incorporated. Suture thread diameters and needle swage and point design have also been modified to meet working needs associated with delicate tissue manipulation and tensionless wound edge approximation.

Training facilities and educational curriculum development followed to instruct and capacitate microsurgeons across all medical disciplines [14]. Exercises have been developed in different models, both in vitro and in vivo that prepare the microsurgeon in training to think, visualize, and execute the different steps associated with microsurgical performance prior to being exposed to the patient population in need of this expert delivered therapy [15, 16] (Fig. 1).

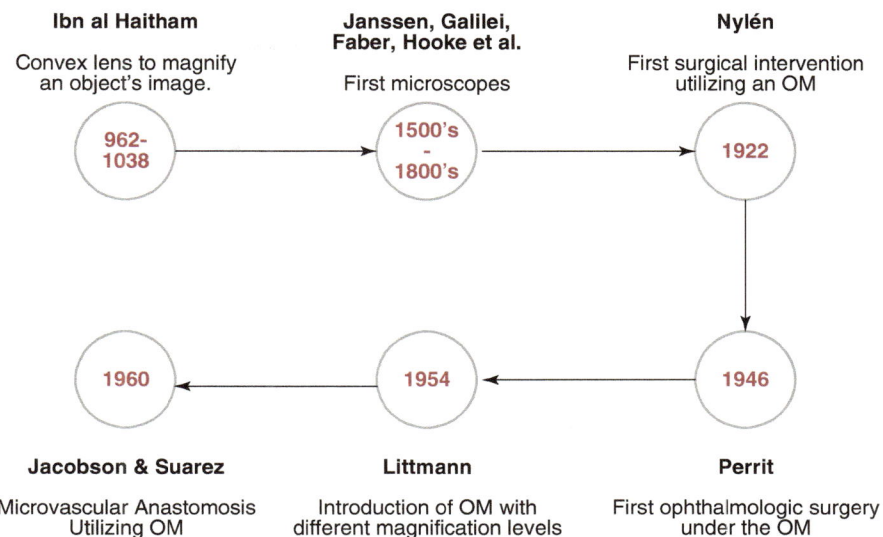

Fig. 1 Timeline landmark events: OM in medicine

3 History of Operating Microscope in Dentistry

Although at first glance the utilization of the OM in the dental field seems to be a relatively new discipline, when compared to historic events in the scientific and medical fields, the first steps toward incorporating this technology in dentistry date back to 1907 when Bowles presented a binocular, bi-objective (Greenough type stereoscopic visual device) microscope to be used in the dental operatory. This device came equipped with an electrical light/reflector combination that illuminated the working field [17]. The mechanical and functional shortcomings of this early model stagnated the interest and adoption of this technology into clinical applications.

In 1975, an otorhinolaryngologist suggested the use of the microscope as a practical tool in dentistry [18]. A few years later, efforts of a dentist and an otorhinolaryngologist, Drs. Apotheker and Jako, lead to the development of the first modern microscope equipped with accessories to allow for documentation (via still pictures and videotapes) and a CO_2 laser [19]. This instrument offered stereoscopic and binocular vision, magnification of 5–10× with high resolution, working distance between the object and the microscope of 200–300 mm, several options to mount it either to the dental chair, floor or ceiling, and independent source of illumination. In spite of having a well thought out product, the commercial enterprise supporting this innovation in the dental field did not prosper.

The dental world had to wait for efforts led by individual clinicians practicing endodontics in the early 1990s who demonstrated the undeniable advantages of incorporating microscopy in their field, for this technology to gain significant traction in the dental profession [20, 21]. Endodontic therapy is mostly performed on individual teeth, usually with operator–patient movements constricted to single planes and minimal engagement of axes of rotation (predominantly occlusal access for non-surgery and buccal access for surgical interventions) which facilitates task execution under the microscope. This simplistic kinematic interaction has been fundamental in the adoption of the OM by this dental discipline. The support of this novel approach to endodontics led to the celebration of the first symposium on microscope endodontic surgery which was held at the University of Pennsylvania School of Dental Medicine in 1993. In view of the interest aroused among the endodontic community, The American Association of Endodontists (AAE) sponsored a workshop on microscopy for endodontic program directors. This event was the catalyst that led to include microscopy training in the accreditation standards for advanced specialty education programs in endodontics in 1998 [22]. Within eight years, from 1999 to 2007, the use of microscopes by endodontists went from 52% to 90% [23].

The remaining dental specialties have not followed in unison the path blazed by the endodontic community. Isolated efforts have been showcased in pediatric dentistry, oral and maxillofacial surgery, prosthetic and restorative procedures and periodontal and implant therapy.

Chou and Pameijer demonstrated the significant benefits of utilizing stereomicroscope in the dental prosthetic laboratory in processes that require precision such as die trimming, wax pattern seals, and finishing and polishing both metal and porcelain materials [24]. Martignoni and Schonenberger showcased the microscope in fixed prosthodontics as an essential tool to execute work demanding high precision in tooth preparation, margin definition, and preservation of soft tissue integrity when working with the natural dentition [25].

Microscope-assisted exodontia has been documented and its merits illustrated by Schmidt and Boudro, emphasizing the reduction in morbidity and avoidance of undesirable sequelae when magnification and optimal field illumination are combined and made available with the use of the OM. Procedures such as teeth subluxation, elevation, and alveolar socket debridement and preservation can be performed with minimal trauma when the OM is incorporated as part of the surgeon's armamentarium [26] (Fig. 2).

4   History of OM in Periodontology and Implant Dentistry

Microscope-assisted periodontal therapy was introduced to the specialty of periodontology in 1992 by Shanelec and Tibbetts during the 78th American Academy of Periodontology annual meeting in Orlando, Florida. Since then, several publications have been made available defining the clinical philosophy behind this approach, describing the armamentarium required to perform microscope-assisted periodontal surgical procedures and spelling the benefits associated with the adoption of this way of clinical practice [27–35]. The current existing evidence supports the benefits

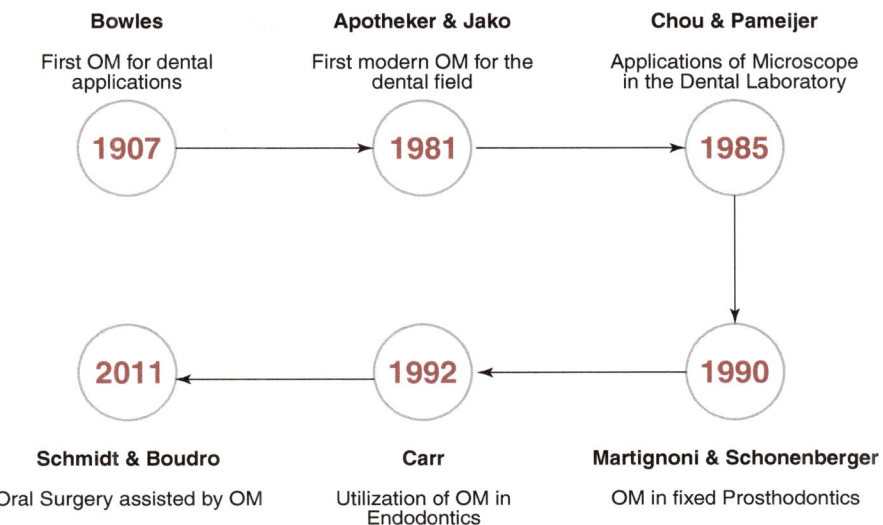

Fig. 2 Timeline landmark events: OM in Dentistry

and superiority of outcomes when utilizing the OM for surgical periodontal therapy geared toward regenerative and root coverage procedures.

The benefitting effects of high degrees of magnification provided by the OM in non-surgical periodontal therapy have also been documented. Facilitating the detection of calculus and its differentiation with tooth structures, while at the same time allowing for the identification of anatomical contours that ultimately lead to accurate access and efficient cleaning of radicular and dental surfaces while scaling and root planing remains as a landmark benefit of incorporating this technology into the non-surgical periodontal practice [28].

When it comes to surgical periodontal therapy, the utilization of the OM has been documented mainly in two clinical arenas: regenerative therapy and mucogingival therapy. These treatment scenarios and their respective historical backgrounds will be covered in finer detail in individual chapters of this textbook.

Published material and professional anecdotes share a common recurring theme: when performing periodontal surgical procedures aided by an OM, visual acuity is enhanced by both magnification and illumination. This translates into enhanced and controlled manipulation of soft and hard tissue structures that make up the periodontium. From incision to final closure of the surgical wound, microsurgical procedures are framed by gentle and accurate soft tissue manipulation, less extensive flap designs, enhanced vision field that facilitates identification of defects, anatomical landmarks like furcations, cemento-enamel projections, anatomical grooves, and others such as accretions, defective restorative margins, caries lesions, etc. Tissue trauma is reduced when smaller suture thread diameter in combination with complementary smaller needles is used. In an in vitro experiment, it was shown that finer suture diameter (7-0) leads to thread breakage rather than tissue rupture when compared to wider diameter suture threads (3-0, 5-0) [37].

When treating periodontal disease and specifically handling pathology affecting interproximal spaces, the OM greatly facilitates access and visibility to execute incisions, delicate flap elevation, removal of granulation tissue, root surface planing, placement of biomaterial and tissue approximation to obtain primary closure thus achieving blood clot stability which is the foundation for a successful regenerative outcome.

Surgical therapy utilizing advanced flap designs without the utilization of an OM allows stable primary closure of the flap in the interdental space in 67 to 70% of the treated sites [30–32]. The incidence of primary closure when performing surgical regenerative therapy aided by an OM reached 92.3% in one study [28], This is a significant difference that translates into an equally significant improvement of the clinical parameters evaluated and relevant to reversing the deleterious effects of periodontal disease.

When it comes to mucogingival surgical applications and the execution of these procedures utilizing an OM, the test groups (OM aided) consistently showed higher root coverage and superior complete root coverage when compared to procedures performed without assistance of the OM [33–35].

It is evident that the scientific literature behind the utilization of the OM in periodontal surgical procedures is constituted mainly by opinion papers, anecdotal case reports, and technical essays illustrating operational procedures. These types of publications are meritorious and form an important segment of the evidence-based-tiers of publications and clinical expertise that guide clinical care [33]. The cohort studies and randomized controlled trials, albeit scarce, seem to consistently suggest the superiority of the outcomes when the OM is utilized to assist surgical periodontal therapy procedures.

The application of the OM in implant therapy has been documented by Shanelec in 2005 showcasing a case series of 100 dental implants in the anterior maxilla placed under the microscope in extraction sockets with immediate fabrication of implant supported fixed interim restorations [42]. In the words of Dr. Shanelec, acknowledged as the father of microscopy in periodontics and implant dentistry, "Microscopy has the potential to advance dentistry from an era of traumatic tooth loss to one of exact and seamless replacement of a failing anterior tooth with an esthetic implant supported crown." Another visionary example of Dr. Shanelec's vibrant legacy in anticipation of what has become routine treatment executions with the assistance of the OM Fig. 3.

5 Advantages of Using OM in Surgical Dentistry

Table 1 summarizes the advantages of using OM in surgical dentistry. The most obvious advantage that OM has over surgical loupes is higher and adjustable magnification [2, 14, 15]. The magnification of a typical OM is adjustable, ranging from

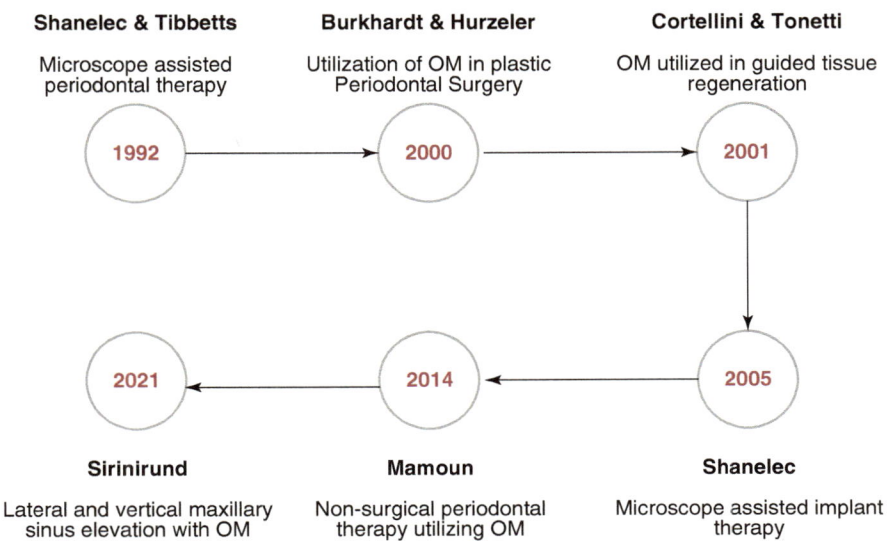

Fig. 3 Timeline landmark events: OM in Periodontics and Implant Dentistry

Table 1 Summary of advantages of using OM in surgical dentistry

At device/instrument level
- Provide higher magnification
- Provide coaxial illumination
- Facilitate use of microinstruments/microsutures
- Improve ergonomics

At provider level
- Enhance precision
- Achieve higher visual acuity and fine motor skills
- Improve tactile sensation

At pre-clinical level
- Induce less surgical trauma
- Achieve faster vascularization
- Provide wound stability

At clinical level
- Improve surrogate/true endpoints
- Improve patient centered outcomes

3.5× to approximately 30× [27–31]. Because of optical principles, higher magnification is at the expense of a narrower field of view. With OM, the surgeon can easily balance between magnification and field of view with magnification changers that are in steps or in continuous fashion. Comparing to most surgical loupes, which have fixed magnification of 2.5×, 3.0× or 3.5×, OM provides versatility and high image resolution of the region of interest (~30–50 line pairs/mm for 8× to 20×) [27–31]. Versatility in selecting the degree of magnification is advantageous because certain procedures require a high magnification (10× and higher), e.g., examination of a root fracture, debridement of calculus in the furcation, sinus membrane integrity evaluation, manage of thin phenotype tissues, etc. Lower magnification (~6×) could be used during suturing when a larger field of view may be needed. Coaxial illumination is another feature of OM that gives brightness to the surgical field, especially confined structures without obstructive shadowing. This built-in function is nowadays provided through LED optical fibers with long life span (~5000 h) and low maintenance [27–31]. It is very useful when examining intraosseous defects during minimally invasive regenerative procedures around teeth and implants, sinus membrane integrity during vertical sinus augmentation, and during socket debridement that is close to the maxillary sinus or at the furcation septum. Additionally, under magnification, now fine surgical instruments, sutures, and needles can be used for delicate soft tissue handling and to introduce less trauma [30–33]. Sutures smaller than size of 6-0 can only be operated efficiently under higher magnification provided by OM.

Improved ergonomics is another distinct advantage of working with an OM. Numerous pairs of lenses in OM direct light in the way the surgeon's eyes can see directly forward with the neck and head staying in a neutral position (straight) during patient treatment. This unique design reduces musculoskeletal stresses significantly compared to what is experienced when working without magnification and with surgical loupes. The delicate yet heavy optical structures that OM is composed of are connected to a supporting arm, which is then attached to a ceiling, a wall, or a pole with a base on wheels (a floor mounted design). Unlike surgical loupes that is mounted on the surgeons' body, the weight of OM does not rest on the surgeon. This ergonomic advantage provides comfort and stability to the surgeon who can perform surgeries for prolonged periods of time experiencing minimal, if any, fatigue, and muscle soreness.

The abovementioned technical advantages inherited to OM have opened opportunities for surgeons to improve visual acuity, surgical precision, and tactile sensation, which eventually convert to optimized pre-clinical and clinical outcomes [38–40]. A series of studies have shown a significant increase in visual acuity with OM in a pre-clinical experimental design [27–30]. Surgical precision and tactile sensation vary drastically among practitioners but can be improved with use of OM [27–30]. In the literature, few studies have shown use of OM is related to reduced surgical trauma by a minimally invasive flap design, faster vascularization, and improved wound stability [38–40]. Improved incision designs accompanied by use of OM have resulted in a higher incidence of primary wound closure, a prerequisite for predictable periodontal regeneration [38–40]. A recent systematic review showed microsurgery significantly achieved a higher percentage of root coverage and prevalence of complete root coverage in periodontal plastic surgeries [43]. Given the obvious technical advantages and promising pre-clinical as well as clinical evidence, it is the prime time for the surgical dental community to revisit the benefits of using OM in periodontal and implant surgeries and design well-structured clinical studies to validate use of OM.

6   Current Trends that Favor Using OM

Table 2 summarizes the current trends that are in favor of using OM. We have witnessed a paradigm shift to practicing regenerative medicine from tissue resection in terms of the therapy approach [38–40]. More procedures are performed with the regenerative concept, in lieu of a resective approach, if the indication allows. Common tissue regeneration therapy includes guided tissue regeneration, guided bone regeneration, sinus augmentation, and periodontal/peri-implant soft tissue augmentation. These procedures require accurate and gentle hard and soft tissue handling and will benefit tremendously from use of OM. Following the same line, over the past few decades, minimally invasive approach emerges as a preferred treatment modality [38–40]. This development in dentistry aligns well with what has occurred in medicine, where laparoscopy, Da Vinci surgery, and minimally invasive endovascular surgeries have been widely used nowadays. The surgical site is exposed by flap reflection "as little as possible, and as large as necessary" for improved wound stability and reduced postoperative morbidity. We anticipate seeing a continuous progression in this direction and a vital role of OM in this development. As for the surgical indications in periodontal and implant field, we are experiencing a decline in the number of patients in need of full mouth surgeries to control periodontal disease and an increase in esthetic demands and use of dental implants [31, 33–35]. These indications are all in favor of use of OM. Use of OM in the esthetic zone, edentulous sites for implant placement, and periodontal surgery involving 1–3 teeth are less challenging, which can reduce the learning curve of using OM. The acceptance rate of adapting this technology could be increased. More and more Millennials and Generation Z are graduating from dental schools and joining our community as dentists. They are technology savvy and willing to embrace technology for patient care. They are enthusiastic to learn about and incorporate new gadgets in the care of their patients and share their user experience through social media. OM is an excellent device to document cases in video formats for knowledge dissemination [34–36]. Last, the cost to invest in OM has decreased in the recent years because many new companies are competing in this market now. OM has low maintenance need; therefore, the recurring expenses are negligible. The cost–benefit ratio of using OM is becoming more favorable, allowing more

Table 2   Current trends in surgical dentistry that favor use of OM

	Current trends	Tradition
Paradigm shift	Tissue regeneration	Tissue resection
Approach	Minimally invasive	Macrosurgery
Focus	Esthetics	Disease control/function restoration
Surgical extent	1–3 teeth	Quadrant
Surgical site	Edentulous sites as well as dentate sites	Predominantly dentate sites
Clinician generation	Millennials and generation Z	Boomers and generation X
Investment costs	Lower cost, more options	High costs, fewer options

practitioners to consider purchase of this useful device. Using OM may improve practitioners' quality of life, prolong the dental career by establishing ergonomically healthy postures while seeing patients, and decrease missing workdays due to musculoskeletal problems.

7 Future Directions

Ultimately, it will be the goal for the periodontal and implant community to consider embracing this useful technology for patient care. Table 3 summarizes the efforts that are required to reach this end. The top priority is to encourage high-quality research to study the differences in wound healing and tissue behaviors with and without using OM. Admittedly, more evidence is much needed of using OM for improved wound healing and surgical outcome [41]. Studies evaluating the influence of minimally invasive approach and use of fine instruments on clinical outcomes will enhance our understanding and provide future directions. The adoption of the OM in endodontic specialty is a successful story that could be duplicated in periodontal and implant dentistry [23]. Nowadays OM use is an essential part of daily endodontic practice, mainly attributing to the inclusion of microscopic training in graduate endodontic curriculum in the USA [23]. Oral and maxillofacial surgery (OMFS) residency programs incorporate microsurgery training in their curriculum as well. OM is mainly used for vascular anastomosis in free grafts in reconstructive procedures [44]. It will be valuable to study how OM training has been developed in the endodontic and OFMS fields. Therefore, these lessons can be learned and implemented in periodontal and implant field. It would be the first logical step to include microsurgery lectures and hands-on exercises as elective periodontal courses. Ultimately, it is the authors' opinion that OM training should become a required course in graduate periodontal curriculum. At the same time, training programs in which the trainees spend 1 to 2 years of undivided efforts to master microsurgery should be developed and eventually accredited. These subspecialty programs can effectively train surgeons who can then become seed coaches to promote microsurgery and to fulfill the increased training demands. At the predoctoral level, an elective program should be rolled out so dental students can be exposed to this technology in their early learning stage. Interested students can be identified and advanced trainings provided. Finally, it is essential to engage related industry and corporations for providing funding and equipment to support training courses, research, and for product development.

Table 3 Efforts and plans to implement OM in surgical dentistry

Encourage research to study the benefits of using OM
Collaboration with other dental specialties, e.g., oral surgery, endodontics, etc.
Consider inclusion of microsurgical training in postgraduate periodontal curriculum
Consider formation of periodontal and implant microsurgical subspecialty
Promote microsurgical training at the predoctoral level
Collaborate with industry/corporation

Taking the University of Michigan as an example, we have been offering microsurgery training in the forms of lectures, hands-on exercises, and in the clinics for patient care to our periodontal residents since 2018 with enormous support from Dr. Laurie McCauley, Dean of the University of Michigan School of Dentistry, Dr. William Giannobile, Department Chair, now Dean of the Harvard University School of Dental Medicine, Dr. Rogerio Castilho, Interim Department Chair, Dr. Hom-Lay Wang, Graduate Periodontal Program Director, and many others. Lectures related to microsurgery are given annually in Classic Literature Review, Periodontal Therapy, Current Literature Review, Implant Literature Review, and Implant Therapy. Currently our clinic is equipped with OM for students to use. The Periodontics, Implant, and Microsurgery Academy (PiMA) at the University of Michigan was established in 2018 with a mission to "achieve minimally invasive, precise, and predictable intraoral soft and hard tissue surgical outcomes by promoting periodontal and implant microsurgery through education, hands-on trainings, and research to predoctoral students, postgraduate students, general dentists, and specialists" (https://www.dent.umich.edu/education/periodontal-and-implant-microsurgery-academy-pima). The first achieved outcome of this Academy is the formation of a 6-month and a12-month dental postgraduate programs in periodontal and implant microsurgery (DPP-PIM) in 2020 (https://dent.umich.edu/education/periodontal-and-implant-microsurgery). Recently, microsurgery webinars with 7 series covering a broad spectrum of periodontal and implant indications were successfully launched during Feb–May 2021 (PiMA webinar 2021).

The PiMA is continuously adding didactic and hands-on courses and research projects to its curriculum and activities. During 2021, two scientific articles from our outstanding periodontal residents were published, Dr. Sirinirund [45] about a case series on microsurgical maxillary sinus augmentation and Dr. Di Gianfilippo [43] about a systematic review on periodontal plastic surgery outcomes with microsurgery. Both articles aimed to bring awareness of the potential benefits of using OM for periodontal and implant-related surgeries. These exciting programs and initiatives are just the beginning of the journey. We are extremely passionate about the minimally invasive concept and microsurgical approach and welcome individuals who share similar dreams to work together toward these goals!!

8 Conclusion

OM has been widely used in medicine for improving surgical outcomes and reducing patient morbidity. The use of this device has contributed to thorough examinations, precise tissue management, and removal of etiologic factors. In dentistry, endodontists have found indications for using OM and adopted this technology in the 1990s. The search for periodontal and implant-related applications started about the same time by an enthusiastic group led by Dr. Shanelec, based in Santa Barbara, California, USA. The paradigm shift to surgical regeneration, higher esthetic standard, increased indications in focal zone (1–3 teeth), and increased number of younger and technology-savvy dentists joining our specialty will propel adoption of this useful technology. It is our primary responsibility and mission to conduct high-quality research to understand therapeutic benefits of the OM, disseminate microsurgical knowledge through educational platforms involving masterly lectures and hands-on workshops, and collaborate with the industry to develop user-friendly and efficient devices and instruments.

9 Key Points

1. In medicine, the OM was first adopted for surgeries in early 1922 by an otolaryngologist, followed by an ophthalmologist in 1946, a plastic surgeon for vascular anastomosis in 1960 and by many other specialties now.
2. In periodontics and implant therapy, Drs. Shanelec and Tibbetts piloted microscope assisted periodontal therapy in 1992, followed by Drs. Burkhardt and Hurzeler for plastic periodontal surgery, Drs. Cortellini and Tonetti for periodontal regeneration, and Dr. Sirinirund for sinus augmentation.
3. OM can provide higher and adjustable magnification, coaxial illumination, ergonomics, and video documentation, etc.
4. Paradigm shifts to regenerative procedures, esthetic-driven surgeries, localized (1-3 teeth) periodontal procedures, in addition to younger technology-savvy dentists joining our community and cost reduction of the OM, favor adoption of the OM in periodontal and implant field.
5. Increased use of the OM among periodontists and implant surgeons relies on fundamental research on the benefits of using the OM for optimal wound healing, inclusion of OM education in the periodontal postgraduate curriculum, focused continuing education programs, and collaboration with the industry.

References

1. Bradbury S. The evolution of the microscope. Oxford: Pergamon; 1967.
2. Fanibunda U, Meshram G, Warhadpande M. Evolutionary perspectives on the dental OM: a macro revolution at the micro level. Int J Microdent. 2010;2:15–9.
3. Dohlman GF. Carl Olof Nylén and the birth of the otomicroscope and microsurgery. Arch Otolaryng. 1969;90:161–5.
4. Perritt R. Superficial keratectomy. J Int Coll Surg. 1952;17:220–3.
5. Barraquer JI. The history of the microscope in ocular surgery. J Microsurg. 1980;1:288–99.
6. Littmann H. Ein neues operations-mikroskop. Klin Monbl Augenheilkd Augenarztl Fortbild. 1954;124:473–6.
7. Jacobson JH, Suarez EL. Microsurgery in anastomosis of small vessels. Surg Forum. 1960;11:243–5.
8. Lee S, Frank DH, Choi SY. Historical review of small and microvascular vessel surgery. Ann Plast Surg. 1983;11:53–62.
9. Kurze T, Doyle JBL. Extradural intracranial (middle fossa) approach to the internal auditory canal. J Neurosurg. 1962;19:1033–7.
10. Gropper PT, Kester DA, McGraw RW. Introduction to microsurgery. Clin Obstet Gynecol. 1980;23:1145–50.

11. Yasargil MG, Krayenbuhl H, Jacobson JH. Micro-neurosurgical arterial reconstruction. Surgery. 1970;67:221–33.
12. Daniel RK. Microsurgery: through the looking glass. N Engl J Med. 1979;300:1251–7.
13. Serafin D. Microsurgery: past, present and future. Plast Reconstr Surg. 1980;66:781–5.
14. Kriss TC, Kriss VM. History of the OM: from magnifying glass to microneurosurgery. Neurosurgery. 1998;42:899–908.
15. Miko I, Brath E, Furka I. Basic teaching in microsurgery. Microsurgery. 2001;21:121–3.
16. Ilie VG, Ilie VA, Dobreanu C, Ghetu N, Luchian S, Pieptu D. Training of microsurgical skills on nonliving models. Microsurgery. 2008;28:571–7.
17. Bowles SW. A new adaptation of the microscope to dentistry. Dental Cosmos. 1907;49:358–62.
18. Baumann RR. What is the use of the microscope for the dentist? Quintessenz. 1975;26:33–4.
19. Apotheker H, Jako GJ. A microscope for use in dentistry. J Microsurg. 1981;3:7–10.
20. Carr G. Microscopes in endodontics. Calif Dent Assoc J. 1992;11:55–61.
21. Pecora G, Andreana S. Use of dental operation microscope in endodontic surgery. Oral Surg Oral Med Oral Pathol. 1993;75:751–8.
22. Selden HS. The dental OM and its slow acceptance. J Endod. 2002;28:206–7.
23. AAE special committee to develop a microscope position paper. AAE position statement. Use of microscopes and other magnification techniques. J Endod. 2012;38:1153–5.
24. Chou TM, Pameijer CH. The application of microdentistry in fixed prosthodontics. J Prosthet Dent. 1985;54:36–42.
25. Martignoni M, Schonnenberger A. Precision fixed prosthodontics: clinical and laboratory aspects. Chicago, Ill: Quintessence Publishing Co Inc; 1990.
26. Schmidt R, Boudro M. The dental microscope. Why and how. Medford, OR: S&B Publishing; 2011.
27. Shanelec DA. Periodontal microsurgery. J Esthet Restor Dent. 2003;15:402–8.
28. Tibbetts LS, Shanelec DA. An overview of periodontal microsurgery. Curr Opin Periodontol. 1994;187–93.
29. Tibbetts, LS, Shanelec D. Principles and practice of periodontal microsurgery. Int J Microdent 2009;1:13–24.
30. Sitbon Y, Attathom T. Minimal intervention dentistry II: part 6. Microscope and microsurgical techniques in periodontics. Br Dent J. 2014;216:503–9.
31. Burkhardt R, Hurzeler MB. Utilization of the surgical microscope for advanced plastic periodontal surgery. Pract Periodontics Aesthet Dent. 2000;12:171–80.
32. Charles A, Freed H. The surgical microscope in the periodontal practice. Pract Periodontics Aesthet Dent. 2004;16:suppl 8–9.
33. Nordland WP. The role of periodontal plastic microsurgery in oral facial esthetics. J Calif Dent Assoc. 2002;30:831–7.
34. De Campos GV, Bittencourt S, Sallum AW, et al. Achieving primary closure and enhancing aesthetics with periodontal microsurgery. Pract Proced Aesthet Dent 2006;18:449–54.
35. Belcher JM. A perspective on periodontal microsurgery. Int J Periodontics Restorative Dent. 2001;21:191–6.
36. Mamoun J. Use of high-magnification loupes or surgical OM when performing prophylaxes, scaling and root planing procedures. NY State Dent J. 2013;79:48–52.
37. Burkhardt R, Preiss A, Joss A, Lang NP. Influence of suture tension to the tearing characteristics of the soft tissues: an in vitro experiment. Clin Oral Impl Res. 2008;19:314–9.
38. Cortellini P, Pini-Prato G, Tonetti M. The simplified papilla preservation flap. A novel approach for the management of soft tissues in regenerative procedures. Int J Periodontics Restorative Dent. 1999;19:589–99.
39. Cortellini P, Pini-Prato G, Tonetti M. The modified papilla preservation technique. A new surgical approach for interproximal regenerative procedures. J Periodontol. 1995;66:261–6.
40. Cortellini P. Minimally invasive surgical techniques in periodontal regeneration. J Evid Base Dent Pract. 2012;12(3 Suppl):89–100.
41. Nevins M. Editorial: limitations of evidence-based dentistry. Int J Periodontics Restorative Dent. 2017;37:779.

42. Shanelec DA. Anterior esthetic implants: microsurgical placement in extraction sockets with immediate provisionals. J Calf Dent Assoc. 2005;33:233–40.
43. Di Gianfilippo R, Wang I-C, Steigmann L, Velasquez D, Wang H-L, Chan H-L. Efficacy of microsurgery and comparison to macrosurgery for gingival recession treatment: a systematic review with meta-analysis. Clin Oral Investig. 2021;25:4269–80. https://doi.org/10.1007/s00784-021-03954-0.
44. Kansy K, Mueller AA, Mücke T, et al. A worldwide comparison of the management of surgical treatment of advanced oral cancer. J Craniomaxillofac Surg. 2018;46:511–20. https://doi.org/10.1016/j.jcms.2017.12.031. Epub 2018 Jan 8. PMID: 29395993.
45. Sirinirund B, Chan H-L, Velasquez D. Microscope-assisted maxillary sinus augmentation: a case series. Int J Periodontics Restorative Dent. 2021;4:531–7. https://doi.org/10.11607/prd.5407. PMID: 34328471.

The Impact of a Minimally Invasive Approach on Oral Wound Healing

Rino Burkhardt

Contents

R. Burkhardt (✉)
Private Practice, Zurich, Switzerland

Center of Dental Medicine, University of Zurich, Zurich, Switzerland

Prince Philip Dental Hospital, The University of Hong Kong, Hong Kong, SAR, China

Department of Periodontics & Oral Medicine, University of Michigan, Ann Arbor, MI, USA

© The Author(s), under exclusive license to Springer Nature Switzerland AG 2022
H.-L. (A.) Chan, D. Velasquez-Plata (eds.), *Microsurgery in Periodontal and
Implant Dentistry*, https://doi.org/10.1007/978-3-030-96874-8_2

Abstract

Wound healing is a spontaneous occurring process in a state of hemostasis. Surgical interventions rely on the stages and processes naturally orchestrated by the host and influenced by the operator in the surgical theater.

Biological pathways to mucosal wound repair and regeneration are staged and defined as a preamble to the impact of the microsurgical technique on healing processes of oral wounds, emphasizing the relevancy of incision tracing and flap design.

Micromechanical aspects of the blood clot during wound healing of oral mucosal tissues are defined under the symbiotic interaction of microsurgically controlled instrument handling and its impact on tissue mechanotransduction is elucidated and discussed.

Keywords

Wound healing · Angiogenesis · Microsurgery · Mechanotransduction

1   Introduction

Writing a book chapter about oral wound healing and how it is affected by a microsurgical approach is a challenging task for various reasons. Firstly, our understanding of wound healing has vastly increased in the last decades, a fact which was accompanied by an explosion in the number of publications, ranging from basic science to clinical studies. A recent literature search in PubMed with the terms "wound healing" resulted in almost 200,000 publications, with an upward tendency of more than 10,000 new articles annually. Such a dramatic rise in new knowledge makes it very difficult to select the relevant information and to process and condense it into meaningful concepts.

Secondly, wounds in the oral cavity are common manifestations, intentionally caused by surgical procedures or unintentionally, when, for example, pulp tissues are injured during tooth preparation. Depending on the intraoral area and the type and composition of the tissues, the healing characteristics of the different sites may vary substantially. Conversely, oral wound healing processes such as mucosal healing, regeneration of periodontal structures, healing of bone and extraction sockets, and healing around oral implants have also many basic features in common. To investigate the effects of a microsurgical approach on the healing processes and postsurgical results, we have to distinctly determine the intraoral area and define the tissues of interest and whether we focus on biological outcomes (cellular and molecular), clinical results, and/or the patient-reported outcome measures.

Thirdly, for the presentation of scientific findings and a critical discussion of the results in a book chapter, it is necessary to be precise in the wording because the reader does not have a direct chance to check the meaning and may come from a totally different background where the same term has another connotation. Therefore, definitions of terms matter, because concepts, and thus definitions, are shaped by the perceptions of the readers, and these perceptions might differ as a result of language, education (especially the education of a health professional), and the cultural differences [1]. As a consequence, we have to define the periodontal key terms used in the present chapter and contextualize them with each other.

Commonly, the definition of *periodontal microsurgery* refers to a refinement in surgical technique by which normal vision is enhanced through magnification [2]. Such attempts of definition emphasize the importance of the technical equipment, including surgical microscopes and loupes, the utilization of ergonomic microinstruments, and the inclusion of fine suture materials. In a broader sense, however, microsurgery implies an extension of surgical principles by which gentle handling of tissues is of paramount importance. This relates to the invasiveness of the surgical procedure which comprises the experience, expertise, and motor skills of the surgeon and depends on how tissues react on the application of physical forces. According to the National Institute of Health (NIH Cancer Institute), *minimally invasive surgery* is defined as "*...surgeries that encompass surgical techniques that limit the size of incisions needed and so lessen wound healing time, associated pain, morbidity and risk of infection.*" Minimally invasive surgical procedures have been enabled by the advance of various medical technologies (microsurgery, laparoscopic surgery, robotic surgery, augmented-reality surgery) and are summarized in the scientific literature under the abbreviation MIS (minimally invasive surgery).

In periodontal and periimplant surgeries, a technique or procedure should be regarded as *minimally invasive* when its effectiveness is combined with the attempt to minimize the extent of surgical trauma (e.g., accelerating early wound healing), minimizing the need for additional surgical sessions and in some specific tasks as well as reducing chair time needed for each session, eliminating or minimizing the need for reconstructive devices such as membranes or graft materials through maximizing the inherent healing potential of the treated lesion, limiting intraoperative morbidity, with lower incidence and severity of intra-surgery complications and adverse events, limiting postoperative morbidity, with lower incidence and severity of postsurgery complications and adverse events, including higher patient acceptance, tolerance, and satisfaction, and maintaining or improving pre-existing esthetics (e.g., limited to no scarring and/or gingival recession). In the following, we will use the term *minimal invasiveness* when at least one of the above-mentioned criteria is fulfilled and, by mutual agreement, we take it for granted that a microsurgically modified procedure aims at reducing the invasiveness.

Since a comprehensive description of the different clinical wound healing processes in the oral cavity would go beyond the scope of the present chapter, we will focus on the impact of minimal invasiveness on the healing of mucosal flaps and grafts, the regeneration of periodontal structures, and the interface between mucosal flaps and root surfaces.

The present chapter about wound healing of oral tissues after microsurgical interventions is organized into four sections. The first one reviews the fundamentals of current knowledge in mucosal wound healing and offers the surgeon a practical guide as the outcome ultimately depends on uncomplicated procession through normal wound healing.

The second section gives an overview of the available literature data regarding the results of periodontal and periimplant plastic and reconstructive microsurgeries and depicts how the minimally invasive modification may impact on the clinical outcome. As wound healing is one of the most complex biological processes and in order to understand how a microsurgical approach can trigger the wound healing phases, it is important to additionally evaluate the potential interfaces in the daunting array of mechanical and biochemical factors on a cellular and molecular level.

Section 3 sheds light on the clinical aspects of microsurgery and tries to identify how applied mechanical forces can be used as effective control levers to positively influence the molecular interplay during wound healing and, thereby, improve the clinical outcomes.

In the last section, a summary of the key relevant aspects of periodontal microsurgery, and how they are interconnected with the complex process of wound healing, is provided. It serves as a guidance for the clinicians how to learn the correct surgical techniques, emphasizing the most critical details, and on what they have to focus in order to achieve the well described beneficial clinical effects of a microsurgically modified intervention.

2 An Overview of the Biological Pathways to Mucosal Wound Repair and Regeneration

Understanding mucosal wound healing today involves much more than simply stating that there are three phases. Although a simplification, the classic division of wound healing into inflammatory, proliferative, and remodeling phases is still useful in understanding both routine and pathologic wound healing. Given the complexity of the mucosal wound repair process, it is remarkable how uneventful intraoral wounds heal and that, in general, they rarely become uncontrolled.

The oral mucosa is composed of a dense network of collagen fibers [3], the extracellular matrix (ECM), which provides the mucosal tone and is connected to a high number of embedded cells [4]. In health, together they maintain a tensional homeostasis which is crucial to keep the cells alive. After injury when tissue boundaries are disintegrated, the mechano-protective architecture of the ECM is disturbed and, in addition to these mechanical changes, bleeding occurs and cells come exposed to an overwhelming cocktail of cytokines initiate and orchestrate the process of wound healing.

Similar to other organ systems, the mucosal response to injury occurs in the same three overlapping but distinct wound repair stages which will be described in the following subsections.

2.1 Inflammation Phase (First Stage of Mucosal Wound Healing)

In all kind of wounds, the precondition for the initiation of the inflammatory phase is the control and stop of bleeding, known as coagulation, which however is just one part of the complex hemostatic process (for overview see [5]). During clotting, thrombin converts fibrinogen, an abundant plasma protein, into fibrin [6]. When fibrin molecules align to protofibrils and grow sufficiently long, they aggregate laterally to form fibers. These fibers, together with entrapped red blood cells and platelets, form the thrombus, or the blood clot. For clinicians it is important to know that blood clots are not uniform, homogenous structures but differ substantially based on individual patients. They are characterized by a great diversity of structural, biological, physical, and chemical properties, depending on the conditions of formation [7]. The resistance of the clot to mechanical and fibrinolytic dissolution, for example, plays an important role for early wound stability, a fact that might have an impact on the healing process when macroscopic physical forces are applied on mucosal flaps.

Immediate vasoconstriction upon wounding and the fibrin clot formation are the first sequences of healing and, thus, paving the way for appropriate inflammation. Besides its mechanical function, the blood clot and surrounding tissue release pro-inflammatory cytokines and growth factors. Once bleeding is controlled, inflammatory cells migrate into the wound (chemotaxis) and promote the inflammatory phase [8].

The first inflammatory cells infiltrating the wound are neutrophils. Their main function is considered to be prevention of infection by clearance of bacteria, foreign body materials, and damaged cells in the wound by phagocytosis [9]. Actual studies emphasize the importance of a balanced neutrophil recruitment to limit their tissue-destructive potential [10]. In the absence of microbial contamination, neutrophils may be even detrimental to tissue repair [11].

In the early wounds, likewise, the macrophages release cytokines which promote the inflammatory response. In the later stages, the same cells undergo a phenotypic transition to clear apoptotic cells (including neutrophils) and to ingest wound debris. Their critical role in non-specific defense and their recruitment of other immune cells such as lymphocytes (specific defense) underline the importance and multiple functions of this cell type in the inflammatory stage. Additionally, by the stimulation of keratinocytes, fibroblasts and the angiogenic potential [12], macrophages promote the transition to the proliferative phase of healing [8]. Figure 1 provides an overview of the timely occurrence and quantity of the different cells, interacting with each other in the wound healing process.

phases of wound healing (with involved cell types)

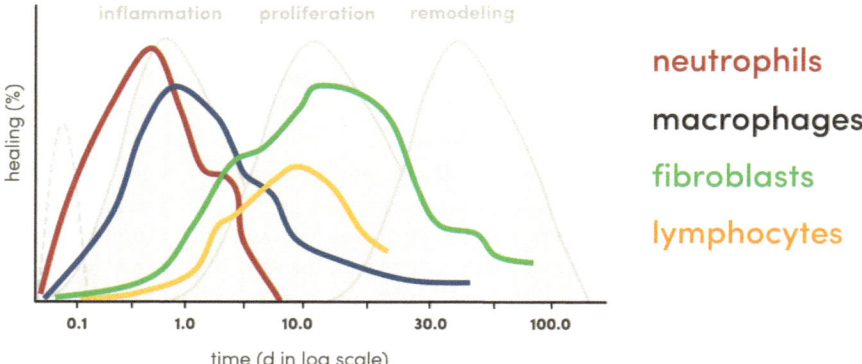

Fig. 1 Presentation of the main wound healing cell types (temporal occurrence and quantity) in relation to the classical wound healing stages. Despite many similarities in the healing characteristics of skin and oral mucosal wounds, it should be noted that mucosal wounds heal faster and with lower complication rates. Most of what we know about wound healing has been investigated in skin models. The present graphic representation is adapted to the healing process of the oral mucosa. Temporal occurrence and quantity of individual cells might differ depending on wound size and modality of healing (primary or secondary intention)

2.2   Proliferation Phase (Second Stage of Mucosal Wound Healing)

The proliferative phase is overlapping the previous one and characterized by angiogenesis, collagen deposition, granulation tissue formation, epithelialization, and wound contraction. While in the early wound healing stages the blood clot served as a temporary shield protecting the denuded wound tissues and as a reservoir of cytokines, the provisional matrix of the clot now builds the scaffold through which cells can migrate during the repair process.

2.2.1   Epithelialization

For proper wound healing, the process of re-epithelialization has to be initiated rapidly after injury in order to form a protective barrier against fluid losses and further bacterial invasion and to re-establish mucosal integrity (for overview see [4]). The first migratory cells derive from the suprabasal layer of the residual epithelial structures in the wound margins. These epithelial cells have to dissolve their hemidesmosomal connections, to detach from the basement membrane and to proliferate, which takes time and lasts about 24 h, corresponding with the observed lag phase between injury and cell migration [13]. During migration, most of the basement membrane components underneath the keratinocytes are missing and the cells move forward on the exposed connective tissue matrix underneath the fibrin clot [14]. In small gingival wounds (2–3 mm between wound margins), however, the high phagocytic activity of the keratinocytes allows them to directly penetrate through tissue debris and the clot without interacting with the connective tissue matrix. With a forward movement of about 1 mm per day, the keratinocytes continue migration until they are stopped moving by mechanical cues. They change their gene expression and become basal stationary keratinocytes. There is evidence that keratinocytes themselves are capable of making extracellular matrix that they can use to support or modulate their own migration if the provisional matrix is not permissive to migration [15]. Once changed into a stationary phenotype, the keratinocytes contribute to the regeneration of the basement membrane even if a significant portion of the basement membrane components is synthesized by the wound fibroblasts [16]. There is no doubt that the interaction between the wound keratinocytes and the underlying fibroblasts, described as cross-talk, influences and regulates the healing process of re-epithelialization [17]. The complete reorganization of the basement membrane is complete at 4 weeks. It is well recognized that epithelial cells have a crucial function in the healing process of the injured oral mucosa. Even in healthy periodontal tissues, keratinocytes are not just passive bystanders, but rather are metabolically active and capable of reacting to external stimuli by synthesizing a number of cytokines, adhesion molecules, growth factors, and enzymes.

2.2.2 Angiogenesis

Macroscopically, the granulation tissue of the healing mucosal wound gets its granular, pink appearance by the numerous capillaries that invade the newly formed connective tissue matrix. Many studies from the second half of the last century document the course of new vessel formation after injury of the oral mucosa and periodontal tissues on a light microscopic base [18–22]. The advent of molecular biology in the last decades enabled a deeper insight into the mechanism of vasculogenesis (de novo formation of capillaries deriving from the hematopoietic system), arteriogenesis (formation of a collateral circulation by arterial assembly), and angiogenesis (sprouting of new capillaries from already existing blood vessels), the latter being the predominant modality of revascularization in mucosal wound healing.

The uneventful and quick re-establishment of the vasculature of the injured mucosal area is of importance as nutrients and oxygen supply to the newly formed tissues are mainly provided by a functional blood perfusion [23]. The complex process of capillary sprouting, originating from vessels of the wound bed and neighboring tissues, is precisely regulated and strongly modulated by mechanical and chemical factors, with the vascular endothelial growth factor (VEGF) family as the main regulator (for overview see [24]).

There are some controversies in the literature about the angiogenic regulation and the promotion of wound healing. While some authors state that blocking angiogenesis does not have a significant influence on wound healing [25, 26], others document that the inhibition of angiogenesis significantly delays wound repair [27, 28].

The contradictory results can be explained on the one hand by the fact that most of the studies evaluated angiogenesis by counting the number of blood vessels and not the functionality of the vessels. In fact, many blood vessels formed during wound repair are not perfused [29], thus, the decrease in blood vessels density by the selective elimination of non-perfused blood vessels may not have a significant effect on wound healing.

On the other hand, angiogenesis correlates with the inflammatory process as inflammatory cells release proangiogenic factors [30]. In skin wounds, angiogenesis produces an up to ten times more dense network of capillaries than exists in unwounded tissue. In the consecutive healing stages, the density of capillaries returns to that of normal by selective apoptosis of many of the recently formed blood vessels [31].

Comparing skin and mucosal wounds, the intraoral wound, similar to the fetal one, seems to be a privilege site of healing with reduced scar formation and less inflammation [32, 33]. During the initial wound healing stage in skin, stimulated macrophages and keratinocytes produce high levels of proangiogenic factors such as VEGF which are much less pronounced in the oral mucosa. As a consequence, oral mucosal wounds seem to circumvent the development of excess vasculature, proceeding directly to a well-formed vascular network. Therefore, both decreased inflammation and well regulated, refined angiogenesis are features of optimal healing after injury of the intraoral mucosa. It has to be noted that the density of vascular capillaries and blood flow in healthy oral mucosa is significantly higher compared to healthy skin [34].

2.2.3   Granulation Tissue Formation

Collagen, produced by fibroblasts, is the main structural protein in the extracellular matrix and the repaired mucosal wound. In healthy tissues, fibroblasts reside in a quiescent state and have a slow proliferation rate and metabolic activity. Upon wounding they become activated and attracted from the wound margins by chemotactic cues and start to initially synthesize and deposit a primitive, unorganized, and structurally weak ECM. The major fibrillar collagen produced early in the granulation tissue is type III. Later on, type I collagen production speeds up, accounting for at least 75% of the whole collagen content in the granulation tissue after the first postoperative week [35, 36]. The first secretion of new extracellular matrix proteins in the granulation tissue seems to occur approximately two to four days after wounding. In this stage of wound healing, the primary role of the fibroblasts is to rapidly produce new connective tissue in the ECM to re-establish tissue strength and function [37].

In the second half of the proliferation stage, around the seventh postoperative day, when granulation tissue is well established, some of the fibroblasts differentiate into myofibroblasts [38], cells with contractile elements that bring collagen fibrils together and reorganizes them, thus promoting wound closure and increasing the mechanical strength of the wound [39]. Based on more actual data, myofibroblasts seem to originate not only from fibroblasts but other cells such as mesenchymal stem cells, endothelial cells, pericytes, and epithelial cells [40].

Exposure of fibroblast to serum that is present in the blood clot in the wound initiates not only a rapid general stimulus for cell proliferation but also a more specific gene expression that controls function of other cells involved in inflammation, angiogenesis, and re-epithelialization.

Therefore, it is likely that fibroblasts and their subsets or fibroblast-like cells originating from various sources play a more important role in the physiology of wound repair than has been previously realized (for overview see [37]).

2.3   Remodeling Phase (Third Stage of Mucosal Wound Healing)

Tissue maturation and remodeling of mucosal wounds begin at approximately seven to ten days after injury and can last up to several months. But the start of tissue remodeling is individual and depends on the size of the wound. In surgical wounds caused by a small releasing incision and healing by primary intention, only very little granulation tissue is formed so that wound contraction can already occur at day three post-wounding, followed by an early balance between ECM production and degradation. In larger excisional wounds such as those left in the hard palate after harvesting a free masticatory mucosal graft, more granulation tissue is accumulated and it may take more than two weeks until remodeling commences [38]. In the remodeling phase, the number of cells secreting the ECM is reduced and their secretion downregulated. Additionally, the components of the ECM are reorganized and the stability of the ECM is increased by appropriate cross-linking of the collagen. Optimal mucosal wound healing leads to an early qualitatively and quantitatively normal connective tissue with re-establishment of a quiescent fibroblast phenotype responsible for tissue maintenance and homeostasis.

Wound healing is a complex biological process and the ideal outcome strongly depends on timing, duration, and the well-coordinated interactions of inflammatory and tissue resident cells, structural molecules, and mechanical forces generated in the wound environment (Fig. 2). The notion among clinicians that wounds in oral mucosa heal fast and with low complication rates has been supported by systematic studies [32, 33, 41]. Nevertheless, with few exceptions, wounds of the oral mucosa rather heal in tissue repair than regeneration, including complete restoration of the tissues in form and function. When the application of a microsurgical technique has been shown to improve the clinical results of traditional periodontal surgical interventions, it might be reasonable to assume that a change in the incision design and/or the modification of the exerted forces on the tissues (interface instrument–tissue) interfere with the biological processes of wound healing. Therefore, in the following sections, we try to identify the surgically accessible and controllable lever arms and to discover how one can intentionally interfere with the wound healing process in order to achieve the aforementioned improved surgical results.

timing of wound healing stages with their histological characteristics

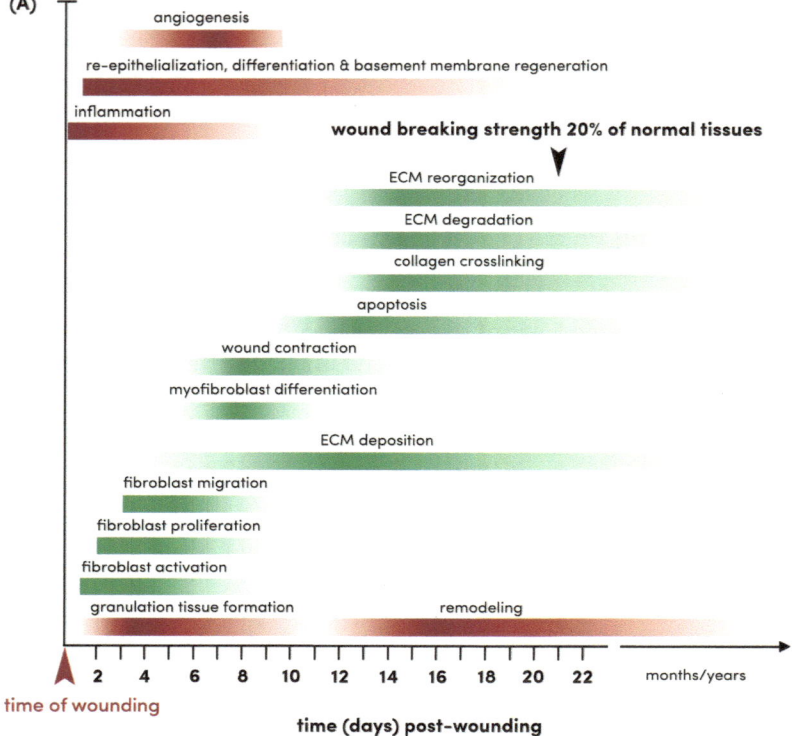

Fig. 2 Schematic presentation of timing of the wound healing stages and the corresponding histological characteristics (**A**) after full-thickness excisional skin wounds in pig. Red color indicates the chronological sequences of the different wound healing stages. Green color depicts the histological events in relation to the wound healing stages (figure adapted from Häkkinen et al. 2012)

3 Impact of the Microsurgical Technique on the Healing Process of Oral Mucosal Wounds: Clinical Results and Potential Triggers for Enhanced Healing

3.1 Scientific Evidence of Improved Outcomes After Periodontal Plastic Microsurgeries: Some Critical Comments about the Clinical Relevance of the Results

A considerable amount of data, published in the last decade, document the beneficial impact of a microsurgical approach on the clinical postoperative results after periodontal plastic surgical interventions. Additionally, the patient-reported outcome measures also favor microsurgery with improved esthetics, patient's satisfaction, and reduced pain (for review see [42]). Some of the articles, investigating the application of a microsurgical technique in periodontal surgery, rank high in the evidence pyramid and underline the sound documentation of the procedures. There is no doubt that clinical practice guidelines based on the principles of evidence-based medicine (EBM) build the basement for teaching and implementing available knowledge about microsurgery into clinical workflows.

Nevertheless, since the introduction of EBM in the mid-nineties, we have learned that, despite the considerable benefits of EBM, there have also been unintended consequences and the evidence-based "quality mark" has been misappropriated and distorted by vested interests [43–46].

On one side, the energetic intellectual EBM community, committed to making clinical practice more scientific and thereby achieving safer, more consistent clinical results, underestimated the time, effort, and skills needed on part of the clinicians, to access the right information among the massive volumes of research. Furthermore, many practitioners did not learn how to interpret and use scientific evidence in their daily practice and how to amalgamate it with their clinical experience and expertise as a basis for good clinical decisions in each individual patient. Without knowledge dissemination and implementation, evidence derived from systematic reviews only improves the dentist's knowledge but does not change their clinical performance by establishing a relevant improvement of their technical skills and/ or clinical decision-making competences [47].

Conversely, and apart from the fact, that surgeons not always apply to the existing evidence when making their treatment plans, for a large number of clinical problems, there is simply not enough practice-related evidence available. The fact that in periodontal microsurgery the influencing factors are numerous and interconnected with each other, underlines the difficulty to find the relevant, practice-related evidence.

Along with the different levels of technical skills, there is an entire array of nontechnical skills such as teamwork with the chairside assistant, the quality of intraoperative decision-making, and the ability of self-reflection, which influence the quality of the microsurgical results and which are described in the specialist literature as *center-*, or more precise, *provider-effect* [48, 49]. It is therefore not surprising that a Cochrane review including endodontic surgery, a closely related specialty to periodontal microsurgery, ended up with the conclusion that "there is no evidence to support or refute a difference in clinical outcomes when either a microscope, endoscope or surgical loupes are adopted during endodontic surgery" [50]. The authors justified the findings with the low number and average quality of the included articles as well the high number of factors that might have an impact on the success of the surgical therapy.

As it is the goal of the present book to provide interested clinicians with an overview of the current state of knowledge in periodontal microsurgery and thus help them to improve performance and reduce errors, it becomes obvious that these goals cannot be achieved by summarizing the actual evidence-based literature about microsurgery. There would be too many important questions remaining unanswered by just choosing this approach. In the following section we will direct attention to the surgical technical variables such as applied physical forces and incision design, their interconnectedness with each other, and how they may interfere with the wound healing process.

3.2   The Interconnectedness of the Microsurgical Technique with the Healing Process of Mucosal Wounds

The biological concept of regenerative periodontal surgery has been developed in the last decades of the twentieth century (for overview see Chap. 9). The results from multiple animal studies strongly suggested that the exclusion of epithelial and gingival connective tissue cells from the healing area by the use of a barrier membrane may allow (guide) periodontal ligament cells to repopulate the detached root surface (for overview see [51]). This observation provided the basis for the clinical application of the principle termed "guided tissue regeneration" (GTR) which, in those times, was perceived as a paradigm shift. The prospects of achieving a healing result that includes a reconstruction of lost or injured tissues in such a way that the architecture *and* function of the involved tissues are completely restored led to an eruption of enthusiasm in the worldwide community of periodontists, which soon after was followed by a great deal of frustration. The reason was that the promising results of GTR described in the early animal studies [52] and first clinical case reports on human teeth [53] could not be duplicated with just approximately sufficient prognosis in the clinical settings. There were simply too many interconnected factors, systemic-, site- and surgeon-related ones, that influenced the outcome and thus increased the technical complexity of GTR interventions. It took almost another decade to unravel the critical influencing factors and make GTR a reliable treatment option with predictable prognoses (for overview see [54]). Among other aspects, the maintenance of wound integrity turned out to be a major problem as bacterial contamination of the exposed non-resorbable membranes often led to infections [55]. The systematic assessment of the relevant surgical factors associated with variability of clinical attachment gain provided evidence that minimal-invasive and low traumatic soft tissue manipulation have the potential to substantially decrease the risks for wound dehiscences and, thus, having a great impact on the wound healing processes.

3.2.1   Influence of Modified (Minimal-Invasive) Incision Designs on Wound Stability and Wound Integrity

Clinical reports from the nineties emphasized the importance of flap and incision designs in order to maintain primary soft tissue closure after regenerative periodontal surgeries in the course of time [56, 57]. In this context, the preservation of the interdental gingiva and the papillary structures gained more and more importance and gave rise to redesigning the surgical approaches following the guidelines of minimal invasiveness. In the first decade of the current century, the modified (MPPF) and simplified (SPPF) papilla preservation flap [58, 59], the single flap approach (SFA) [60], and the papilla amplification flap (PAF) [61] were generally regarded as the golden standards of flap design when it came to guided regenerative therapies. Despite the many published clinical trials, documenting the beneficial effects of the above-mentioned flap designs on the results after GTR treatments (for overview see [54]), one has to critically comment that a statistically significant influence of such minimally invasive approaches on clinical attachment gain could not be confirmed by a high ranking Cochrane systematic review [62]. Again, the findings from the meta-regression analyses regarding a potential influence of the surgical procedure on the outcome were explained by the many influencing variables and the troubling extent of clinical heterogeneity, which not only existed between studies but also within multicenter trials.

Nevertheless, the efficacy of GTR therapies was scientifically proven and in compliant, non-smoking patients with good oral hygiene and presenting with a narrow, angular defect with an infrabony component of three and at least six millimeters of probing pocket depth, probing attachment level gains of four to five millimeters after one year of healing were more the rule than the exception [63]. In those times, the materials used for space provision and cell occlusion were either non- or bioresorbable barrier membranes and the flaps were raised according to the above described designs extended at least one tooth unit mesially and distally to the defect area of the affected tooth. Buccal releasing incisions were chosen on the surgeon's discretion when either flap mobilization was impaired or visual access to the defect site was restricted.

At the turn of the century, enamel matrix derivatives (EMD) extended the spectrum of regenerative therapies [64], but despite the lower risks for postoperative mucosal dehiscences, probing attachment level gains in sites with similar defect morphologies were substantially lower in the ones treated with enamel matrix derivatives compared to those treated with GTR [65]. The predominant flap designs used for regenerative periodontal surgeries with EMD were congruent with the above described and extensively documented ones for GTR therapies.

Within the scope of a lively stream of publications on regenerative periodontal procedures, all of a sudden, the outcome of surgical therapies combined with EMD dramatically increased to a level that could not anymore be explained by the learning curve and increased skills of the individual clinicians. The unexpected improvement of clinical attachment gain after regenerative surgeries with EMD can be attributed to the continuous modifications of flap design. By using barrier membranes which itself are characterized by a certain thickness of the material and which are indicated to provide space, flaps had to be mobilized and advanced in order to achieve primary wound closure. In contrast, EMD is applied in a gelform and, thus, adds much less to the volume of the defect site when a three-wall, self-containing bony defect has to be covered with the local mucosal flap. Attentive surgeons soon became aware of this fact and started to modify the already existing papilla preservation flaps, following the concepts of MIS [66, 67]. Modifications directed at the reduction of the number and the extension of incisions at the expense of impaired visual accessibility of the defect site. To overcome the disadvantage, high-power magnification devices such as loupes or surgical microscopes were recommended and became indispensable components of the surgical equipment.

The development of flap designs in the field of regenerative surgery nicely documents how the waiver of releasing incisions and the reduction of tissue elevation to a minimum required for visual and instrumental access to the root surfaces positively affect the patient morbidity, improve the prognosis for wound integrity and stability and, thus, the regenerative result of the surgical intervention. Surprisingly, split-mouth design studies of regenerative treatments of three-wall infrabony defects even proved that the minimal invasiveness of the approaches and gentle handling of the soft tissues, in some specific clinical circumstances, have a more pronounced impact on the healing capacity of the tissues than the use of any biomaterial [68].

The above summarized scientific data paired with personal experience perfectly illustrate the effectiveness and external validity of minimal-invasive flap designs applied in regenerative therapies. Additionally, they indirectly confirm the clinically observed positive impact of MIS on the wound healing process. A paradigm shift from a conventional to a less invasive approach, using magnification aids, newly designed instruments, and fine suture materials can be observed in many different indications of periodontal plastic surgery (e.g., tunnel techniques for recession coverage which, at least partly, replaced the conventional coronally advanced flaps with releasing incisions or in implant surgeries, the flapless approaches for implant placement). So far, it is still unclear to what extent the magnification influences the wound integrity and the subsequent clinical results after healing. One might speculate that in periodontal plastic surgeries at sites with unproblematic visual access and limited to buccal or oral surfaces, high-power loupes might be sufficient to duplicate the good results from randomized trials. When it comes to modern, minimally invasive regenerative surgeries (modified minimally invasive surgical technique, m-MIST) where root surfaces have to be accessed via a small keyhole [68], it is evident, even without scientific evidence, that surgical access and light transmission to the root surface and bottom of the bony defect is impossible without a coaxial light direction and, thus, the aid of a surgical microscope.

Periodontal plastic surgeries are characterized by a high biocomplexity as hard, acellular, non-vascularized, and non-shedding surfaces of teeth or implants with their components might be included in the wound area and constitute parts of the wound boundaries. Therefore, it is difficult to isolate single factors such as the number and the extension of the incisions and directly relate them to wound stability and the final clinical outcome. A reduction of the incision design to maintain mucosal blood perfusion might also present a higher risk for residual flap tension with all the negative consequences.

The fact that already minor incisions have a substantial negative impact on the vascularity of the gingiva has been shown in a study on humans [19]. By injecting a fluorescent dye, it could be observed how lengths of mucoperiosteal flaps directly correlate with the reduction of blood perfusion in the flaps. Even more negative impact on the vascularity of the mucosal tissues than flap design could be registered for advanced flaps, stabilized, and sutured under residual tension.

A conventional flap and incision design for periodontal surgery (control site) was compared with a minimally invasive approach (test site) by histological assessment in an animal experiment [69]. The sites treated with different levels of invasiveness were followed up with particular focus on the distribution of type III collagen, which plays a crucial role in the early wound healing phases and provides a scaffold required for angiogenesis and the migration of various types of cells. The histological and immunohistochemical analyses revealed a higher type III collagen content in the experimental sites compared with the conventionally treated ones, reaching statistical significance on day 3 and 5. The results from this study, comparing the early wound healing processes after conventional and minimally invasive flaps by histological analyses, clearly documented that a reduction of the surgical tissue trauma positively interferes with the wound healing process by markedly less neutrophils in the infiltration area and a timely acceleration of the healing phases, resulting in earlier tissue maturation.

From a clinician's perspective, there is no doubt that the application of MIS techniques in periodontal plastic surgery results in increased wound stability, faster tissue maturation, less scar formation, reduced patient morbidity, better esthetic appearance, and overall improvement of the healing outcome. However, it should be noted that most of these findings evolve from studies based on clinical measurements or subjective observations of the surgeons. Scientific evidence based on direct comparisons of healing processes after the application of different incision designs on the level of inflammatory cellular composition, blood microcirculation, or wound fluid cytokine levels is still scarce and needs further elucidation.

3.2.2 Healing of Periodontal Wounds Created by Traditional, but Microsurgically Modified Flap Designs

While in the previous section we shed light on the impact of applied MIS techniques (fewer incisions and restricted soft tissue elevations) on the clinical results and documented their overall beneficial effects, it is the goal of the subsequent one, to evaluate if, and if yes, how the application of a microsurgically modified technique influences the healing process and clinical outcome of traditional flaps. The modification consists of the use of high-power magnification (surgical microscope), microsurgical instruments, and fine suture materials while the flap design and extension of the incisions remain unchanged and correspond to those of traditional approaches.

Referring to the scientific literature of regenerative periodontal therapies, wound integrity seems to be a crucial aspect for undisturbed healing and is considered as a requirement for clinical success. As reported above, mucosal dehiscences with denudation of non-shedding surfaces such as roots, implant components, or inserted biomaterials are prone to bacterial colonization and, thus, once exposed to the oral cavity, promoting infections [55]. It has been documented that such adverse events are highly prevalent [62] and still remain a problem that is difficult to circumvent in many clinical situations [70]. The difficulty lies in the primary closure of the interdental soft tissues and its maintenance over the first postoperative weeks, especially if accesses are restricted by tooth proximities or locations in the posterior area of the dental arch. With traditional incision designs (access flaps), dissecting the interdental gingiva in the mid-col area, it is almost impossible to closely adapt the mucosal flaps with reliable prognosis for primary intention healing. The prevalence of dehiscences, reported in published studies, decreased when papilla preservation techniques have been introduced [58, 59, 71, 72]. Nevertheless, mucosal dehiscences remained predominant complications after GTR therapies, even in the hands of skillful, experienced surgeons.

In a patient cohort study, investigating the probing attachment level gains after GTR therapies, the application of a simplified papilla preservation flap (SPPF) provided a complete primary wound closure in all treated sites at the end of the surgical procedure [59]. Six weeks postoperatively, clinical examinations have shown that only 67% of the originally completely closed wounds could be maintained intact, indicating the fragility of the interdental tissues in response to surgical manipulation and the difficulties to avoid partial necrosis of the col. area.

In patients with more favorable papillary morphologies, ideally treated with modified papilla preservation flaps (MPPF), primary interdental wound closures could be achieved in 93% of all treated sites and 73% remained completely closed for the entire observation period of six weeks [58].

When the same, previously mentioned clinicians modified their clinical approach and accessed the interdental area by using a surgical microscope and corresponding instruments, all treated sites could be completely closed after the intervention and mucosal closures were maintained in 92.3% of all treated defects for the entire follow-up period [73].

These results clearly documented that the use of a surgical microscope, provided that the surgeons are familiar with the characteristics of the microsurgical technique, allowed a much more accurate and less traumatic manipulation of the interdental tissues compared to conventional approaches performed without magnification aids. It is reasonable to assume that primary wound closures stabilized the underlying blood clot, sealed the environment from bacterial invasion and, thus, had a substantial impact on the healing processes and final clinical outcome.

The impact of a microsurgical modification on mucosal healing and clinical outcome was evaluated for another periodontal plastic indication, namely the coverage of gingival recessions [74]. In split-mouth design, bilateral symmetric mucosal dehiscences were randomly treated with either a double pedicled flap or the corresponding flap design but microsurgically modified. The influence on healing was assessed by angiographic techniques, measuring the mucosal blood perfusion on a previously defined, squared area in the center of the covered recession. The vascularity of the treated sites was recorded immediately after the surgery and three and seven days postoperatively (Fig. 3). Clinical parameters were evaluated before and several times, up to 12 months, after the interventions.

The results have shown that the use of a surgical microscope, corresponding instruments and 9–0 sutures had a substantial impact on the mucosal blood perfusion of the treated sites, reaching statistical significance on the third and seventh postoperative day. Interestingly, the sites with a very good vascularity in the early wound healing stages were the ones presenting with the highest percentage of root coverage at the end of the one year follow-up period. The positive impact of a microsurgical approach on the clinical outcome after the surgical coverage of mucosal dehiscences has been documented in several other studies (for review see [42]).

clinical snapshots with corresponding angiograms

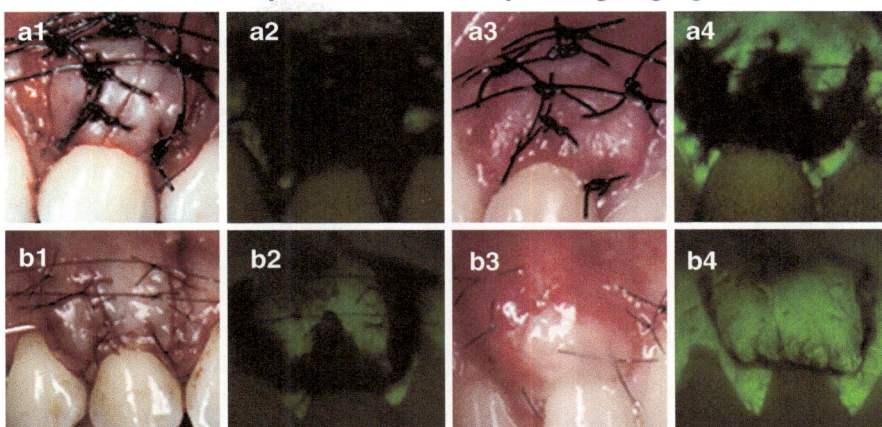

Fig. 3 Micro- (b1-4) and macrosurgically (a1-4) treated mucosal recessions with corresponding angiograms. a1/b1 depict the surgical sites immediately after the interventions; a2/b2 angiograms representing the blood perfusion of the treated sites immediately after the interventions (green = perfused); a3/b3 surgical sites, 7 days postoperatively; a4/b4 corresponding angiograms at day 7 postsurgery

Despite the documented promising results of microsurgically modified interventions, it is still unclear how visual enhancement can influence the instrument–tissue interface and how the applied physical forces can trigger the wound healing processes. In the following section, we try to shed light on the questions raised above and, based on findings from basic research, to substantiate the hypothesis that the magnitude of mechanical forces applied on mucosal tissues directly affects the wound healing process on a cellular and molecular level.

4   How to Translate Findings from Basic Research into Clinical Success?

4.1   Incision Design and Wound Healing from a Histological and Physiological Perspective

To plausibly explain the mechanisms how a microsurgical modification of a traditional flap approach can positively interfere with the wound healing processes, we first have to focus on the single aspects of the microsurgical technique and equipment. The surgical microscope, widely considered as the core component of the microsurgical technique, can just have an indirect impact as there is no direct interface between the visual acuity and the tissue trauma. The magnified vision and bright illumination of the surgical site might enhance the detection of tissue microstructures and, after appropriate clinical training, help the surgeon to improve bimanual control and fine motor skills. One can only speculate how an utmost careful manipulation of the oral mucosa during flap preparation has the potential to minimize the reduction of the presurgically existing blood perfusion and the amount of cellular debris caused by tissue damage and, thus, paves the way for an uneventful healing. In fact, animal studies have shown that the size of the surgical site characterized by an extension of the incision design positively correlates with the size of the infiltration area of neutrophils [69], which partly explains the faster wound healing after MIS interventions. These findings were supported by another animal study on skin wounds [75], documenting that all inflammatory mediators, tested in serum of the operated animals, and immune reactions induced by skin surgical trauma are closely correlated to the length of the skin incisions. The presented results from clinical studies on patients and animals are concordant with the common sense that a minimally invasive surgical approach, with limited incisions and accesses via keyholes, positively affects the wound healing process, resulting in better final outcome and reduced patient morbidity. Nonetheless, it does not explain if the use of a surgical microscope, combined with corresponding instruments and fine suture materials, has a beneficial effect on the outcome likewise, when flap preparation, mobilization, and fixation are technically executed in the same manner, macro- and microsurgically.

When similar surgical approaches were directly compared from which one was microsurgically modified, such immediate postsurgical trauma reduction could not be confirmed, at least for the vascular blood supply in the treated areas [74]. This, in turn, and as the initial impairments of blood supply after macro- and microsurgical operations were relatively similar, might be an indicator that the true microsurgical control lever that triggers wound healing must be searched elsewhere.

In most periodontal surgical procedures, after flap preparation and flap elevation, the mucosal tissues must be mobilized, advanced, stabilized, and fixed in a new position. In the last stage of the surgery, when flaps have to be firmly stabilized and closed, a passive adaptation of the flap margins seems to be an indispensable prerequisite for uneventful healing and the maintenance of wound integrity during the entire postoperative period. Tensionless or *passive wound closure* became a tenet in periodontal and implant surgery since long ago and its importance is emphasized in numerous clinical studies, articles, and book chapters. This is somewhat surprising as a digital search in the Medline database, entering key terms related to passive wound closure, provided only very few studies including clinical measurements of flap tension after periodontal and implant surgeries [76–78]. Current findings document that the available scientific evidence of the concept of *passive wound closure* is relatively scarce and its validity in periodontal surgery may at least be questioned. Additionally, it must be noted that almost none of the authors stressing the tenet of *passive wound closure* ever defined the term and explicitly described their ideas about it.

Studies on patients have shown that residual flap tensions tend to impair blood supply [19] and increase the risk for wound dehiscences, especially when forces beyond 0.1 N are applied [77]. It is important to note that the experienced periodontal surgeon who treated the sixty patients in the just mentioned study did not perceive any differences in residual flap tension and prepared all the flaps in good faith of complete passivity (personal comment of the author). Interestingly, in the group of low residual tensions, between 0.01 N and 0.05 N, none of the 25 patients exhibited a mucosal dehiscence—a finding which was independent of flap thickness.

The fact that uneventful healing with maintenance of wound integrity is compatible with residual flap tensions was confirmed in another clinical study on patients treated with bone grafts [78]. The authors defined a wound closure with a residual flap tension of up to 0.05 N as completely passive and did not observe any adverse healing outcome in the group of patients with low-tension flap closures. Data from animal studies confirmed the above-mentioned findings and, surprisingly, even proved that some soft tissue wounds closed under tension showed significantly higher tensile strength between one and three weeks postoperatively [79, 80] compared to wounds which were passively closed.

These observations raise an important question, namely how much tension, applied to the wound margins, is compatible with an uneventful mucosal healing? Or more provocative: Is there a range of applied minimal tension that has a beneficial effect on the wound healing process compared to a completely passively closed wound?

4.2 Micromechanical Properties of the Extracellular Matrix of the Oral Mucosa and the Blood Clot after Wounding

4.2.1 Micromechanical Aspects of Oral Mucosal Tissues

In health, the fibroblasts as the predominant cell type of the oral mucosa are connected to the dense network of collagen fibers, the main structural element of the extracellular matrix (ECM) [3, 81]. Under physiological conditions, the ECM maintains a tensional homeostasis which is crucial to keep the embedded cells alive. That means, in concrete terms, residing fibroblasts experience, and vitally need, specific mechanical signals within a distinct range of magnitude, caused by gravity [82], tension [83], compression [84], shear stress [85], and osmosis [86].

After injury when tissue boundaries are disintegrated, the mechano-protective architecture of the ECM is disturbed and, in addition to the mechanical changes, cells become exposed to an overwhelming cocktail of cytokines [87]. Little was known about how cells convert mechanical signals into a chemical response, named mechanotransduction, and how these signals are integrated with other signals, until a group of researchers, almost two decades ago, presented reliable models. These models were based on experimental findings which documented that cells are hard-wired to respond immediately to mechanical stresses transmitted over cell surface receptors that physically couple the cytoskeleton to the extracellular matrix or to other cells [88, 89]. We now have evidence from numerous studies that mechanical stimuli are transduced into a biochemical response through force-dependent changes in scaffold geometry (for overview see [81, 90]). The molecular signaling pathways of applied mechanical forces are described for the biological processes in the ECM [91], the cell membrane [90] as the interface between the ECM and the cell, for the intracellular mechanical force transmission via the cytoskeleton [41] and even the interface between the cytoplasm and the nucleus of the cell [92].

While the research community, interested in wound healing and for a long time, was focused on identifying the molecular components that trigger wound healing processes, it is now clear that there is more to the equation: the whole is truly greater than the sum of its parts. Today, we know on a solid base of evidence-based research, that mechanical forces, rather than chemicals cues, act as biological regulators and have a substantial impact on embryogenesis [93], the function of organs [94], the growth of skin and muscles [95], but also the etiology of many debilitating diseases [96] and last but not least on wound healing of the oral mucosa [81]. Additionally, the cells of the oral mucosa and the periodontal ligament, such as fibroblasts and keratinocytes, have been shown to be highly mechanosensitive [97] which underlines the potential role of applied mechanical forces in the wound healing process when flaps are manipulated and sutured under tension of different magnitudes.

An excellent way to illustrate the applied principle of mechanotransduction in a therapeutical concept is the orthodontic movement of teeth. As most dentists might have observed in everyday clinical practice, by just applying a small mechanical force on a macroscale within a range of few grams, after an initial lag phase of about one month the teeth start to move, indicating that the mechanical impulse has been transmitted into biochemical signals and activating the genetic machinery of the ligament cells, changing their phenotype and starting with a new behavior [98].

4.2.2 Micromechanical Aspects of the Blood Clot during Healing

Referring to the beginning of the present chapter and the illustration of the different wound healing stages (Fig. 2), we have seen that blood clot formation to prevent local hemorrhage and to build a provisional matrix for wound healing is one of the first processes to take place after wounding [36]. Blood clots can best be described as branched three-dimensional networks of taut fibrin fibers with entrapped blood cells. But the heterogeneity of fibrin as a main component of the fibrin fiber results in blood clots which are characterized by different viscoelastic properties such as rigidity and elasticity. Immediately after clot formation, stability means the resistance of the clot to mechanical stress which is essential to withstand arterial pressure and to stabilize the early wound [99]. After surgical wound closure, the viscoelastic properties of the blood clot might determine how it responds to treatment. A stiff or brittle clot might have a greater tendency to disrupt from a root surface or other wound beds, while those that are more viscous or plastic might deform and maintain their mechanical function [100]. Although not much is known about the relationship between mechanical properties of fibrin and its impact on clinical wound stability, it has been documented on periodontal wounds in an animal experiment that the tissue characteristics of the wound bed have a substantial effect on blood clot stability and adherence. Interfaces between a non-shedding avascular surface, such a dentin, and the blood clot were more prone to disruption when forces were applied in the early wound healing phases than those consisting of mucosal connective tissues and blood clots [101].

In the subsequent wound healing phases, blood clot stability refers more to the fibrinolytic properties of fibrin and the balanced equilibrium between clotting and the lytic susceptibility of the clot [99] than purely mechanical aspects. To reinforce the wound and initiate wound contraction, fibroblasts have to migrate into the provisional matrix and deposit collagen which requires a local dissolution of the blood clot. Research findings from a study on human blood clots revealed that mechanically stretched fibrin fibers in the blood clot (e.g., by increased wound tensions) are more resistant to proteolytic dissolution, which again documents the biological mechanisms of mechanotransduction and the interconnectedness of applied mechanical forces with undisturbed wound healing [102]. In this regard it has to be noted that the above-mentioned findings must be viewed from a qualitative perspective than being judged on the basis of absolute numbers and the magnitude of the actually exerted mechanical forces.

The biocomplexity of wound healing is mirrored in the fact that uneventful healing depends on finely balanced mechanical forces in the microenvironment of the wound. While excessive mechanical stress in the granulation tissue and early connective tissue matrix leads to a delay in healing and increases the risks for adverse outcome, an insufficient amount of mechanical force can have a similar effect, well documented by the phenotypic changes of fibroblasts. Few days after injury, fibroblasts in the wound area undergo a phenotypic change into myofibroblasts, cells that are significant for wound contraction and characterized by de novo development of in vivo stress fibers and contractile forces [83]. The transition of fibroblasts into proto- and fully differentiated myofibroblasts requires, along with a cocktail of cytokines (TGF-ß, fibronectin), mechanical tension. Without an appropriate mechanical wound environment, fibroblasts do not undergo the phenotypic changes, or comparably, when fully differentiated myofibroblasts are cultivated in collagen gels, kept under tension, and tensions are suddenly released, the cells will undergo apoptosis (for review see [103]).

A last example of mechanotransduction and its importance in the wound healing process is the morphogenesis of new capillaries. Since the 1990s, a sound basis of scientific evidence documents and explains the mechanisms of angiogenesis [104] and how surgically injured tissues are newly revascularized [105]. After migration of endothelial cells into the wound area, it is the mechanical configuration of the fibrin clot that mainly determines the capillary morphogenesis driven by local thinning of the ECM which results in local cell distortions. These well-coordinated changes in cell and cytoskeletal form with consequent changes in the cellular biochemistry result in cell growth and motility that drive morphogenesis and lumen formation of the new capillary [89, 93] (Fig. 4).

Findings from the above-mentioned basic research document how mechanically exerted forces, on a microscale, may influence the wound healing sequences and provide new insights into the complexity of the biological processes of mucosal healing. Additionally, the findings are confirmed by clinical observations on a macroscale, which corroborate the hypothesis that, firstly, applied mechanical forces on flap margins which exceed a certain magnitude

lumen formation of a new capillary in in the wound healing process

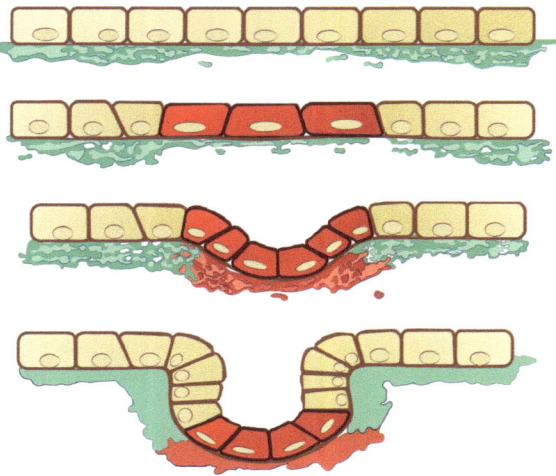

Fig. 4 Schematic representation how local changes in the extracellular matrix (ECM) may guide morphogenesis of a new capillary. Local accelerated turnover of the ECM results in local cell distortions with consequent coordinated changes in cell and cytoskeletal form. The latter produce changes in cellular biochemistry that result in cell proliferation and motility. Cell growth and migration are constrained to the small group of cells (red) that is underlined by the thinned region of the basement membrane (green). Outward budding results when red cells extend and grow because neighboring cells along the same basement membrane do not experience the stress and hence remain quiescent (white cells). (Graphic adapted from Ingber 2003)

can have a deleterious effect on soft tissue healing and, secondly, that residual flap tensions within a very low range of force are fully compatible with an uneventful healing.

4.3   Microsurgically Controlled Instrument Handling and its Impact on Tissue Mechanotransduction

The remaining question now still is how a microsurgical modification of a traditional flap approach can have the potential to positively interfere with the wound healing process in a way that blood perfusions of the microsurgically treated sites, just few days postoperatively, are significantly better compared to those treated by a conventional approach without a surgical microscope [74].

Keeping in mind that mechanical forces applied on wound margins play a pivotal role in the course of healing, and remembering the technical core components of the microsurgical technique (surgical microscope, fine suture materials, and micro instruments), one can safely assume that the lever arm for recorded improved outcome after microsurgical interventions has to be looked for in the quality of the suture materials.

In the previously mentioned randomized clinical trial, comparing macro- and microsurgical techniques in the coverage of mucosal recessions, suture diameters of either 9-0 (micro) or 4-0 (macro) were used which obviously are characterized by different mechanical properties such as rigidity and breaking strength of the threads.

An in vitro study on mucosal samples harvested from pig jaws, fixed in an apparatus with suture materials of different diameters (3-0, 5-0, 7-0) and continuously loaded with increasing forces has shown that, in fact, tissue trauma could be reduced just by choosing finer suture diameters. While 3-0 sutures mainly led to tissue breakage at an average of 13.4 N, the corresponding 7-0 ones only resulted in breakage of the thread at a mean applied force of 3.7 N [106]. As thinner sutures lead to thread breakage rather than tissue breakage, fine suture materials can be considered as the weakest link in the transmission of macroscopically applied forces and, thus, limiting the application of excessive forces. For better illustration, a 4-0 suture with a diameter of 0.2 mm and a resulting breaking strength of 1540 g (straight pull) is faced with a 9-0 suture of 0.04 mm diameter and a corresponding breaking strength of 60 g.

Focusing on mechanotransduction from applying a surgical force to the ECM to the genome and asking if all the pieces are now in place, we can state that in the last decade, basic research has proven that oral mucosal tissues are susceptible to externally applied physical forces [81] and that such forces, by the communication of mechanical cues between the ECM and the cells, can directly influence gene expression [87]. The fact that a surgically applied force on flap margins is transferred to the cytoskeleton of the involved cells, which, in turn, change their phenotype and function [107], might be used as an ideal biomechanical model to explain the beneficial impact of the microsurgical technique on wound healing. That the magnitude of applied tensional forces on flap margins trigger wound healing can also be observed clinically by inspecting the dimension of the scar when wound healing is completed. Both, skin and mucosal wounds, closed and healed in the presence of tension, end up in significantly more scarring and fibrosis [87, 108], the latter being slightly less prone to fibrosis because of the different biochemical environment [32].

The above-mentioned scientific findings paired with the clinical observations of improved healing pattern after microsurgical interventions suggest that a mechano-modulatory approach might be a promising way to address the multiple pathways involved in the healing response, at least in the oral mucosal wound healing setting. A better understanding of the microenvironmental cues within mucosal wounds and how they influence the behavior of cells and tissues in the healing process would help to identify therapeutic targets for mechanomodulatory approaches in periodontal surgery. The microsurgical modification of traditional surgical interventions might have the potential to be identified as such novel mechanosensitive approach and, thus, open the door for innovative surgical orientations. Until the regulatory mechanisms of applied surgical forces in periodontal surgery are better understood and surgeons trained in fine motor touch perception, the traditional tenet of passive wound closure is still justified.

5 Closing Remarks

Mucosal wound healing is a complex process, which is dependent on many cell types and mediators interacting in a highly sophisticated temporal sequence. Usually, wounds in the oral mucosa heal fast and with low complication rates.

For many years, efforts to modulate wound healing focused on the biochemical mechanisms, while more recent research has revealed a central role for mechanical forces in triggering these pathways. Mechanotransduction, which refers to the mechanisms by which mechanical forces are converted to biochemical stimuli, has been closely linked to inflammation, angiogenesis, wound contraction, collagen synthesis, and scar formation.

In the periodontal surgical setting, minimally invasive surgical procedures have shown to minimize the extent of surgical trauma, limit patient's morbidity and improve the esthetic results. Most of these beneficial effects can be explained by miniaturized flap designs and its consequent impact on blood clot stability and wound integrity.

When traditional surgical techniques have been compared with microsurgically modified ones, faster wound healing and better revascularization of the injured tissues could be observed. The underlying biological mechanisms that explain the substantial positive impact of a microsurgical modification on wound healing still are a subject of speculation. Nevertheless, the model of mechanotransduction might explain, at least partly, how microsurgery affects the microenvironmental cues that trigger cell behavior and, as a consequence, the wound healing process.

6 Key Points

1. **Mucosal wound healing**

   Mucosal wound healing after periodontal surgical interventions occurs through a complex cascade of carefully orchestrated biochemical and cellular events in overlapping phases, namely hemostasis, inflammation, proliferation, and ultimately remodeling.

2. **Minimally invasive surgical (MIS) techniques in periodontal therapy**

   From a clinical perspective, microsurgical modifications of periodontal surgical interventions minimize the trauma, limit intra- and postoperative patient morbidity, and improve the surgical outcome regarding esthetics and the quality of healing (regeneration rather than repair).

3. **Effects of MIS on the biological processes of wound healing**

   Microsurgically executed periodontal interventions limit the size of incisions needed and alter the magnitude of applied forces on the oral soft tissues (bioengineering interface between instrument and mucosal tissues), two surgical key factors which have a mechanomodulatory influence on the wound environment.

4. **Mechanotransduction**

   Mechanotransduction is defined as a biological process which refers to the mechanisms by which mechanical forces, applied on a macroscale, are converted to biochemical stimuli which substantially influence the behavior of the cells participating in wound healing.

References

1. van Mil JF, Henman M. Terminology, the importance of defining. Int J Clin Pharm. 2016;38(3):709–13.
2. Shanelec DA, Tibbets LS. A perspective on the future of periodontal microsurgery. Periodontol. 2000;1996(11):58–64.
3. Cromar GL, Xiong X, Chautard E, Ricard-Blum S, Parkinson J. Toward a systems level view of the ECM and related proteins: a framework for the systematic definition and analysis of biological systems. Proteins. 2012;80:1522–44.
4. Häkkinen L, Uitto VJ, Larjava H. Cell biology of gingival wound healing. Periodontol. 2000;2000(24):127–52.
5. Oakley C, Larjava H. Hemostasis, coagulation and complications. In: Larjava H, editor. Oral wound healing. Cell biology and clinical management. Oxford: Wiley-Blackwell; 2012. Chapter 2.
6. Mosesson MW. Fibrinogen and fibrin structure and functions. J Thromb Haemost. 2005;3(8):1894–904.
7. Weisel JW. Structure of fibrin: impact on clot stability. J Thromb Haemost. 2007;5(Suppl.1):116–24.
8. Guo S, DiPietro LA. Factors affecting wound healing. J Dent Res. 2010;89(3):219–29.
9. Robson MC, Steed DL, Franz MG. Wound healing: biologic features and approaches to maximize healing trajectories. Curr Probl Surg. 2001;38(2):71–141.
10. Liew XP, Kubes P. The neutrophil's role during health and disease. Physiol Rev. 2019;99:1223–48. Available from: https://journals.physiology.org/doi/full/10.1152/physrev.00012.2018
11. Dovi JV, Szpaderska AM, DiPietro LA. Neutrophil function in the healing wound: adding insult to injury? Thromb Haemost. 2004;92:275–80.
12. Mosser DM, Edwards JP. Exploring the full spectrum of macrophage activation. Nat Rev Immunol. 2008;8:958–69.
13. Woodley DT. Reepithelialization. In: Clark RA, editor. The molecular and cellular biology of wound repair. New York: Plenum Press; 1996. p. 339–54.
14. Oksala O, Salo T, Tammi R, Hakkinen L, Jalkanen M, Inki P, Larjava H. Expression of proteoglycans and hyaluronan during wound healing. J Histochem Cytochem. 1995;43:125–35.
15. Larjava H, Salo T, Haapasalmi K, Kramer RH, Heino J. Expression of integrins and basement membrane components by wound keratinocytes. J Clin Invest. 1993;92:1425–35.
16. Fischer D, Brown-Ludi M, Schulthess T, Chiquet-Ehrismann R. Concerted action of tenascin-C domains in cell adhesion, anti-adhesion and promotion of neurite outgrowth. J Cell Sci. 1997;10:1513–22.
17. Ghaffari A, Kilani RT, Ghahary A. Keratinocyte-conditioned media regulate collagen expression in dermal fibroblasts. J Invest Dermatol. 2009;129:340–7.
18. Cutright DE. The proliferation of blood vessels in gingival wounds. J Periodontol. 1969;40:137–41.
19. Mörmann W, Ciancio SG. Blood supply of human gingiva following periodontal surgery. A fluorescein angiographic study. J Periodontol. 1977;11:681–92.
20. Caffesse RG, Castelli WA, Nasjleti CE. Vascular response to modified Widman flap surgery in monkeys. J Periodontol. 1981;51:2–7.
21. Caffesse RG, Kon S, Castelli WA, Nasjletil CE. Revascularization following the lateral sliding flap procedure. J Periodontol. 1984;55:352–8.
22. Kon S, Caffesse RG, Castelli WA, Nasjleti CE. Revascularization following a combined gingival flap-split thickness flap procedure in monkeys. J Periodontol. 1984;55:345–51.
23. Li WW, Talcott KE, Zhai AW, Kruger EA, Li VW. The role of therapeutic angiogenesis in tissue repair and regeneration. Adv Skin Wound Care. 2005;18:491–500.
24. Guerra A, Belinha J, Natal JR. Modelling skin wound healing angiogenesis: a review. J Theor Biol. 2018;459:1–17.

25. Lange-Asschenfeldt B, Velasco P, Streit M, Hawighorst T, Detmar M, Pike SE, Tosato G. The angiogenesis inhibitor vasostatin does not impair wound healing at tumor-inhibiting doses. J Invest Dermatol. 2001;117:1036–41.
26. Roman CD, Choy H, Nanney L, Riordan C, Parman K, Johnson D, Beauchamp RD. Vascular endothelial growth factor-mediated angiogenesis inhibition and postoperative wound healing in rats. J Surg Res. 2002;105:43–7.
27. Streit M, Velasco P, Riccardi L, Spencer L, Brown LF, Janes L, Lange-Asschenfeldt B, Yano K, Hawighorst T, Iruela-Arispe L, Detmar M. Thrombospondin-1 suppresses wound healing and granulation tissue formation in the skin of transgenic mice. EMBO J. 2000;19:3272–82.
28. Rossiter H, Barresi C, Pammer J, Rendl M, Haigh J, Wagner EF, Tschachler E. Loss of vascular endothelial growth factor a activity in murine epidermal keratinocytes delays wound healing and inhibits tumor formation. Cancer Res. 2004;64:3508–16.
29. Bluff JE, O'Ceallaigh S, O'Kane S, Ferguson MW. The microcirculation in acute murine cutaneous incisional wounds shows a spatial and temporal variation in the functionality of vessels. Wound Repair Regen. 2006;14:434–42.
30. Koh TJ, DiPietro LA. Inflammation and wound healing: the role of the macrophage. Expert Rev Mol Med. 2011;13:e23.
31. DiPietro LA. Angiogenesis and wound repair: when enough is enough. J Leukoc Biol. 2016;100(5):979–84.
32. Szpaderska AM, Zuckerman JD, DiPietro LA. Differential injury responses in oral mucosal and cutaneous wounds. J Dent Res. 2003;82(8):621–6.
33. Szpaderska AM, Walsh CG, Steinberg MJ, DiPietro LA. Distinct patterns of angiogenesis in oral and skin wounds. J Dent Res. 2005;84(4):309–14.
34. Canady JW, Johnson GK, Squier CA. Measurement of blood flow in the skin and oral mucosa of the rhesus monkey (Macaca mulatta) using laser Doppler flowmetry. Comp Biochem Physiol. 1993;106(1):61–3.
35. Hering TM, Marchant RE, Anderson JM. Type V collagen during granulation tissue development. Exp Mol Pathol. 1983;39(2):219–29.
36. Laurens N, Koolwijk P, De Maat MP. Fibrin structure and wound healing. J Thromb Haemost. 2006;4:932–9.
37. Häkkinen L, Larjava H, Koivisto L. Granulation tissue formation and remodeling. In: Larjava H, editor. Oral wound healing. Cell biology and clinical management. Oxford: Wiley-Blackwell; 2012. Chapter 6.
38. Gurtner GC, Werner S, Barrandon Y, Longaker MT. Wound repair and regeneration. Nature. 2008;453(15):314–21.
39. Tomasek JJ, Gabbiani G, Hinz B, Chaponnier C, Brown RA. Myofibroblast and mechano-regulation of connective tissue remodelling. Nat Rev. 2002;3:349–69.
40. Hinz B, Gabbiani G. Fibrosis: recent advances in myofibroblast biology and new therapeutic perspectives. Biol Rep. 2010;11:78. https://doi.org/10.3410/B2-78.
41. Wong VW, Akaishi S, Longaker MT, Gurtner GC. Pushing back: wound mechanotransduction in repair and regeneration. J Invest Dermatol. 2011;131:2186–96.
42. Di Gianfilippo R, Wang I, Steigmann L, Velasquez D, Wang HL, Chan HL. Efficacy of microsurgery and comparison to macrosurgery for gingival recession treatment: a systematic review with meta-analysis. Clin Oral Investig. 2021;25:4269–80.
43. Pope C. Resisting evidence: the study of evidence-based medicine as a contemporary social movement. Health. 2003;7:267–82.
44. Popelut A, Valet F, Fromentin O, Thomas A, Bouchard P. Relationship between sponsorship and failure rate of dental implants: a systematic approach. PLoS One. 2010;5:e10274. https://doi.org/10.1371/journal.pone.0010274.
45. Greenhalgh T, Howick J, Maskrey N. Evidence based medicine: a movement in crisis? BMJ. 2014;348:g3725. https://doi.org/10.1136/bmj.g3725.
46. Probst P, Knebel P, Grummich K, Tenckhoff S, Ulrich A, Büchler MW, Diener MK. Industry bias in randomized controlled trials in general and abdominal surgery. An empirical study. Ann Surg. 2016;264:87–92.

47. van der Sanden WJ, Mettes DG, Plasschaert AJ, Grol RP, Mulder J, Verdonschot EH. Effectiveness of clinical practice guideline implementation on lower third molar management in improving clinical decision-making: a randomized controlled trial. Eur J Oral Sci. 2005;113:349–54.
48. Nguyen N, Elliott JO, Watson WD, Dominguez E. Simulation improves nontechnical skills performance of residents during the perioperative and intraoperative phases of surgery. J Surg Educ. 2015;72(5):957–63.
49. Saposnik G, Redelmeier D, Ruff CC, Tobler PN. Cognitive biases associated with medical decisions: a systematic review. BMC Med Inform Decis Mak. 2016;16:138. Available from: https://bmcmedinformdecismak.biomedcentral.com/articles/10.1186/s12911-016-0377-1
50. Del Fabbro M, Taschieri S, Lodi G, Banfi G, Weinstein RL. Magnification devices for endodontic therapy. Cochrane Database Syst Rev. 2015;12:CD005969. Available from: https://www.cochranelibrary.com/cdsr/doi/10.1002/14651858.CD005969.pub3/full.
51. Karring T, Lindhe J. Concepts in periodontal tissue regeneration. In: Lindhe J, Lang NP, editors. Clinical periodontology and implant dentistry. 6th ed. Oxford: John Wiley & Sons, Ltd.; 2015. p. 521–55.
52. Gottlow J, Nyman S, Karring T, Lindhe J. New attachment formation as the result of controlled tissue regeneration. J Clin Periodontol. 1984;11:494–503.
53. Nyman S, Lindhe J, Karring T, Rylander H. New attachment following surgical treatment of human periodontal disease. J Clin Periodontol. 1982;9:290–6.
54. Cortellini P, Tonetti MS. Regenerative periodontal therapy. In: Lang NP, Lindhe J, editors. Clinical periodontology and implant dentistry. 6th ed. Oxford: John Wiley & Sons, Ltd.; 2015. p. 901–68.
55. Mayfield L, Söderholm G, Hallström H, Kullendorff B, Edwardsson S, Bratthall G, Brägger U, Attström R. Guided tissue regeneration for the treatment of intraosseous defects using a bioabsorbable membrane. A controlled clinical study. J Clin Periodontol. 1998;25(7):585–95.
56. Harrel S. A minimally invasive surgical approach for periodontal regeneration: surgical technique and observation. J Periodontol. 1999;70:1547–57.
57. Harrel S, Nunn ME, Belling CM. Long-term results of a minimally invasive surgical approach for bone grafting. J Periodontol. 1999;70:1558–63.
58. Cortellini P, Pini-Prato GP, Tonetti M. The modified papilla preservation technique. A new surgical approach for interproximal regenerative procedures. J Periodontol. 1995;66:261–6.
59. Cortellini P, Pini-Prato GP, Tonetti MS. The simplified papilla preservation flap. A novel surgical approach for the management of soft tissues in regenerative procedures. Int J Periodontics Restorative Dent. 1999;19:589–99.
60. Trombelli L, Farina R, Franceschetti G, Calura G. Single-flap approach with buccal access in periodontal reconstructive procedures. J Periodontol. 2009;80(2):353–60.
61. Zucchelli G, De Sanctis M. The papilla amplification flap: a surgical approach to narrow interproximal spaces in regenerative procedures. Int J Periodontics Restorative Dent. 2005;25(5):483–93.
62. Needleman I, Tucker R, Giedrys-Leeper E, Worthington H. Guided tissue regeneration for periodontal intrabony defects – a Cochrane systematic review. Periodontol. 2000;2005(37):106–23.
63. Cortellini P, Tonetti MS. Focus on intrabony defects: guided tissue regeneration. Periodontol. 2000;2000(22):104–13.
64. Craig RG, Kallur SP, Inoue M, Rosenberg PA, LeGeros RZ. Effect of enamel matrix proteins on the periodontal connective tissue-material interface after wound healing. J Biomed Mater Res A. 2004;69(1):180–7.
65. Esposito M, Coulthard P, Worthington HV. Enamel matrix derivative (Emdogain®) for periodontal tissue regeneration in intrabony defects. Cochrane Database Syst Rev. 2003;2:CD003875. https://doi.org/10.1002/14651858.CD003875.pub2/full.
66. Cortellini P, Tonetti MS. A minimally invasive surgical technique (MIST) with enamel matrix derivate in the regenerative treatment of intrabony defects: a novel approach to limit morbidity. J Clin Periodontol. 2007;34:87–93.

67. Cortellini P, Tonetti MS. Improved wound stability with a modified minimally invasive surgical technique in the regenerative treatment of isolated interdental intrabony defects. J Clin Periodontol. 2009;36:157–63.
68. Cortellini P, Tonetti MS. Clinical and radiographic outcomes of the modified minimally invasive surgical technique with and without regenerative materials: a randomized-controlled trial in intra-bony defects. J Clin Periodontol. 2011;38:365–73.
69. Azuma H, Kono T, Morita H, Tsumori N, Miki H, Shiomi K, Umeda M. Single flap periodontal surgery induces early fibrous tissue generation by wound stabilization. J Hard Tissue Biol. 2017;26(2):119–26.
70. Burkhardt R, Hämmerle CHF, Lang NP. How do visual-spatial and psychomotor abilities influence clinical performance in periodontal plastic surgery? J Clin Periodontol. 2018;46(1):1–14.
71. Evian CI, Corn H, Rosenberg ES. Retained interdental papilla procedure for maintaining anterior esthetics. Compend Contin Educ Dent. 1985;58:58–64.
72. Takei HH, Han TJ, Carranza FA, Kenney EB, Lekovic V. Flap technique for periodontal bone implants. Papilla preservation technique. J Periodontol. 1985;56(4):204–10.
73. Cortellini P, Tonetti MS. Microsurgical approach to periodontal regeneration. Initial evaluation in a case cohort. J Periodontol. 2001;72(4):559–69.
74. Burkhardt R, Lang NP. Coverage of localized gingival recessions: comparison of micro- and macrosurgical techniques. J Clin Periodontol. 2005;32:287–93.
75. Ioannidis A, Arvanitidis K, Filidou E, Valatas V, Stavrou G, Michalopoulos A, Kolios G, Kotzampassi K. The length of surgical skin incision in postoperative inflammatory reaction. JSLS. 2018;22(4):e2018.00045.
76. Pini-Prato G, Pagliaro U, Baldi C, Nieri M, Saletta D, Cairo F, Cortellini P. Coronally advanced flap procedures. Flap with tension versus flap without tension: a randomized controlled clinical study. J Periodontol. 2000;71:188–201.
77. Burkhardt R, Lang NP. Role of flap tension in primary wound closure of mucoperiosteal flaps: a prospective cohort study. Clin Oral Impl Res. 2010;21:50–4.
78. De Stavola L, Tunkel J. The role played by a suspended external-internal suture in reducing marginal flap tension after bone reconstruction: a clinical prospective cohort study in the maxilla. J Oral Maxillofac Implants. 2014;29:921–6.
79. Morin G, Rand M, Burgess LP, Voussoughi J, Graeber GM. Wound healing: relationship of wound tension to tensile strength in rats. Laryngoscope. 1989;99:783–8.
80. Pickett B, Burgess LP, Livermore GH, Tzikas TL, Vossoughi J. Wound healing: tensile strength versus healing time for wounds closed under tension. Arch Otolaryngol Head Neck Surg. 1996;122:565–8.
81. Hinz B. Matrix mechanics and regulation of the fibroblast phenotype. Periodontol. 2000;2013(63):14–28.
82. Blaber E, Sato K, Almeida EA. Stem cell health and tissue regeneration in microgravity. Stem Cells Dev. 2014;23(Suppl 1):73–8.
83. Hinz B, Phan SH, Thannickal VJ, Prunotto M, Desmoulière A, Varga J, De Wever O, Mareel M, Gabbiani G. Recent developments in myofibroblast biology. Am J Clin Pathol. 2012;180(4):1340–55.
84. Chu EK, Cheng J, Foley JS, Mecham BH, Owen CA, Haley KJ, Mariani TJ, Kohane IS, Tschumperlin DJ, Drazen JM. Induction of the plasminogen activator system by mechanical stimulation of human bronchial epithelial cells. Am J Respir Cell Mol Biol. 2006;35(6):628–38.
85. Gemmiti CV, Guldberg RE. Shear stress magnitude and duration modulates matrix composition and tensile mechanical properties in engineered cartilaginous tissue. Biotechnol Bioeng. 2009;104(4):809–20.
86. Gulino-Debrac D. Mechanotransduction at the basis of endothelial barrier function. Tissue Barriers. 2013;1(2):e24180.

87. Duscher D, Maan ZN, Wong VW, Rennert RC, Januszyk M, Rodrigues M, Hu M, Whitmore AJ, Whittam AJ, Longaker MT, Gurtner GC. Mechanotransduction and fibrosis. J Biomech. 2005;27(9):1997–2005.

88. Ingber DE. Tensegrity: the architectural basis of cellular mechanotransduction. Annu Rev Physiol. 1997;59:575–99.

89. Ingber DE, Tensegrity II. How structural networks influence cellular information processing networks. J Cell Sci. 2003;116:1397–408.

90. Wong VW, Longaker MT, Gurtner GC. Soft tissue mechanotransduction in wound healing and fibrosis. Semin Cell Dev Biol. 2012;23:981–6.

91. Hynes RO. Extracellular matrix: not just pretty fibrils. Science. 2009;326:1216–9.

92. Wang N, Tytell JD, Ingber DE. Mechanotransduction at a distance: mechanically coupling the extracellular matrix with the nucleus. Nat Rev Mol Cell Biol. 2009;10:75–82.

93. Mammoto T, Mammoto A, Ingber DA. Mechanobiology and developmental control. Annu Rev Cell Dev Biol. 2013;29:27–61.

94. Hahn C, Schwartz MA. Mechanotransduction in vascular physiology and atherogenesis. Nat Rev Mol Cell Biol. 2009;10:53–62.

95. Zöllner AM, Buganza A, Kuhlb T, Kuhlb E. On the biomechanics and mechanobiology of growing skin. J Theor Biol. 2012;297:166–75.

96. Dieffenbach PB, Maracle M, Tschumperlin DJ, Fredenburgh LE. Mechanobiological feedback in pulmonary vascular disease. Front Physiol. 2018;9:951. https://doi.org/10.3389/fphys.2018.00951/full.

97. Van Beurden HE, Snoek PA, Von den Hoff JW, Torensma R, Maltha JC, Kuijpers-Jagtman AM. In vitro migration and adhesion of fibroblasts from different phases of palatal wound healing. Wound Rep Reg. 2006;14:66–71.

98. Chukkapalli SS, Lele TP. Periodontal cell mechanotransduction. Open Biol. 2018;8:180053. https://doi.org/10.1098/rsob.180053.

99. Weisel JW. Stressed fibrin lysis. J Thromb Haemost. 2011;9:977–8.

100. Liu W, Carlisle CR, Sparks EA, Guthold M. The mechanical properties of single fibrin fibers. The mechanical properties of single fibrin fibers. J Thromb Haemost. 2010;8:1030–6.

101. Burkhardt R, Ruiz Magaz V, Hämmerle CH, Lang NP. Interposition of a connective tissue graft or a collagen matrix to enhance wound stability – an experimental study in dogs. J Clin Periodontol. 2016;43:366–73.

102. Varjú I, Sótonyi P, Machovich R, Szabó L, Tenekedjiev K, Silva MM, Longstaff C, Kolev K. Hindered dissolution of fibrin formed under mechanical stress. J Thromb Haemost. 2011;9:979–86.

103. Darby IA, Laverdet B, Bonté DA. Fibroblasts and myofibroblasts in wound healing. Clin Cosmet Investig Dermatol. 2014;7:301–11.

104. Nehls V, Herrmann R. The configuration of fibrin clots determines capillary morphogenesis and endothelial cell migration. Microvasc Res. 1996;51:347–64.

105. Knapik A, Hegland N, Calcagni M, Althaus M, Vollmar B, Giovanoli P, Lindenblatt N. Metalloproteinases facilitate connection of wound bed vessels to pre-existing skin graft vasculature. Microvasc Res. 2012;84:16–23.

106. Burkhardt R, Preiss A, Joss A, Lang NP. Influence of suture tension to the tearing characteristics of the soft tissues: an in vitro experiment. Clin Oral Impl Res. 2008;19:314–9.

107. Gieni RS, Hendzel MG. Mechanotransduction from the ECM to the genome: are the pieces now in place? J Cell Biochem. 2008;104:1964–87.

108. Sorg H, Tilkorn DJ, Hager S, Hauser J, Mirastschijski U. Skin wound healing: an update on the current knowledge and concepts. Eur Surg Res. 2017;58(1):81–94.

Fundamentals of the Operating Microscope

Irene Marron-Tarrazzi

Contents

I. Marron-Tarrazzi (✉)
Private Practice, Miami, Florida, USA

Adjunct Clinical Professor, Department of Periodontics, Nova Southeastern University, Fort Lauderdale, FL, USA
e-mail: marron@nova.edu

Abstract

The surgical microscope offers the periodontist increased illumination and enhanced visualization of small anatomical structures. It allows the surgeon to perform procedures with greater precision than with other methods of magnification.

This chapter provides an overview of magnification in dentistry, reviews the basics of the different instruments of optical magnification currently available. It compares the use of loupes with the operating microscope, describing the history, types of loupes, visual acuity, advantages, and disadvantages of each magnification system. The section describes in detail the parts and components of a surgical microscope: including the body of the microscope, light source, and supporting structures.

The improved visual acuity of microsurgery provides significant advantages for surgeons. These advantages include tremendously increased visibility and lighting, enhanced ergonomics and posture, ease of documentation, and improved precision in the delivery of surgical skills. The use of an operating microscope grants the periodontist the ability to perform minimally invasive procedures more accurately in less time.

Keywords

Operating microscope · Lenses · Microscopy · Microscopy/instrumentation · Microsurgery/history · Dental equipment/design · Loupes

1   Introduction

Minimally invasive surgery has revolutionized the field of surgery, including periodontics and implant dentistry and these procedures demand more precision. Periodontal microsurgery involves the use of adequate magnification and proper illumination for enhanced visualization of anatomical details and fine structures. For these reasons surgical microscopes have become an essential device for such surgical procedures [1]. Operating microscopes (OM) offer three distinct advantages to the clinician: illumination, magnification, and increased precision in the delivery of surgical skills [2]. With the advent of microscopes, it became easier for surgeons to perform minimally invasive procedures more accurately in less time.

Using a microscope initially will be challenging, there will be a steep learning curve when transitioning from other magnification systems. With constant use, the OM will become an indispensable tool for your clinical practice.

Operating microscopes have improved tremendously since they first entered the market. Today they offer good magnification without significant aberrations, sufficient illumination without excessive heat, and satisfying stability without sacrificing operational flexibility [3].

2 Magnification

The use of magnification devices in dentistry has become more and more common, with the objective of improving the quality of treatment [4]. Research shows that magnification combined with illumination improves visibility, diagnostic ability, operator ergonomics, and treatment outcome. Magnification enhances the visual acuity and supports more precise treatment [5–7]. In periodontics and implant dentistry we can find a variety of simple and complex magnification systems such as loupes, OM (Fig. 1), endoscopes, and videoscopes. Endoscope technology aids periodontal diagnosis and therapy by providing indirect visualization and magnification of the soft tissues of the sulcus, as well as the tooth surface [8, 9]. The dental videoscope has a camera at the end of the scope that transmits the digital image to a monitor [10].

The resolving power of the unaided human eye is only 0.2 mm. In other words, most people who view two points closer than 0.2 mm will see only one point. A common operating microscope can raise the resolving limit from 0.2 mm to 0.006 mm (6 microns) or well beyond the resolving power of the naked eye. Clinically, most dental practitioners routinely perform procedures requiring resolution well beyond the 0.2 mm limit of human sight [11]. For periodontics, the optimal magnification factors range from 5× to 12× [2].

Fig. 1 Operator's working position with the OM

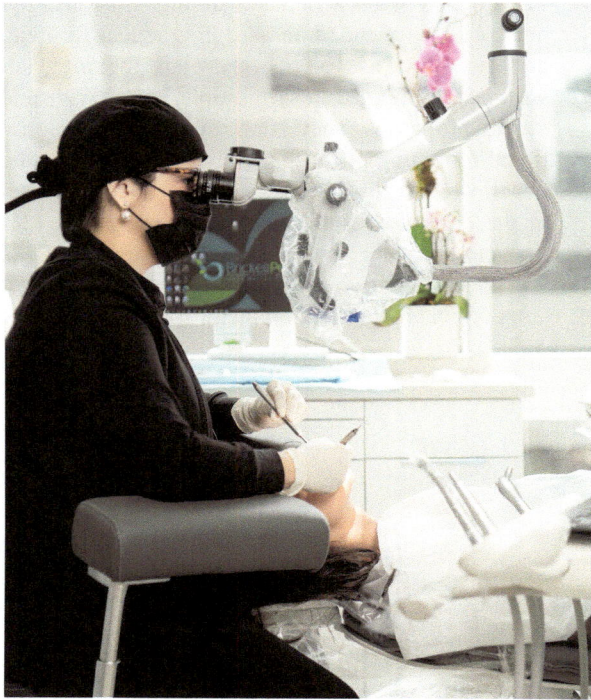

3 Loupes

Loupes, the most common magnification system used in dentistry today, were introduced to medicine in 1876 by Saemisch, a German physician [2]. Magnifying loupes were developed to address the problem of proximity, decreased depth of field, and eyestrain occasioned by moving closer to the subject [11]. All loupes employ convergent lenses (Greenough optics) [12], to form a magnified image with stereoscopic properties [11, 12]. Loupes are essentially two monocular microscopes, with lenses side by side and angled to focus on an object [12]. Basically, their lens convergence is the source of eyestrain and fatigue that dentists often experience from wearing loupes [12].

Loupes are classified by the optical method in which they produce magnification [11]. Dependent on the optical construction, different magnification factors are possible. Loupes are classified according to their different optical construction into simple loupes (single lens loupes), compound loupes (Galilean loupes), and Prismatic Loupes (Keplerian loupes) [7].

There are three types (Fig. 2) of binocular magnifying loupes:

1. **Simple Loupes**: consist of a single pair of positive, side-by-side meniscus lenses. Each simple lens has two refracting surfaces. They tend to be primitive magnifiers with limited capabilities. Their magnification can only be increased by increasing the lens diameter and thickness. The working distance and depths of field are compromised and are highly subject to optical aberrations, therefore are not recommended and are impractical for dental applications [7, 12]. They are also known as a diopter, flat-plane, or single lens loupe [11].
2. **Compound Loupes**: use multiple lenses with intervening air spaces to adjust optical properties. They offer a substantially improved optical design; with additional refracting power, magnification, working distance and depth of field can be adjusted to clinical needs without excessive increase in size or weight. Some of these loupes can be achromatic, not all are [12]. They are also known as a surgical telescope with a Galilean system configuration (the pairing of convex and concave lens elements) [3, 11].

A typical magnification factor for Galilean loupes is 2.5× with an upper limit of 3.2× [7].

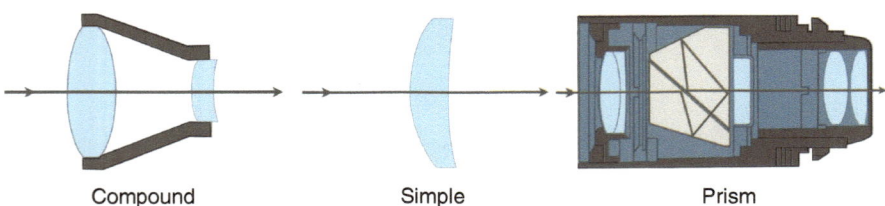

Compound   Simple   Prism

Fig. 2 Types of Loupes

3. **Prismatic Loupes**: are the most optically advanced type of loupe magnification, are actually low power telescopes. They contain Schmidt, or roof-top prisms that lengthen the light path through a series of mirror reflections within the loupes. Prism loupes produce better magnification, larger field of view, wider depths of field, and longer working distances than other loupes types. These loupes are also known as a surgical telescope with a Keplerian system configuration (prism roof design that folds the path of light) [11]. They allow a free choice of the magnification factor, commonly between 3.5× and 4.5×. The Keplerian loupe with a magnification of 4.3× achieved the best visual acuity at the typical working distance for all dentists [7]. Currently available up to 10× magnification. Only the operating microscope can provide better magnification and optimal characteristics than prismatic loupes [12].

Comparison of dental loupes		
Simple loupes	Compound loupes (Galilean system)	Prism telescopic loupes (Keplerian system)
Single pair of side-by-side meniscus lenses	Multiple lenses	Schmidt, or roof-top prisms lengthen the light path through a series of mirror reflections within the loupes
Their magnification can only be increased by increasing the diameter and thickness of the lens	Magnification can be increased by lengthening the distance between the lenses	Wider field of view, longer depth of field, better working distance
Subject to optical aberrations Impractical for magnification beyond 1.5	Some can be achromatic Inefficient above 3×	Achromatic Highest magnification: From 2.5× to 10×

4 Loupes Versus Operating Microscope

Initially, all microscopes previously developed were monocular instruments. Surgeons tried to magnify their operating field with optical aids. By the end of the nineteenth century, loupes with a ten-fold magnification and 7 cm object distance were created. The first binocular loupes were initially mounted with a light source on a headband (the Westien's double loupes with headband). In 1912, the Zeiss Company presented a binocular loupe system that was ten-fold lighter than the Westien system and had a working distance of 25 cm. These "Zeiss loupes" opened the door to modern microsurgery and are still in use. Another remarkable innovation, the von Eicken–prismatic loupe, was introduced by the Leitz Company in 1923 [13].

The use of loupes and microscopes has been shown to improve visual acuity, the clinicians' working posture, ergonomic comfort, and efficiency by increasing the working distance and therefore reduce the occurrence of repetitive stress injuries related to bad posture [14–16].

Conversely, loupes with improper working distances and/or looking-down angles (called "declination angles") can actually cause chronic neck and upper back pain [17].

There is a strong relationship between the working angle of the head (i.e., head tilt angle) and neck muscle fatigue or discomfort (Fig. 3); if the head tilt angle increases, the neck muscle fatigue is more rapid [17].

Many studies have reported presbyopia and a loss of visual acuity with increasing age. The usage of magnification devices, such as loupes, can compensate for presbyopic deficiencies [7, 18–20]. The presbyopic decrease of visual performance is inevitable and a progressive limitation of the near vision that starts at an age of around 40 years [21, 22].

Without magnification devices, visual acuity can be improved by moving closer to the object being examined. But moving closer alone is not good enough for many finely detailed clinical procedures [17]. Younger dentists can profit from natural magnification by reducing the eye-object distance, with a linear relationship between distance and magnification. This is biologically not possible for older dentists as a result of their presbyopia [18–20]. It involves not only reduced accommodation, but also more sensitive to glare, a reduced ability to recognize contrasts, and an increased need for light [22]. Studies assessing the near vision of dentists have shown that a simple test to reveal our visual deficiencies, such as the undetected beginning of presbyopia, is reading the very small print on a US $5 bill (the words of the Lincoln Memorial have to be read from a distance of 300 mm). The difference between the performance of subjects <40 years and those aged ≥40 years was highly significant [21].

Visual performance is also influenced by the type of loupe and by the practitioners' age [22]. When selecting a proper pair of surgical telescopes, one must consider many factors. These factors can be divided into two major categories: optical-performance and ergonomic [17].

Compound (Galilean) and Prism (Keplerian) loupes are the main two loupe systems used in dentistry. Studies indicate that discrimination between Galilean and Keplerian loupes is important in a clinical context and especially for dentists over 40 years of age [23].

Galilean loupes are the most popular due to their light weight, but their magnification factor is limited to 2.5× by physical constraints [23]. Keplerian loupes are sophisticated optical systems with an open magnification factor. This factor is generally limited to between 3.5× and 4.5× for ergonomic reasons. Keplerian loupes are less popular with dentists owing to their heavier weight [23].

Fig. 3 Head positioning during training exercise with prismatic loupes

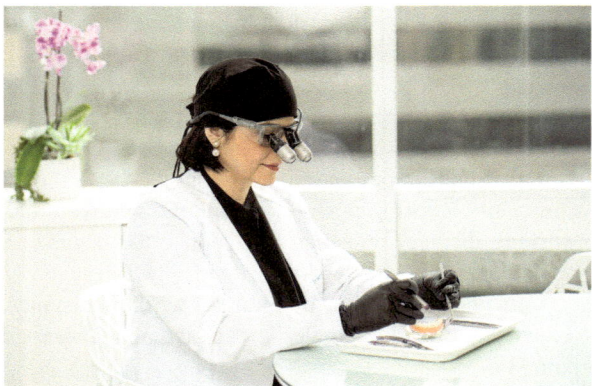

Dentists ≥ 40 years using Galilean loupes (2.5×) can achieve a visual performance similar to younger dental professionals without magnification aids [18].

When comparing these loupes, the highest visual acuity was obtained with the Keplerian loupes, followed by the Galilean loupes, due to their higher magnification [7, 19, 23].

Moreover, it was found that Keplerian loupes and the OM enhance the visual performance of dentists independent of their age [7, 19–21].

The use of high-level magnification (6–10× loupes magnification) (Fig. 8) or higher degrees of magnification provided by the OM (2.5–25×) (Fig. 9) combined with head-mounted, coaxial lighting improves the ability of the operator compared to the performance of the same task using aided vision or entry-level (2.5×) magnification, combined with overhead operatory lighting [24].

Parallel magnification protects the operator's eyes against eye fatigue and tiredness (Fig. 4). The OM allows the operator's eyes to be parallel to the object. Loupes allow for a convergent vision of the object.

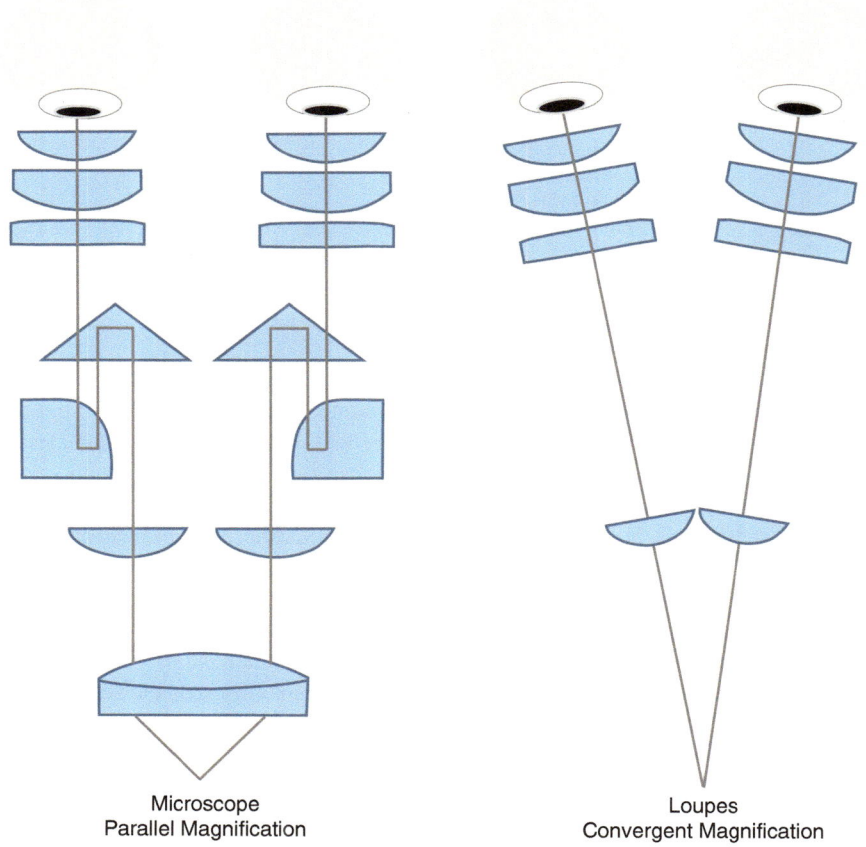

Fig. 4 Parallel magnification versus convergent magnification

Medical loupes are available with a fixed magnification between 2 and 5 times. The magnification factor of an OM is variable between approximately 1.5 and 30 times [5].

A common limitation for both loupes and the OM, of magnification in general, is that the higher the magnification, the narrower will be the field of vision and the smaller the depth of field.

There are a few advantages and disadvantages to each system:

	Loupes	Microscope
Advantages	More portable	Parallel optical path
	Initially easier to use	Binocular vision-stereopsis
	Wide field of view	Wide range of magnification
	Less expensive	Better illumination-coaxial light
	Rapidly change the working position	Better ergonomics
	Do not require space (small in size)	Better visualization (visual acuity)
	No need for higher maintenance	Wide range of documentation
		Improved precision of treatment
Disadvantages	Converging optical path (eyestrain and fatigue)	Challenging learning curve
	Unfavorable posture	New ergonomics
	The higher the magnification the heavier they become	Initial investment cost[a]
	Maximum magnification 4–5–10×	Bulkier and difficult to fit in smaller dental operatories
	Does not provide depth perception due to the lack of stereoscopic view	Provides narrower field of vision
	No documentation	
	Nonadjustable focus (or fixed magnification)	

[a]The initial investment is higher. The long-term return may not be an obstacle, if the utilization of this tool can prevent musculo-skeletal disabilities (nourished by poor ergonomics) that could lead to early retirement. The loss of production due to a shortened career would be of gigantic proportions compared to the initial price tag.

Telescopic loupes combined with a head-mounted and battery-powered lighting are more portable and allow the dentist greater freedom while working. Loupes are less expensive and initially easier to use. They can overcome the bulk of a microscope [3] and less likely to breach a clean operating field [16].

The disadvantage of loupes is that the practical maximum magnification is only about 4.5 diameters [11]. They are limited by their nonadjustable focus [3]. Another disadvantage of loupes is that the eyes must converge to view an image and the prolonged use of poorly fitted loupes can result in eyestrain, fatigue, and vision changes [12]. Loupes with increased magnification introduce the problem of stability because even slight movements of the surgeon's head will cause the surgical field to be out of focus [3].

The higher the magnification of loupes, the heavier they become and therefore potentially more uncomfortable [5, 11]. Using computerized techniques, some manufacturers can provide magnifications from 2.5× to 10× with an expanded field, such loupes require a constrained physical posture and cannot be worn for long periods of time without producing significant head, neck, and back strain [11].

Magnification in general (loupes and the OM) has several disadvantages: a restricted area of vision and loss of depth of field as magnification increases, loss of visual reference points, and a steep learning curve [16].

The OM offers the greatest flexibility and comfort in optical magnification. Loupes cannot compare to the versatility, illumination, and visual acuity offered by the microscope [16]. Unlike overhead lighting, coaxial illumination provided by the OM does not cast shadows on teeth [24].

An additional advantage for the OM is the clinicians' working posture and overall better ergonomics.

Studies have shown that the precision of tooth preparations was significantly outstanding and highly superior when using an OM compared with loupes [6, 23].

The OM has the availability of numerous accessories for digital still case documentation [16]. Also, integrated cameras or with video cameras attached to the OM, images, or video recordings of exceptional quality can be obtained while the treatment is being carried out [5].

Among the disadvantages of the OM, it can be mentioned: treatment at the beginning might be slightly slower, extra time is needed to develop an experienced team approach for planning and practice to avoid errors in positioning instruments and placement of sutures, also accentuated physiologic tremor must be controlled for fine movements.

Making manual adjustments to focus a basic microscope is time consuming, and this is a disadvantage if we compare it with more high-end OM that use a motorized zoom system.

The future development of technologies such as surgical instrument tracking autofocus will thus have the potential to significantly decrease surgical duration and also increase the performance of the surgeon [3].

5   Parts and Functions of a Surgical Microscope

The operating microscope consists of three primary components: the body of the microscope, the light source, and the supporting structure [11].

5.1   The Body of the Microscope

The binocular tube head is placed on the OM body and contains 2 eyepieces, the tube head, the magnification changer, and lens (Fig. 5).

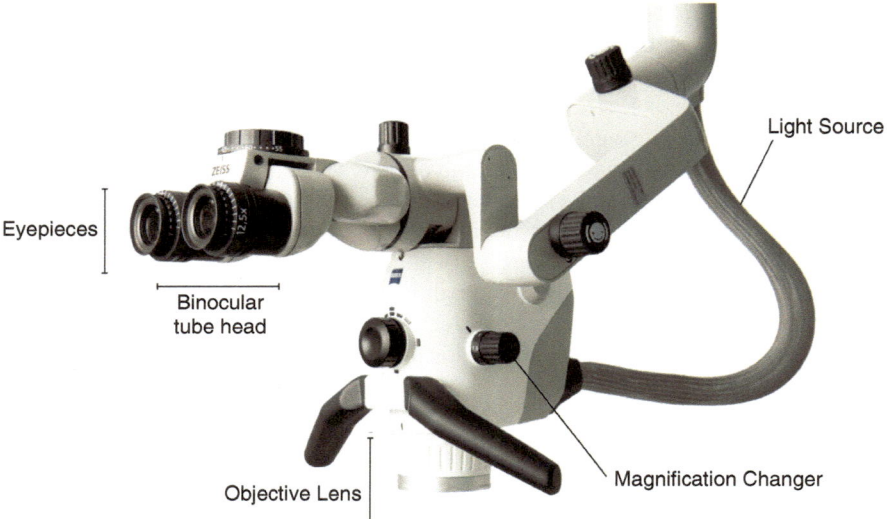

Fig. 5 Parts of an operating microscope

5.1.1 Microscope Eyepieces

The left and right optical paths in the OM view different angles of the object which creates the impression of a three-dimensional image (the stereoscopic image impression). Eyepieces are fitted with a ring for dioptric adjustment. This means that dentists with perfect or impaired vision can use the OM [5]. The eyepieces have to be adjusted to the correct interpupillary distance of the operator, so that the two eyepiece images merge into one. The distance between the pupils varies from person to person and ranges from 54 to 76 mm. It is essential to set the correct individual distance; otherwise, the eyes quickly become fatigued and 3D perception is lost [5].

5.1.2 Binocular Tube Head

The tube head also uses the stereoscopic principle of the left and right optical path for a three-dimensional image. The binocular tube head contains a lens and has a defined focal distance. Prisms inside the tube head create an upright, accurate image. There are several designs:

An inclinable tube head (0–180°) allows the dentist to alter the angle of the eyepiece holders by 180°. That means that the viewing angle of the tube can be adjusted to the position of the OM in such a way that the dentist's head can remain upright and the dentist does not have to lean backwards or forwards. A foldable tube head, even more flexible and adaptable because it accommodates different ergonomics of different operators or different positions of the patient [5]. The use of these tilting binoculars facilitates the use of the OM.

5.1.3 Co-Observation

Observation ports can be added to the microscope and it enables a second person to look into the OM. The co-observation tube can be connected via an optical splitter between the OM body and the binocular tube (Fig. 6).

The optical splitter splits the image information from one of the observation optical paths and redirects it into the co-observation tube [5]. Multiple optical ports are available on the microscope for assistant observers or adaptation of video cameras [25].

Usually, a camera is used to show the live image on a monitor. The advantage of a camera-based co-observation is that one or more persons can follow the treatment without directly looking through the OM [5]. The video image on the screen is two-dimensional and has no depth. To achieve 3D perception for the co-observer it is possible to mount a co-observation tube on the OM. There are two kinds of co-observation tubes:

The stereoscopic co-observation tube. The co-observer looks into a binocular tube with both eyes and has the same view of the treatment area as the dentist. This tube adds weight to the OM and it is important to check whether the suspension system can carry the additional weight.

The monocular co-observation tube. This offers the co-observer a view with only one eye [5].

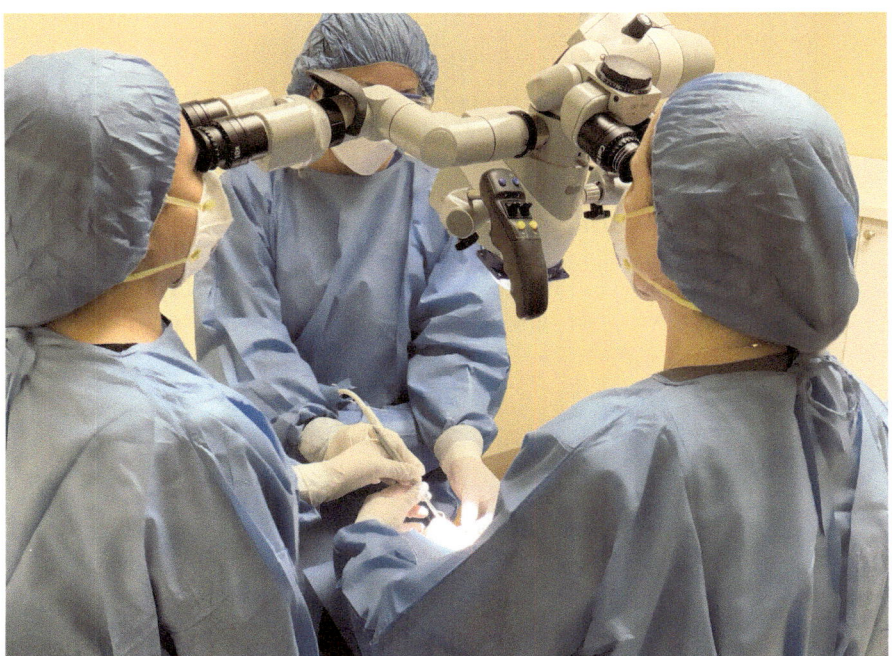

Fig. 6 Use of co-observation tube during periodontal microsurgery. (Source: Image courtesy of Dr. Lizette Llamosa)

5.1.4 Microscope Objective Lens

The objective lens is the final optical element, and its focal length determines the working distance between the microscope and the surgical field [11]. It can have a fixed focal length or a variable focal length. An OM with a fixed focal length would need to be moved up or down to obtain focus [5]. The range of focal length varies from 100 mm to 600 mm. A 200 mm focal length allows approximately 20 cm (8 in.) of working distance [11]. A working distance of 500–600 mm allows you ample space from the face of the patient for long instruments for example.

The adjustment of the focal plane within the working distance range can be performed manually, it can be controlled by turning a knob. With this system focus is obtained by turning the focus knob, this speeds up the workflow [5].

In some OM by unlocking the magnetic clutches on the handgrip, you can maneuver easily into the desired working position. This offers smooth movement and precise, stable positioning. The push of a button on the handgrip releases the magnetic brakes.

5.1.5 Microscope Magnification Changer or Zoom system

The magnification changer magnifies or minimizes the image by a given factor [5]. The magnification factor could be altered during treatment and this provides flexibility to work at a lower or higher magnification if more detail is necessary. Two systems are available: the stepless zoom system and the magnification changer (a step system, Galilean changer).

1. **Magnification Changer**: The majority of OM are fitted with a manual magnification changer (or manual zooming option, Fig. 7a). The most common magnification changer has 5 steps, and it is composed of a turret with two telescope systems of different magnification factors. By turning the turret, the telescopic systems can be viewed in either direction to achieve different magnification factors. The optical principle is an astronomical telescope, called the Galilean telescope after its inventor. This system has a compact construction with low technical complexity. The view of the treatment area is blocked while the turret is being turned manually [5].

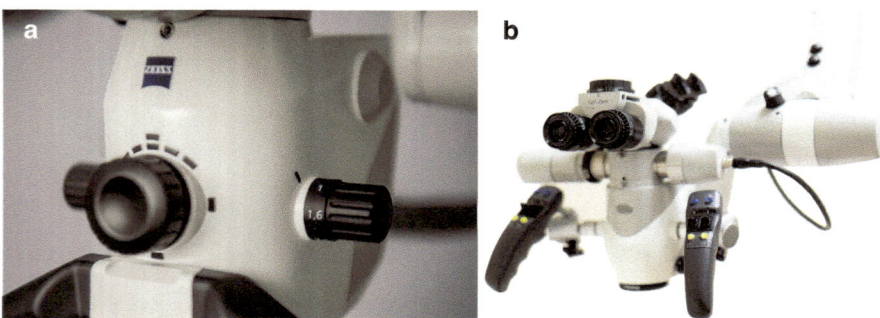

Fig. 7 (a) Magnification changer . (b) Stepless zoom system

2. **Zoom System:** It is a motorized magnification changer (Fig. 7b) and considerably more convenient [5]. The zoom changer is either a series of lenses moving in and out of the viewing axis or a system that changes the relative positions of lens elements [26]. Focusing with a power zoom microscope is performed by a foot control or by a manual control knob (handgrips/Joystick) located on the head of the microscope. The advantage of the power zoom changers is that they avoid the momentary visual disruption or jump that occurs with manual step changers as the clinician rotates the turret and progresses up or down in magnification [11]. In most OM the handgrip or joystick may control the zoom, focus, light intensity, and magnetic break or clutch.

In some OM the brightness setting adjusts automatically as you increase or decrease magnification levels.

The total magnification (M_{total}) of a surgical microscope is determined or calculated by the four optical components in the microscope, namely the focal length of the objective lens (f_{OBJ}), zoom value (M_{ZOOM}), the focal length of binocular (f_{TUBE}), and the magnifying power of eyepieces (M_{EP}) [26]. The total magnification can be represented by the following formula:

$$M_{total} = \frac{f_{TUBE}}{f_{OBJ}} \times M_{EP} \times M_{ZOOM}$$

For example:

f_{TUBE}: The focal length of binocular (binocular focal length) = 125 mm

f_{OBJ}: The focal length of the objective lens (objective lens focal length) = 250 mm

M_{EP}: Magnifying power of eyepieces (eyepiece magnification) = 10×

M_{ZOOM}: Zoom value or magnification factor = 0.5.

Total magnification = 125/250 × 10 × 0.5 = 2.5× [11]

Some operating microscopes with zoom system can calculate the total magnification automatically and display it (Figs. 8 and 9).

5.1.6 Focusing

Microscopes need to be well focused (Fig. 10) before their operation, and when the position of the OM is adjusted during surgery, refocus is needed. A fast focusing capability can save setup time for surgery [25]. During a procedure, because of the shape of the teeth and other structures it is very difficult for the whole surgical site to be perfectly on the focal plane. Depth of focus, in other words, depth of field (DOF), is a term that indicates the area in front of and behind the point of perfect focus where the sharp focus is maintained. It depends on many factors, including but not limited to the quality of optical design, the size of objective lens aperture relative to the focal length of the objective lens, and the magnification of the object, and it is reciprocal of the resolution [26].

Another important term is parfocal, which means an optical system can stay in focus even with magnification changes. Due to the need of switching magnification during surgery, a surgical microscope being parfocal saves surgeons from repeated refocusing [25].

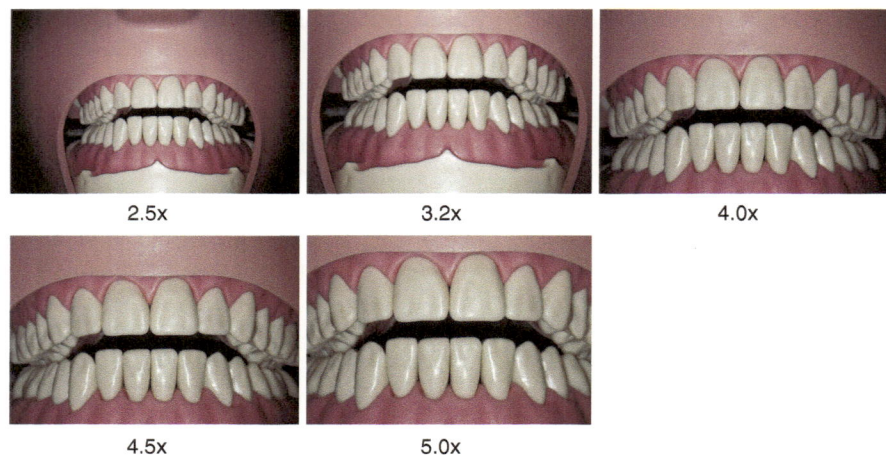

| 2.5x | 3.2x | 4.0x |

| 4.5x | 5.0x |

Fig. 8 Different magnification levels using loupes. (Source: Image courtesy Carl Zeiss Meditec AG)

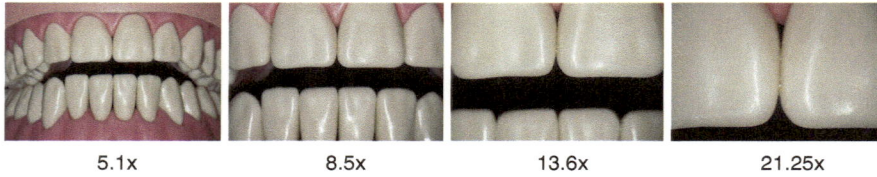

| 5.1x | 8.5x | 13.6x | 21.25x |

Fig. 9 Different magnification levels under a microscope. (Source: Image courtesy Carl Zeiss Meditec AG)

Fig. 10 Adjusting the interpupillary distance

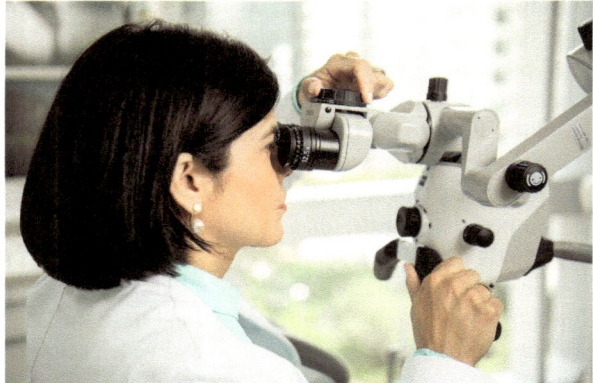

To parfocal decide if you will use the OM with glasses or not. Then set both of the oculars to zero (+/−). Focus the left and right eyepieces, one at a time, by turning the diopter ring until the image is clear and sharp. Starting with your dominant eye, then bringing the image into decent focus at first, second to highest magnification.

5.2   Light Source

5.2.1   Illumination

Illumination is another key factor besides the optical system for the imaging quality of a microscope. Successful surgical illumination has four key factors, namely the luminance, shadow management, volume of light, and heat [25].

Initially microscopes only had externally mounted independent illuminators but this created shadows.

Currently, illumination is provided through a light source on the rear side of the OM which beams the light in through the objective lens onto the treatment area. The light is integrated coaxially via the lens. This means that the light from the illuminator bulb is re-routed to a point very near the viewing axis of the microscope and is projected down through the same objective lens used for viewing [26]. Coaxial illumination, which means the light line is parallel to the sight line, provides clinicians with shadow-free images, it minimizes shadows and focuses on the operating field [17].

The tissue surface being viewed under a surgical microscope during operation is usually wet and highly reflective. The light that comes from an angle can be easily reflected away and cause a dark view [25]. The coaxial light (fiber-optic cable) is the solution to this, unlike overhead lighting, the built-in coaxial illumination does not cast shadows on teeth; [24] it provides shadow-free illumination [5, 16]. Coaxial illumination matches the optical axes of the illumination and visualization (lens) [27]. Some microscopes have slit illumination or oblique illumination.

A desirable illumination for OM should provide a stable brightness for the viewing area regardless of the change of working distance or magnification [25]. As the level of magnification increases (the larger the working distance), the field of view becomes darker because light has to travel further. If the working distance is doubled (e.g. if a working distance of 400 mm is selected instead of 200 mm), then the intensity of light at the object is reduced to a quarter. With increasing magnification, brightness also decreases at the viewer's eye [5]. The OM automatically compensate for this by adapting the light intensity to the selected magnifications, in most OM the operator can adjust the brightness manually. The advanced light management ensures stability of illumination as well as the safety of tissue. Commonly used light sources for surgical microscope are (Fig. 11) halogen light bulbs, xenon light bulbs, or light-emitting diodes (LED) [25].

1. **Halogen**: Compared to LED and xenon, halogen has a lower color temperature and thus appears yellowish to the eye (3200 to 5000 K). It can provide stable

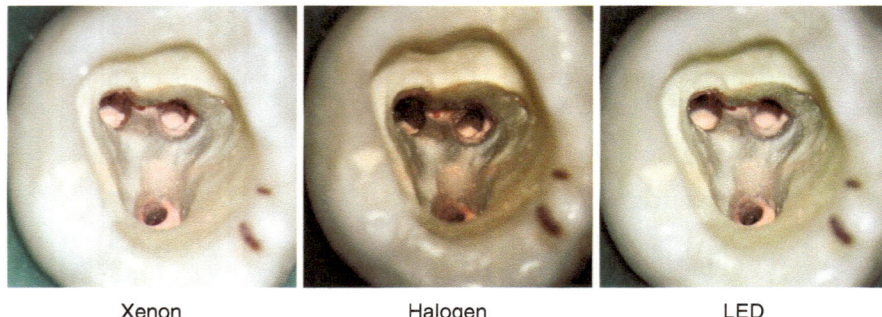

Xenon   Halogen   LED

Fig. 11 Source: Image courtesy Carl Zeiss Meditec AG

illumination. The life of a halogen lamp (e.g., 50 hours) is also much shorter than that of a xenon lamp or LED [5].

2. **Xenon**: Xenon light has the advantage that its color temperature is similar to that of daylight (white light −4000 to 6000 K). It gives the viewer the impression that the object looks natural and also provides true-color reproduction for documentation. The intensity of xenon lamps is 180 watts (higher than conventional 100-watt halogen light). Light intensity is important when working at high magnification, especially if using a SLR camera to keep exposure times short and obtain a sharp image. The life of a xenon lamp is defined by the manufacturer (e.g., 500 h) [5].

3. **LED** (light-emitting diode). LED can provide illumination in the visible wavelength range with good brightness, good stability, less power consumption, and extremely low heat [25]. The intensity of an LED light source is lower compared to xenon. The big advantage of LED is its considerably longer lifetime, usually specified at 70000 h [5]. LED as a surgical light source also has disadvantages: the higher color temperature and narrower wavelength range make the light not as close to sunlight; its spectrum is insufficient for fluorescence-guided applications; moreover, it is not easy to replace [25]. It consumes 90% less energy and generates 90% less heat than halogen. LED Expected Lifetime: 80% original brightness at 88,500 h.

4. **TriLED**. It is a maintenance-free light source that provides natural colored light at high intensities (xenon like intensities).

The light source location also impacts the level of light that reaches the clinician. Ideally, the light source should be installed away from the optics, clinician, and the patient. This light source will generate heat, so there typically is a fan by the light source to keep it cool. Most clinicians do not want the heat near them or the patients, nor do they want the fan near them because of the noise and the fact that the fan can be dispersing particles that are aerosolized from the work being done in the patient's mouth. The weight of the light source and the fan also add more weight to the suspension arm which puts more wear and tear on the suspension system.

HALOGEN	LED	XENON	TriLED
Lower color temperature	Intensity is lower (not as close to daylight)	Color temp is similar to daylight	same intensity as xenon
Appears yellowish to the eye	Not easy to replace	True-color reproduction for documentation	
Lifetime is shorter (50 H)	Lifetime: 70000 hours	Lifetime (500 H)	Maintenance free light source

5.2.2   Augmented Visualization

Contemporary surgical microscopes are enriched with various intraoperative imaging modules (Fig. 12) such as standard non-cure composite light, fluorescence imaging [25], multispectral mode (increases tissue contrast), polarized light (suppresses light reflections). Technology like Fusion Optics, where one eyepiece provides high resolution and the second eyepiece an enhanced depth of field.

Furthermore, high-definition (HD) display and three-dimensional (3D) display facilitate better visualization of both the surgical field and the multimodality images.

5.3   The Suspension System

Mechanical stability is the second most important criteria when selecting an OM. The supporting structure has the fundamental task for supporting structure to keep the microscope stable [25] and it has precision motorized mechanics so the microscope can be balanced easily and adjusted flexibly to the right position. The drift or vibrating of a microscope after positioning distracts surgeons' focus on the surgical site. Therefore, superior suspension and balancing mechanisms are important [25].

When getting a dental microscope, it is also important to consider the functionality. Space management is crucial when making a decision on how to incorporate the OM to the operatory. This means that it should be easy to integrate the microscope into the practice environment so as to enhance workflow. The ideal design should be easy to work with.

There are four types of platforms that support the OM based on its configuration (Fig. 13): (i) on casters, (ii) wall mounted, (iii) table top, and (iv) ceiling mounted.

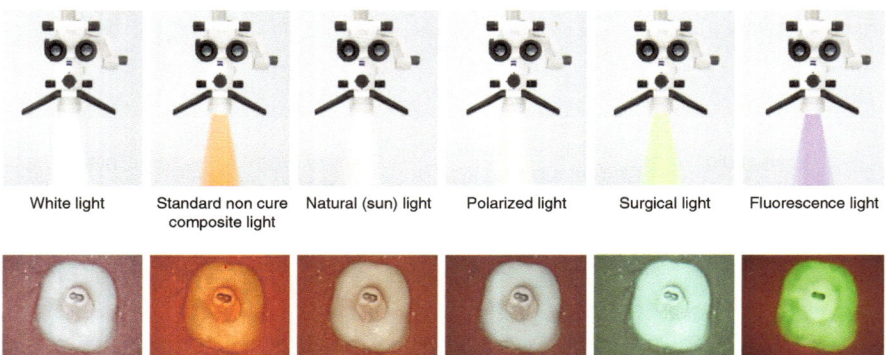

Fig. 12 Augmented visualization modes. (Source: Image courtesy Carl Zeiss Meditec AG)

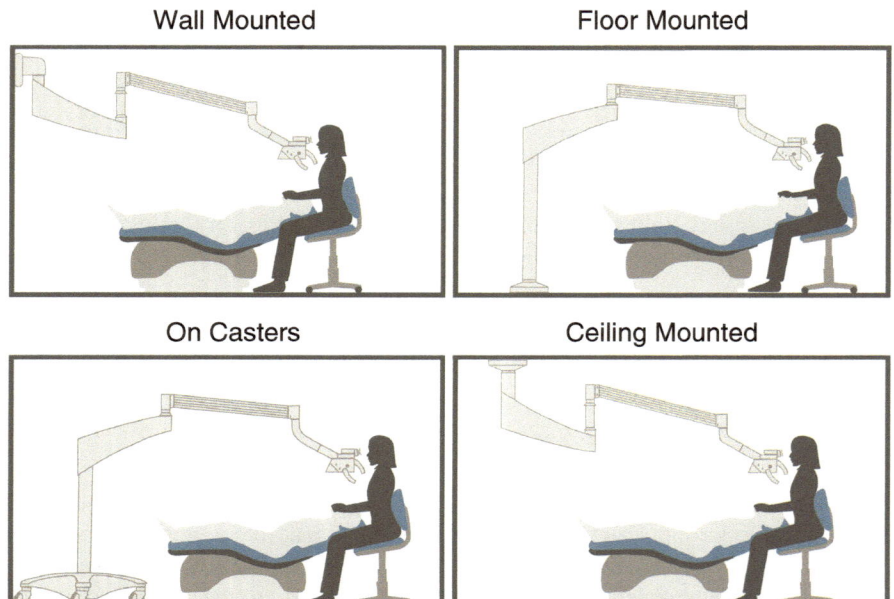

Fig. 13 Types of platforms that support the OM

The on-caster stand is the most popular supporting structure due to its better mobility, but a ceiling mount or wall mount can help with space management [1].

On-casters microscopes are floor-mounted devices that have retractable casters with single, double, or compound wheels. The caster is specifically designed to provide absolute equilibrium, allowing free movement of the balanced microscope. It provides the user with portability and flexibility capabilities. This category held the largest share of 79.5% in 2019 and is anticipated to expand at the highest annual growth over the incoming years [1].

5.4 Imaging Systems and Documentation Devices

The ease of documentation is a key benefit of the microscope. You can take high quality photos and videos without stopping the workflow. All microscopes have a way to connect a camera and video through internal optics or a beam splitter. Cameras (SLR), integrated HD video cameras, or other imaging systems can also be adapted to the OM optical ports for video recording (Fig. 14) or photography of the ongoing surgery, allowing for real time video. Some OM brands offer other visual methods, such as using smartphones, tablet applications for camera control including recording, voice recording, and media data management.

HD display and 3D display [28] have been employed in the surgical microscope for sharing of the view with high resolution and enlarged stereoscopic images [25]. The weight of the imaging system can also add more weight to the suspension arm which puts more wear and tear on the suspension system.

Imaging recording and display make it easier when training the dental team and sharing the clinician's expertise; it can also aid in patient consultation by enhancing understanding and trust.

To facilitate the use of the OM and to free the surgeons' hands during surgery contemporary surgical microscopes are often equipped with different controlling devices. We can mention foot pedals, joystick controls [5] for highly precise micropositioning, touch-screens for operation mode selection, or switching images intraoperatively [25].

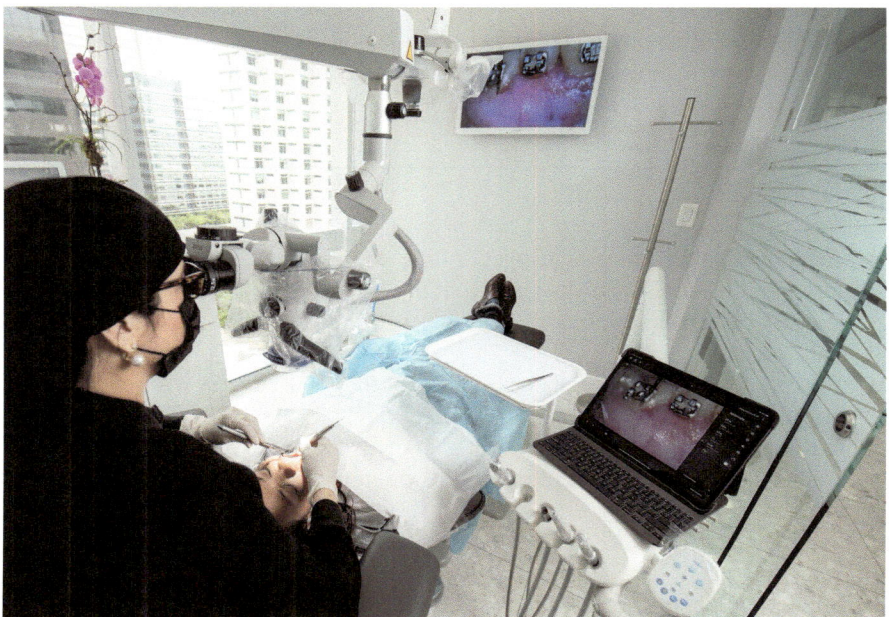

Fig. 14 Documentation using integrated HD video cameras

Emerging technologies such as wide-angle illumination, red reflex illumination, and automation and augmented reality microscopy are expected to boost the market growth [1].

The introduction of technologically advanced products is driving the demand for surgical microscopes as they are more precise, offer better illumination sources, and provide options for customization and technology integration based on the complexity of the procedures [1].

6 Conclusions

Operating microscopes (OM) offer three distinct advantages to the clinician: illumination, magnification, and increased precision in the delivery of surgical skills [2].

The visual performance is influenced by magnification devices as well as by the dentist's age. Even at low magnification, the OM provides better image quality, depth of field, illumination, and visual acuity than the naked eye or loupes. It also prevents eye fatigue and tiredness.

Choose the microscope that fits your demands. A microscope's design does not only have the esthetics in mind, but also the functionality. A carefully considered design should make it easy to integrate the microscope into the practice environment and even improve the workflow.

Among the factors to take into account when considering adding a microscope to your practice, especially in periodontics are the quality of the lens, quality of the light, depth of field, maneuverability to optimize your dental workflow, and range of movement.

Adequate magnification and proper illumination are key for the success of periodontal surgery for these reasons surgical microscopes have become an essential device for such surgical procedures.

7 Glossary

- Accommodation: is the adjustment of the optics of the eye to keep an object in focus on the retina as its distance from the eye varies.
- Depth of field: When focusing an object in the OM, we focus on a particular focal plane.
- We can also see an area above and below the focused area with equal clarity. These areas are referred to as the depth of field.
- Parfocality: an optical system can stay in focus even with magnification changes. Achieving the same focal plane on the video monitor and in both eyepieces at the same.
- Presbyopia: A gradual, age-related loss of the eyes' ability to focus actively on nearby objects.
- Stereoscopic properties: The left and right eyes perceive a particular object from two different angles (parallax). The brain then puts these two slightly different sets of visual information together to form a 3D image.

8 Key Points.

1. The operating microscopes offer the greatest flexibility and comfort in optical magnification. It provides the clinician with two distinct advantages: illumination and magnification.
2. Most loupes are available with a fixed magnification between 2 and 5 times. The magnification factor of an OM is variable between approximately 1.5 and 30 times. For periodontics, the optimal magnification factors range from 5× to 12×.
3. Coaxial illumination provides clinicians with shadow-free images. Research shows that magnification combined with illumination improves visibility, diagnostic ability, operator ergonomics, and treatment outcome.
4. The visual performance is influenced by magnification devices as well as by the dentist's age. Even at low magnification, the OM provides better image quality, depth of field, illumination, and visual acuity than the naked eye or loupes. It also prevents eye fatigue and tiredness.
5. Among the factors to take into account when considering adding a microscope to your practice, especially in periodontics are the quality of the lens, quality of the light, depth of field, mechanical stability, maneuverability to optimize your dental workflow and range of movement.

References

1. Grand View Research Smms, share and trends analysis report by type (on caster, wall-mounted), by application (oncology, ophthalmology, neurosurgery and spine), by end-use, and segment forecasts, 2018—2025," https://www.grandviewresearch.com/industry-analysis/surgical-microscopes-market. Accessed, 2020.
2. Belcher JM. A perspective on periodontal microsurgery. Int J Periodontics Restorative Dent. 2001;21:191–6.
3. Uluç K, Kujoth GC, Başkaya MK. Operating microscopes: past, present, and future. Neurosurg Focus. 2009;27:E4.
4. Del Fabbro M, Taschieri S, Lodi G, Banfi G, Weinstein RL. Magnification devices for endodontic therapy. Cochrane Database Syst Rev. 2015;2015:Cd005969.
5. Zeiss. Microscopic dentistry: a practical guide: Carl Zeiss; 2014. Available from: https://www.zeiss.com/meditec/us/c/dental-book-form.html.
6. Eichenberger M, Biner N, Amato M, Lussi A, Perrin P. Effect of magnification on the precision of tooth preparation in dentistry. Oper Dent. 2018;43:501–7.
7. Eichenberger M, Perrin P, Neuhaus KW, Bringolf U, Lussi A. Influence of loupes and age on the near visual acuity of practicing dentists. J Biomed Opt. 2011;16:035003–1–5.
8. Graetz C, Schorr S, Christofzik D, Dörfer CE, Sälzer S. How to train periodontal endoscopy? Results of a pilot study removing simulated hard deposits in vitro. Clin Oral Investig. 2020;24:607–17.
9. Kwan JY, Newkirk SM. Ultrasonic Endoscopic Periodontal Debridement. In: Harrel SK, Wilson Jr TG, editors. Minimally invasive periodontal therapy: clinical techniques and visualization technology. Hoboken, NJ: Wiley-Blackwell; 2015. p. 13–53.
10. Wilson TG Jr. The use of the dental endoscope and Videoscope for diagnosis and treatment of Peri-implant diseases. In: Harrel SK, Wilson Jr TG, editors. Minimally invasive periodontal therapy: clinical techniques and visualization technology. Hoboken, NJ: Wiley-Blackwell; 2015. p. 65–75.

11. Carr GB, Murgel CA. The use of the operating microscope in endodontics. Dent Clin N Am. 2010;54:191–214.
12. Shanelec DA. Optical principles of loupes. J Calif Dent Assoc. 1992;20:25–32.
13. Schultheiss D, Denil J. History of the microscope and development of microsurgery: a revolution for reproductive tract surgery. Andrologia. 2002;34:234–41.
14. Perrin P, Jacky D, Hotz P. The operating microscope in dental practice: minimally invasive restorations. Schweiz Monatsschr Zahnmed. 2002;112:722–32.
15. Behle C. Photography and the operating microscope in dentistry. J Calif Dent Assoc. 2001;29:765–71.
16. Tibbetts LS, Shanelec D. Principles and practice of periodontal microsurgery. MICRO: The International Journal of MicroDentistry. 2009;1:13–24.
17. Chang BJ. Ergonomic benefits of surgical telescope systems: selection guidelines. J Calif Dent Assoc. 2002;30:161–9.
18. Eichenberger M, Perrin P, Sieber KR, Lussi A. Near visual acuity of dental hygienists with and without magnification. Int J Dent Hyg. 2018;16:357–61.
19. Eichenberger M, Perrin P, Ramseyer ST, Lussi A. Visual acuity and experience with magnification devices in Swiss dental practices. Oper Dent. 2015;40:142–9.
20. Eichenberger M, Perrin P, Neuhaus KW, Bringolf U, Lussi A. Visual acuity of dentists under simulated clinical conditions. Clin Oral Investig. 2013;17:725–9.
21. Perrin P, Eichenberger M, Neuhaus KW, Lussi A. A near visual acuity test for dentists. Oper Dent. 2017;42:581–6.
22. Perrin P, Bregger R, Lussi A, Vögelin E. A near visual acuity test for hand surgeons. J Hand Surg Eur. 2019;44:326–7.
23. Perrin P, Neuhaus KW, Eichenberger M, Lussi A. Influence of different loupe systems and their light source on the vision in endodontics. Swiss Dent J. 2019;129:922–8.
24. Mamoun J. Use of high-magnification loupes or surgical operating microscope when performing prophylaxes, scaling or root planing procedures. N Y State Dent J. 2013;79:48–52.
25. Ma L, Fei B. Comprehensive review of surgical microscopes: technology development and medical applications. J Biomed Opt. 2021;26:010901.
26. Crain CL, Basic principles of the surgical microscope, https://www.scribd.com/document/358089541/Microscope-Basics/ (2006).
27. KEYENCE. Coaxial illumination. https://www.keyence.com/ss/products/microscope/glossary/cat5/coaxial_illumination/. Accessed 2021.
28. Mendez BM, Chiodo MV, Vandevender D, Patel PA. Heads-up 3D microscopy: an ergonomic and educational approach to microsurgery. Plast Reconstr Surg Glob Open. 2016;4:e717.

Design and Ergonomics of Microsurgical Instruments

Rino Burkhardt

Contents

R. Burkhardt (✉)
Private Practice, Zurich, Switzerland

Center of Dental Medicine, University of Zurich, Zurich, Switzerland

Prince Philip Dental Hospital, The University of Hong Kong, Hong Kong, SAR, China

Department of Periodontics & Oral Medicine, University of Michigan, Ann Arbor, MI, USA

© The Author(s), under exclusive license to Springer Nature Switzerland AG 2022
H.-L. (A.) Chan, D. Velasquez-Plata (eds.), *Microsurgery in Periodontal and
Implant Dentistry*, https://doi.org/10.1007/978-3-030-96874-8_4

Abstract

Instrument design in microsurgery has evolved mainly as an organic logistic response to the inherent progression in the operational demands by surgeons and their teams across different medical and dental disciplines. The understanding of the function of the human hand and the role played by its complex neuromotor framework, which fuels unparalleled motion and sensory capabilities, have been fundamental to translate the concept behind microsurgical instruments becoming natural extensions of the human body.

A well-designed microsurgical instrument ought to enable a stable grip, facilitate fine rotatory movements, provide feedback of the position of the instrument and how it is interacting with the elements of the surgical field, and minimize triggering tremors due to operational fatigue. Quality of materials utilized for crafting these instruments, along with the size, shape, and texture of the handle will ultimately determine the quality of that symbiotic relationship that exists between the hand and the instrument itself.

Understanding the intricacies of instrument design and how it interacts with the gloved hand of the microsurgeon ought to help make decisions relevant to acquisition and care of armamentarium that will ultimately facilitate the execution of tasks and enhance surgical performance when utilizing the operating microscope.

Keywords

Microsurgery · Touch Perception · Touch Ergonomics

1 Introduction

Despite the promising results of periodontal microsurgery and unlike in other specialties in dentistry, there is a slow acceptance of the surgical microscope in the periodontal community [1]. This might be explained by the fact that the novice has to overcome considerable psychomotor and perceptual problems before even learning to perform periodontal microsurgery safely. Human factors (HF), a discipline of study that deals with the human–instrument interface, is at the core of learning microsurgery and, therefore, has to be addressed when writing about microsurgical instrument design. HF is a multidisciplinary field incorporating contributions from psychology, engineering, industrial design, operations research, and others [2]. To understand the impact and the importance of instrument design on surgical performance, we have to focus on behavioral psychophysics and neurophysiology in order to explain how the use of instruments extends the internal representation of the surgeon's hand and how haptic feedback is task-specifically processed to the hand and fingertips of the surgeon. Once familiar with these aspects of HF, this knowledge helps us to improve the quality and efficiency of the microsurgical training and education.

The present chapter about design and ergonomics of microsurgical instruments is organized into four sections. The first one reviews the human hand function. It begins with describing the hand's anatomy, mechanics, and skin structure. It then examines human hand function from a neurophysiological perspective and finally, it considers manual behavioral tasks that require tactile and haptic feedback, respectively. The second section addresses ergonomics of microsurgical instruments related to instrument design and its impact on prehensile skilled movements of fingers and hands. The third section describes a basic set of innovative instruments for periodontal and periimplant microsurgery, including information about the correct use and adequate protection in the sterilization processing. Section 4 draws some conclusions about ergonomics of microsurgical instruments and offers a guideline for the proper selection of microsurgical instruments.

2 From Touch Perception to Prehensile Skilled Movements in Periodontal Microsurgery

2.1 Anatomy and Neurophysiology of the Human Hand

There is no doubt that the human hand, from a biomechanical point of view, is the most complex body part and one of the most remarkable adaptations in the history of evolution. Not surprisingly, the study of human hand function derives its historical roots from multiple sources such as anthropology, paleontology, psychology, psycholinguistics, philosophy, and neurosciences (for overview see [3]). Darwin was credited with the first formulation of the potential impact of an upright walking posture: a hand freed of the obligation to support body weight can take on other tasks. Evolutionary researchers confirm that the acquisition of new hand functions such as tool use and throwing motion required enormous changes in visual-motor and tactile-motor connections [4, 5]. Biogenetically, these are closely related to the development of primate brains and, as a consequence, to certain behavioral traits which are distinctively and exclusively human, namely: language, reason, and self-consciousness.

The human hand from an anatomical and biomechanical perspective consists of 27 single bones which are interconnected with a complicated network of ligaments and tendons. This mechanical masterpiece is operated by the muscles of the forearm and the 29 muscles of the hand itself [6]. In total, the human hand, including the wrist, has 27 degrees of freedom of movement. If we had to count the number of possible hand positions and just take the two end and one middle position of each degree of freedom, we would get the enormous number of 3^{27} positions (a 7 followed by twelve 0). Compared to the average duration of a human life of approximately 3 billions of seconds, it is obvious that we can just use a small fraction of all possible hand positions. Based on the principle of economics, it makes sense to unite degrees of freedom of movements to frequently applicable motion synergies.

The muscles and skin of the hand are innervated by the radial, median, and ulnar nerves but the pattern of sensory and motor innervation does vary considerably across individuals. From the perspective of the functional use of the hand, the median nerve is the most important in that it conveys information from a large area of skin on the palmar surface of the hand and innervates the intrinsic muscles controlling the thumb (for overview see [7]). From all the five fingers of each hand, the thumb of the dominant hand plays the most critical role in the "grasping repertoire of the hand" or as John Napier [6] had put it: "Without the thumb, the hand is put back 60 million years in evolutionary terms to a stage when the thumb had no independent movement and was just another digit." If following amputation a thumb is missing, one estimates that there is a 40% loss in the functional capacity of the hand, which might be a reason for musicians or surgeons to take out an insurance, at least for the loss of a thumb [8]. There are different features that distinguish the human hand from nonhuman primates species, noting that these morphological features allow different kinds of precision grips and precise handling of tools [9].

To unravel the complexity of precise hand movements we have to shed light on the soft tissue covering of the hand, and especially, on the anatomical features of its volar aspect and the skin of fingers and fingertips [10]. The skin on the volar surface of the hand is described as "glabrous" in contrast to hairy skin, which is found on the dorsal surface of the hand. The skin on the volar aspect is relatively thick and is capable of bending along the flexure lines of the hand when objects are grasped (Fig. 1). These folds enhance the security of the grasp and demarcate the areas of the hand where the skin is mobile as compared to the adjacent areas that are tightly bound to the underlying tissue and bones. Like all skin, the soft tissue covering of the palmar surface of finger and fingertips consists of two histological subdivisions, namely the epidermis and the dermis. The former provides a protective barrier to prevent loss of moisture and intrusion of bacteria and appears as unique fingerprint patterns (epidermal raised ridges and recessed furrows) on fingers and thumb (Fig. 2) (for overview see [11]). These characteristic patterns are mirrored in the papillary layer of the underlying dermis [12, 13]. The functional tasks of the dermis, consisting of a papillary (upper) and an elastin rich reticular (lower) layer [14], comprise the nourishment of the epidermis through its extensive network of blood vessels and capillaries (Fig. 1) and the formation of a strong and supportive structure. The fibrillar network of the dermis is housing the key anatomical elements for touch perception, the mechanoreceptors, as well as the sweat glands ($>300 \text{ cm}^{-2}$) (Fig. 3). The numerous eccrine sweat glands of the skin of the hand assist in controlling body temperature and regulate the moisture secreted by the sweat pores. This phenomenon is of utmost importance when gripping an instrument with ungloved hands. As the keratin of the skin outer layer is relatively stiff and rough at a small scale, the actual contact area between the fingerpad ridges and the impermeable metal surface is initially small as is friction. Because the keratin softens when it is hydrated by the sweat moisture, it requires many seconds for the contact area to increase to the value reached almost instantaneously with a soft material. That is why gripping a handle coated with a rubbery material is instantaneously more stable than grasping a metal instrument [15].

A good deal of what is known about hand function originally derived from two separate but related scientific disciplines, namely psychophysics and single-unit

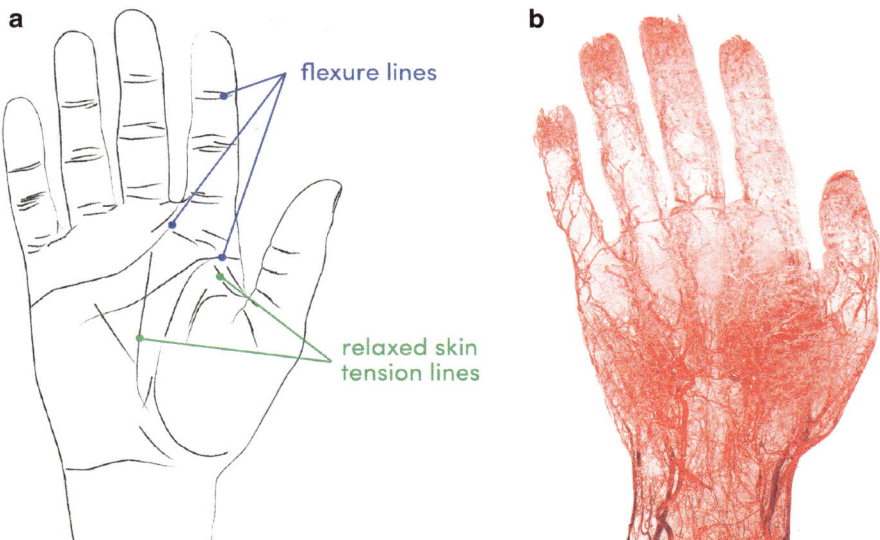

Fig. 1 Volar aspect of the human hand with the hairless skin described as "glabrous," in contrast to hairy skin on the dorsal face of the hand. (**a**) Three types of lines can be distinguished in the hand: *flexure lines* are permanent skin creases that open and close during grasping and gripping following the movements of the underlying joints. They are lines of skin stasis produced by an anchoring of the skin to the deep packing tissues. Flexure lines define the principal axis of movements of the hand. *Relaxed skin tension lines* (RSTL; Langer's lines) are topological lines drawn on a map of the human hand indicating the direction of the least flexibility of the palmar skin. They are parallel to the natural orientation of collagen fibers in the dermis and perpendicular to the underlying muscle fibers. *Papillary ridges* are explained in Fig. 2. (**b**) Corrosion specimen (epoxy resin) of the vessels of the human hand (palmar aspect). The vascular supply of the hand is a complex network of vessels derived from the radial and ulnar arteries. Two longitudinal lateral arteries on either side of each digit split up into a dense network of capillaries and anastomoses which characterize the good blood supply of the pulp of the distal phalanges of the digits

neurophysiology. Most of the research findings in the latter have been based on anesthetized animals, whereas the psychophysical work has been based on the responses of alert humans. This gap was bridged with the introduction of microneurography (recording from a single afferent unit) and microstimulation (stimulation of the same afferent), within an attentive human observer (for overview see [16–18]).

The four basic kinds of cutaneous sensations are pressure (touch/tactile sensing), warmth, cold, and pain, while other more complex sensory experiences such as itching, wetness, or tickling are based on combinations of all of these four sensations [19]. Tactile sensing activates a variety of tactile units, each consisting of an afferent fiber and its (presumed) ending. The four different types of endings in the glabrous skin of the human hand are (1) Merkel cells, (2) Meissner's corpuscles, (3) Ruffini endings, and (4) Pacinian corpuscles. The location in the glabrous skin and structural form of the four mechanoreceptors can be seen in Fig. 3. Although all populations of these endings respond to mechanical stimulation, they may be characterized

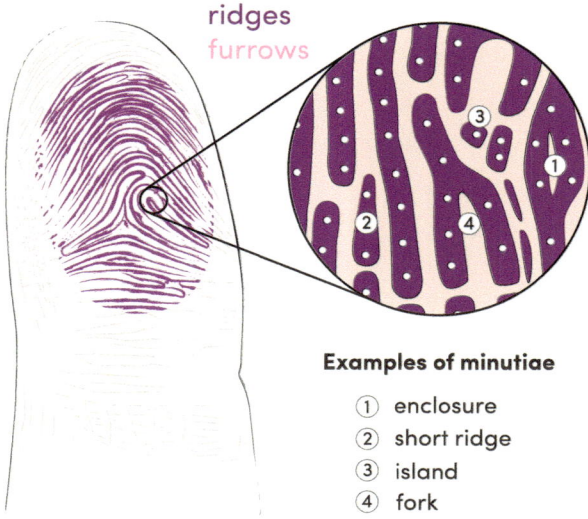

ridges
furrows

Examples of minutiae

① enclosure
② short ridge
③ island
④ fork

Fig. 2 Fingerprint structure, formed by the interconnection of epidermis and dermis via a series of papillary folds, characterizes the palmar skin areas which are involved in grasping. Fingerprint pattern exhibits many defects, called *minutiae* in fingerprint literature. Such defects include dislocations, island ridges, and incipient ridges. Sweat pores (white dots) on the ridges finely regulate the moisture in the furrow that maximizes the friction irrespective of whether a finger pad is initially wet or dry

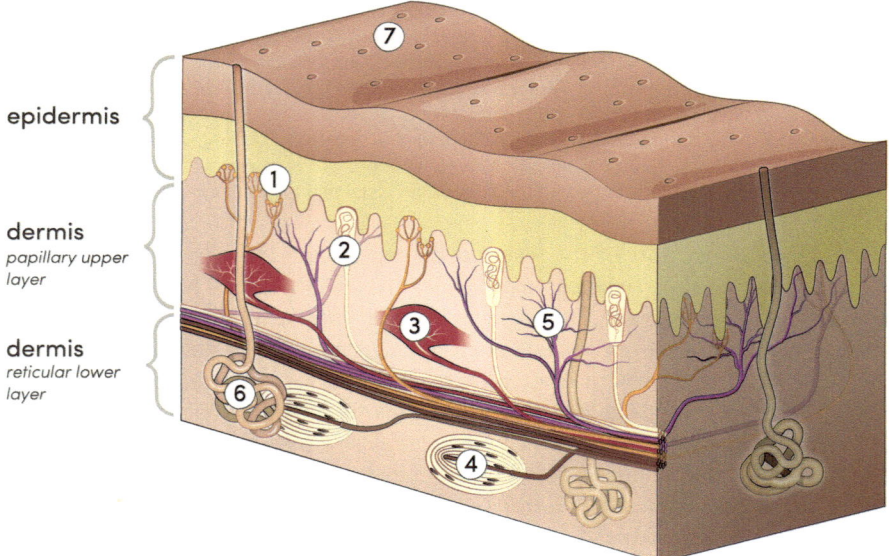

epidermis

dermis
papillary upper layer

dermis
reticular lower layer

Fig. 3 Vertical section through the glabrous skin of the human hand. Locations of the different nerve terminals and other structural elements: (1) Merkel cell neurite complex (slowly adapting type I, SAI), (2) Meissner corpuscle (fast adapting type I, FAI), (3) Ruffini corpuscle (slowly adapting type II, SAII), (4) Pacinian corpuscle (fast adapting type II, FAII), (5) free nerve endings (nociception), (6) sweat glands, (7) sweat pores

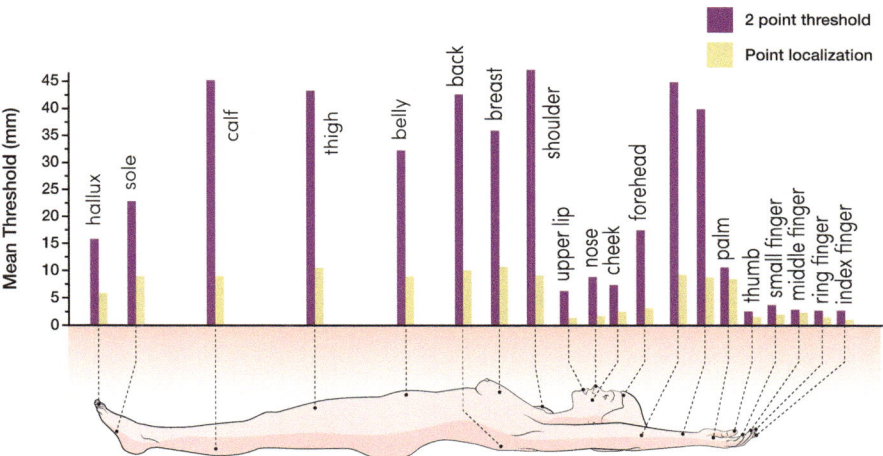

Fig. 4 Touch perception is mediated by mechanoreceptors, located in the dermis of the skin. Depending on the distribution of the different types of mechanoreceptors, two-point touch and point localization thresholds differ from various body sites. Although the threshold values of the latter are usually lower than the corresponding former ones, the measures are highly correlated. The results indicate that the more distal parts of the body are more spatially acute. The most sensitive areas for point localization are the distal phalanges of the thumb and index finger and the lips (figure adapted from [47])

by different afferent fibers. Slowly adapting afferents with a highly dynamic sensitivity (SA I) end in Merkel cell neurite complexes, however, SA II afferents with a less pronounced dynamic sensitivity and very regular sustained discharge terminate in the Ruffini type endings. The fast adapting units, preferentially sensitive to the rate of skin indentations (FA I type) are presumed to end in Meissner corpuscles, whereas the FA II units, which are highly sensitive to acceleration and respond not only when indentation is increased, but also when the stimulus is retracted, end in Pacinian corpuscles [7].

The more than 17,000 mechanoreceptive units innervating the glabrous skin of the human hand make the fingers and fingertips to the most pressure sensitive parts of the human body (Fig. 4) and, as hand and brain are close partners in two important and closely interconnected functions, to the best represented body part in the sensory cortex of the brain [20]. How touch perception and tactile tasks have an impetus to the redesign, or reallocation, of the brain's circuitry and capacity to respond to experienced demands, has been described in numerous studies about cortical plasticity [21, 22]. An adequate model to study such human experience-related cortical plasticity is musical training [23, 24]. Similar to minimally invasive surgeons who operate at the very edge of their perceptual, cognitive, and psychomotor faculties, learning and playing an instrument involves several sensory systems and the motor system and requires fine-grained perception and motor control that is unlike other everyday activities. Magnetoencephalography (MEG) studies demonstrated how intensive music training has been associated with an expansion of the functional representation of finger or hand maps. For example, the somatosensory representation of the lower lip in clarinetists or the left fifth digit in string players was found to be larger than in non-musicians [25]. Violinists who had begun training early in life (<13 years) demonstrated larger cortical representation of this digit compared to those who started to play their instrument later. This finding is reflected at a behavioral level in much lower two-point discrimination thresholds at the fingertip of musicians who started their training earlier [26].

Besides the tactile feedback of fingers and hands, the kinesthetic sense, allowing for control of muscle and tendon tension as well as joint positions, constitutes another basis for refined somatosensory perception and enables continuous monitoring of fine finger and hand movements during high-level performances such as microsurgical interventions.

2.2   Tactile Sensing and the Threshold Concept

Even if tactile sensing is essentially sensory in nature and serves to effect contact between the passive hand and an object which may or may not be moving, it provides certain information about the properties of the object (e.g., surface texture) and, therefore, is important for fine tactile acuity, which allows us to manipulate microsurgical instruments with high precision. From the different areas of the glabrous skin of the hand, the fingertips show the highest density of the four types of mechanoreceptive units compared to the remaining part of the finger and the palm (Fig. 5). The receptive fields of SA I units (Merkel cell neurite complexes) are relatively small, about 2–3 millimeters in diameter, with local areas within the receptive field that are highly sensitive. They constitute the only receptor population that responds linearly (without adaptation) to skin indentations up to about 1500 μm, making them very sensitive to vibrotactile stimulation, decoding form, texture, and curvature very well. With 1.5 units per mm^2 in the fingertip, the FA I units (Meissner cell neurite complexes) are even more densely distributed than the SA I units. They respond well to transient skin deformation and low-frequency vibration which occurs during initial contact between skin and an instrument [27]. They are activated by the application of normal force and are most sensitive to tangential force components, providing critical feedback for precise grip control. As FA I units also signal forces that act suddenly on an instrument grasped in the hand, they are important to detect both actual slip between skin and an instrument and local microslip [28]. Type 1 receptors are located near the surface of the skin (Fig. 3) and responsible for the detection of the smallest intensity of pressure (absolute pressure threshold). For men, the normal mean values for absolute tactile sensitivity average about 0.158 g on the palm and about 0.055 g on the fingertip, while the corresponding values for women are consistently lower with 0.032 g and 0.019 g, respectively [29]. The traditional test to evaluate spatial acuity of the touch sense, known as the two-point discrimination, measures the smallest gap between two points contacting the skin that are experienced as two separate tactile sensations. The threshold values tend to be about 2–4 mm on fingertips and about 10–11 mm on the palm [29]. In

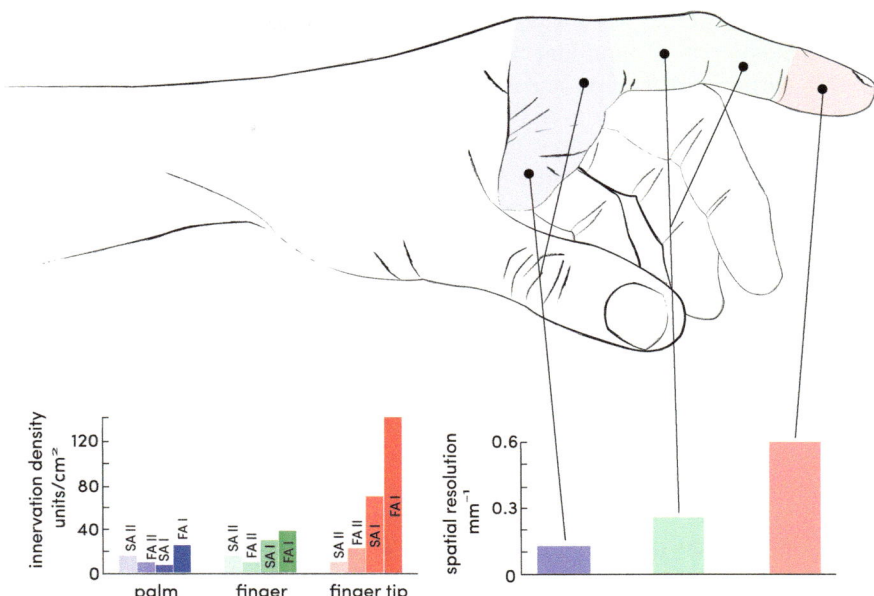

Fig. 5 The spatial resolution of different skin areas of the hand correlates with the distribution of the four types of mechanoreceptor units. Right graphic: Spatial resolution in a psychophysical test of two-point discrimination. The height of the columns gives the inverse of the two-point threshold in units of mm^{-1}. Left graphic: Histogram showing the density of innervation of the mechanoreceptive units of the glabrous skin. The spatial resolution increases roughly in parallel with the increase in density of FAI and SAI units (SAI, Merkel cell neurite complex; FAI, Meissner corpuscule; SAII, Ruffini corpuscule; FAII, Pacinian corpuscule)

general, tactile acuity of individuals is influenced by skin mechanical properties such as fingertip size [30], epidermal stiffness [31], and the spacing of fingerprint ridges [32] and declines of almost 1% per year from 12 to 85 years [33].

Type II receptors (Ruffini and Pacinian), located deeper beneath the skin in the dermis, are less densely distributed in the hand (about 350 per finger and 800 in the palm) with larger receptive fields compared to type I receptors. Hence, they are not useful to detect fine spatial details. However, as they are exquisitely sensitive to transient stimulation such as skin stretch, including vibration, SA II units play an especially important role in perceiving hand configuration and finger position and FA II units are very important for detecting more remote events, for example, those that occur with handheld instruments [17].

2.3 Dynamic Touch and Precision Grips in Periodontal Microsurgery

In contrast to the mainly sensory *touch perception*, with the fingers completely passive, active exploration of objects (*haptic touch*) and manipulation with instruments (*dynamic touch* as a subsystem of haptic touch) often result in flexed and extended fingers and palms so that the dorsal skin becomes stretched, providing additional information in the form of kinesthetic inputs. The activation of the mechanorecep-tors in the muscles, tendons, and joints of the hand, together with the type II units of the palmar skin creates movement-related skin-strain cues which may be used to assess the geometric properties of objects such as the handle of a surgical instru-ment [34]. Unlike tactile sensing, whole-hand haptic and dynamic exploration pro-duces faster and more accurate identification of objects classified by their geometric properties than does manual exploration that is limited to a single finger [35]. That is why a discussion of haptic sensory feedback in the context of manipulating surgi-cal instruments has to include prehensile activities involving grasping a handle. The properties of the instrument handle (e.g., size, weight, texture, and shape) and the task objective usually determine how the instrument is held, the contact between the handle and the hand, and the number of digits involved in the grasp (see Sect. 3). When, for example, both the thumb and index fingerpads are simultaneously used to explore a surface actively, the magnitude of sensory input perceived with the index finger is greater when two fingers are stimulated than when the index finger-pad is stimulated on its own [36]. These results suggest that a perceptual enhance-ment effect occurs due to spatial summation at these sites.

In general, there are two dominant prehensile postures, that is, the power grip and the precision grip (for taxonomy of grasps see [37]). The former is character-ized by a large area of contact between the grasped object and the palmar surfaces of the fingers and palm and used when force is the primary objective (Fig. 6). In contrast, the precision grip involves grasping an object between the tips of the thumb and index finger, and sometimes also the middle finger, in such a way that there is precise control of the position of the object and the grasping forces. Related to the task and geometry of the object, different types of precision grip are com-monly distinguished, characterized by the opposition of the thumb to one or more

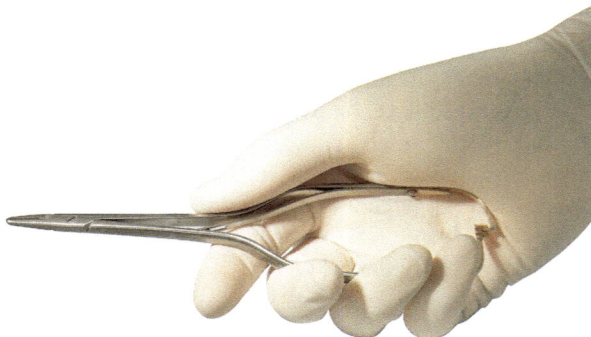

Fig. 6 Mathieu needle holder fixed in the power grip, characterized by a large area of contact between the grasped instrument and the surfaces of the fingers and palm and by little or no ability to impart motions with the fingers. Hence, power grasps do not allow fine and accurate finger and hand motions. It is primarily the instrument design which dictates how an instrument is grasped and ideally manipulated according to its function

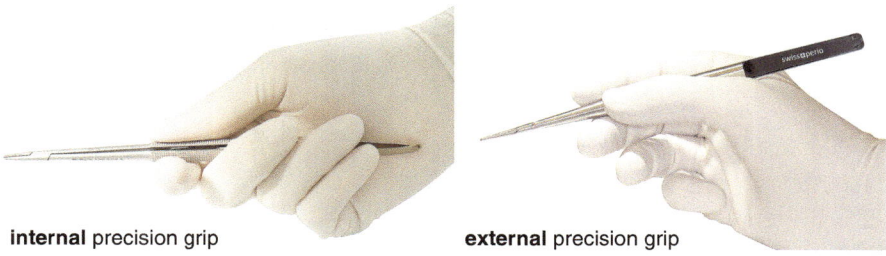

internal precision grip   external precision grip

Fig. 7 Prismatic precision grips (taxonomy revised from [37]) are characterized by the opposition of the thumb to the index and sometimes the middle finger. Such grips allow precise control of grasping forces and the position of small objects such as microsurgical instruments. In the internal variant, the instrument handle is held by the tips of the thumb, index, and middle fingers, parallel to the work surface rather than at an angle to it. The hand is steadied by the little finger edge of the hand and perhaps knuckles resting or moving on the work surface. There is only a small range of movement (protraction and retraction) in using the instrument because of its angle, its butt hitting the palm, and the middle finger not being free to flex and extend. The external precision grip starts off with a pinch grip but has the two extra components of support for the instrument in the cleft of the thumb and support for the whole hand along its medial edge. It is of special importance for microsurgery

other fingers (tip, lateral and palmar pinch). In microsurgery, where instruments are manipulated by a grasped handle of well-defined shape, only one choice between two basic types of precision grip has to be made, namely between the internal and external precision grip (Fig. 7). The latter is the common and important one for all kind of microsurgery. It is characterized by at least three separate components, each worth considering in detail because of its implication for instrument design. These components are: (1) the tips of the semiflexed index and middle fingers, and thumb, providing grip and also rotation, (2) a knowledgeable patch of skin at the apex of the thumb cleft and along the side of the index finger, providing antitremor support, guidance, and information by touch and pressure about the position of the instrument and how much force it is exerting, and (3) support from the edge of the ring and little fingers, edge of the hand, wrist, and forearm, as they rest on a stable surface providing control of tremor.

For most tasks in periodontal microsurgery, grip forces generated at the fingertips securing an instrument handle in the precision grip should be very low. Higher forces (>1 N) increase the hand tremor and continuously degrade the fine sensory experience [38]. At very low forces, the fingertip contact area increases sharply with increasing normal force, but by 1 N it is almost 70% of the contact area at 5 N [39]. This means that the contact area increases rapidly with relatively small changes in grip force (Fig. 8). At force levels of around 0.5 N, it has been estimated that the receptive fields of approximately 350 tactile units would be stimulated, and about 66% of these would be FA I units. At 1 N, approximately 450 tactile units would be stimulated, most of them extremely sensitive to small skin deformations [40]. As the grip force increases further, there is little additional change in the contact area, and so the FA I and SA I units would be less effectively stimulated.

Remember that the extensive area of contact between the fingerpads of the thumb and index finger and the dense distribution of tactile units is a uniquely human

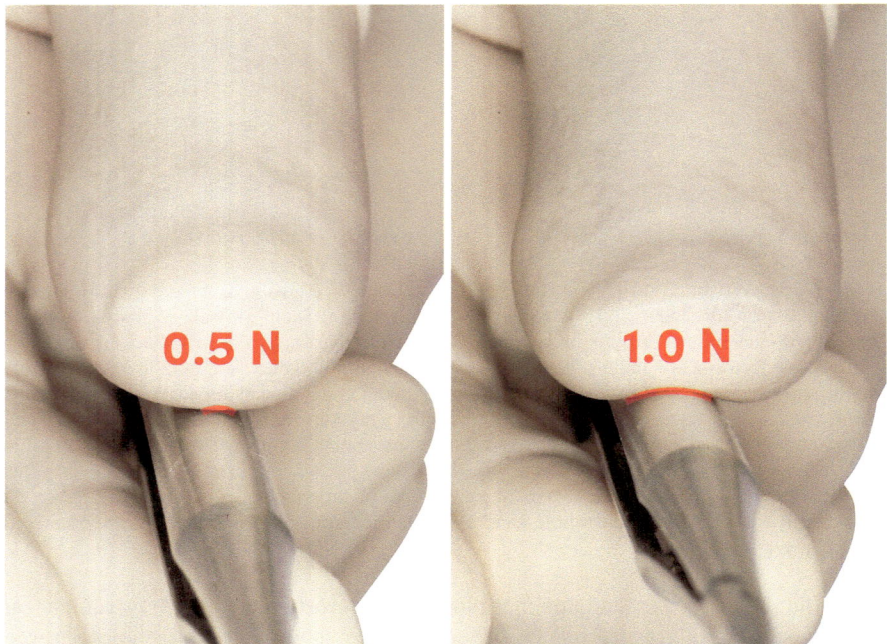

Fig. 8 Friction control, besides other variables, depends on handle curvature and fingerpad grip force which, at low levels (≈0.3–1.0 N), is directly related to an increase of the contact area. By 1 N grip force, when most of the tactile units are stimulated, the contact area is almost 70% of the one at 5 N. For most of the manipulations in periodontal microsurgery, grip forces between 0.5 and 1 N seem to be ideal. Higher forces increase hand tremor and do not help to control friction nor improve the perception in the receptive fields

characteristic, however, it is the development and elaboration of the central nervous system and not the specialization of the hand that provides the substrate for human manual skill [41].

Most manipulative surgical tasks require precise coordination of forces generated at the fingertips in order to hold the instrument in a stable grasp or to manipulate it with the required accuracy. As the intrinsic properties of the instrument (e.g., its geometry, mass, and surface texture) influence the grasping forces and the perceived instrument stability, the discussion of dynamic touch will continue in the following section about instrument design.

3   Instrument Design

3.1   Ergonomics of Microsurgical Instrument Handles

The room for error in microsurgery is so much less than in work on larger structures that it is necessary to look in critical and practical terms at the whole process of work by the periodontal surgeon. A simplified model of the surgeon at work shows three primary components—the operator, the instrument, and the tissue. These three components determine two interfaces. The first of these is ergonomics, mainly dealing with the relation between hand and handle. Ergonomics, actually a subset of HF, is a term scarcely known to most surgeons, defined as the science of the interaction between humans and their working environment [42]. The second interface, between instruments and tissue, is closely related but can be separated as the study of bioengineering. This is concerned with the physical properties of tissue and how they relate to applied physical forces. An obvious example is the unwanted crushing effect of an occluding surgical forceps on the delicate papilla of an elevated buccal flap. The distinction is a useful one in sorting out a large number of interlocking factors so that they can be analyzed and managed one at a time. This section will refer to ergonomics of microsurgical instruments, while the aspects of the bioengineering interface will be discussed later on. Instrument properties may be hierarchically organized into two major categories, namely (1) material (e.g., texture, compliance, and thermal properties) and (2) geometry (e.g., size and shape), which occurs at both micro (fingertip) and macro (larger than fingertip) levels. Weight reflects the contribution of both material and geometric features since it is partly determined by object mass (product from object density and volume) [35].

3.1.1   Instrument Handle's Shape and Size

The adoption of an external precision grip as the predominant hand posture in periodontal microsurgery requires a certain instrument length so that the instrument can lie in the surgeon's saddle between the thumb and the index finger (Fig. 7). Ideal instrument length, based on an average hand length of 19.3 cm for males and corresponding 17.2 cm for females [43], ranges from 12 cm to 24 cm, depending on the field of application. Such a size enables a primary support by the distal phalange of the middle finger and a secondary one on the base of the thumb in order to overcome gravity and stabilize the instrument without generating load between the thumb and index finger (Fig. 9). Shorter instruments are grasped with the fingertips of the thumb and the index finger and as there is no secondary support, a certain grip force must be exerted and maintained, approximately proportional to the weight of the instrument, to prevent the instrument from slipping between the fingers. These grip forces must be controlled at a constant ratio which requires a coordinated pattern of muscle activation in the hand and arm muscles [44]. The forces have to be large enough to prevent the instrument handle from slipping but not excessive, as this may cause muscle fatigue and tremor.

Besides good instrument support, the external precision grip allows fine motor manipulation of the instrument handle. Depending on the form of the handle, flat or cylindrical, rotational movements can be executed, known as one of the most precise movements that the human hand is able to perform. To precisely rotate the handle of a microsurgical instrument, the applied grip force must be minimal but exceed the slip force, defined as the minimum force at which the handle begins to slip. The slip force, in turn, is proportional to the load (tangential) forces and varies as a function of the friction between the instrument handle and the skin, or intraoperatively, the surgical glove. The friction between the glove and the instrument being grasped depends on the material of the handle, the amplitude of the grip force

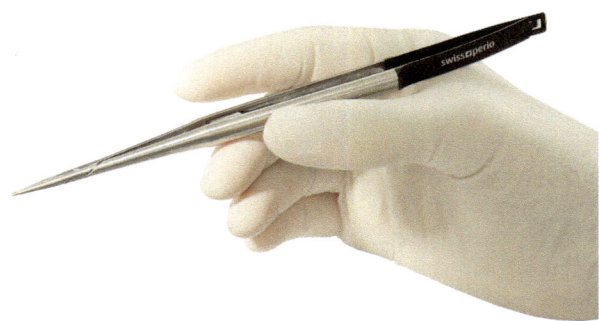

Fig. 9 The external precision grip is characterized by the support of the instrument by the middle finger and the cleft of the thumb. In this way, the instrument is stable in the hand without applying any force between the thumb and index finger to overcome gravity. Such a grip allows the best possible control of grip force to finely sense the vibrations transferred from the tip of the instrument to the receptive fields of the fingerpads. Such a size enables a primary support by the distal phalange of the middle finger and a secondary one on the base of the thumb in order to overcome gravity and stabilize the instrument without generating load between the thumb and index finger. Shorter instruments are grasped with the fingertips of the thumb and the index finger, and as there is no secondary support, a certain grip force must be exerted and maintained, approximately proportional to the weight of the instrument, to prevent the instrument from slipping between the fingers. These grip forces must be controlled at a constant ratio which requires a coordinated pattern of muscle activation in the hand and arm muscles [44]. The forces have to be large enough to prevent the instrument handle from slipping but not excessive, as this may cause muscle fatigue and tremor

at low forces (<1 N), and the contact area [45]. For cylindrical instruments, the curvature of the handle, inversely related to the radius, directly influences the contact area between handle and fingertip (Fig. 8). Measures for handle diameter providing good tactile sensing and fitting within the fingertips range from 7 mm to 12 mm [46–48]. A handle diameter of about 10 mm reveals ideal shape by skin indentations so that responses of adapting mechanoreceptors (FA I, SA I units) are directly mapped to the pressure gradient on the skin [49]. A thinner handle may allow more sensitivity because the feedback of touch is not diluted over as large an area, but there is loss of control of position within the fingertips. Wider handle diameters offer only reduced tactile feedback and shape perception reflects more the contribution of kinesthetic inputs.

To summarize the geometric features of an ideal microsurgical instrument handle: The shape should be cylindrical with a diameter of approximately 10 mm. Even if the curvature has little or no effect on the magnitude of the grasping force, it influences the safety margins that are used to prevent microslip. A handle diameter of 10 mm provides an ideal curvature to prevent slips by minimally applied grip forces. Slip responses are detected by FA I and SA I mechanoreceptors and if an instrument begins to slip between the fingers, there is an automatic increase in grip force, which occurs within 70 ms of the slip, resulting in a more stable grasp [27]. Thereby, it does not matter if the shape of the handle consists of a convex or concave surface as compared to those with flat surfaces which provide much lower safety margins related to slip prevention [50]. Besides the poor control of rotational movements, another reason why surgical blade holders with flat surfaces should be considered as obsolete.

3.1.2   Materials and Weight of Microsurgical Instruments

The predominant material for microsurgical instruments from a metallurgical point of view is martensitic stainless steel. Just for needle holders, forceps, and scissors there is an ongoing discussion about whether the instruments should be made of stainless steel or titanium, the latter being harder, lighter, and capable of being anodized to reduce glare, but more brittle, expensive, and difficult to machine. Titanium instruments tend to maintain their fine tips even after long and intense use. Additionally, they are lighter in weight than equivalent stainless steel instruments and as titanium is a nonmagnetic metal, they do not cause the light microsurgical needles to dance about. Thus, stainless steel instruments periodically need to be demagnetized by passing the instrument through a specially designed electrical coil. Despite some apparent advantages of titanium, many operators like the feel of a stainless steel instrument as titanium needle holders very often have not the same ease and smoothness of movement as steel has.

The weight of the instruments should not be so great that they dilute what feel is available to the fingers from tissue resistance. As previously described, the fingertips can sense a force down to about half a gram (an olive pip weighs about a gram), and instruments weighing less than about 40 g (the weight of a ballpoint pen) will allow an appreciation of tissue resistance that would be lost with heavier ones [38]. Both materials, stainless steel and titanium, allow the fabrication of microsurgical instruments within this low level of weight.

Regarding ergonomics, researchers have demonstrated that haptic weight perception is strongly influenced by the instrument's size and shape, which are geometric properties. This distortion of weight perception is known as the size-weight illusion [51], including both visual and haptic inputs. With low-mass objects, such as microsurgical instruments are, haptic weight perception is also influenced by object material, although less than previously noted with object size. This material-weight illusion is the result of using the cutaneous inputs to judge instrument material, which in turn influences judgments of weight [52]. Such illusions of perception might play a role when comparing and selecting surgical instruments but have a minor effect on performance in the surgical theater when the surgeon's hands are gloved.

More important than the subjective weight perception is the instrument's center of mass as it has an impact on ergonomics [53]. An instrument hold in the external precision grip is supported by the distal phalange of the middle finger and a knowledgeable patch of skin at the apex of the thumb cleft. As the center of mass lies on the grip axis, there is no torque tangential to the grip surface, and consequently, no risk for instrument rotating in the hand. To provide instrument stability, the center of mass has to be between the two supporting areas; otherwise, the instrument will tilt to either one or the other of its ends. Depending on the application requiring different instrument lengths distal from the handle, the center of mass can be adapted

Fig. 10 Examples for manufacturer-specific instrument designs, influencing weight distribution, and handling characteristics. (**a**) Proximal counterweight of a surgical forceps (S&T AG, 8212-Neuhausen, Switzerland). (**b**) Proximal stiffness adapter in microsurgical needle holder (Geister Medical Technology, 78532-Tuttlingen, Germany). (**c**) Distal counterweight of a blade holder (American Dental Systems GmbH, 85591-Vaterstetten, Germany)

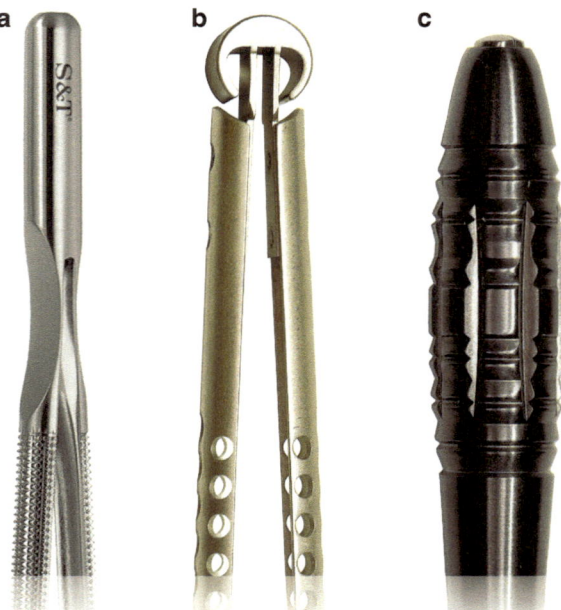

to the preference of the surgeon by instrument design, thereby influencing the weight distribution of the instrument held in the precision grip (Fig. 10). In periodontal surgery, some specific intraoperative tasks such as tissue manipulation in posterior aspects do not allow perfect hand support and thus, a slightly tip heavy balance of the instrument facilitates the precise manipulation of the instrument in the oral cavity.

3.1.3 Fine Surface Texture and Roughness of the Instrument Handle

Surgical instruments are not only passively supported in static hand positions but must be firmly stabilized in different kinds of manipulations. During rotational movements such as penetrating coarse tissues with a curved needle, fixed in the needle holder, the grip forces have to be large enough to prevent the instrument from slipping between the fingers. To penetrate the oral mucosa with a microsurgical needle, depending on the size and configuration of the needle and the site specific properties of the soft tissues, very low forces are needed (<1 N). As mentioned above, the minimum force at which the instrument handle begins to slip between the fingers, known as the slip force, varies as a function of the friction between the fingers (or gloves) and the instrument handle. Thereby, the term "safety margin" describes the difference between the slip and the grip force. If an adjustment in grip force is required due to instrument microslip, there is a delay of about 70 ms which represents about half the latency of a voluntarily initiated change in force that can be elicited by cutaneous stimulation of the fingers and twice the latency of the fastest spinal reflex in intrinsic hand muscles [54]. In general, there are large interindividual differences in grip force even if the corresponding slip forces are equivalent. The safety margins tend to be smaller the more dexterous the surgeons are and represent an important aspect in the microsurgical training.

Friction between fingers and the instrument handle plays crucial role as decreasing frictions require higher normal forces to maintain instrument stability, which in turn decrease haptic perception such as, e.g., sensing tension applied to the wound margin is. Additionally, low frictions not only influence the dynamics of prehensile force control as described above, but also affect the more proximal musculature in the arm, such as the elbow and shoulder muscles that are involved in fine motor movements during microsurgical interventions [55].

In the clinical setting, surgeons rely on friction of the instrument handle against the skin to optimize grip force, independent of whether the friction comes from macroscopic or microscopic features of the handle or a coating between the handle's surface (water, saliva, talc) and the skin [56]. Basic research in ergonomics has been done to evaluate how friction is influenced by surface parameters (dot width, interelement spacing, spatial period, ratio of element width to gap width) and the manner in which the surfaces contact the skin (force, relative speed) [36, 57, 58]. Results have shown that people are remarkably good at fine texture perception (dots and bars only a fraction of a micron high) which is mediated by vibration (PC channels; Pacinian corpuscles), whereas coarse texture (roughness) perception is not. Macrotextures are mediated by the volumetric deformation of the skin and seem to have a minor influence on friction. For a set of incised metal gratings varying in groove width from 0.123 to 1 mm (constant ridge width of 0.25 mm) no effects were found related to friction when the surfaces were either dry or lubricated with detergent [59].

To summarize the surface characteristics of an ideal instrument handle and how it affects friction: For stainless steel or titanium surfaces of a cylindrical instrument of a given diameter of around 10 mm, friction mainly depends on the contact area between the fingers and the instrument. Surface structures such as grooves or dots reduce the contact area and thus have a negative impact on friction (grip forces <1 N). Ideal microsurgical instrument handles are macroscopically smooth. Different microscopic surface textures comparable to silk, suede, and sandpaper may increase friction but the main effect is reduced to the rate with which the normal force changes during preload and loading phase (grasping the instrument), whereas the time course of the change in tangential force is similar for all surfaces [40].

3.2   Influence of Surgical Gloves on Tactile Sensitivity, Finger Pad Friction, and Surgical Performance

The manner in which the hand makes contact with the environment affects the type of information that can be extracted and the actions that can be performed. It is therefore important to expand the discussion of instrument design now to consider the impact of surgical gloves and how they affect ergonomics.

The most prominent material used for glove production is natural rubber latex, a highly deformable elastomer, allowing easy conformation to the shape of the hand [60]. The most common alternative is nitrile, characterized by a different elastic loading response which means that the conformability to the hand is perceived to be inferior to that of rubber latex. Until 2000, powder was used to coat the interior surface of gloves, allowing a reduced friction coefficient for donning. However, due to the rise in the incidents of latex allergies, there have been concerns over the proteins in latex rubber being airborne upon the removal of the glove. Consequently, in 2010 the National Health Services in the UK and many other countries released guidelines stating that rubber latex gloves must be free of powder.

3.2.1 Touch Sensation and Haptic Perception Thresholds

The literature regarding the influence of gloves on touch sensation is conflicting as between the studies many variations in the methodology are present. While some authors report a reduced tactility when gloves are worn compared to the bare hand, some others found that there was no change in the sensitivity (for overview see [61, 62]). Besides the distinction of two different points as a method to assess touch sensation, sandpaper was used to evaluate the detection of surface roughness [63]. It was shown that subjects could perceive roughness differences when moving their gloved fingers across sandpaper, but not when statically pressing. Conversely, in both the dynamic and the static tests, there was a significant difference in perceived roughness between the ungloved condition and the two gloved conditions (thickness of a single glove of 0.27 mm). Thereby, glove thickness positively correlated with a loss of cutaneous sensibility. Such increase in sensory thresholds may be explained by a disruption of the FA I mechanoreceptor function [64] which, together with SA I afferents, are important in precision grip control [28]. Interestingly, even if latex rubber is damping the vibrations caused by dynamic touch and weaken the signals to the FA I receptors, SA I mechanoreceptor function was not disrupted [64]. Traditional views of the segregated role of FA I mechanoreceptors in precision grip have been challenged and there is increasing evidence that cortical integration is multimodal, involving inputs from multiple receptor types [65]. Accordingly, the contributions of FAI and SAI afferents to grip control may overlap and involve complex interactions with other afferent subtypes [66].

In general, it is not well investigated as to how much surgical gloves affect the tactile sensitivity of a microsurgeon in different specific tasks, but it is clear they are having a negative effect. When comparing glove thickness, studies have found that the thinner gloves provide more sensitivity [67–69]. That is why gloves marketed as microsurgical gloves have a thickness of about 0.17 mm in the fingertips and 0.14 in the palm.

3.2.2 Fingerpad Friction and Grasp Force

As described above, latex rubber gloves reduce the tactile sensation, which unconsciously has an impact on grip force, which in turn is imperative for instrument control. Many of the mentioned studies appear to see an increase in grip force as beneficial, but do not look at the effects of this increase in grip, however slight, on hand fatigue and reduction in the stimulation of tactile units. Such over-gripping effect could be due to a reduced friction coefficient between the instrument and the hands when gloves are introduced [70] and has a psychophysical impact on manipulative tasks in which force control is required. Gloved hands employ a higher safety margin above the minimum force required to hold the instrument. With the use of thinner gloves a relatively low grip force level is maintained for slippery and non-slippery surfaces and a better efficiency of force and temporal control in precision handling of small objects is provided [71].

Reliable information from studies regarding frictions and slip control between gloved fingers and the instrument is scarce. Intraoperatively, surgical gloves act as a barrier to protect from bodily fluids such as blood, saliva, and water. None of the frictional tests incorporates simulative bodily fluids into the systems to assess how frictional properties may change, which will affect sensitivity and dexterity. Including fluids into assessments would provide a greater significance to the results of any of the friction and grip studies being conducted.

There is just one study found, investigating static friction of wet latex rubber gloves on a variety of dental tool patterns [72]. Greater friction coefficients for tools with medium to coarse knurled surface patterns were observed compared to annular or macroscopically smooth instrument surfaces. As the goal of the study was to determine whether a modified instrument surface texture could reduce the high pinch forces required to perform root scaling, an applied force of 40 N between gloved fingertip and instrument handle was chosen for study purposes. Such an amount of force is far above the required ones for precise manipulations in periodontal surgery, and therefore, the conclusion that knurled surfaces provide more friction cannot be used to design ideal surface textures of microsurgical instruments (Fig. 11).

3.2.3 Influence of Gloves on Surgical Performance

Surgeons express criticism for glove materials that are different from their preferred choice by claiming that the gloves are too thick, slippery, and ill fitting [62]. Most studies suggest that sensitivity, friction, and grip are affected when medical gloves are worn but, surprisingly, objective performance perception does not [73–75]. Further study is needed to understand these results, to isolate the effects of material, fit, and thickness, and to identify the critical factors in glove design which affects clinicians' ability to perform dexterous tasks [63].

As mentioned above, no major differences regarding performance could be noted for normal surgical tasks with gloved compared to bare hands, tested in laboratory conditions. Nevertheless, there is a tendency for improved performance in microsurgical tasks when thin elastic latex rubber gloves are worn instead of thicker ones or those made of nitrile [76].

3.3   Instrument use and How it Affects Hand Representation in the Brain

Instrument manipulation in periodontal microsurgery represents complex tool use that converts movements of the hands into qualitatively different mechanical actions (e.g., rotating hand into penetrating needle through mucosal tissues).

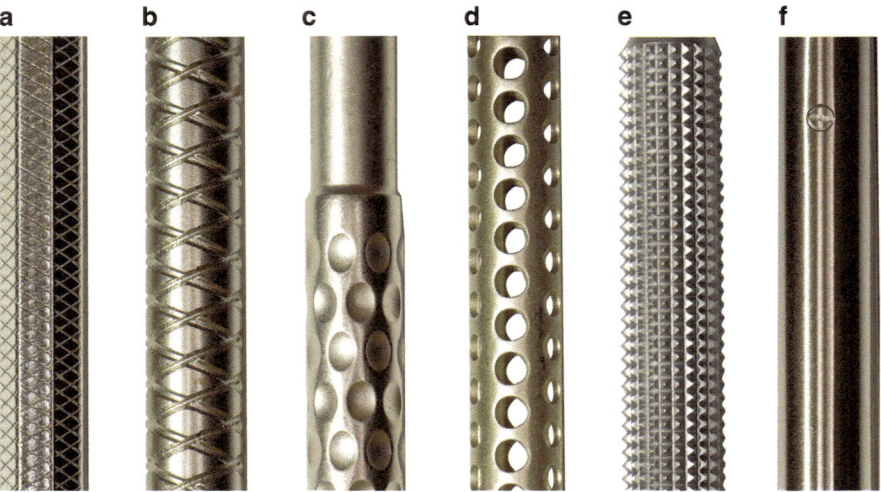

Fig. 11 Different macro- and microtextures of microsurgical instrument handles. (**a**) Hexagonal cross-section of the handle with micro furrows (Deppeler, 1180-Rolle, Switzerland), (**b**) annular crossed furrows (Hu-Friedy, 60618-Chicago, United States), (**c**) macro indents (Hu-Friedy, 60618-Chicago, United States), (**d**) perforations for friction control and additional weight reduction (Geister Medical Technology, 78532-Tuttlingen, Germany), (**e**) medium knurled surface pattern (Aesculap, 34212-Melsungen, Germany), (**f**) fine smooth surface (Hu-Friedy, 60618-Chicago, United States). The surface designs (**a**) to (**d**) seem to have no substantial positive impact on friction dynamics under wet gloved conditions. Medium to coarse knurled surface patterns (**e**) increase the friction between gloves and handle when very high grip forces are applied (<30 N). Smooth handles (**f**) provide the largest contact area between finger and handle when low grip forces are applied and, thus, the best precondition for friction control

Recent studies with "proficient" tool users such as amputees with prosthetic arms [77] and "non-proficient" tool-users such as healthy but blind-folded subjects using a blind cane to explore the environment [78] have proposed different concepts of tool-use and its modifications on the sensorimotor system and the plastic changes at the level of the body representation (for review see [79]). In general, tool-mediated sensing still is a poorly understood aspect of the daily human experience. Nevertheless, it might be of importance when surgical instruments are newly designed, in order to optimize the information process through the instrument at the sensory and motor level.

Instrument use extends the peripersonal space (PPS), defined as the space immediately surrounding the body, now generally accepted as a region of integration of somatosensory, visual, and auditory information [80]. It is a privileged interface for goal-directed actions with nearby objects such as tissue manipulation during microsurgical intervention is.

Different than the PPS and other body representations (body image, body structural description), which are conceptually and functionally difficult to disentangle, the body schema (BS), essentially *sensimotor* in nature, seems to be universally accepted and well described, with a relatively unifying definition. BS is defined as a highly plastic representation of the body parts (including hands), in terms of posture, shape, and size, that can be used to execute or imagine executing movements accurately [81]. The BS allows for execution and constant monitoring of our actions and appears to be fed mainly by proprioceptive, but also tactile and kinesthetic, information [82]. It is interesting to discuss the concept of BS in the context of surgical instrument use as it has been shown that, comparing the activity of parietal bimodal cells (i.e., cells responding to both tactile and visual stimuli) before and after instrument use, after tool use, the visual receptive fields were enlarged along the tool axis (from the hand to the working end of the instrument). Thanks to the BS we are capable of locating our hands in space, knowing exactly where the fingers are, without vision. This information is refreshed instantaneously at every single movement of the hands. A rich array of vibratory signals from the instrument are transduced by mechanoreceptors (Pacinian corpuscles) into neural response patterns that preserve the location-specifying information. The population response starts within milliseconds, which means that this time course is in line with responses of mechanoreceptors during object manipulation with the hand, suggesting that the nervous system can extract sensory information from an instrument with a similar speed as the hand itself [83, 84]. These results clearly show that a handheld instrument functions as a sensory extension of the user's body and point to the existence of an embodiment of the instrument, rather than sensory distalization or sensory projection [84]. Nevertheless, full embodiment requires the existence of three layers, namely the affective one (individual shows the same affective reactions as for his/her own body), the motor one (moves as a body part and is perceived as under one's control), and the spatial one (the space it is located in is processed as body space) [85]. The use of the above described microsurgical instruments fulfills at least the latter two criteria of embodiment. But it is important to mention that different tools or the way how they are held in the hand or how the functional end of the instrument looks like extend the BS in different ways [86]. This, in turn, underlines the importance of instrument design in order to refine the functional coupling between the instrument and the surgeon's hand.

Scientists have only recently begun investigating how handheld instruments are treated by the nervous system as sensory extensions of the body. Actual data confirm that effective motor control of instruments involves both a tool-specific expansion of the body schema (BS plasticity), and a mapping that captures how movements of the hands are transformed into actions of the instrument's end-effector (representations of the so-called motor-to-mechanical transformation). By working surgically with handheld instruments we turn from grasping the instrument to using the instrument to manipulate the tissues, while at the same time, many neurons code the movements of the end-effector of the instrument, rather than that of the hand.

To further elucidate how haptic feedback to the operator's hand can be improved by instrument design and at the same time be perfectly associated with the tissues of his or her visual attention, in depth research is needed, including specialists in manufacturing instruments, behavioral psychophysics, structural mechanics, and neuronal modeling.

4   Basic Set of Instruments for Periodontal Microsurgery

4.1   Description of Microsurgical Instruments

An ideal basic set of instruments for periodontal (plastic) microsurgery is depicted in Fig. 12. Even if at the first glance, many instruments from different manufacturers have a similar look, they widely vary in quality, price, delivery times, and back-up services. The instruments presented here are characterized by high quality standards, which not only refer to instrument design but equally to high precision in product fabrication. As many surgeons have their own preferences in instrument design and decisions to buy are often made on the basis of the catalogue price alone, it is important to have objective standards for assessing instruments for purchase. The sharpness of scissors can be tested by trying to cut thin gauze or glove rubber with them, and their stiffness can be tested by pressing them onto a simple scale for weighing letters. In a similar way forceps and needle holders can be checked for their stiffness and grip. The SwissPerio instrument set contains two scissors, one for soft tissue dissection and one for cutting threads (Fig. 13). The inclined working ends of the latter one have smooth cutting edges and allow access to difficult areas even far distal to molars in posterior zones. The tissue scissor is finely serrated which improves the cutting properties when mucosal tissues tend to slip sideways.

The needle holder, characterized by non-serrated, smooth working ends and optimal stiffness, is unmatched in its precision. It allows a firm seat for smaller needles

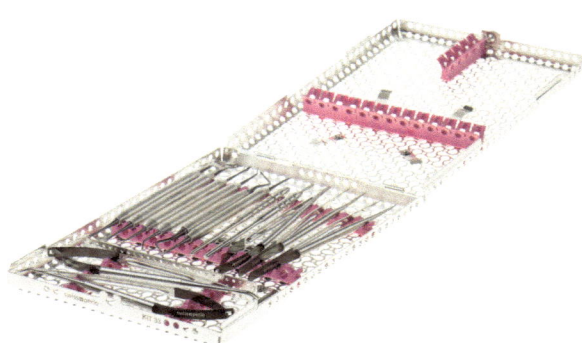

Fig. 12 Basic set of microsurgical instruments (SwissPerio, Hu-Friedy, 60618-Chicago, United States) with needle holder, forceps, scissors, and different elevators, designed for minimal traumatic flap mobilization and retraction in the palatal, buccal, and interdental areas of the oral cavity. The design of the instruments fulfills the criteria for optimal ergonomic handling, and even if the instruments are offered as microsurgical tools, they are equally suitable for interventions on a macrosurgical basis, using suture materials in the sizes of 5-0 and 6-0

Fig. 13 Two scissors for different applications, cutting threads and tissues, belong to the SwissPerio basic instrument set. One cutting edge of the tissue scissor is finely serrated to avoid mucosal slips sideways (**a**). The suture scissor with inclined working ends allows easy access to all areas of the oral cavity (**b**). The distance between the two branches of the opened suture scissor is less than 3 mm which improves instrument stability when sutures have to be removed. Both the instruments have rounded edges and are handmade with highest precision

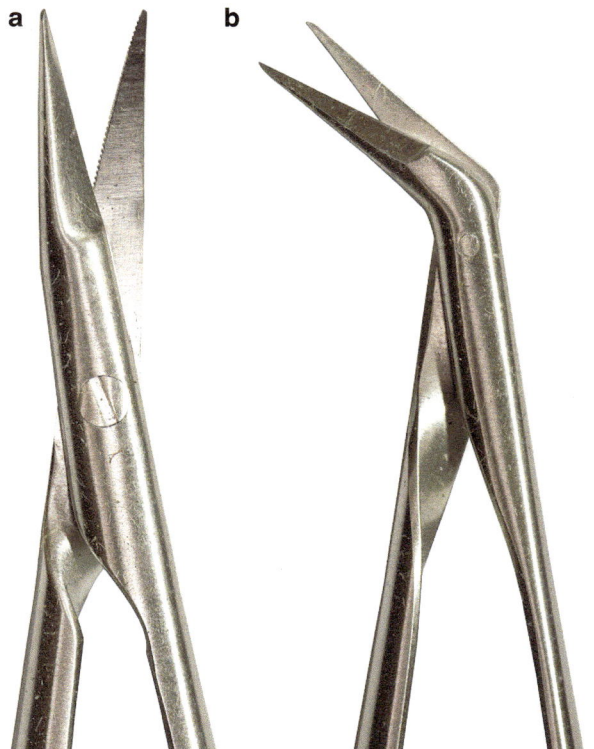

and provides an easy handling of suture diameters in a range of 5–0 to 9–0 (Fig. 14). The instrument is equipped with a lock that facilitates finger rotation without applying pressure, leading to a more precise execution of finger and hand movements. Additionally, the low locking forces reduce hand tremor while grasping the needles.

Two different types of forceps (surgical one with micro teeth/anatomical one with smooth surfaces), both configured with very fine working ends, allow firm grasping of the oral mucosa without traumatizing flaps unnecessarily, precise tissue manipulation, and fluent suturing with knot tightening.

The set is completed with four different kinds of elevators, whereof one is specifically designed as a double-end instrument to elevate papillae and interdental tissues under ultimate controlled conditions (i.e., pulling the papilla with the stiff, sharp microelevator and pushing the col. tissues with the dull pushing end). All SwissPerio instruments are coated for a harder, smoother surface for optimal edge retention and enhanced lubricity. The distinct black finish enriches the contrast and the visual acuity at the surgical site. Additionally, in the highly illuminated surgical working area, the light reflection of the instruments is reduced by matte finished handles and the black working ends.

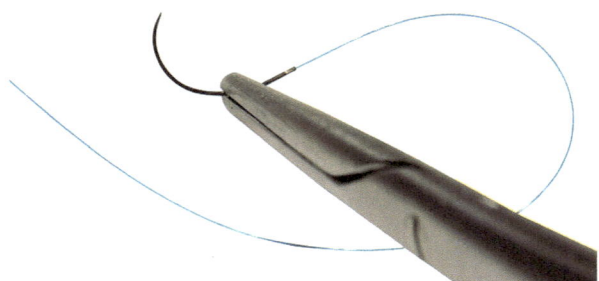

Fig. 14 The needle holder with its requirement for functionality and ergonomics is a key instrument in periodontal microsurgery as suturing has an important impact on wound stability and integrity. The instrument has smooth working ends which provide a firm seat of the grasped threads and needles. Equipped with a lock, the instrument allows finely controlled rotating movements. The lock opens and closes by just applying a minimal amount of finger pressure which contributes to good hand stability. It is suitable for the manipulation of sutures in the range of 5-0 to 9-0

4.2 Sterilization Process and Caring for Microsurgical Instruments

In order to prevent damage, microinstruments should be stored in a special perforated sterile container or tray. The tips of the instruments must not touch each other during sterilization procedures or transportation (Fig. 12). The practice staff should be thoroughly instructed about the cleaning and maintenance of such instruments, as cleaning microinstruments in a thermodisinfector without fixing them in place may cause irreparable damage to their tips. It is highly recommended to follow the manufacturer's instructions for instrument cleaning.

The ease of cleaning is also affected by the surface characteristics of the instrument. That is why overall smooth surfaces and only minimally knurled or as well smooth handles have a positive impact on the cleaning process. During surgeries, tissue fluids should not be allowed to dry on instruments and assistants must keep the instruments moist and frequently clean them with sterile watery solutions or mineral-free distilled water.

Before sterilizing the instruments and re-use, a regular general check-up is recommended to guarantee the perfect functionality of the microsurgical instruments. Such a list includes the following checkpoints: (1) General appearance. The surfaces should be clean and smooth, and edges well finished without burrs. (2) Joints should work easily. It should not take more than 100 g applied to the fingerpads to close the instruments. (3) The tip of the instrument should not be hooked nor snag. They should meet accurately before the rest of the jaws when inspected against the light and preferably using a magnifier. (4) Locking and unlocking forces of needleholders should not exceed 150 g until the ratchet is locked.

Provided that the rules and recommendations for proper instrument handling and care are followed, microsurgical instrument keep their functionality and high quality properties over a long period of time independent of the frequency of use.

5   Conclusions

Periodontal microsurgery is performed by means of surgical microscopes or high magnifying loupes which guarantee an ideal visual presentation of the structures to deal with. Besides the visual sensory inputs, the tactile signals from the whole hand and their transfer to the brain in millisecond precision are of utmost importance as meticulous execution of precise hand movements depends on corresponding haptic sensory inputs.

The interface between the instrument and the gloved surgeon's hand is primarily influenced by the design and the surface characteristics of the microsurgical instrument and especially the handle of the instrument. That is why microsurgical instruments must meet the criteria to be held and manipulated in the external precision grip. Rounded handles of about 10 mm diameter seem to ideally transfer mechanical forces into vibratory stimuli, decoded by the mechanoreceptors of the skin of fingertips and palm. Additionally, smooth rounded handles provide best friction control when low gripping forces are applied. It should be noted that literature findings regarding microslips between gloved hands and microsurgical instruments under clinical conditions are scarce.

Similar to other medical faculties, in periodontal surgery the tasks dictate the design of the instruments which has been previously described. But as the oral mucosa is a very delicate soft tissue, all surgical manipulations on the oral masticatory, lining and specialized mucosae should follow the rules of minimal invasiveness and, as such, there should be no distinction between macro- and microsurgical instrument design. The only differences consist in the configuration of the working ends of anatomical forceps and needle holders when very fine suture materials are preferred or in the surface textures of instrument handles when higher gripping forces are required such as the ones for scaling and root planing. Otherwise, the instruments for periodontal microsurgery are equally suitable for periodontal and periimplant surgeries applied in a conventional manner. Or expressed in a better way, in periodontal and periimplant surgeries, an approach based on magnified vision and executed with microinstruments, providing the best tactile feedback and optimal transfer of motor activity into mechanical action, should be the rule rather than the exception.

6   Key Points

1. **The sense of touch of the human hand**

   In periodontal microsurgery, the interface of the human hand and the instrument is of utmost importance (discipline of human factors). To understand the essence of the sensory feedback for precise instrument manipulation, firstly, we must be familiar with the anatomical features of the hand and the psychophysics of touch, tactile, and haptic sensing.

2. **Instrument design**

Psychomotor execution of precise hand movements depends on visual and tactile sensory inputs. The latter ones are transferred via the instrument to the surgeon's skin. That is why instrument characteristics from a macroscopic (e.g., form, size, weight) and microscopic (e.g., texture, surface roughness) perspective are important features when it comes to ergonomy in periodontal microsurgery.

3. **Precision grip in microsurgery**

In surgery, the tasks dictate the instrument designs and the way the instruments are held in the hand. In the taxonomy of grips, the external precision grip is the dominant hand position in periodontal microsurgery. It is characterized by at least three separate components, each worth considering in detail because of its implication for instrument design.

4. **Instrument use and brain plasticity**

Instrument use seems to extend the peripersonal space, defined as the space immediately surrounding the body, now generally accepted as a region of integration of somatosensory, visual, and auditory information. Findings from recent studies support the hypothesis that handheld instruments function as a sensory extension of the hand and point to the existence of an embodiment of the instrument.

5. **Surgical gloves and their impact on precise hand movements**

Surgical gloves interfere with the transfer of mechanical stimuli to the mechanoreceptors of the fingers and the palm of the gloved hand, thereby, impairing friction control. It is important to discuss the factors which influence the control of microslips between instrument and fingers and how ergonomy can be maintained even with gloved hands.

6. **Basic instrument set for periodontal microsurgery**

The basic instruments are described and recommendations for selection are given. Additionally, there are guidelines and checklists how to care for the instruments and how to avoid damage.

Acknowledgments The support in photography and the expertise in graphic design of Mrs. Idoia Felis as well as her meticulous preparation of the figures are highly appreciated. Likewise, the personal communications with Dr. Susan Lederman and Dr. Lynette Jones helped to find the relevant basic literature and are highly acknowledged. Thanks to their recommendations, the contact to the currently leading researchers in the field was possible.

References

1. Atkins JL, Kalu PU, Lannon DA, Green CJ, Butler PE. Training in microsurgical skills: does course-based learning deliver? Microsurgery. 2005;25:481–5.
2. Gallagher AG, Smith CD. From the operating room of the present to the operating room of the future. Human-factors lessons learned from the minimally invasive surgery revolution. Semin Laparosc Surg. 2003;10:127–39.
3. Wilson FR. The hand. How its use shapes the brain, language, and human culture. 1st ed. New York: Vintage; 1999. p. 15p.

4. Marzke MW, Marzke RF. Evolution of the human hand: approaches to acquiring, analysing and interpreting the anatomical evidence. J Anat. 2000;197:121–40.
5. Young RW. Evolution of the human hand: the role of throwing and clubbing. J Anat. 2003;202:165–77.
6. Napier JR. The human hand. Burlington, NC: Carolina Biological Supply; 1976. p. 16p.
7. Jones LA, Lederman SJ. Human hand function. Oxford, NY: Oxford University Press; 2006. p. 18p.
8. Reid DA. Reconstruction of thumb. J Bone Jt Surg. 1960;42B:444–65.
9. Marzke MW. Precision grips, hand morphology, and tools. Am J Phys Anthropol. 1997;102:91–110.
10. Abdo JL, Sopko NA, Milner SM. The applied anatomy of human skin: a model for regeneration. Wound Med. 2020;28:1–10.
11. Küken M, Newell AC. Finger print formation. J Theor Biol. 2005;235:71–83.
12. Misumi Y, Akiyoshi T. Scanning electron microscopic structure of the finger print. Anat Rec. 1984;208:49–55.
13. Petrovic A, Petrovic V, Milojkovic B, Nikolic I, Jovanovic D, Antovic A, Milic M. Immunohistochemical distribution of Ki67 in epidermis of thick glabrous skin of human digits. Arch Dermatol Res. 2017;310:85–93.
14. Thomine JM. The skin of the hand. In: Tubiana R, editor. The hand. Philadelphia: Saunders; 1981. p. 107–15.
15. Dzidek B, Bochereau S, Johnson SA, Hayward V, Adams MJ. Why pens have rubbery grips. Proc Natl Acad Sci U S A. 2017;114:10864–9.
16. Johansson RS, Vallbo AB. Tactile sensory coding in the glabrous skin of the human hand. TINS. 1983;6:27–32.
17. Johnson KO. The roles and functions of cutaneous mechanoreceptors. Curr Opin Neurobiol. 2001;11:455–61.
18. Vallbo AB, Johansson RS. Properties of cutaneous mechanoreceptors in the human hand related to touch sensation. Hum Neurobiol. 1984;3:3–14.
19. Cevikbas F, Lerner EA. Physiology and pathophysiology of itch. Physiol Rev. 2020;100:945–82.
20. Sutherling WW, Levesque MF, Baumgartner C. Cortical sensory representation of the human hand: size of finger regions and nonoverlapping digit somatotopy. Neurology. 1992;42:1020–8.
21. Buonomano DV, Merzenich MM. Cortical plasticity: from synapses to maps. Annu Rev Neurosci. 1998;21:149–86.
22. Schmidt-Wilcke T, Wulms N, Heba S, Pleger B, Puts NA, Glaubitz B, Kalisch T, Tegenthoff M, Dinse HR. Structural changes in brain morphology induced by brief periods of repetitive sensory stimulation. NeuroImage. 2018;165:148–57.
23. Herholz SC, Zatorre RJ. Musical training as a framework for brain plasticity: behavior, function, and structure. Neuron. 2012;76:486–502.
24. Münte TF, Altenmüller E, Jäncke L. The musician's brain as a model of neuroplasticity. Neuroscience. 2002;3:473–8.
25. Elbert T, Pantev C, Wienbruch C, Rockstroh B, Taub E. Increased cortical representation of the fingers of the left hand in string players. Science. 1995;270:305–7.
26. Ragert P, Schmidt A, Altenmüller E, Dinse HR. Superior tactile performance and learning in professional pianists: evidence for meta-plasticity in musicians. Eur J Neurosci. 2004;19:473–8.
27. Johansson RS, Westling G. Roles of glabrous skin receptors and sensorimotor memory in automatic control of precision grip when lifting rougher or more slippery objects. Exp Brain Res. 1984;56:550–64.
28. Macefield VG, Häger-Ross C, Johansson RS. Control of grip force during restraint of an object held between finger and thumb: responses of cutaneous afferents from the digits. Exp Brain Res. 1996;108:155–71.
29. Weinstein S. Intensive and extensive aspects of tactile sensitivity as a function of body part, sex, and laterality. In: Kenshalo DR, editor. International symposium on the skin senses. Springfield: C.C. Thomas; 1968. p. 195–222.

30. Peters RM, Hackeman E, Goldreich E. Diminutive digits discern delicate details: fingertip size and the sex difference in tactile spatial acuity. J Neurosci. 2009;29:15756–61.
31. Scheibert J, Leurent S, Prevost A, Debrégeas G. The role of fingerprints in the coding of tactile information probed with a biomimetic sensor. Science. 2009;323:1503–6.
32. Gerling GJ, Thomas GW. Fingerprint lines may not directly affect SA-I mechanoreceptor response. Somatosens Mot Res. 2008;25:61–76.
33. Stevens JC, Patterson MQ. Dimensions of spatial acuity in the touch sense: changes over the life span. Somatosens Mot Res. 1995;12:29–47.
34. Edin BB, Johansson N. Skin strain patterns provide kinaesthetic information to the human central nervous system. J Physiol. 1995;487:243–51.
35. Klatzky RL, Loomis JM, Lederman SJ, Wake H, Fujita N. Haptic identification of objects and pictures of objects. Percept Psychophys. 1993;54:170–8.
36. Verrillo RT, Bolanowski SJ, McGlone FP. Subjective magnitude estimate of tactile roughness. Somatosens Mot Res. 1999;16:352–60.
37. Cutkosky MR, Howe RD. Human grasp choice and robotic grasp analysis. In: Venkataraman ST, Iberall T, editors. Dextrous robot hands. 1st ed. New York: Springer; 1990. p. 5–31.
38. Patkin M. Ergonomics in microsurgery. In: Olszewski WL, editor. CRC handbook of microsurgery. Boca Raton (FL): CRC Press; 1989. Chapter 1, p. 13–26.
39. Serina ER, Mote CD, Rempel D. Force response of the fingertip pulp to repeated compression: effects of loading rate, loading angle, and anthropometry. J Biomech. 1997;30:1035–40.
40. Westling G, Johansson RS. Responses in glabrous skin mechanoreceptors during precision grip in humans. Exp Brain Res. 1987;66:128–40.
41. Lemon RN. Neural control of dexterity: what has been achieved? Exp Brain Res. 1999;128:6–12.
42. Stone R, McCloy R. Ergonomics in medicine and surgery. BMJ. 2004;328:1115–8.
43. Tubiana R, Thomine JM, Mackin E. Examination of the hand and wrist. 2nd ed. London: Martin Dunitz Ltd; 1998. p. 402.
44. Johansson RS, Westling G. Programmed and triggered actions to rapid load changes during precision grip. Exp Brain Res. 1988;71:72–86.
45. Buchholz B, Frederick LJ, Armstrong TJ. An investigation of human palmar skin friction and the effects of materials, pinch force and moisture. Ergonomics. 1988;31:317–25.
46. Goodwin AW, Wheat HE. Magnitude estimation of contact force when objects with different shapes are applied passively to the fingerpad. Somatosens Mot Res. 1992;9:339–44.
47. Lederman SJ, Klatzky RL. Haptic perception: A tutorial. Atten Percept Psychophys. 2009;71:1439–59.
48. Adams MJ, Johnson SA, Lefèvre P, Lévesque V, Hayward V, André T, Thonnard JL. Finger pad friction and its role in grip and touch. J R Soc Interface. 2012;10:20120467.
49. Goodwin AW, Macefield VG, Bisley JW. Encoding of object curvature by tactile afferents from human fingers. J Neurophysiol. 1997;78:2881–8.
50. Jenmalm P, Goodwin AW, Johansson RS. Control of grasp stability when humans lift objects with different surface curvatures. J Neurophysiol. 1998;79:1643–52.
51. Charpentier A. Experimental study of some aspects of weight perception. Arch Physiol Norm Path. 1891;3:122–35.
52. Ellis RR, Lederman SJ. The material weight illusion revisited. Percept Psychophys. 1999;61:1564–76.
53. Salimi I, Hollender I, Frazier W, Gordon AM. Specificity of internal representations underlying grasping. J Neurophysiol. 2000;84:2390–7.
54. Matthews PB. The contrasting stretch reflex responses of the long and short flexor muscles in the human thumb. J Physiol. 1984;348:545–58.
55. Saels P, Thonnard JL, Detrembleur C, Smith AM. Impact of the surface slipperiness of grasped objects on their subsequent acceleration. Neuropsychologia. 1999;37:751–6.
56. Cadoret G, Smith AM. Friction, not texture, dictates grip forces used during object manipulation. J Neurophysiol. 1996;75:1963–9.

57. Hollins M, Risner SR. Evidence for the duplex theory of tactile texture perception. Percept Psychophys. 2000;62:695–705.
58. Monzée J, Lamarre Y, Smith AM. The effects of digital anesthesia on force control using a precision grip. J Neurophysiol. 2003;89:672–83.
59. Taylor M, Lederman SJ. Tactile roughness of grooved surfaces: a model and the effect of friction. Atten Percept Psychophys. 1975;17:23–36.
60. Yip E, Cacioli P. The manufacture of gloves from natural rubber latex. J Allergy Clin Immunol. 2002;110(2):s3–s14.
61. Mylon P, Lewis R, Carré MJ, Martin N. A critical review of glove and hand research with regard to medical glove design. Ergonomics. 2014;57:116–29.
62. Preece D, Lewis R, Carré MJ. A critical review of the assessment of medical gloves. Tribol—Mater Surf Interfaces. 2021;15:10–9.
63. Mylon P, Buckley-Johnstone L, Lewis R, Carré MJ, Martin N. Factors influencing the perception of roughness in manual exploration. Do medical gloves reduce cutaneous sensibility? Proc Inst Mech. Eng., Part J. 2015;229:273–84.
64. Park SB, Davare M, Falla M, Kennedy WR, Selim MM, Wendelschafer-Crabb G, Koltzenburg M. Fast-adapting mechanoreceptors are important for force control in precision grip but not for sensorimotor memory. J Neurophysiol. 2016;115:3156–61.
65. Saal HP, Bensmaia SJ. Touch is a team effort: interplay of submodalities in cutaneous sensibility. Trends Neurosci. 2014;37:689–97.
66. Johansson RS, Flanagan JR. Coding and use of tactile signals from the fingertips in object manipulation tasks. Nat Rev Neurosci. 2009;10:345–59.
67. Kopka A, Crawford JM, Broome IJ. Anaesthetists should wear gloves – touch sensitivity is improved with a new type of glove. Acta Anaesthesiol Scand. 2005;49:459–62.
68. Han CD, Kim J, Moon SH, et al. A randomized prospective study of glove perforation in orthopedic surgery: is a thick glove more effective? J Arthroplast. 2013;28:1878–81.
69. Hatzfeld CH, Dorsch S, Neupert C, Kupnik M. Influence of surgical gloves on haptic perception thresholds. Int J Med Robotics Comput Assist Surg. 2017;14(2):e1852. https://doi.org/10.1002/rcs.1852.
70. Rock KM, Mikat RP, Foster C. The effects of gloves on grip strength and three-point pinch. J Hand Ther. 2001;14:286–90.
71. Kinoshita H. Effect of gloves on prehensile forces during lifting and holding tasks. Ergonomics. 1999;42:1372–85.
72. Laroche CH, Barra A, Dong H, Rempel D. Effect of dental tool surface texture and material on static friction with a wet gloved fingertip. J Biomech. 2007;40:697–701.
73. Nelson JB, Mital A. An ergonomic evaluation of dexterity and tactility with increase in examination surgical glove thickness. Ergonomics. 1995;38:723–33.
74. Fry DE, Harris WE, Kohnke EN, Twomey CL. Influence of double-gloving on manual dexterity and tactile sensation. J Am Coll Surg. 2010;210:325–30.
75. Mylon P, Lewis R, Carré MJ, et al. A study of clinicians' views on medical gloves and their effect on manual performance. Am J Infect Control. 2014;42:48–54.
76. Sawyer J, Bennett A. Comparing the level of dexterity offered by latex and nitrile safe skin gloves. Ann Occup Hyg. 2006;50:289–96.
77. Romano D, Caffa E, Hernandez-Arieta A, Brugger P, Maravita A. The robot hand illusion: inducing proprioceptive drift through visuo-motor congruency. Neuropsychologia. 2015;70:414–20.
78. Serino A, Bassolino M, Farnè A, Làdavas E. Extended multisensory space in blind cane users. Psychol Sci. 2007;18:642–8.
79. Martel M, Cardinalic L, Roy AC, Farnè A. Tool-use: an open window into body representation and its plasticity. Cogn Neuropsychol. 2016;33:82–101.
80. Graziano MS, Cooke DF. Parieto-frontal interactions, personal space, and defensive behavior. Neuropsychologia. 2006;44:845–59.

81. Medina J, Coslett HB. From maps to form to space: touch and the body schema. Neuropsychologia. 2010;48:645–54.
82. Shenton JT, Schwoebel J, Coslett HB. Mental motor imagery and the body schema: evidence for proprioceptive dominance. Neurosci Lett. 2004;370:19–24.
83. Saal HP, Delhayea BP, Rayhauna BC, Bensmaia SJ. Simulating tactile signals from the whole hand with millisecond precision. Proc Natl Acad Sci U S A. 2017;114:E5693–702.
84. Miller LE, Montroni L, Koun E, Salemme R, Hayward V, Farnè A. Sensing with tools extends somatosensory processing beyond the body. Nature. 2018;561:239–42.
85. de Vignemont F. Embodiment, ownership and disownership. Conscious Cogn. 2011;20:82–93.
86. Arbib MA, Bonaiuto JB, Jacobs S, Frey SH. Tool use and the distalization of the end-effector. Psychol Res. 2009;73:441–62.

The Science and Art of Microsuturing

Diego Velasquez-Plata and J. David Cross

Contents

Supplementary Information The online version contains supplementary material available at [https://doi.org/10.1007/978-3-030-96874-8_5].

D. Velasquez-Plata (✉)
Private Practice, Fenton, MI, USA

Adjunct Clinical Assistant Professor, Periodontics and Oral Medicine Department,
The University of Michigan School of Dentistry, Ann Arbor, MI, USA
e-mail: dvelasq@umich.edu

J. D. Cross
Private Practice, Springfield, IL, USA

© The Author(s), under exclusive license to Springer Nature Switzerland AG 2022
H.-L. (A.) Chan, D. Velasquez-Plata (eds.), *Microsurgery in Periodontal and Implant Dentistry*, https://doi.org/10.1007/978-3-030-96874-8_5

Abstract

Technically speaking, approximation of wound margins is the last step to be executed during a surgical procedure. Practically speaking, soft tissue approximation and closure of the open wound should have been visualized and planned before the first incision has been traced. The microsurgeon must become knowledgeable on biological and physiological concepts that define wound healing, must develop competent skills in handling hard and soft tissues, must have a clear understanding of the different biotextiles and biomaterials available to utilize when performing microsurgical procedures in periodontal and dental implant related therapy.

This chapter covers the historical background and evolution of surgical biotextiles and needles, principles of wound closure, technical details of the armamentarium utilized while suturing, elaborates on the geometry of suturing emphasizing biomechanical aspects of suture performance and offers resources to develop suturing skills under the operating microscope (OM). All these concepts are delivered and supported with photographic material and videos to facilitate the understanding and application of principles related to the science and art of microsuturing.

Keywords

Wound Healing · Microsurgery · Suture Techniques · Sutures · Needles

1 Introduction

Wound closure can be achieved by using sutures, adhesives, tapes, staples, and laser tissue welding. Sutures are the most common method to achieve such task. Suture has been defined as a strand or fiber used to sew parts of the living body [1]. Accurate and secure approximation of the wound edges is of paramount importance to procure stability of tissues while healing. Maintaining wound margins approximated facilitates clot maturation, protects underlying tissues, and maintains biomaterials protected and isolated. Passive and precise wound margin approximation promotes closure by primary intention and contributes to prevent scar formation.

Suture materials should remain functional until the tensile strength of the wound is adequate to withstand passive and functional stress. Considering that all suturing processes inflict tissue trauma (starting with the piercing action inflicted by the needle and continued by the presence of the foreign material that facilitates bacterial penetration by means of the perisutural cuff), it is important to follow practices that can minimize these deleterious effects such as implementing an adequate suturing technique (tight sutures can impair blood flow and impair host defenses), selecting small suture diameters (starting with 7-0 suture diameter), and utilizing low infection-potentiating material types (chemical composition/origin) [2–6].

2 Historical Background of Suture Materials, Needles/ Evolution

Medically implantable biotextiles have been utilized by men as early as 4000 years ago with linen being the material of choice for wound closure. Other materials followed such as iron, gold, silver wire, dried gut, tendon, horsehair, bark fibers, cotton, and silk. Both natural and synthetic polymers and copolymers were then utilized to fabricate suture fibers. These materials have unique physical properties that in conjunction with the complexity of the wound itself, with different layers and types of tissue (each exhibiting unique physical and biomechanical features), dictates what suture composition is the most appropriate for the task. As time went on and different surgical applications required different conditions and technical performance standards, it became evident that not all materials delivered similar results. There are materials that are not homogenous in their composition influencing the variability of its resorption time, and materials that create friction, are porous, or lack smoothness which facilitate wicking of bacteria into the wound, therefore causing a significant adverse inflammatory reaction that is deleterious to healing. Coatings such as wax, oils, silicone, and Teflon are some examples of attempts to reduce friction and wicking. The incorporation of the operating microscope made palpable the disadvantages of needles and suture materials utilized prior to this point in time. Therefore during the 1950s braided silk and gut in 5-0 to 6-0 thread thickness were the most used materials for surgical applications. Once the 1960s arrived, the incorporation of finer threads (9-0, 10-0) in monofilament suture materials (nylon) became a trend that remains strong to these days.

The development of needles was also greatly impacted by the incorporation of the microscope as a surgical tool across medical disciplines. Eyed needles were identified as being impractical for the execution of fine, delicate maneuvers and overly traumatic due to its increased bulk which was necessary to accommodate the double strand of suture material used to fixate the suture material to the body of the needle. Microsurgical driven procedures demanded consistently sharp needles, flexible enough so fractures would not occur under pressure, featuring drilled (using mechanical or laser driven tools) shafts that accommodated a single suture strand, with tips that rendered customized cutting ends, different sizes and circumferential designs that would facilitate their utilization by the microsurgeon.

Suture materials are no longer packaged in glass vials embedded on some antiseptic solution. Sutures are sterilized by radiation or chemical means such as ethylene oxide, depending on the compatibility of these methods with the structural properties of the different biotextiles utilized to fabricate suture materials. The fine needle tips are protected in a foam casing to prevent them from being damaged during packaging, shipping, and handling. The symbiotic evolution on needles and suture materials has been modulated under the auspices of surgical panels constituted by members of the medical profession and industry. The open dialogue has been the key for the constant enhancement of the materials being utilized nowadays in microsurgery.

3 Wound Closure: Principles

The principle of wound closure is achieved by the approximation of similar tissues in the same plane, accompanied by intimate apposition of appropriate cell phenotypes. Relevant knowledge pertaining to the anatomical and physiological repair processes is fundamental in achieving the desired wound closure outcome [7]. The main objectives are to reduce healing time, prevent infection, and preserve the appearance and function of the treated area [8]. Wound healing has four phases as follows: Phase I hemostasis immediately follows injury and is characterized by a hemostatic plug developing into a fibrin scaffold with platelets releasing multiple growth factors. Phase II inflammation occurs from days 0 through 5. The plug transforms into a complex extracellular matrix with molecular chemo-attractants directing leukocytes to the area. Phase III proliferation occurs from days 5 through 10 and involves the formation of granulation tissue, concluding with the formation of an immature scar. Phase IV remodeling occurs from day 10 to 2 years, involving a change from disorganized and weak Type III collagen to an organized Type I collagen matrix metalloproteinases [9]. Factors that influence wound healing include wound closure. Primary wound closure is the optimal healing method as it minimizes infection risk and scarring [9]. In periodontal and peri-implant microsurgeries, the clinician may mobilize the flap by including releasing incisions to extend the flap laterally and coronally, thus, allowing stabilization and adaptation of the flap [10].

Gingival flaps may be designed to allow passive wound closure that promotes ideal healing with successful functional and esthetic results [11]. Primary wound closure through an appropriate flap design is essential for successful results. Several studies and clinicians have advocated both a decision tree for flap design based on the vertical ridge augmentation and anatomical considerations and a series of layered incisions for releasing flaps to allow for passive wound closure [11–13]. Using both vertical releasing incisions and internal incisions, buccal and lingual flaps may be split several times, allowing for coronal positioning of gingival tissues. The visual information and guidance obtained from the microscope guide atraumatic flap elevation and precise closure without tension [14]. Releasing full thickness flaps may also be accomplished by releasing the periosteum. Microsurgical flap designs and releasing incisions allow for wound closure in a multilayered approach, without tension or with a significant reduction in tension.

Passive flap adaptation allows for suture placement without tension. These principles are directly related to each other and form the end goal of primary microsurgical wound closure and healing [7, 15]. When sutures are placed under tension, complications such as ischemic tissue necrosis, infection, and wound dehiscence can arise [16, 17]. Moreover, the use of multiple sutures with variable tension can result in tissue deformation and secondary wound healing [7, 15].

4   Armamentarium

For a desirable wound closure, the surgeon must select the appropriate instruments for a particular suture placement. The armamentarium for wound closure includes needle holders, tissue forceps, tying forceps, and micro-scissors.

Microsurgical instruments are made from stainless steel, carbon steel, and titanium. Titanium instruments have several distinct advantages over traditional dental instruments, as they are light-weight, corrosion-resistant, durable, and non-magnetic [18, 19].

Needle holders vary in their design by length, diameter, jaws, and locking mechanism. Selecting the correct needle holder for a particular suture needle plays a direct role in the ergonomics and success of wound closure.

Needle holders have lengths ranging from 16 to 20 cm and their curved or straight jaws are usually tapered and flat on the inside. Toothed or grooved jaws can affect and deform the needle [20]. The locking mechanism may be present or absent, which can sometimes cause uncontrolled movement of the needle holder tip [20].

Tissue forceps also come in similar lengths of 15–20 cm. They have two basic designs, smooth and toothed. The toothed forceps can have teeth with a 90-degree angulation and varying degrees of tooth angulation. The choice of instrument is based on the surgeon's discretion after evaluation of the tissue being treated. Smooth forceps are considered in the management of delicate tissue, while the selection of toothed forceps is largely determined by tissue toughness and degree of manipulation necessary [20].

Tying forceps have different lengths, designs, and angulations. This instrument should have no teeth or serrations. The surgeon should be aware that over-compression of the instrument will cause the working surface to gape or open up [20].

Micro-scissors should be designed with a squeeze handle, allowing for greater control when cutting the suture. Additionally, the design may include both straight and curved styles. When using the curved style, the sharp end should be directed away from the tissue for increased visualization and safety [20].

Proper hand–instrument relationship begins with comfort and stability of both the upper body and resting of the wrist on a stable surface [21, 22]. This position allows the forearm to rest. The working position of both hands can be further refined by resting the hand down with the tip of the middle finger on a stable surface or stacked on top of the two ulnar fingers. Curling fingers 4 and 5 underneath the hand provides stability and balance. The important digits are the thumb and the index and middle fingers. When grasping the instrument, these fingers should neither be hyper-flexed nor hyper-extended; the three digits should be semi-flexed [21, 83].

Approximately 1 in. of the instrument should project beyond the tips of the fingers. If the instrument is excessively extended beyond the tips of the fingers, it is difficult to rest and stabilize the hand. The instrument can then rest in the metacarpophalangeal joint [19, 83].

Another important factor is grasping the instrument with the thumb and index and middle fingers in contact with one another to aid in instrument stabilization. Non-contact of the thumb with the other fingers may result in unwanted tremors of the thumb [19, 83]. This type of instrument grasp allows the microsurgeon to accurately and precisely rotate the needle through the oral tissues. The addition of bimanual balancing and support can supplement suturing precision [19, 23].

5 Sutures and Needles

5.1 Suture Classification

Suture classification can be grouped into four main categories defined by origin, size, physical configuration, and speed of degradation (Table 1). According to their origin, sutures could be natural or synthetic. Size describes the diameter of the suture utilizing two standards: the USP (United States Pharmacopeia) and the EP

Table 1 Suture Classification. * = United States Pharmacopeia. ** = European Pharmacopeia

Category	Origin	Speed of Degradation	Size	Physical Configuration
Division	Natural	Absorbable	USP*	Monofilament
				Multifilament
	Synthetic	Non-absorbable	EP**	Braided
				Twisted

(European Pharmacopeia). Physical configuration will characterize sutures as monofilament, multifilament, braided, or twisted [24]. Depending on the speed of degradation in tissues with its consequent loss of tensile strength, sutures have been allocated to two groups: absorbable and nonabsorbable [25].

Absorbable suture: These materials generally lose their entire or most of their tensile strength within 3 months. Nonabsorbable suture: These materials maintain their initial strength longer than 2–3 months.

Absorbable sutures are derived either from collagen that can be in its natural state (gut: bovine/ovine submucosal layer of the small intestine) or coated with chemicals to delay the absorption rate (chromium trioxide is added to gut to form chromic gut) or synthetic polymers.

Synthetic materials for absorbable sutures contain one or a combination of the five basic building blocks: glycolide, L-lactide, p-dioxanone, ε-caprolactone, and trimethylene carbonate. The first two are the most rigid and the latter three are the most flexible [26]. Among synthetic absorbable polymers, polyglycolic acid sutures are the most commonly used substitutes to the collagen derived suture materials. This braided material is absorbed by chemical hydrolysis, in contrast to collagen derived materials which are digested by invading macrophages [27]. As an alternative to braided sutures, a glycolide derived (poly-p-dioxanone) monofilament resorbable suture is available offering flexibility and ease of handling with the inherent advantages of having less tissue dragging, tearing, and minimizing capillary wicking when compared to braided sutures.

Nonabsorbable sutures are divided into natural (silk, cotton, and linen) and synthetic fibers. Synthetic suture materials have been derived from polyamides (nylon), polyolefins (polypropylene), and polytetrafluoroethylene.

Nylon is the best-known polyamide that has high tensile strength and low tissue reactivity. It is available in monofilament and multifilament presentations [28]. The most common types of Nylon for suture making are Nylon 66 (made from adipic acid and hexamethylene diamine and most commonly used in the USA) and Nylon 6 (made from caprolactam and most commonly used in Europe). It is pliable and easier to manipulate than polypropylene, although Nylon is known for losing strength after implantation [29]. Polypropylene is the most commonly used polyolefin-based suture. It presents a low coefficient of friction which facilitates knot construction and suture passage through tissues. This material is highly inert [30]. Polypropylene sutures are the standard to which other suture materials are compared in vascular and cardiac surgery, in part due to its long-term tensile strength retention (as long as two years).

Expanded polytetrafluoroethylene (ePTFE) suture material is supple and has no plastic memory. It has been modified to produce a porous microstructure ranging from 30 to 100 µm rendering its structure to approximately 50% air by volume [31]. This may explain that bacterial adherence to ePTFE suture material although slightly lower did not show large differences when compared to silk suture [32]. Something worth noting is that due to the air by volume content (>50%) of the ePTFE sutures, the size of this material (measured in its pre-expanded form) does not follow the USP size classification. For example, a CV-4 ePTFE suture has a similar diameter (0.35 mm) to a 2–0 Prolene (0.303 mm) [33]. Figures 1 and 2 show scanning electron microscope images of some absorbable and nonabsorbable sutures available as of 2022.

The information above has been limited to the most used microsurgical suturing materials in periodontics and implant dentistry (Table 2).

For a broader review on biomaterials of different implantable biotextiles, the reader is referred to the following source: Chu CC, von Fraunhofer JA, Greisler HP. Wound closure biomaterials and devices. 1st. ed. Boca Raton: CRC Press; 1996 [34].

Sutures have been categorized by the United States Pharmacopeia according to their thickness as shown in Table 3.

Microsutures are considered by the authors as any non-collagenous material exhibiting a diameter thread finer or equal to 0.050–0.069 mm (7-0). When the clinician is working with materials of this diameter, visual control takes over tactile sensations for their manipulation. This statement is based on the research by Burkhardt et al. [35] in which it was illustrated that 7-0 sutures broke before tissues were torn in every instance with forces not exceeding 5 N without a difference in tissue characteristics (mucosa or gingiva) or thickness. Choosing 7-0 sutures allows for passive wound closure, thus reducing tissue trauma.

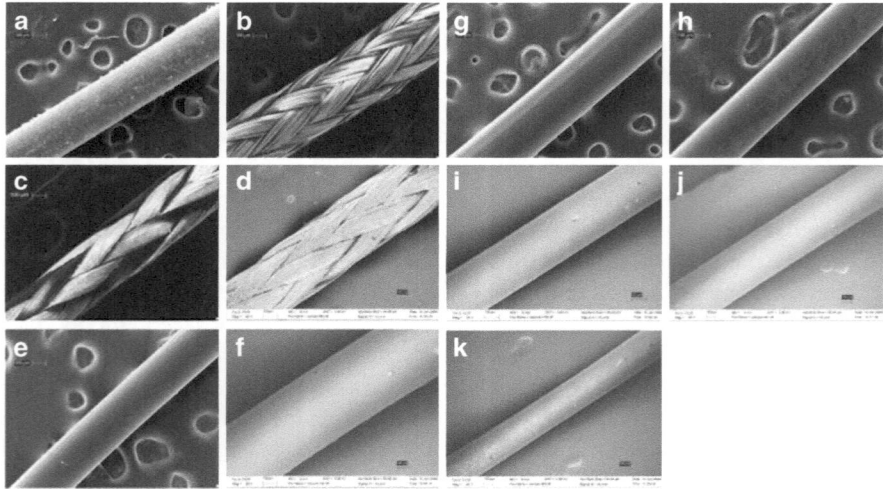

Fig. 1 Scanning electron images of some commercial absorbable sutures: (**a**) Chromic catgut: polyglycolic acid family; (**b**) Dexon: poly(glycolide/L-lactide) copolymer or polyglactin 910 family; (**c**) Vicryl; (**d**) Vicryl Plus: poly-p-dioxanone family; (**e**) PDSII; (**f**) MonoPlus: poly(glycolide/trimethylene carbonate) copolymer or polyglyconate family; (**g**) Maxon: poly(glycolide/ε--caprolactone) copolymer or poliglecaprone 25 family; (**h**) Monocryl: poly(glycolide/trimethylene carbonate/dioxanone) or Glycomer 631 family; (**i**) Biosyn: poly(glycolide/trimethylene carbonate/ε-caprolactone) copolymer or Glyconate family; (**j**) Monosyn: poly(glycolide/trimethylene carbonate/lactide/ε-caprolactone) copolymer or polyglytone 6211 family; and (**k**) Caprosyn. (Reproduced with permission from [85])

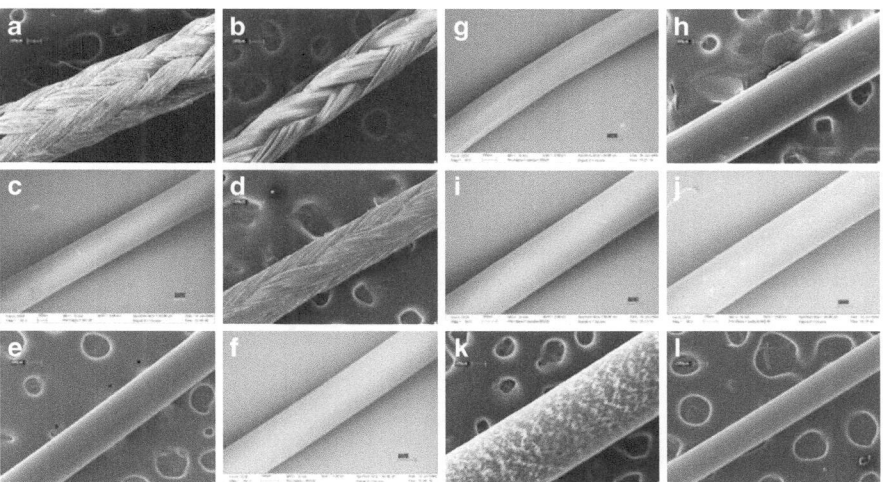

Fig. 2 Scanning electron images of some commercial nonabsorbable sutures (**a**) Silk: polyester family; (**b**) Mersilene; (**c**) Novafil: polyamide family; (**d**) Nurolon; (**e**) Ethilon; (**f**) Dermalon; (**g**) Supramid: polypropylene family; (**h**) Prolene: polyvinylidene fluoride family; (**i**) Pronova: poly(ether ester) family; (**j**) Dyloc: poly(tetrafluoroethylene) family; (**k**) Gore-Tex (**l**) Stainless steel. (Reproduced with permission from [85])

5.2   Suture Biocompatibility

The act of suturing is invasive in nature. Needle piercing and advancement through tissues of the needle–suture complex is traumatic and will trigger an inflammatory host's response. The depth and length of the needle-suture passage, duration of suture material within tissues, and physical and chemical composition of the suture material all play a role in increasing infection risks.

Natural fibers such as silk and cotton elicit high inflammatory reactions. Collagen derived sutures have also been associated with marked host responses due to breakdown mechanisms. Suture materials that trigger the least adverse inflammatory effects are synthetic monofilaments [2–5, 36].

5.3   Needles

Needles are made of stainless steel alloys with a minimal amount of 12% chromium. Depending on the alloy used, other metals such as nickel and titanium will be present. This combination translates into greater resistance to bending and breakage. The most common high nickel maraging stainless steel utilized to develop strong and ductile wires for the manufacturing of surgical needles is S45500. It is composed of 7.5% to 9.5% nickel, 0.8% to 1.4% titanium, and 11% to 12.5% chromium. In contrast, S42000 stainless steel is composed of 12% to 14% chromium without nickel or titanium [30, 37].

Table 2 Commonly used implantable biotextiles in the USA. Adapted from [33].

Generic Name	Trade Name®	Physical Configuration	Surface Treatment	Manufacturer®
Natural absorbable sutures				
Cat gut	Softcat plain or chromic	Monofilament	Plain or chromic	B. Braun
Collagen-beef serosa or sheep submucosa	Surgical gut	Monofilament	Plain or chromic	Ethicon
Cat gut	Palin gut, Chromic gut	Monofilament	Plain or chromic	Unify
Synthetic absorbable sutures				
Polyglycolic acid	Safil	Braided	Coated: dyed or undyed	B. Braun
L-lactide Polyglactin 910	Vicryl	Braided or monofilament	Dyed violet or undyed	Ethicon
Polyglycolic acid	PGA surgical suture	Braided	Dyed violet or undyed	Unify
Poly (glycolide/trimethylene carbonate/ε-caprolactone)	Monosyn	Monofilament	Dyed violet or undyed	B. Braun
Poly (glycolide/ ε-caprolactone)	Monocryl	Monofilament	Violet dyed or undyed	Ethicon
Poly (glycolide/ ε-caprolactone)	PGCL	Monofilament	Violet dyed or undyed	Unify
Poly-p-dioxanone	Monoplus		Dyed violet	B. Braun
Poly-p-dioxanone and Irgacare	PDSII	Monofilament	Violet dyed or undyed	Ethicon
Poly-p-dioxanone	PDO	Monofilament	Violet	Unify
Synthetic non-absorbable				
Polyamide Family				
Ployamide 6.6	Dafilon	Monofilament	Dyed black	B. Braun
Nylon 6	Ethilon	Monofilament	Dyed green/black or undyed (clear)	Ethicon
Ployamide	Nylon	Monofilament	Dyed black	Unify
Polyamide (ether ester) family				
Polypropylene	Premilene	Monofilament	Dyed blue	B. Braun
Polypropylene	Prolene	Monofilament	Dyed blue	Ethicon
Polypropylene	Polypropylene	Monofilament	Dyed blue	Unify
Polytetrafluoroethylene-based				
E-polytetrafluoroethylene	Gore-Tex	Monofilament	White	Gore-Tex
Polytetrafluoroethylene	PTFE	Monofilament	White	Unify
Polytetrafluoroethylene	Cytoplast	Monofilament	White	Osteogenics

Table 3 Suture diameter: classification

Diameter of thread (mm)	USP size codes		EP size codes
Min.-Max.	All materials except collagen	Collagenous materials	All materials
0.01–0.019	11/0		0.1
0.02–0.029	10/0		0.2
0.03–0.039	9/0		0.3
0.04–0.049	8/0		0.4
0.05–0.069	7/0	8/0	0.5
0.07–0.099	6/0	7/0	0.7
0.10–0.14	5/0	6/0	1
0.15–0.19	4/0	5/0	1.5
0.20–0.24	3/0	4/0	2
0.25–0.29	2/0	3/0	2.5
0.30–0.39	0	2/0	3
0.40–0.49	1	0	4
0.50–0.59	2	1	5
0.60–0.69	3	2	6
0.70–0.79	4	3	7
0.80–0.89	5	4	8
0.90–0.99	6	5	9
1.00–1.09	7	6	10

5.3.1 Needle Parts

All needles have three components: swage (site of attachment to the suture thread material), body, and point (Fig. 3).

The swage of modern needles has been laser (Yttrium-aluminum-garnet: YAG) drilled providing shorter, smaller, and smoother swage configurations that translate into minimal mechanical dragging and trauma to tissues. A shorter swage enables the surgeon to grab the needle closer to the needle end, thus having better control when advancing the needle through tissue.

The body is the area where the needle holder comes in contact with the needle. Its cross-sectional area varies and so does the stability of the grip with the needle holder. This cross-sectional design can be circular, rectangular, triangular, and trapezoidal [30].

The curvature of the needle is described by the radius of its arc. The radius is the distance from the center of the needle to the body of the needle as if the body intended to form a full circle. It ranges from 90° (1/4), to 135° (3/8), 180° (1/2). The most common needle configurations utilized in periodontics and implant dentistry are the 135° and 180° Fig. 4.

Other elements of the body are the chord length (distance from the central point of the swage to the point of the needle), the needle diameter (width of the wire used to make the needle).

The needlepoint extends from the tip of the needle to the maximum cross section of the body [38].

Fig. 3 Needle parts

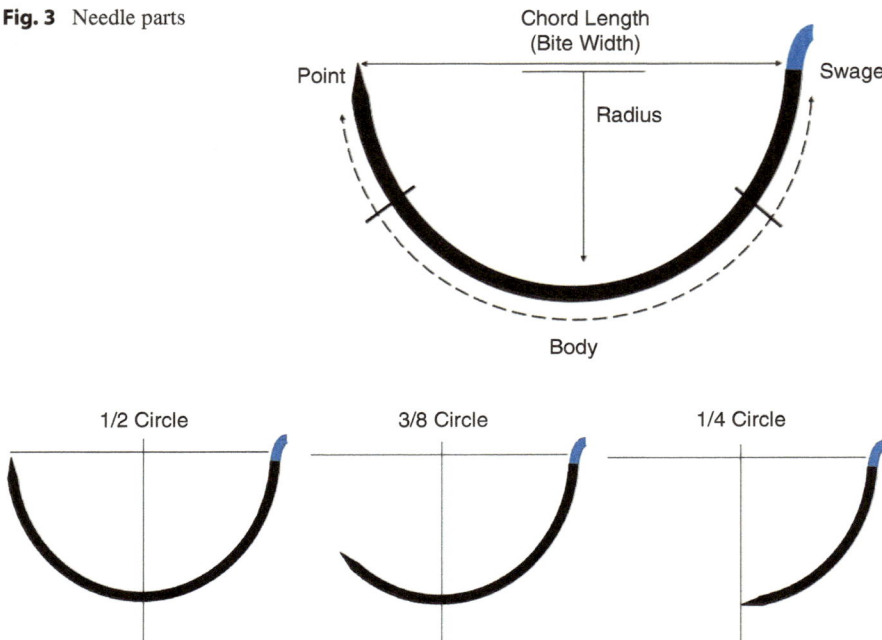

Fig. 4 Needle curvatures

5.3.2 Needle Designs/Geometry

There are three cutting edges. Two on the sides of the point, and depending on the location of the third one, a needle can have a conventional cutting edge (located in the concave, inner part of the needle) or a reverse cutting edge (located in the convex, outer part of the needle). Needles have also been flattened (spatula needles) eliminating inner and outer cutting edges, leaving the cutting edges on the sides. Taper point needles taper off to a sharp tip. This needle displaces tissue without cutting it. Taper cut needles have their cutting edge in a short distance from the tip to the round tapered body of the needle and these cutting surfaces reduce the penetration forces [39–42] Fig. 5.

5.3.3 Needle Color Innovations

When it comes to needle colors, there are two main options: Silver needles and black needles. Black needles reflect less light and are easier to visualize in well illuminated fields such as those encountered when working under high magnification and coaxial illumination proper of the operating surgical microscope. Silver needles can reflect light from the light source of the OM and from surrounding tissues. When black needles are utilized, these instruments are easy to see and manipulate by the microsurgeon [43].

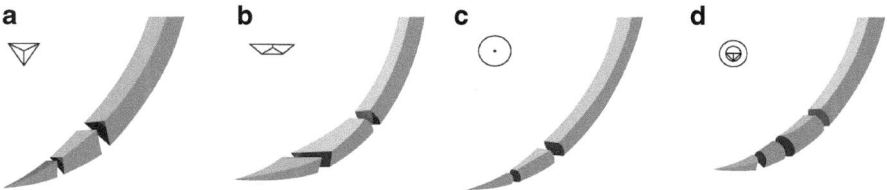

Fig. 5 Needle points. (**a**) Reverse cutting. (**b**) Spatula (**c**) Taper point. (**d**) Taper cut

6   The Geometry of Suturing

The geometry of suturing was developed and taught by Dennis Shanelec at the Microsurgery Training Institute known as MTI, founded in 1990 in Santa Barbara, California. This technique and its philosophy were taught at MTI until 2017. The protocol and components can also be found in other training institutes and literature [20, 83]. Microsurgical training requires a low instructor to student ratio (1:1 to 1:4) along with continuous practice and reevaluation of techniques [14].

The initial step of wound closure is acquisition of the correct needle. The surgical needle has three areas: the sharp point, the middle-third, and the swagged end (Fig. 3). The needle is picked up in the middle-third at an angle perpendicular to the needle holder. This position allows the surgeon to rotate the needle accurately while also not damaging the sharp or swagged end from the pressure of the needle holder [14, 83].

The needle holder is held in the dominant hand, while the tissue and tying forceps are held in the nondominant hand. Both instruments are held in the external precision grip using the three-point tip pinch, involving the thumb and the index and middle fingers [14, 83] (Figs. 6, 7 and 8).

The geometry of suturing has six components as follows:

- Bite size.
- Angle of entry and exit.
- Direction of passage.
- Symmetry.
- No tension.
- Frequency.

Prior to initiating the entry and passage of the needle, it is critical to evaluate the tissue thickness that determines the bite size. The tissue thickness at the needle entry and exit points should be approximately 1.5 times the tissue thickness from the margin of the incision [14, 83] (Figs. 9, 10, 11 and 12).

The angles of entry and exit are at 90-degrees to the surface of the tissue, allowing for the positioning of similar tissue layers in a butt joint closure [14, 83] (Figs. 13 and 14).

Fig. 6 Needle holder being held in the dominant hand

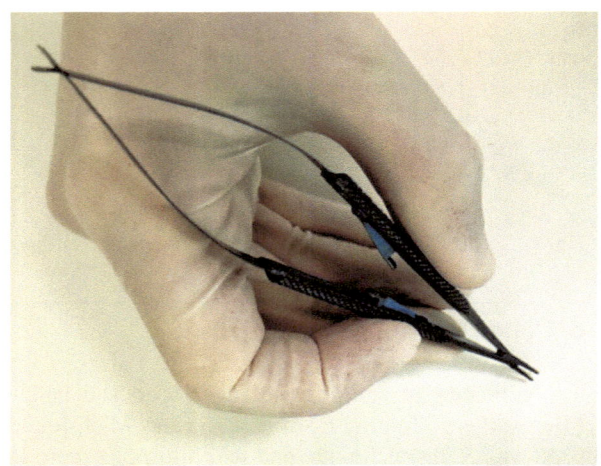

Fig. 7 Tissue and Tying forceps held in non-dominant hand

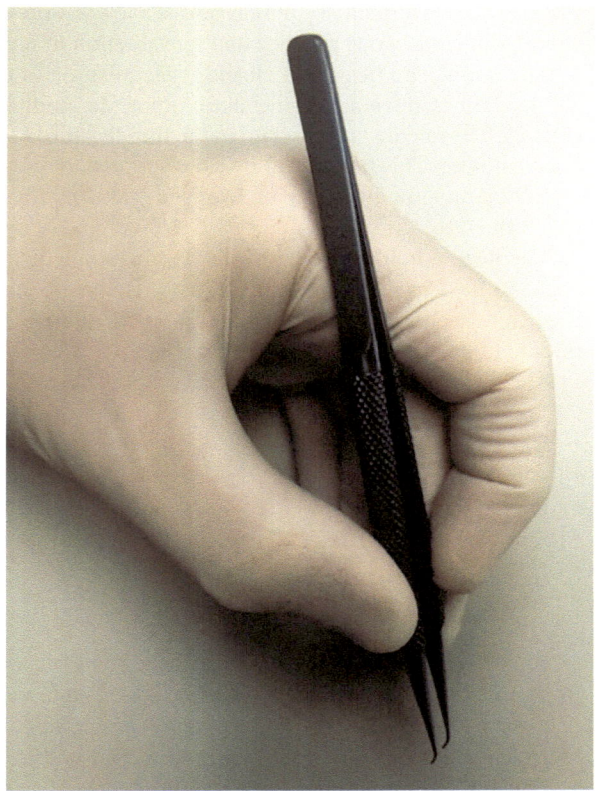

Fig. 8 Needle holder and tissue/tying forceps are held in the external precision grip

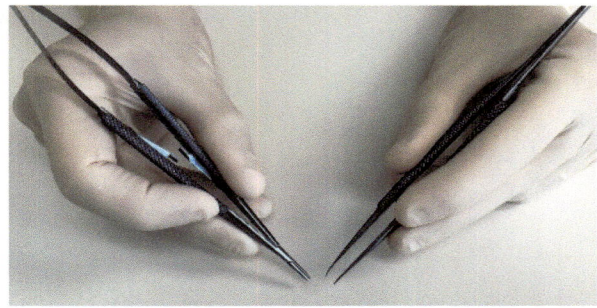

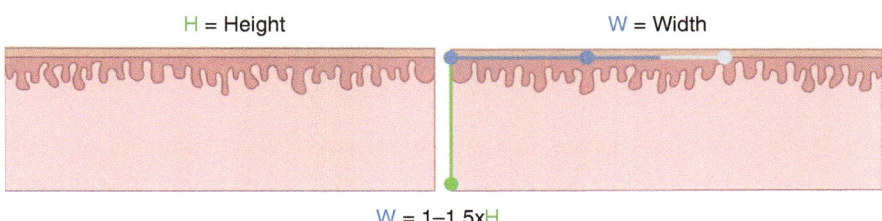

H = Height   W = Width

W = 1−1.5xH

Fig. 9 Bite size: Tissue thickness (height) determines the bite size (width)

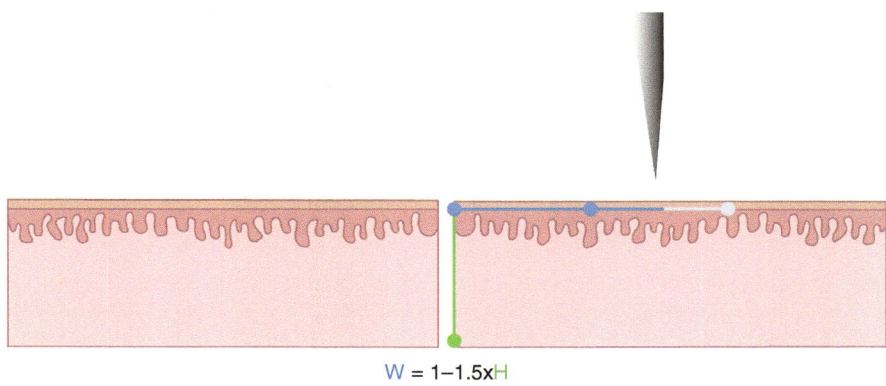

W = 1−1.5xH

Fig. 10 Bite size: Needle entry point should be close to 1.5 times the tissue thickness measured from the margin of the incision

As the needle enters the flap, the gingival tissue is elevated by the tissue forceps and is rotated through the entry-side; as it progresses to the exit side, a counter pressure is placed on the exit side of the flap by the tissue forceps. This counter-pressure aids in allowing the exit of the needle to be at 90-degrees to the surface of the tissue and guides the needle to the proper exit point positioning [14, 83] (Figs. 15 and 16).

Once the needle is through the exit side of the flap, the surgeon can evaluate and confirm that the direction of passage of the needle is at a 90-degree angle to the

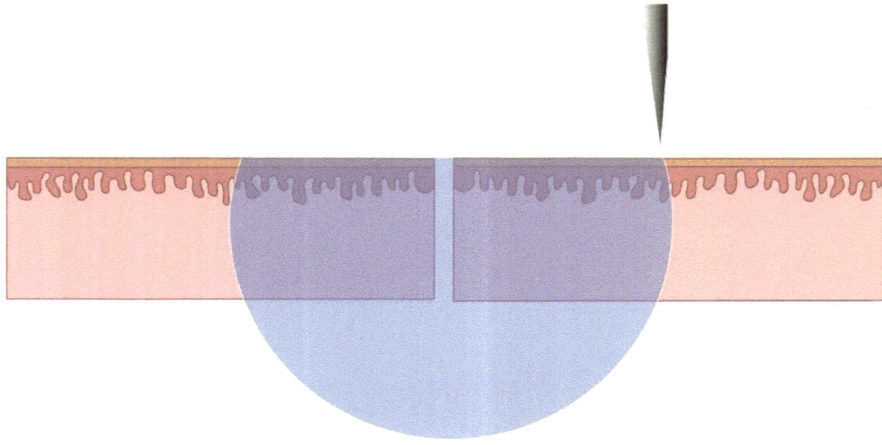

Fig. 11 Bite size: Needle entry and exit point should be equal distance from the incision margin

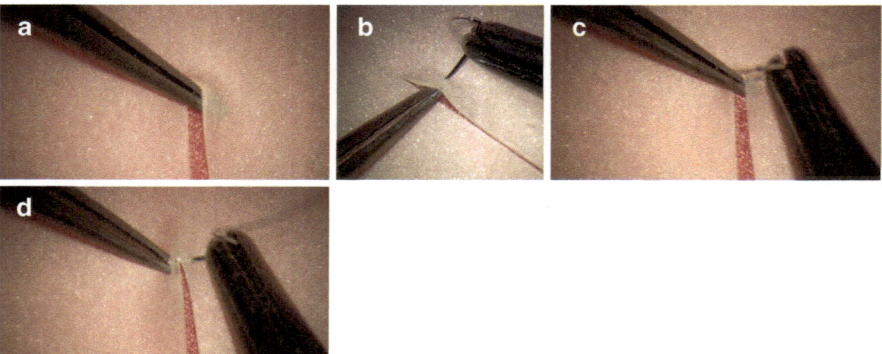

Fig. 12 (**a**) The tissue thickness is evaluated visually by elevating the flap. (**b**) The entry and exit points of the needle are 1.5 times the thickness of the tissue from the incision. (**c**) and (**d**) The needle is rotated as it passes from the entry to the exit point. The gingival tissue is elevated by the tissue forceps and is rotated through the entry-side; as it progresses to the exit side, a counter pressure is placed on the exit side of the flap by the tissue forceps

incision along with the entry and exit points at an equal distance from the incision. If this is not accomplished, unwanted lateral forces on the incision can produce tension or spacing, resulting in non-primary wound closure (Figs. 17 and 18).

The needle is gently rotated through the exit side of the flap, with counter pressure on the exit side gingival tissue. The suture is pulled through until the tail of the suture is sufficient to begin knot tying; this length should be approximately two times the length of the desired final length of the suture tails (Figs. 19 and 20).

For the first throw, the suture is picked up by the needle holder in the dominant hand followed by a clockwise throw of the suture over the tissue/tying forceps in the

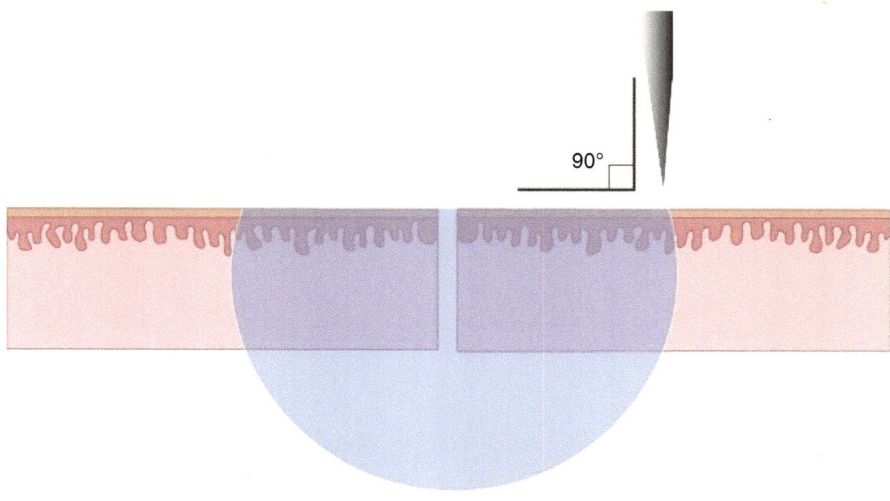

Fig. 13 Entry angle of the needle: 90°

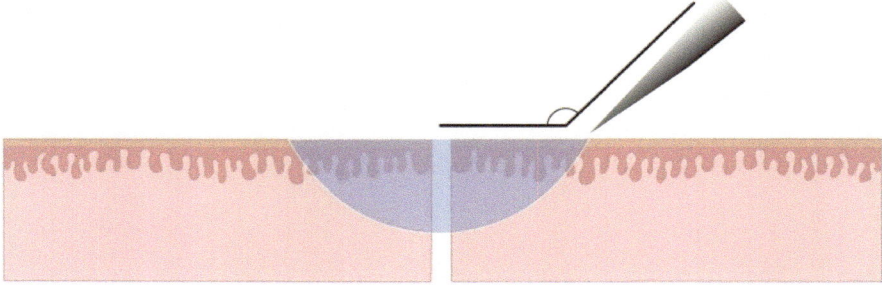

Fig. 14 Entry angles >90° potentially weaken tissue by compromising tissue thickness and blood supply setting the suture for failure either by cutting through tissue or inducing tissue necrosis

Fig. 15 Before completing the passage of the needle, the clinician confirms that the direction of passage is at a 90-degree angle to the incision

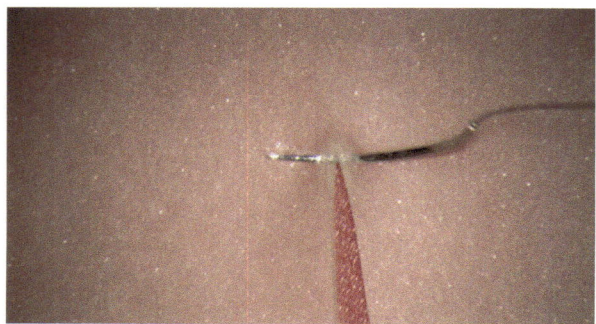

Fig. 16 Tissue forceps are used to create a gentle counter pressure to the needle exiting the gingival tissue. The application of a counter pressure also aids in directing the passage of the needle in a precise position in relation to flap thickness and maintaining a 90-degree angle

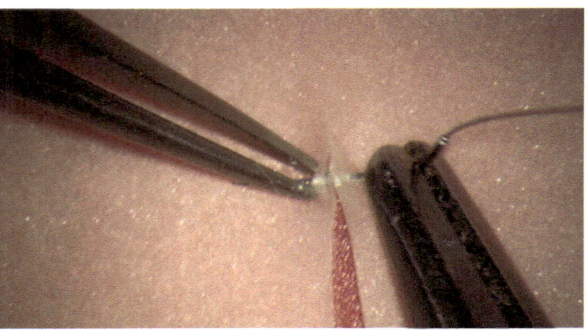

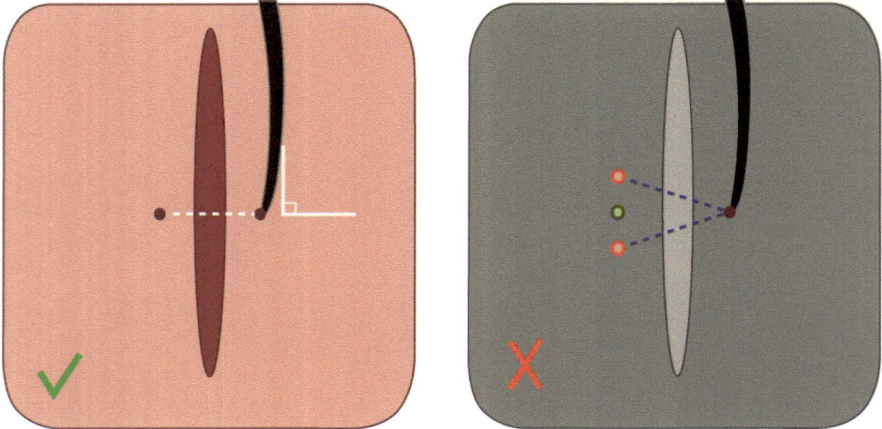

Fig. 17 Confirmation of direction of passage of the needle at 90°. Error to accomplish this may result in non-primary wound closure

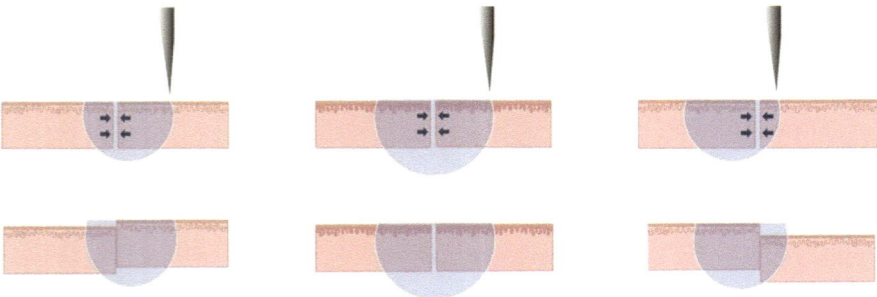

Fig. 18 Consequences of asymmetrical entry/exit needle points: Wound margin eversion and inversion

Fig. 19 Counterpressure being applied on the exit side

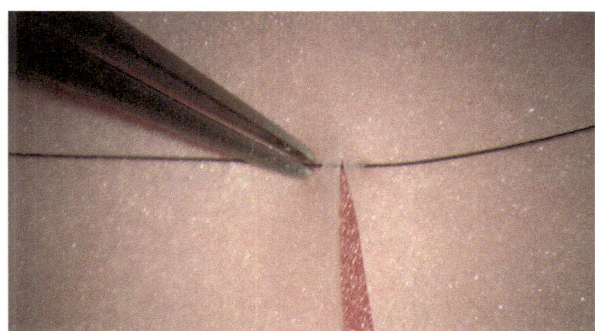

Fig. 20 Pulling of suture getting ready for knot tying

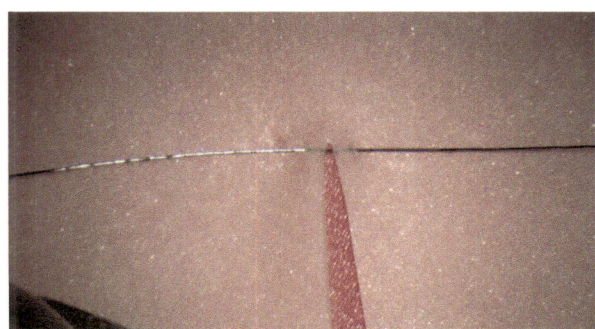

Fig. 21 The tissue forceps cross the incision and position the working tips in close proximity to the tail. A clockwise through is executed by passing the suture around the tissue forceps

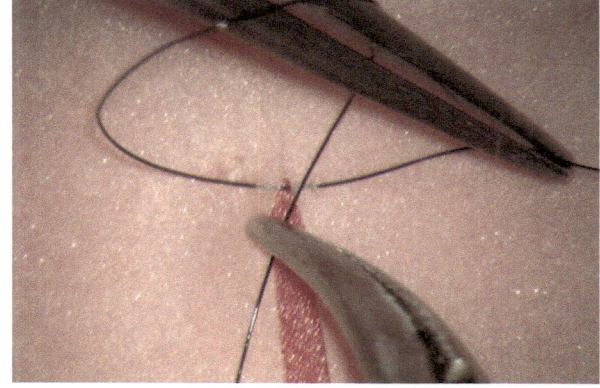

nondominant hand. Both the suture and the tail are pulled with equal pressure and speed at a 90-degree angle to the incision (Figs. 21, 22 and 23).

For the second and final throw, the suture is acquired by the nondominant hand, and a counter clockwise throw is performed over the dominant hand as the needle holder acquires the tail (Figs. 24 and 25).

As the second throw is tightened, the surgeon should keep the first and second throws parallel as the knot is reduced in size (Figs. 26, 27 and 28).

Fig. 22 The tail is brought to the exit side of the flap, while the suture is brought to the entry-side of the flap

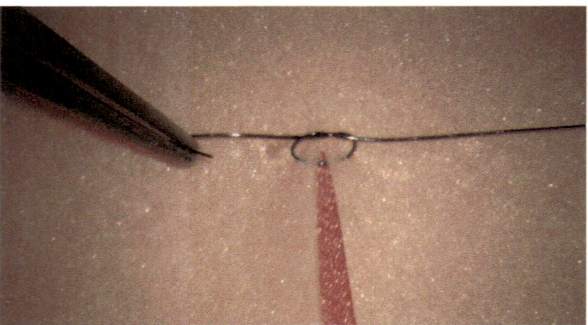

Fig. 23 This is performed while keeping the suture at a 90-degree angle to the incision

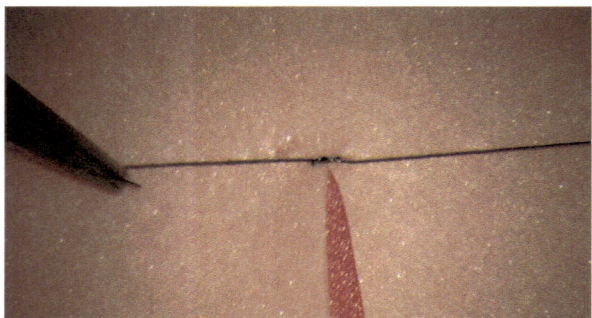

Fig. 24 The second through is executed by bringing the needle holder close to the tail of the suture. A counterclockwise through is performed with the suture over the needle holder

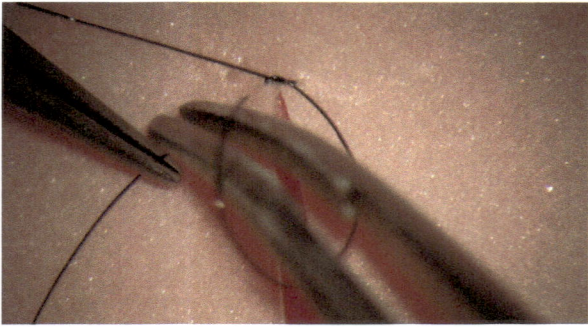

Once the knot is completed, the tails of the knot should be cut at approximately twice the length of the knot (Figs. 29 and 30) (Video 1). Additional throws do not improve the stability of a properly tied knot.

Sutures, including individual sutures, multiple interrupted sutures, and continuous sutures, should be symmetrical. Symmetry refers to regularity and consistent proportions. Balancing the stress distribution surrounding the closure of the incision is fundamental for ideal tissue closure and wound healing.

During suturing, there should be no tension on the flap during closure. Sutures placed under tension may lead to impaired wound healing. For ideal healing to occur, tensionless closure of gingival flaps is required [10, 45]

Fig. 25 The tail is then picked up with the needle holder

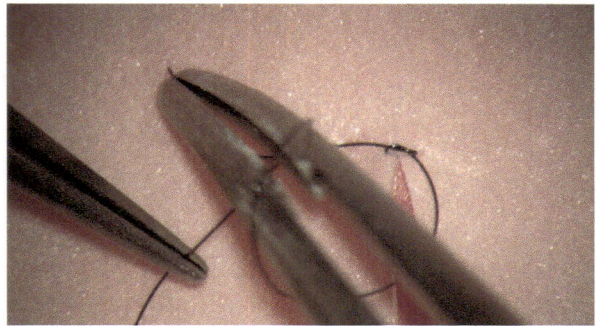

Fig. 26 The needle holder and tissue forceps are used to bring the tail and the suture, respectively, to opposite sides of the incision

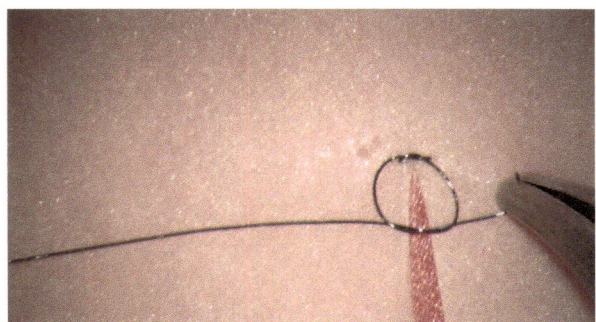

Fig. 27 This movement is important to maintain the second through parallel to the first through as the opening is reduced

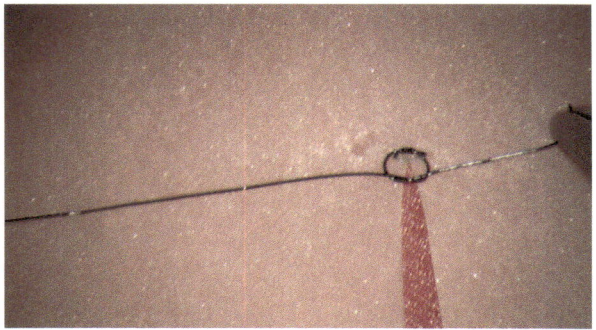

The frequency of sutures is determined by the concept of the load distribution within wound closure, which should be shared equally between each suture, regardless of whether the suture is interrupted or continuous [7]. The length of the suture bites results in different zones of compression. For primary wound healing, the distance between each individual suture should be less than the total length from the point of entry to the point of exit of the individual suture [7] (Fig. 31) (Video 2).

One of the challenges of microsurgery is physiologic tremor. A tremor is a rhythmic and involuntary movement of any body part [46]. Physiologic tremor is mainly produced by the underdamped inertial and viscoelastic properties of the

Fig. 28 The knot is finished by retaining a slight opening between the first and second throughs

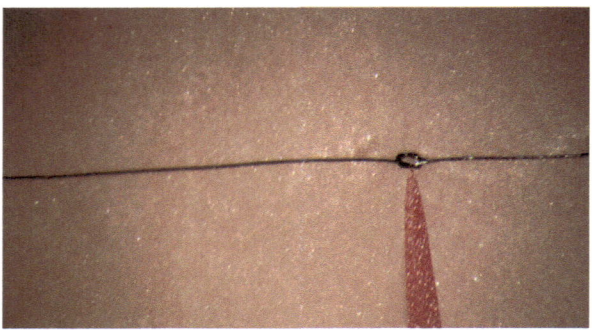

Fig. 29 Preparing to cut the tails of the knot

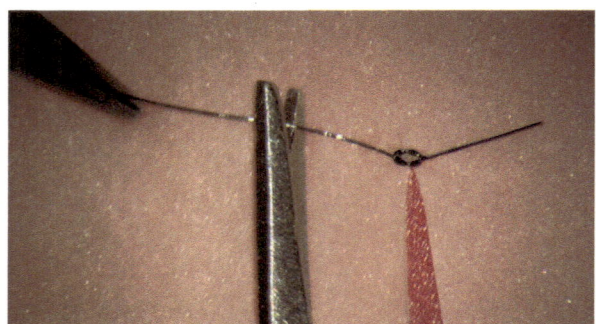

Fig. 30 The tails of the suture are cut at twice the length of the knot

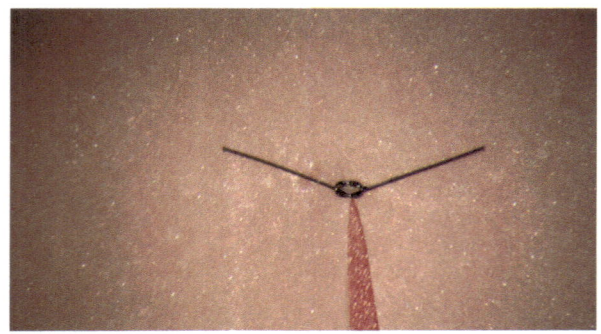

musculoskeletal system. This passive mechanical system is guided by two factors: random irregularities in muscle contraction and the sudden ejection of blood in cardiac systole [47]. Tremor is measured as a frequency (Hz), which is the number of oscillations per second of the affected limb.

Physiologic tremor usually occurs at a high frequency of 8–12 Hz. The frequency of physiologic tremor is directly affected by joint stiffness and inertia. The magnitude of physiologic tremor refers to all errors of movement. The amplitude is the degree of linear and angular movements, with low amplitude in the range of less

Fig. 31 Suture symmetry and frequency present in balanced wound closure, with all sutures having an equal function in wound closure and reflecting a mirror image in different planes around the incision and closure

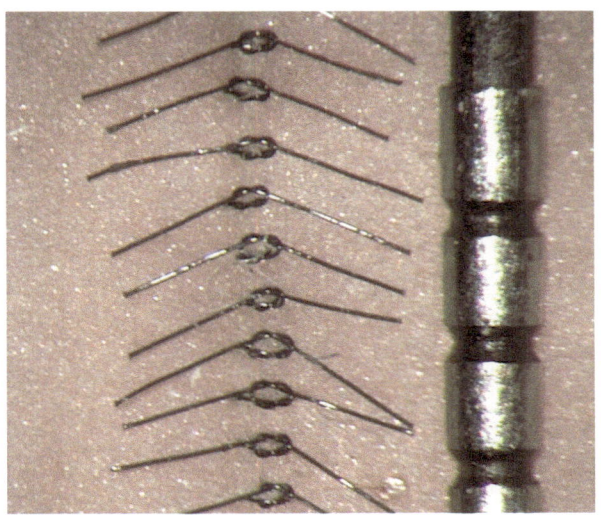

than 0.1 cm to 0.015 cm [44]. The frequency of tremor and the degree or amplitude of tremor are inversely related, meaning the lower the frequency of tremor, the larger the degree of movement that may occur [48–51].

Aperiodic error occurs at 6 Hz or less and plays a major role for microsurgeons. The majority of errors or unwanted movements are not physiologic tremors but aperiodic or arrhythmic errors, and the order of magnitude is greater than that of mechanical-reflex and central neurogenic oscillations [49, 52]. The ability to reduce tremor within the range of 1–3.5 Hz will lead to a reduction in amplitude of displacement by 56% [53].

Understanding normal tremors and methods to control or reduce tremors is helpful for the development of fine motor skills [54]. Physiologic tremor at 8–12 Hz is related to inertia and joint stiffness. A normal elbow tremor (forearm tremor) is at 3–5 Hz, a wrist tremor (hand tremor) is at 7–10 Hz, and a finger tremor is at 17–30 Hz [47, 52, 55, 56]. Surgeon chairs with arm supports or rests improve accuracy in tasks involving fine manipulation by a frequency reduction of 2–8 Hz [57]. Moreover, magnification up to 10× is critical for detailed and accurate micromanipulations [57].

Physiologic tremor may become more pronounced during periods of stress, anxiety, post-exercise, and following the use of caffeine or stimulants [48]. The use of certain beta-blockers, Propranolol has shown benefit in tremor reduction [23, 48, 58]. Tremors can also impact performance and can be reduced with experience, practice, and increased confidence [59]. Furthermore, maintaining mental and physical balance can be beneficial to surgeons in this aspect [57], such as relaxed diaphragmatic breathing, a comfortable physical position with minimal muscle recruitment and activation, and a relaxed mental concentration [14, 21, 22] (Fig. 32).

Fig. 32 A proper physical posture is essential for precision

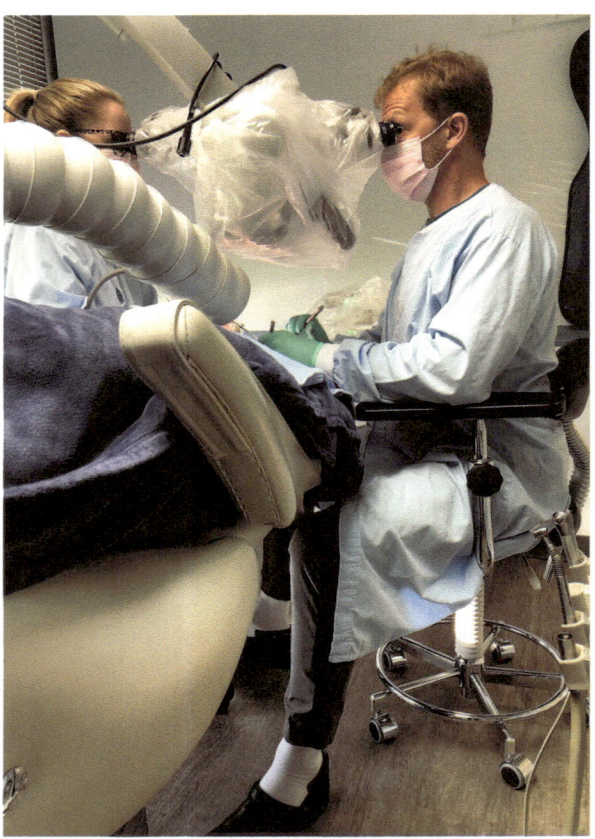

7   Knots

7.1   Knot Coding/Nomenclature

Tying a secure knot is key when it comes to tissue approximation in periodontal and implant surgery. A slipping knot may become loose or completely untied, thus failing to perform its job which is relieving tensional forces associated with healing processes while soft tissues recover their inherent physico-mechanical properties conducive to wound stability.

A knot is formed by tying together suture ends in order to bring closely wound edges or secure biomaterials to a substructure.

When working with a thread of suture material, a loop is formed and geometrically closed with a knot which at its turn is composed by a series of throws snugged against each other. Throws are formed by weaving suture strands together. The residual ends of the loop secured by the knot are called tails and when trimmed at the right length, these tails prevent untying of the knot by slippage [60] (Fig. 33).

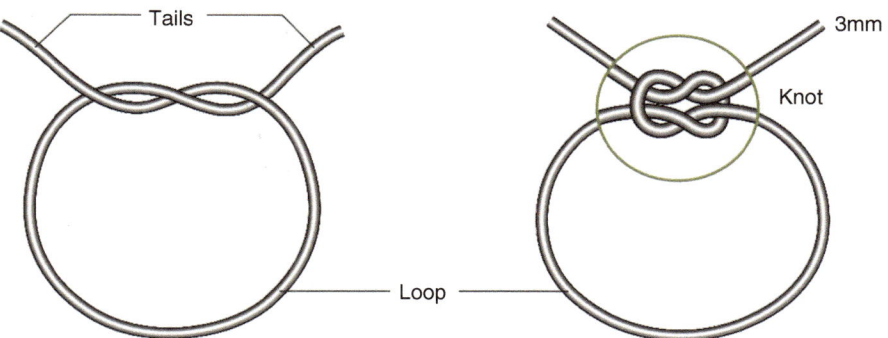

Fig. 33 Suture parts: knot, tails. 3 mm of length for the tails are recommended to prevent slippage

Throws can be single, double, triple, or (rarely) quadruple. A single throw is formed by weaving two strands around each other in a 360° formation. A double throw is formed by weaving these strands twice on a 720° formation. Triple and quadruple throws follow the same sequence ending with 1080° and 1440° formations, respectively.

In order to define, reproduce, and facilitate communication, when working with knots, a nomenclature system code was proposed by Tera et al. in 1976 [61]. For a knot to stay tied, it must have at least two throws superimposed on each other. Each throw consists of 1, 2, 3, or more turns (the number of times the thread ends are weaved around each other). In this code, the number of throws is assigned an Arabic number. Each throw may be combined with the next in either a crossed or a parallel fashion which is illustrated as "X" or "=" respectively.

"The symbol = shows that the thread entering and leaving the knot between two throws, seen by the side of the knot, passes on the same side of the other thread, such as in a reef [square] knot or a surgical knot. Such knots are paralleled knots. In a granny knot these two threads pass crosswise between the first and second throws, again seen from the side. They are therefore indicated by the symbol X between two Arabic figures and are classed as crossed knots" [61].

The three most common knots in periodontal and implant surgery are the square knot, the granny knot, and the surgeon's knot [62].

7.1.1 Square Knot
A square (reef) knot has been formed when the right ear and loop of the two throws exit on the same side of the knot are parallel to each other. The nomenclature used to describe this type of knot formation is: 1 = 1, Fig. 34.

7.1.2 Slip Knot
A slip (granny) knot has been formed when the right ear and loop of the two throws exit on opposite sides of the knot ending up crossed. The nomenclature used to describe this type of knot formation is: 1 × 1, Fig. 35.

Fig. 34 Square knot

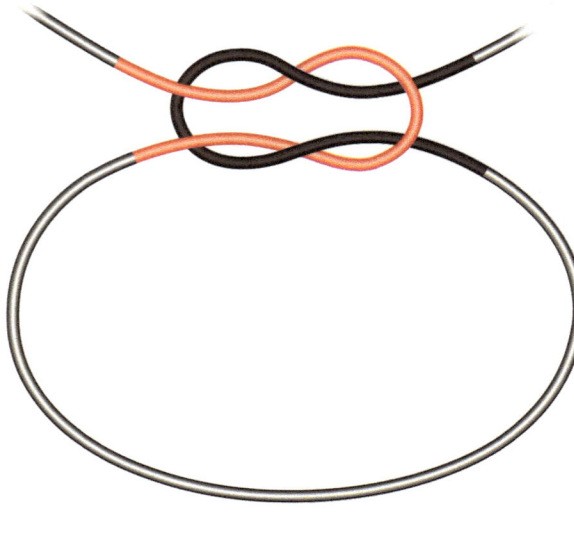

Fig. 35 Slip knot

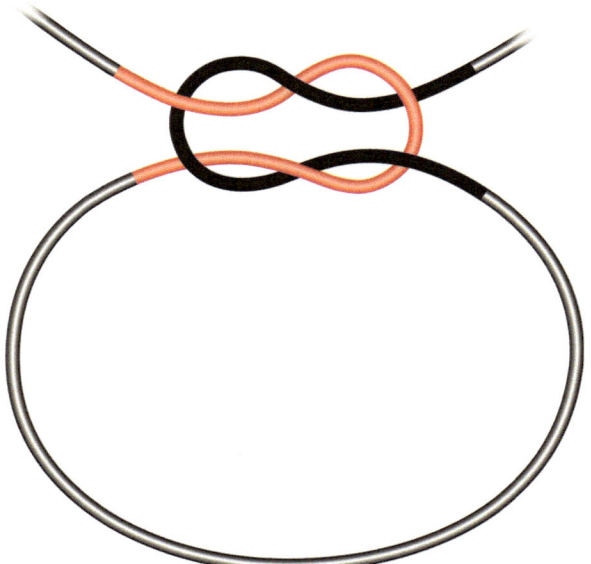

7.1.3 Surgeon's Knot

A surgeon's (friction) knot is constructed by an initial double-wrap throw followed by a single throw. The nomenclature used to describe this type of knot formation is: 2 = 1, Fig. 36.

Fig. 36 Surgeon's knot

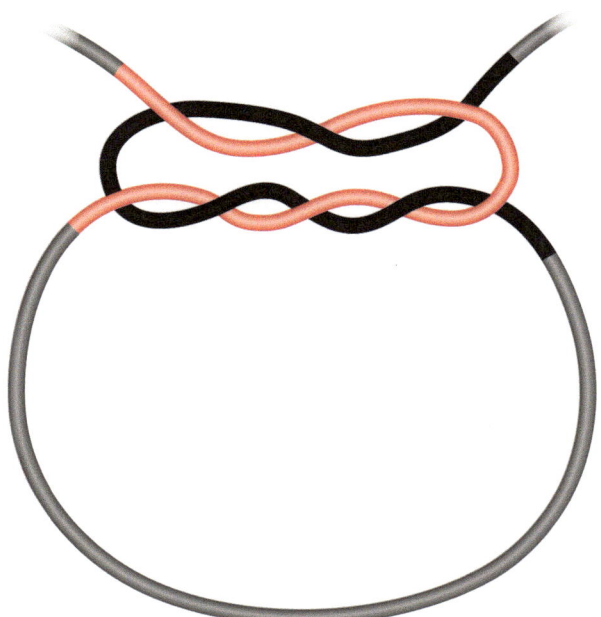

7.2   Knot Tying: Instrument Tie

It is of paramount importance to master instrument tie in periodontal and implant microsurgical procedures. Not only hand tie guided maneuvering will hinder direct visualization of the field but also manipulation of small diameter sutures becomes an optical guided execution rather than a tactile experience. Microsurgical instruments provide access in otherwise difficult to reach areas in the oral cavity when tying knots.

The following sequence illustrates in seven modules the principles of bimanual suturing instrumentation sequence when tying a 1 = 1 = 1 knot utilizing a synthetic flat model (rubber dam) with a 10-0 diameter polyamide suture thread on a 6 mm 3/8 spatula needle. The first four modules depict needle pick up, holding, threading, and finally tying the knot. The remaining three modules exemplify most common mistakes made while handling the needle and knot tying.

Module 1: picking up the needle (Video 3)

1. Pick up the suture thread with the tissue forceps in your nondominant hand and the needle holder with the dominant hand.
2. Manipulate the needle so its body rests against the elastic surface and it is rotated to end up with the needlepoint farthest away from the needle holder jaws.
3. Slightly open the needle holder jaws allowing the back of the needle (closest portion to its swage) to rest against the inner needle holder jaw (white triangle with #1).

4. Once the body of the needle touches the inner jaw, close the needle holder so its outer jaw (black triangle with # 2) clamps down gently on the body of the needle.
5. Once the needle has been captured, straighten it by softening the grip of the needle holder, maintaining the back of the needle in contact with the inner jaw of the needle holder (red triangle) and lightly tapping the portion closest to the needlepoint (white triangle) with the tissue forceps on your nondominant hand.
6. Verify the position of the needle. Its body should be perpendicular to the jaws of the needle holder. This position will facilitate needle advancing/rotation-controlled motions.

Module 2: holding the needle (Video 4)

1. Stay away from the needlepoint (small red rectangle). This area is very delicate and all efforts to prevent damaging it must be made. A damaged tip makes the needle useless.
2. Avoid the swage area (large red rectangle). The swage area is a structurally weak surface since it is hollow. Most swages of microsurgical needles are laser made and the thread is coupled to the needle in this area. Too much pressure will distort the needle and/or break the thread off it, rendering it nonserviceable.
3. The "sweet spot" of the needle is within the green rectangle. That is the target area when grabbing the needle.
4. Ideal point: The middle portion.
5. Holding the needle squarely in the horizontal and vertical axis will allow for a straight tissue penetration and help prevent losing control of the needle.
6. When holding the needle from the closest area of the green rectangle to the swage of the needle, the needle will trend to point upward.
7. When holding the needle from the closest area of the green rectangle to the needlepoint, the needle will trend to point downward. Do not hold it too close to the point, otherwise too little will be projecting out and it is hard to pass it through.

Module 3: needle insertion (Video 5)

1. Holding the needle with the needle holder in the dominant hand, visualize an entry point. The distance from the wound margin (slit in the elastic material) to the entry point should be equal or 1.5× of the thickness of the substrate to be sutured.
2. Tissue holder is being held by the nondominant hand and it is positioned underneath the elastic material everting it to facilitate a bite as close to a 90° angle as possible.
3. Once through, DO NOT let go of the needle. Rotate and advance it forward to an exit point which is equidistant to the entry point.
4. Bring the tissue forceps from above and press down toward the needle so piercing occurs through the substrate being sutured at a 90° angle.

5. Push the needle forward with the dominant hand. Before passing it completely through, evaluate bite size symmetry.
6. Once symmetry is verified, proceed to pull the needle through avoiding grabbing it from the needlepoint and utilizing the tissue forceps to press down on the elastic material to decrease excessive distortive forces as the needle is being manipulated.
7. Pull the needle with the nondominant hand keeping the suture trajectory in a straight line perpendicular to the wound edge and utilizing the needle holder in the dominant hand as a pulley to avoid any suture line angles that could drag and cut through tissues. Stop pulling when the tail measures approximately 2–3 mm. At this point let go of the needle.

Module 4: tying the knot (Video 6)

1. In order to produce a workable loop, make sure that you can see the thread emerging from the side of the tissue holders on your nondominant hand.
2. Once you make a loop, pull the short end of the suture with the tissue holders on your dominant hand thru the loop while pulling the long end with your nondominant hand in the opposite direction to tie the first half square knot.
3. Do not waste your time trying to approximate the "wound edges" at this point.
4. Without letting go of the thread with your nondominant hand, create another loop to tie the second half of the square knot.
5. Now pull first the short end of the thread (1) until "wound edge" approximation occurs and then pull the long end (2) to lock this knot in position.
6. Tie the last security half knot and trim the excess suture leaving both ends at about 2–3 mm in length. If left too long, they will interfere with adjacent suture tying.
7. Pull the needle from the thread dragging it into the visual field. Now you can let go of the thread with your nondominant hand (first time since step 1) and prepare to pick up the needle and start all over again.

Module 5: mistakes when holding the needle (Video 7)

1. Avoid grasping the needle at its swage. This area is hollow and therefore very weak. At best, shape distortion may occur that renders the needle useless.
2. Stay away from the needlepoint. This happens more often when going after the needle and pulling it after incompletely passing it through tissue. Once the fine point is twisted, there is only one thing to do: discard it and get a new one.
3. Again, going after the swage area. Remember, this is a very delicate component. Too much pressure and the suture material may become separated.
4. Holding the needle far away from the edge of the needle holder will decrease its reach, mobility, and accuracy in motion delivery and insertion control.
5. Grabbing the needle too close to the edge of the needle holder will prevent a firm grip and the needle may be ejected and lost.

Module 6: mistakes related to needle insertion (Video 8)

1. Letting go of the needle before advancing/rotating it through tissue to be able to grasp it and pull it out to complete a clean needle insertion movement. It creates unnecessary challenges trying to gain control of the desired angulation, depth, and direction. It can traumatize tissue unnecessarily, slows down the suturing process, and can generate frustration and anxiety on the microsurgical team.
2. Grabbing wound edges with the tissue forceps instead of supporting it as illustrated in module 4. Tissue needs to be gently manipulated and any effort to prevent crushing it needs to be made. Excessive compression can harm delicate capillaries and contribute to compromise vascularization which can escalate to tissue necrosis and wound healing impairment.

Module 7: mistakes during knot tying: (Video 9)

1. Prepare the tissue holder in your dominant hand so its endpoints are facing the tail and are ready to grasp it with a simple opening-closing motion without having to rotate the body of the instrument.
2. If the loop is too small, it will be difficult to get hold of the suture tail.
3. If the loop is too large, the movements will be unnecessarily ample, and this will reduce the efficiency of movements.
4. If the tail is too long, it will be difficult to pull it through the loop in one simple movement.
5. If the tail is too short, it will be difficult to grab it, and very easy to pull it through forcing the whole process to start all over.
6. When tying the second half knot, and both ends (short and long) are pulled at the same time, the knot will be locked (some suture materials slide easier than others and can be more forgiving) preventing border approximation, thus negating primary closure.

7.3   Knot Failure

Failure of a knotted suture loop will be a result of one of the following: knot slippage or breakage, suture cutting through tissue, and mechanical damage of the suture by surgical instruments.

7.3.1 Slippage

All knots slide after tying and left to settle in the recipient tissue. Several factors regulate the degree of slippage: inflammation, friction coefficient of the biomaterial, suture diameter, moisture, knot type, and final geometry. It is known that most parallel knots (i.e. square, surgeons) are more resistant to slippage than crossed knots (i.e. granny). Depending on the suture biomaterial, additional throws prevent failure by slippage. However, additional throws can also lead to know breakage and increased volume has repercussions on plaque accumulation and sensitive disturbance to patients. Choosing the right suture biomaterial is important especially in areas where stretching of the wound via inflammation is anticipated to prevent wound closure failure [63].

7.3.2 Suture Cutting Through Tissue

Tissue phenotype plays an important role in this type of failure. Changes during tissue healing also can influence cutting forces. Adequate distance from the wound edge when entering and exiting with the needle must be observed in order to avoid compromising tissue integrity that may contribute to failure. Needle selection and precise needle insertion will decrease the risk of creating tissue irregularities and introducing tissue defects that may lead to weakening the periphery of the needle-suture passage leading to failure but cutting through tissue [64], Fig. 37.

7.3.3 Mechanical Damage

Fine threads of suture material are susceptible to manipulation related to crushing forces applied by the operator. The configuration of the jaws of the instruments used to tie the knot must be smooth without aggressive topographic features such as teeth as seen in tungsten carbide inserts. While these features provide holding security, breakage and deterioration of physical integrity of delicate suture biomaterials are very likely to happen. Instrument jaws with metallurgically bonded tungsten particles are a compromise and can adequately perform when compared to smooth jaws without any type of surface modification. Compression of the suture material is meant to happen without compromising the suture breaking strength [65].

Fig. 37 Precise needle insertion decreases the risk of adverse wound healing

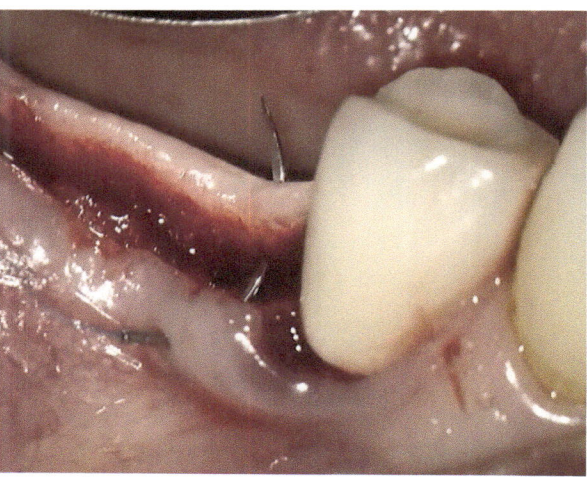

7.4   Biomechanical Properties and Performance

7.4.1 Vectoring/Angulation

A vector of force has two components: direction and magnitude. Vector forces extend in three directions: perpendicular to the wound surface, parallel to the wound margin, and perpendicular to the tissue surface [7]. When closing a simple straight incision line, the forces of approximation must be equal to the forces of separation, Figs. 38, 39 and 40.

Closing forces are applied by the suture which is primarily executed in two ways: interrupted and continuous, Figs. 41 and 42.

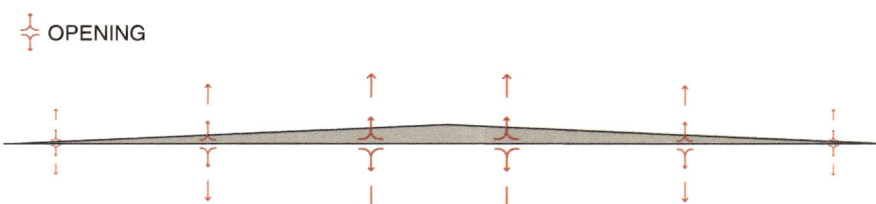

Fig. 38 Forceps of separation of wound margins (red arrows)

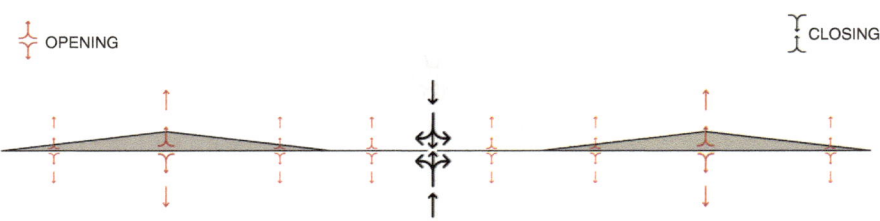

Fig. 39 Single suture counteracting forceps of separation (black arrows)

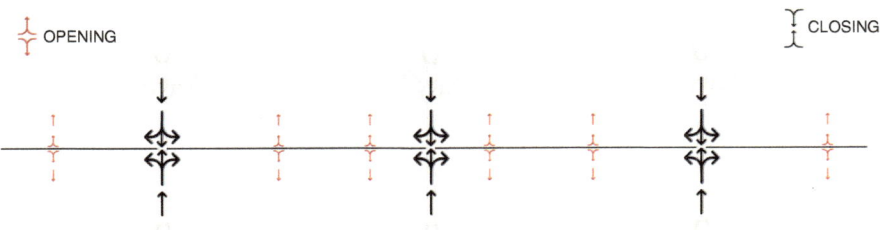

Fig. 40 Forces of separation of wound margins must be matched with equal forces of approximation provided by sutures to achieve primary closure

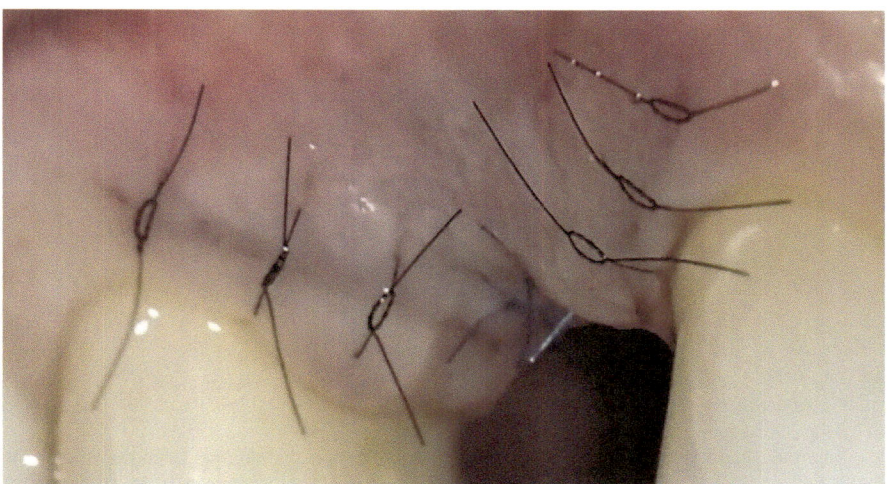

Fig. 41 Interrupted suturing technique

7.4.2 Compression Zones/Frequency/Symmetry

Determining the number of sutures necessary to provide wound closure and stability depends on different factors such as type of tissue being sutured, distance from entry to exit point, space between suture lines, etc. Having the highest number of sutures possible distributed along the wound surface does not guarantee a strong closure. Intact tissue surrounding the entry/exit points remains the strongest biomechanically tissue in the wound zone. It is the intact tissue that provides strength and support during healing. The magnitude of the closing force of one suture is neutralizing an equally opposing opening force. These forces are dissipated within neighboring tissue, thus distributing tension into a broader area. When sutures are placed closer to each other, the buffering area where forces are dissipated onto is reduced and an overlapping of stress points occurs. This phenomenon ultimately weakens this tissue and reduces its capacity to withstand tension. Another negative consequence of placing sutures in close proximity to each other is the blood supply compromise related to the traumatic puncturing of tissues. The principle to keep in mind is that of maximization of healing potential while maintaining tissue strength required to provide wound stability during the healing process [67].

Each interrupted suture is maintaining a balance between eversion and inversion of the wound margin by producing a zone of compression. As referenced above, these tension forces are higher in the trajectory formed by the entry and exit points.

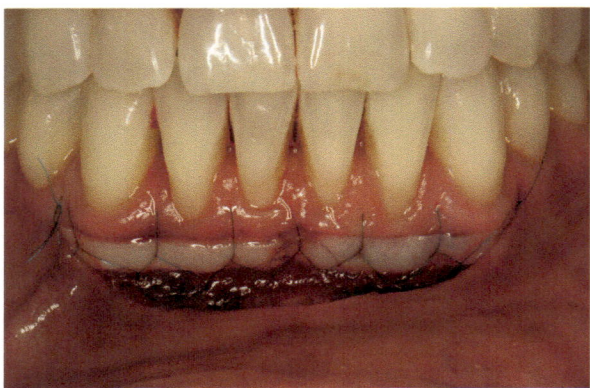

Fig. 42 Continuous suture

In an ideal situation, an interrupted suture is a loop that runs perpendicular to the wound edge with half of the loop above the surface and half of the loop below the surface surrounding the wound edge with an equal tension distribution occurring between these two halves. In this arrangement, the superficial tension equals the superficial closing force and this is mirrored in the subsurface component of the suture loop. This is how primary wound closure is achieved by having equal forces above and below the tissue at the site of incision and closure (the trend for eversion of the wound margin is cancelled by a force inducing inversion with the interrupted suture).

Continuous sutures are more complex due to their arrangement, direction, and distribution above and below the wound surface. In contrast to interrupted sutures, these sutures cannot be placed completely perpendicular to the wound edge since at some point there must be a diagonal component that allows its advancement and coverage over the length of the incision line. There is usually a symmetrically diagonal or an asymmetrical configuration of perpendicular and diagonal patterns in relationship to the wound edge. Due to its oblique component, the vectoring covers an area of the wound surface that leads to a lateral shift of the wound. Based on mathematical models and calculations, Rubinstein and Russell conclude that in order to obtain the same closing force for a continuous suture as for a perpendicular interrupted one, a greater tension is needed in the suture. There are factors that are relevant to the amount of tension inherent to continuous sutures such as the angulation between diagonal sutures and spacing between suture lines. The more distanced sutures are, the more tension to be applied on individual sutures within the continuous arrangement [66], Figs. 43 and 44.

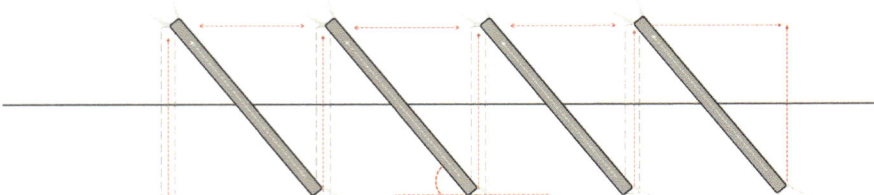

Fig. 43 Oblique nature of the continuous sutures needs greater tension in order to obtain the same closing forces when compared to perpendicular interrupted sutures

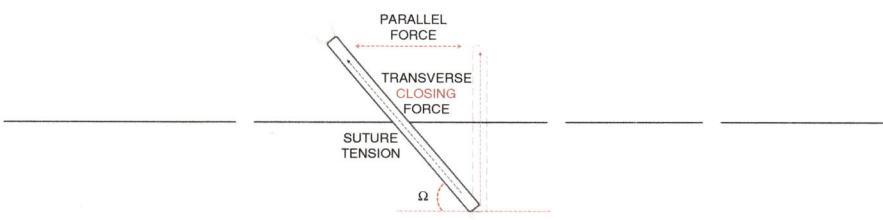

Fig. 44 Angulation between diagonal sutures and spacing between suture lines define the tension of continuous sutures. (Modified from [66])

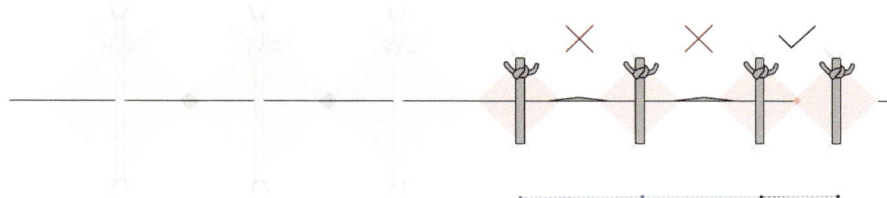

Fig. 45 Compression zones of each interrupted suture are formed by the distance from the wound margin to the exit and entry points after the suture is tightened. (Adapted from [7])

Those forces then dissipate laterally. The extent of the compression zones of each interrupted suture is determined by the distance from the wound margin to the exit and entry points after the suture is tightened. Adequate wound closure occurs when these compression zones overlap each other [7], Figs. 45, 46 and 47.

Symmetrical entry and exit points maintaining an equidistant distance from the wound margin will distribute tension forces in an equal manner, thus neutralizing inversion and aversion trends of the wound edge preventing wound override which can lead to potential scarring due to poor wound edge approximation, Video 10.

7.4.3 Suture Tension on Soft Tissues

There is ample evidence on the effects of tension on cell biomechanical performance, and how wounds closed under high tension are at high risk of impaired healing. The more rigid the fixation of a wound, the longer it takes for a wound to regain its tensile strength [68–70]. Suture placement deals with tension forces that ought to be addressed in order to achieve passive approximation of wound edges that end up facilitating primary closure of the wound. If there is excess pressure being applied to the suture, the suture can break or excess tension builds up on the tissue surrounding the suture which can translate into tissue necrosis which jeopardizes nutrient supplies and may end up in scarring.

Having an overtight suture can deform surrounding tissue and compromise wound closure. It is better to remove it as soon as it is realized that it has occurred rather than to leave it or add additional sutures to correct the existing tissue distortion.

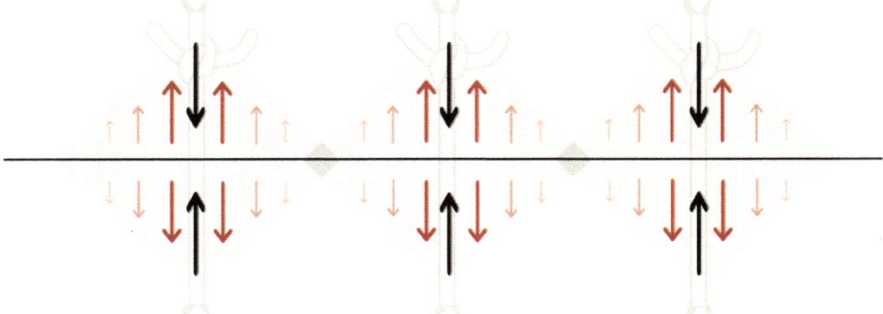

Fig. 46 Adequate wound closure occurs when these compression zones overlap each other

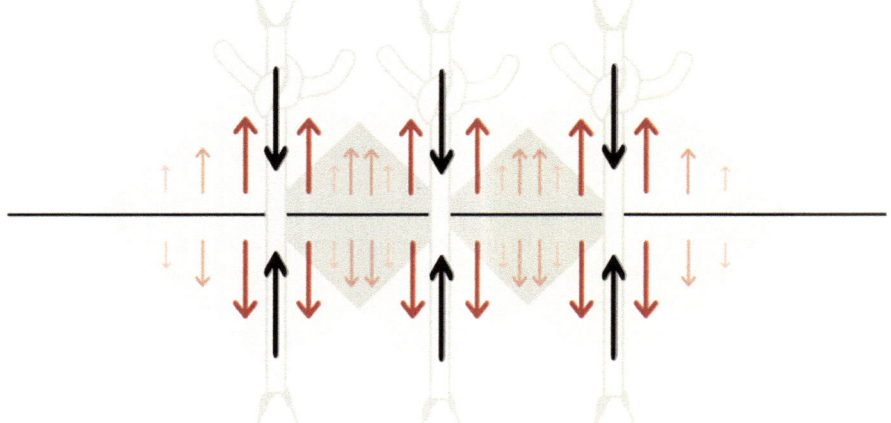

Fig. 47 Forces dissipate laterally. When sutures are too close, higher concentration of forces is confined to tighter spaces interfering with blood flow and potentially weakening tissue integrity

In mucogingival therapy, it has been shown that the higher the flap tension, the lower the recession reduction, with tissue phenotype playing an important role in stability of healing during coronally advanced flap procedures [71].

7.5   Suture Removal

The purpose of sutures is to coalesce wound margins while providing anchor points to release intrinsic tension while fibroblasts realign and collagen gains enough mechanical strength to prevent further opening of the incision line under normal masticatory function within the oral cavity. As reviewed previously, suture spacing, symmetry, and tissue phenotype play an important role in distribution of tension

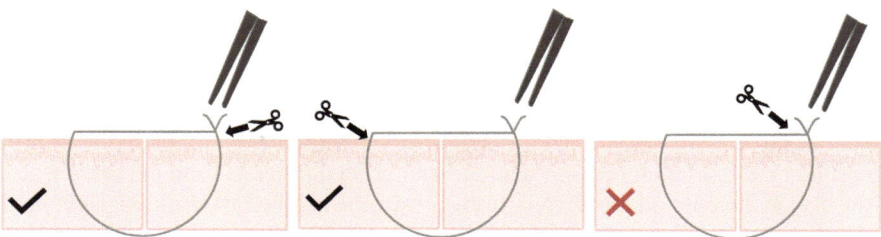

Fig. 48 Correct suture removal avoids pulling the knot and the portion of the suture exposed to the oral cavity through the suture track

related forces in tissues neighboring the wound margins. In a study performed in porcine mucosa investigating tensile strength, elastic modulus, strain at fracture and energy absorption related to areas of the wound maximally influenced by the presence of sutures to those remotely located to sutures, it was shown that when utilizing nylon sutures at 5 and 7 days of healing, the areas closer to the sutures have a lower modulus of elasticity and greater tensile strain than areas farther apart, although the tensile strength is of equal magnitude across the wound site. By day 14 this pattern is no longer present and mechanical behavior on the wound is homogenous, meaning that between 7 and 14 days the presence of sutures is irrelevant to wound strength rehabilitation and protection. What is of interest is that when comparison between sites that had sutures removed at seventh days to those in which sutures were removed at the 14th day was performed, there was a marked increase in tensile strength and energy absorption at suture sites that had early removal of sutures. The authors of this study speculate that it is possible that suture tracks may act as secondary wounds enhancing fibroblast activity and collagen synthesis in this area [72], Fig. 48.

8 Suturing Techniques

Many types of surgical knots exist. Selection of an appropriate knot for wound closure is influenced by suture material and the degree of residual tension in the wound. Out of approximately 3600 types of knots, only a small number of knots are described and used for wound closure [73, 74]. Most techniques have been described for right-handed surgeons. Ideal suture techniques include the least number of throws required to acquire strength and security. Small differences in knot tying techniques have significant negative impact on the performance of the knot. For example, difference of only a single throw exists between a square and a granny knot. Two basic types of knots exist, symmetrical and asymmetrical knots. The symmetrical knots include the square knots. Asymmetrical knots include sliding knots, which involve unequal distribution of friction within the suture [61]. In periodontal microsurgery, the majority of knots utilized are symmetrical.

The square knot (1 = 1), also known as the reef knot, is considered the standard knot. This is due to the fact that this is a very secure knot. In addition, it is considered one of the easiest knots to tie [15, 73]. Once the suture passes through the exit side of the flap, the tissue forceps in the left hand wrap the suture around the needle holder of the right hand in a counter-clockwise direction. The tail is brought to the exit side of the flap by the right hand, while the suture is brought to the entry side of the flap by the left hand. The throw is then tightened to the tissue. For the second throw, tissue forceps in the left hand bring the suture from the entry side of the flap and a clockwise throw is formed over the needle holder in the right hand. The tail of the suture is taken to the entry side of the flap, while the suture is brought to the exit side of the flap, and the throws are tightened. The square knot is the main knot used by surgeons. It has several advantages over other knots owing to its strength, security, and ease of application (Figs. 34 and 49, Video 11). The granny knot (1 × 1) is a variant of the square knot; however, it is a less stable knot that has the tendency to slip under tension [15, 73] (Figs. 35 and 50, Video 12).

The surgeon's knot (2 = 1) is a simple variation of the square knot. This knot includes an extra twist in the first throw. In short, the first throw of this knot has two twists, while the second throw only has one. It is purported that the additional twist in the first throw reduces loosening (Figs. 36 and 51, Video 13).

Fig. 49 The square knot is a standard and frequently utilized knot

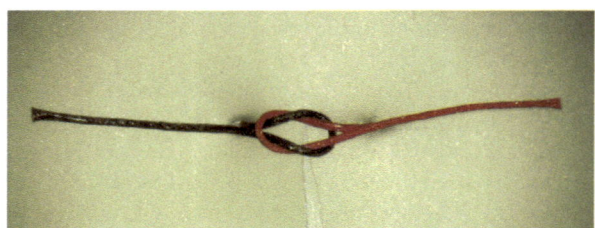

Fig. 50 The Granny knot is a variation of the square knot with a predisposition to loosening

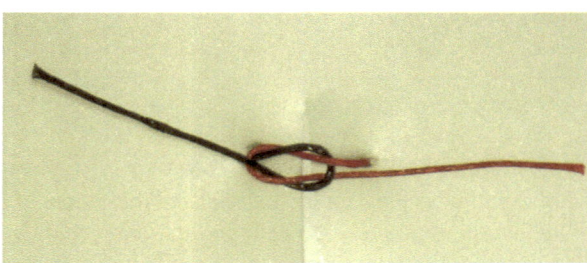

Fig. 51 The surgeon's knot is an asymmetrical knot

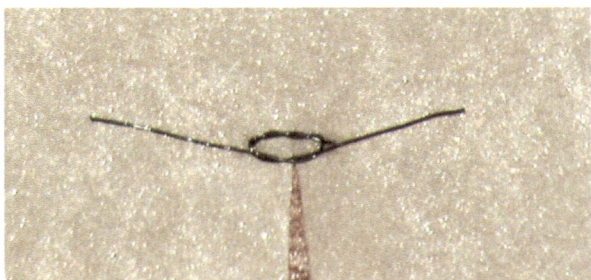

9 The Microsurgical Training Institute

The English Surgeon's Knot (2 = 2) was taught for over 25 years at the Microsurgical Training Institute in Santa Barbara, California founded in 1990 (Figs. 52 and 53, Video 14). This specific knot tying technique is applied at the beginning and end of the continuous suture. It also serves as an excellent suture knot tying technique when the square knot is inadequate, such as the presence of tension. The English Surgeon's Knot consists of two double throws. It was also referred to as the "double knot" or 2 = 2 by Tera and Aberg [61]. The first throw consists of two clockwise twists, using the dominant right hand, over the tissue forceps in the left hand. Once this motion is completed, the tissue forceps acquire the tail, and the first double throw is tightened to the tissue. The second double throw involves performing two counterclockwise twists using the tissue forceps over the needle holder in the right

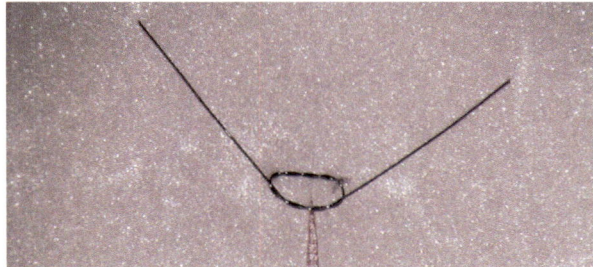

Fig. 52 The English Surgeon's Knot (2 = 2) was taught by Dennis Shanelec and is a fundamental symmetrical knot in microsurgery

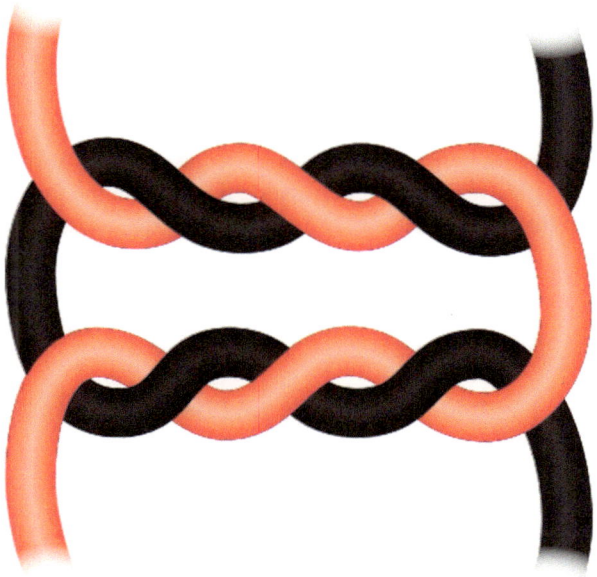

Fig. 53 Diagram illustrating the 2 = 2 knot

Fig. 54 Gingival recession lesion to be surgically corrected

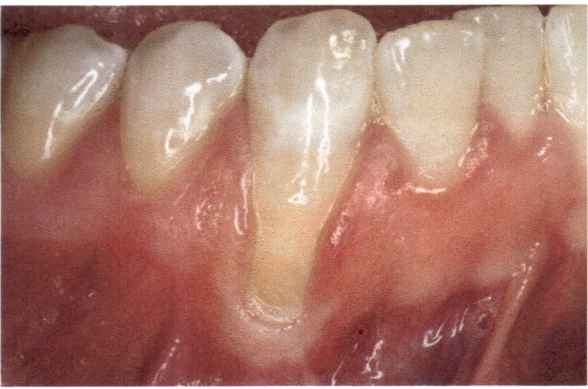

Fig. 55 The application of the English Surgeon's Knot in the Microsurgical Connective Tissue Graft

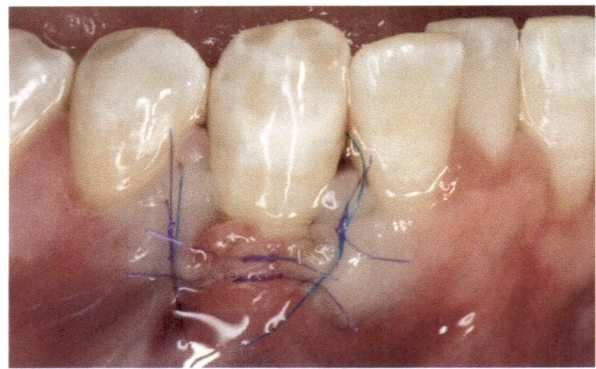

hand. The needle holder then acquires the tail of the suture, which is the closure of the second double throw toward the first double throw while keeping the throws parallel the entire time. A slight space is left open between the two throws to reduce the increase in pressure caused by the swelling of tissues during the inflammatory response and to prevent possible tissue ischemia that can occur with overtightening of the sutures [19] (Figs. 54, 55, 56, 57, 58, 59, 60 and 61, Videos 15, 16 and 17).

10 Methods for Developing Suturing Technique and Practicing

10.1 Training Models and Exercises

Suturing is a skill. Like all skills, it requires continuous, purposeful, and deliberate practice. To maintain the level of skill through which precise, primary wound closure can be achieved consistently, there are several practice tools that have been developed that allow microsurgeons to continue improving their accuracy and precision.

Fig. 56 Postoperative healing of gingival recession lesion depicted in Fig. 54

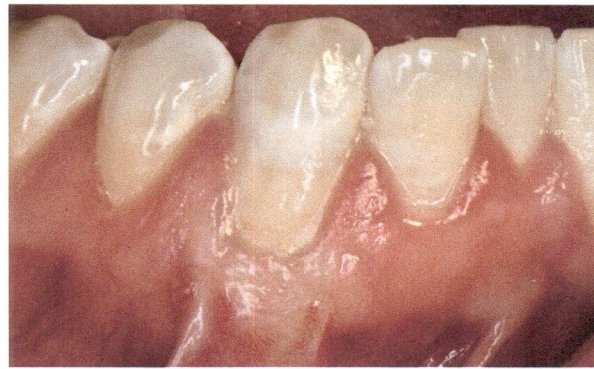

Fig. 57 Initial presentation of patient exhibiting short clinical crowns related to altered passive eruption

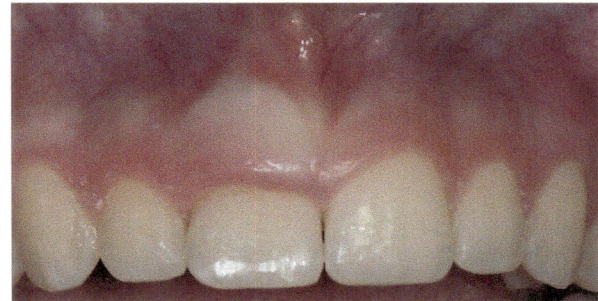

Fig. 58 Clinical application of the English Surgeon's Knot in Microsurgical Esthetic Crown Lengthening

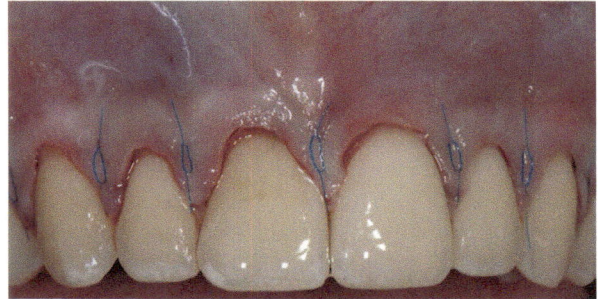

Dental models simulating hard and soft tissues in resin and silicone provide an opportunity, using three-dimensional prototypes, to practice in a setting that resembles clinical scenarios encountered in daily periodontal and implant practice. BoneModels® is a company that manufactures such models and is owned by Fernando-Rojas-Vizcaya, D.D.S., M.S. [18, 75]. The company provides custom-designed soft tissue replicas of varying thicknesses. The microsurgeon can practice all forms of periodontal and implant microsurgery using these models, Fig. 62 (Video 18).

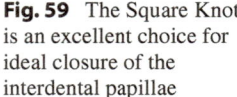

Fig. 59 The Square Knot is an excellent choice for ideal closure of the interdental papillae

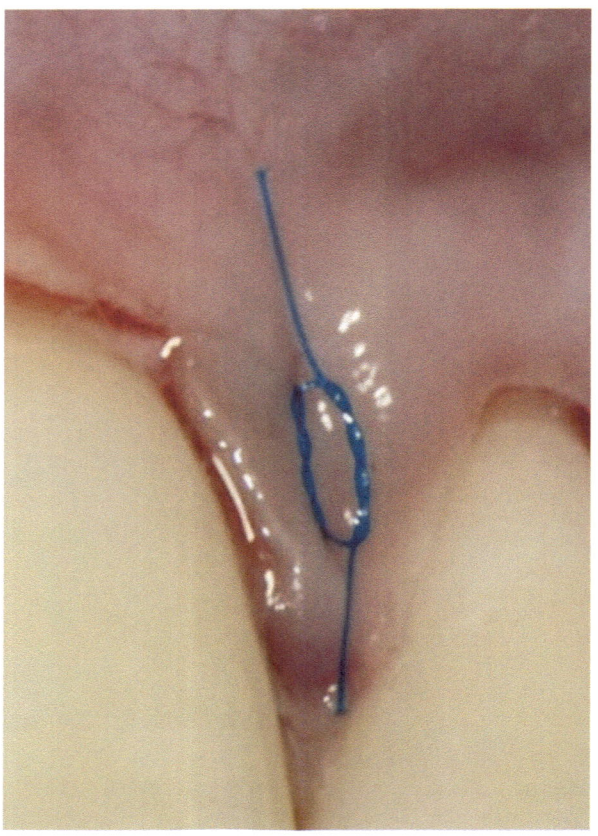

As is necessary for all surgeons, microsurgeons are obligated to commit themselves to maintaining the highest level of hand skills and dexterity. Nowadays, surgeons can avail multiple options through which they can continuously improve their professional skills. Incorporating these techniques into one's weekly practice is considered vital for maintaining and improving one's skill.

Training in microsurgical techniques has become important across all surgical disciplines. These techniques have become routine in otorhinolaryngology, ophthalmology, neurosurgery, trauma, hand, plastic, reconstructive, vascular, orthopedics, gynecology, and urology surgical procedures.

Classical training in microvascular surgery remains a common denominator for all other surgical fields. In vitro models such as plastic tubes allow for practicing correct knotting techniques, instrument handling, and development of inherent finger dexterity before moving onto more complex systems such as animal cadavers and in vivo models.

These exercises offer challenges that continue to develop and refine optical, mechanical, tactile/sensorial, psychomotor, and cognitive skills.

Fig. 60 Postoperative result of patient illustrated in Fig. 57

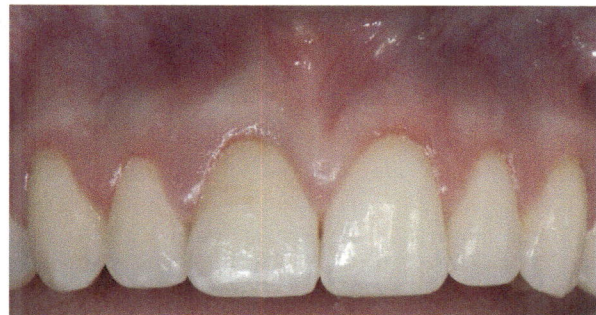

Fig. 61 The continuous suture with the English Surgeon's Knot for precise wound closure

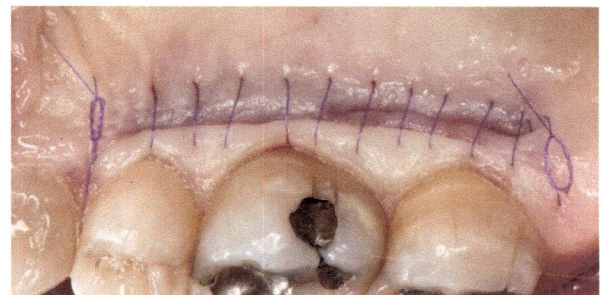

10.1.1 Gauze

This exercise utilizes 100% cotton gauze sponges to familiarize the microscope operator with different magnification levels in a tridimensional model. It starts with low magnification all the way to the highest magnification. Next, the operator is to practice aiming and clamping individual threads utilizing microsurgical tweezers. This helps develop eye–hand coordination at different levels of magnification. Once comfortable with this sequence, threads can be held and cut with curved micro-scissors going at different depth levels of the gauze sponge. This part of the exercise introduces the use of a second hand being brought into the operating field. Threads can then be pulled away and rewoven as desired. The last part of the exercise con-sists in the threading of a needle and suture following the intricacies of the woven mesh practicing holding the needle with both microsurgical tweezers and needle holder [76], Video 19.

10.1.2 Newspaper

This exercise utilizes newspaper to acquaint the microscope operator with different magnification levels and hone tactile skills. In a similar fashion to gauze exercise, it starts by viewing the object with low magnification all the way to the highest mag-nification level. Then, utilizing the tip of a blade (i.e. 15c, 11, or 12) the operator is to choose a letter and scratch the ink off the print without perforating the sheet of paper. This can be done multiple times. The next challenge is to cut out a single let-ter in its entirety with the help of the scalpel blade and microsurgical tweezers.

Eye–hand coordination and utilization of two hands add a level of more advanced complexity. Finesse in movements and force application is tested in this maneuver, Video 20.

10.1.3 Needles

When handling sutures at high magnifications settings working with an operating microscope, it is impractical to handle suture materials with only one instrument. It becomes imperative to utilize instruments in both hands (i.e.: Castroviejo-type needle holder and tissue forceps) that allow for needle and thread manipulation without obstructing the operator's view.

By setting multiple sewing needles with different eye sizes in a circle facing in different directions and at different heights, the operator is challenged to handle the suturing needle simulating clinical situations that require similar maneuvers, Video 21.

10.1.4 Egg

This advanced exercise challenges the operator's tactile sensations and hand–eye coordination at different levels. First, penetration and elevation of the egg shell (average thickness of 0.3 to 0.4 mm) must be accomplished without rupturing the inner egg membranes. Once the inner membranes are exposed, an incision is made. The average thickness of the membranes of the egg ranges from 73 to 114 microns (the average human hair thickness is 100 micros) [77]. Once an opening is accomplished, 10-0 nylon suture material is utilized to approximate the edges of the incision line. Egg membranes (essentially made out of keratin and other proteins) are rather fragile and easy to tear, Video 22.

10.1.5 Eggplant

This exercise utilizes a vegetable model. The uneven contour of the eggplant poses a challenge when harvesting small segments of even thickness.

While advancing the scalpel blade without being able to visualize neither its position nor direction nor range of motion, it forces the operator to enhance a tactile skill by mentally visualizing the desired path, depth, and reach underneath the surface, Video 23.

10.1.6 Tomato-Star

Cherry tomatoes offer a unique opportunity to practice delicate suturing exercises due to the unique composition of their cuticle. Their hydrophobic cuticle limits desiccation, prevents microbial infection, filters damaging UV light, and provides a significant biomechanical support to the pulp. All of that furnished by its single epidermal wall and cuticle complex (~2–9 μm) [78, 79].

Start by outlining a geometrical shape, in this case, a five-pointed star. Utilizing a scalpel blade (15c suggested), dissect the star from the tomato. Once completely removed, place it back and start the fixation process by suturing each point. For further practice, place additional sutures on the intersection points between points. The goal is to try to avoid tearing the cuticle of the tomato, Video 24.

10.1.7 Grass Blade

A blade of grass is a challenging exercise. Getting too close to the edge would not be conducive to maintaining the integrity of the blade since it lacks elasticity and it is not forgiving at all. Utilizing a point tapered needle with a 10-0 polyamide suture and starting away from the edges allowed for the placement of three reef knots. Still, the microtearing of the puncture sites can be observed. After finishing this exercise, the most delicate soft tissue will feel exceedingly thick in comparison, Video 25.

10.1.8 Flower

This exercise has one main goal: to join the base of the petals without tearing them with the needle. The trick is not to move the flower. That way, the operator is forced to engage each entry and exit needlepoint from different positions, most of them rather awkward. This, together with the unsupported flimsiness and delicate consistency of the petals, makes it more challenging, Video 26.

10.1.9 Mushroom

Lamellate manipulation is a delicate exercise that challenges the operator's tactile dexterity. These gills are in charge of producing spores and have a high water content making its paper-like consistency rather fragile under tensile forces [80].

This exercise utilizes an ophthalmic blade. It could also be performed with a fine 15c blade for an extra challenge. Start by removing a set of lamellates to create a clearance space that will allow for access of the remaining lamellates. Utilizing a microsurgical needle (4–6 mm) with a spatula/taper point ending and a 10-0 suture diameter, engage multiple lamellates (3–5) and suture them together at different levels from the external to the most internal (closest to the mushroom stem). Once this is accomplished, proceed to separate a single lamellate and then suture it to another lamellate. The fragility of this fine organic material will force you to hone your skills on delicate manipulation of equally delicate structures, Video 27.

10.1.10 Tissue Paper Box-Silicone/Resin Dental Model

Silicone and resin dental models are fantastic platforms to train. The versatility to mimic angulations and positions that simulate clinical situations is unique. Practicing in flat planes all the time is not conducive to develop spatial accommodations required in the three dimensional theater of the oral cavity, Video 28.

10.1.11 Plastic Micro-tubing

Training in microsurgical techniques has become important across all surgical disciplines. These techniques have become routine in otorhinolaryngology, ophthalmology, neurosurgery, trauma, hand, plastic, reconstructive, vascular, orthopedics, gynecology, and urology surgical procedures.

Classical training in microvascular surgery remains a common denominator for all other surgical fields. In vitro models such as plastic tubes allow for practicing correct knotting techniques, instrument handling, and development of inherent finger dexterity before moving onto more complex systems such as animal cadavers and in vivo models.

These exercises offer unique challenges that continue to develop and refine mechanical, tactile/sensorial, mental, and cognitive skills [81–83], Video 29.

10.1.12 Training Simulators

In efforts to reduce the use of live animals or the expense of working on cadaver-based models, different training simulators have become available over time to help enhance suturing skills. Rubber damn/latex assemblages provide a simple setting to facilitate bimanual instrumentation based suturing exercises under the OM. An advantage of these models is that it allows an evaluation of the working face and its opposite side which is instrumental when evaluating symmetry within the entry and exit point of the suture and in between contiguous sutures, Figs. 63, 64, and 65.

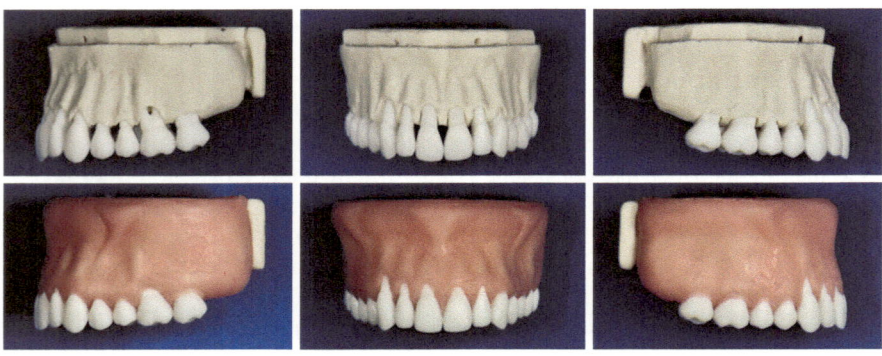

Fig. 62 Dental models simulating hard and soft tissues in resin and silicone. Courtesy of Fernando Rojas-Vizcaya, DDS, MS-BoneModels®

Fig. 63 Latex based simulator

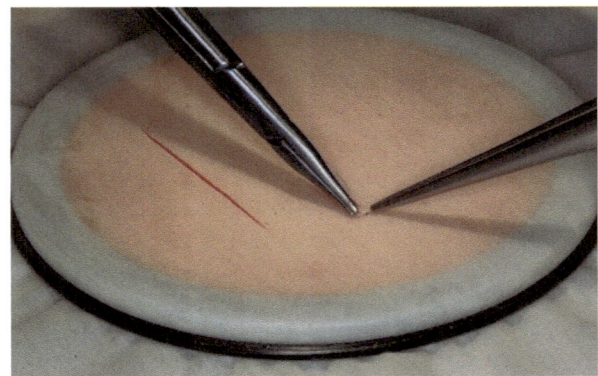

Fig. 64 By utilizing a hollowed rubber damn holder or by detaching the rubber damn material, the front and back surfaces can be evaluated to assess symmetrical suture allocation (front surface view)

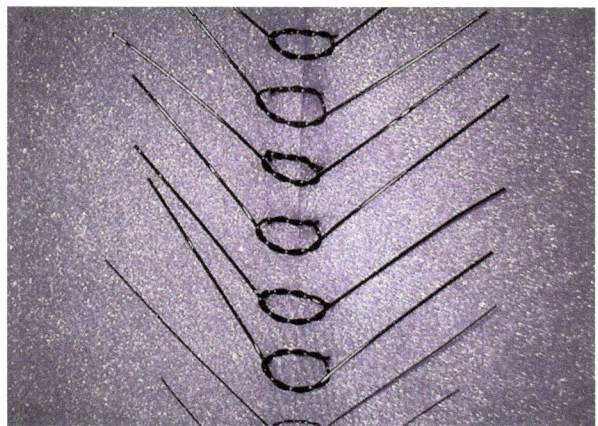

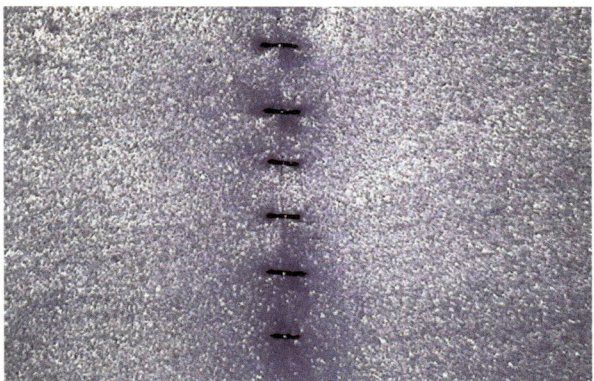

Fig. 65 Evaluation of symmetry of entry and exit points (back surface view of image shown in Fig. 64)

A suture training platform (STP) has been designed by one of the authors (DV-P) in collaboration with BoneModels® to provide a three-dimensional surface to work on flat, convex, and concave surfaces, as well as being equipped with teeth to practice anchoring, sling and other sutures that engage teeth or are performed in the proximity of teeth and its tissue replica structures, Fig. 66.

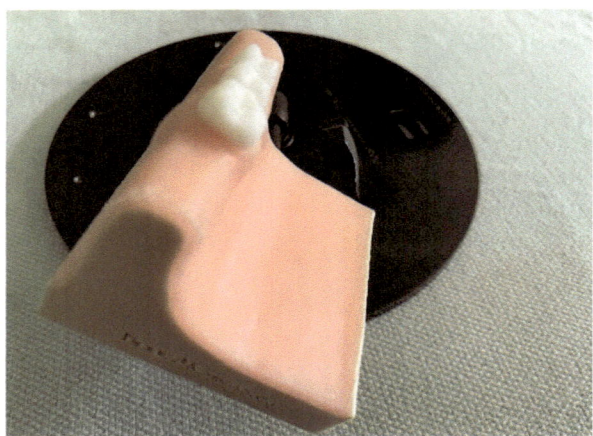

Fig. 66 Suture Training Platform (STP) provides a three-dimensional model with adjustable axial inclinations for practicing suturing techniques

A microsurgical training simulator, "The MicroTrainer" has been designed by Digital Surgicals, a MedTech start-up (www.microsurgical trainer.com). This simulator enables the practice of suturing with the addition of a cloud-based application that provides an objective assessment of performance and allows for longitudinal tracking to monitor progress over time, Figs. 67, 68, 69, 70 and 71.

Fig. 67 The MicroTrainer

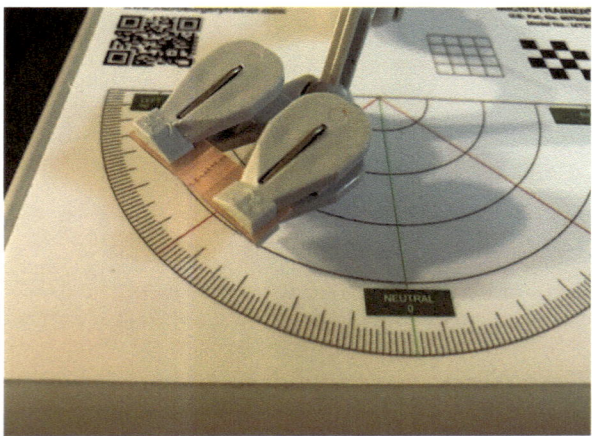

Fig. 68 Latex strips utilized to practice suturing. Back surface

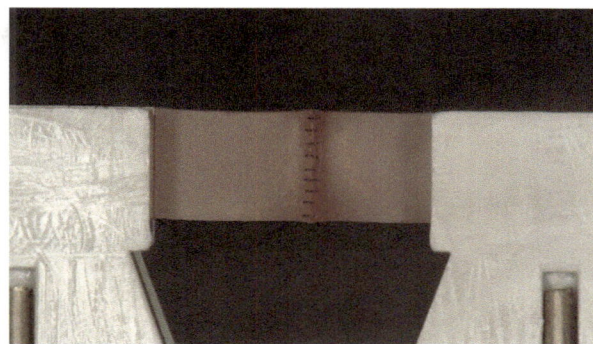

Fig. 69 Latex strips utilized to practice suturing. Front surface

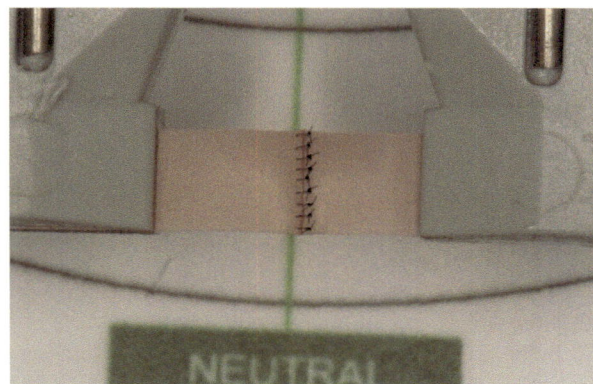

Fig. 70 Digital application assessing performance showing asymmetrical deviations on suturing entry and exit points

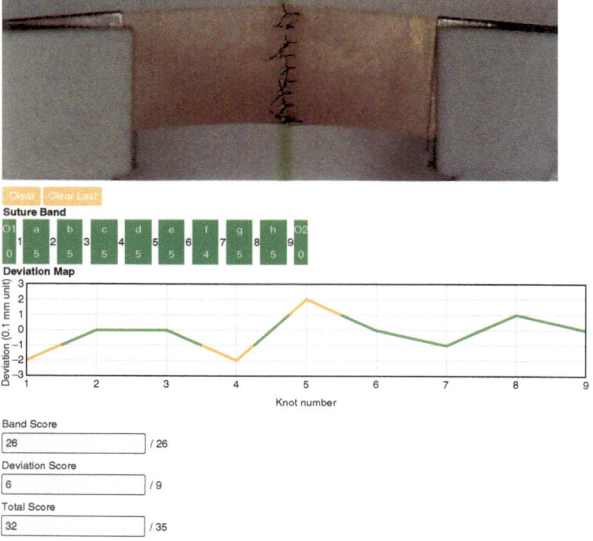

Fig. 71 Digital application assessing performance and tracking progress over time. A perfect score has been registered in this practice

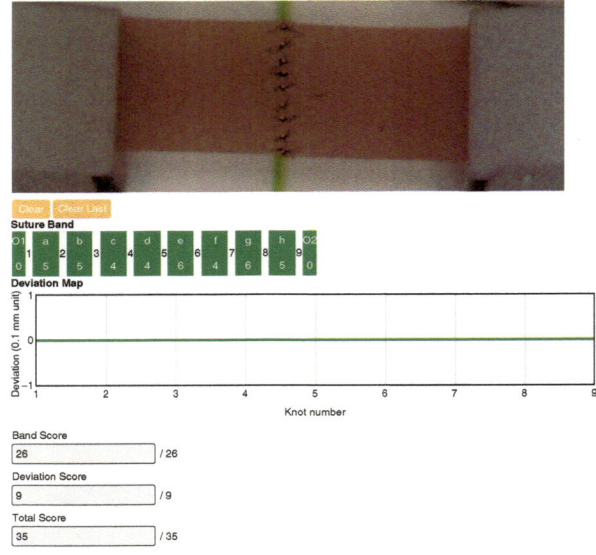

11   Conclusion

"There is the suture that gives a gratifying sense of closure to the activity" stated by Mihaly Csikszentmihalyi in Flow: The psychology of optimal experience [84]. Most surgical periodontal and implant related procedures are technically completed after the last suture is tied. Depending on the nature of the surgery, the microsurgeon will decide, based on formation and experience, what type of bio textile/needle combination to utilize to bring tissue approximation and provide closure and stability to the wound. Suturing is just as important as establishing an accurate diagnosis, tracing well defined incisions, designing biologically sound flaps, and executing the particular task that defines the final objective of the surgical intervention.

The operating microscope and the practice of microsurgery demand a new set of skills from the surgeon and the microsurgical support team. Bimanual instrumentation becomes essential when executing tasks under moderate and high magnification allowing visibility of the operational field without obstructions. Delicate tissue manipulation with precise and symmetrical needle penetration through wound edges must be followed by precise knot tying delivering the right amount of tension that will ultimately be conducive to sustainable primary closure, avoiding tissue "strangulation" under excessive forces that compromise blood flow and ultimately lead to soft tissue necrosis and its inherent negative repercussions. The combination of knowledge and skills is ultimately the defining factors of the science and art of microsuturing.

12 Key Points

1. Sutures remain the most utilized mechanism in microsurgical therapy to accomplish wound closure.
2. The symbiotic relationship between the medical and industrial communities is responsible for the continuous evolution of medically implantable biotextiles.
3. Microsurgical procedures in periodontal and dental implant related therapy requires a specifically designed armamentarium that facilitates performing tasks under the operating microscope.
4. Physiologic tremor can impact performance and can be reduced with experience, practice and physical and mental dispositions that generate comfortable physical positions with minimal muscle recruitment and activation.
5. Bimanual instrument tie is an essential skill when suturing under the operating microscope.
6. Suturing techniques need to be understood, practiced, and mastered to maximize efficiency during microsurgical periodontal and dental implant therapy execution.
7. Suturing is a skill. Like all skills, it requires continuous, purposeful, and deliberate practice.

References

1. Merriam-Webster's Medical Learners Dictionary, S.V. "Suture". Accessed August, 2021. www.merriam-webster.com/dictionary/suture#medicalDictionary.
2. Abi Rahced RSG, Toledo BEC, Okamoto T, Marcantonio E, Sampaio JEC, Orrico SRP, et al. Reaction of the human gingival tissue to different suture materials used in periodontal surgery. Braz Dent J. 1991;2:103–13.
3. Leknes KN, IT RØ, Selvig KA. Human gingival tissue reactions to silk and expanded polytetrafluoroethylene sutures. J Periodontol. 2005;76:34–42.
4. Van Winkle W, Hastings CJ, Barker E, Hines D, Nichols W. Effect of suture materials on healing skin wounds. Surg Gynecol Obstet. 1975;140:7–12.
5. Van Winkle W, Hastings JC. Considerations in the choice of suture material for various tissues. Surg Gynecol Obstet. 1972;135:113–26.
6. Hughes WL, Castroviejo R, Blaydes JE, McPherson SD, Riall CT, Himsel WL, et al. The evolution of ophthalmic sutures. Ann Plast Surg. 1981;6:48–65.
7. Benjamin L. The physics of wound closure. Including tissue tactics. In: Marion M, editor. Ophthalmic microsurgical suturing techniques. Berlin: Springer; 2007. p. 1–7.
8. Breitenbach KL, Bergera JJ. Principle and techniques of primary wound closure. Prim Care. 1986;13:411–31.
9. Panayi AC. Wound healing and scarring. In: Ogawa R, editor. Total scar management. Berlin: Springer; 2020. p. 3–16.
10. Burkhardt R, Lang NP. Fundamental principles in periodontal plastic surgery and mucosal augmentation – a narrative review. J Clin Periodontol. 2014;41:S98–107.
11. Hürzeler MB, Weng D. Functional and esthetic outcome enhancement of periodontal surgery by application of plastic surgery principles. Int J Periodontics Restorative Dent. 1999;19:36–43.
12. Simman R. Wound closure and the reconstructive ladder in plastic surgery. J Am Coll Certif Wound Spec. 2009;1:6–11.

13. Plonka AB, Urban IA, Wang H-L. Decision tree for vertical ridge augmentation. Int J Periodontics Restorative Dent. 2018;38:269–75.
14. Shanelec DA, Tibbetts LS, McGregor A, Cross JD, Pearson BS, Kissel SO, Broline L, Henshaw R. Periodontal Microsurgery. In: Newman MG, Takei HH, Klokkevold PR, Carranza FA, editors. Newman and Carranza's clinical periodontology. 13th ed. Philadelphia: Elsevier; 2019. p. 614–81.
15. Johnson AJ, Stulting RD. Knot tying principles and techniques. In: Macsai M, editor. Ophthalmic microsurgical suturing techniques. Berlin: Springer; 2007. p. 21–8.
16. Cuddy LC. Wound closure, tension-relieving techniques, and local flaps. Vet Clin North Am Small Anim Pract. 2017;47:1221–35.
17. Marsidi N, Vermeulen SAM, Horeman T, Genders RE. Measuring forces in suture techniques for wound closure. J Surg Res. 2020;255:135–43.
18. Brunette DM, Tengvall P, Textor M, Thomsen P. Titanium in medicine. Verlag: Springer; 2012.
19. Shanelec D. (Founder and course director of the microsurgery training institute, Santa Barbara, California). In discussion with author 2002–2017.
20. Smith JH, Macsai M. Needles, sutures, and instruments. In: Macsai M, editor. Ophthalmic microsurgical techniques. Berlin: Springer; 2007. p. 9–20.
21. Coulson CJ, Slack PS, Ma X. The effect of supporting a surgeon's wrist on their hand tremor. Microsurgery. 2010;30:565–8.
22. Hara Y, Goto T, Okamoto J, Okuda H, Iseki H, Hongo K. An armrest is effective for reducing hand tremble in neurosurgeons. Neurol Med Chir (Tokyo). 2015;55:311–6.
23. Mürbe D, Hüttenbrink KB, Zahnert T, Vogel U, Tassabehji M, Kuhlisch E, Hofmann G. Tremor in otosurgery: influence of physical strain on hand steadiness. Otol Neurotol. 2001;22:672–7.
24. Wei H, Benson R. Polymeric biomaterials. In: Kutz M, editor. Applied plastics engineering handbook. 2nd ed. Norwich, NY: William Andrew Publishing; 2017. p. 145–64.
25. Burkhardt R, Lang N. Influence of suturing on wound healing. Periodontol. 2000;2015(68):270–81.
26. Chu CC. Materials for absorbable and nonabsorbable surgical sutures. In: King MW, Gupta BS, Robert G, editors. Biotextiles as medical implants. 1st ed. Oxford: Woodhead Publishing; 2013. p. 277.
27. Gomel V, McComb P, Boer-Meisel M. Histologic reactions to polyglactin-910, polyethylene and nylon microsuture. J Reprod Med. 1980;25:56–9.
28. Kappelhof JP, Swart W, Willekens BL. A comparison between three brands of 10.0 nylon sutures. Doc Ophthalmol. 1989;72:209–13.
29. Chu CC. Materials for absorbable and nonabsorbable surgical sutures. In: King MW, Gupta BS, Robert G, editors. Biotextiles as medical implants. 1st ed. Oxford: Woodhead Publishing; 2013. p. 299.
30. Edlich RF, Gubler K, Wallis AG, Clark JJ, et al. Wound closure sutures and neeles: a new perspective. J Environ Pathol Toxicol Oncol. 2010;29:339–61.
31. Dang MC, Thacker JG, Hwang JC, Rodeheaver GT, et al. Some biomechanical considerations of polytetrafluorethylene sutures. Arch Surg. 1990;125:647–50.
32. Pons-Vicente O, Lopez-Jimenez L, Sanchez-Garces MA, Sala-Perez S, Gay-Escoda C. A comparative study between two different suture materials in oral implantology. Clin Oral Implant Res. 2011;22:282–8.
33. Chu CC. Materials for absorbable and nonabsorbable surgical sutures. In: King MW, Gupta BS, Robert G, editors. Biotextiles as medical implants. 1st ed. Oxford: Woodhead Publishing; 2013. p. 302.
34. Chu CC, von Fraunhofer JA, Greisler HP. Wound closure biomaterials and devices. 1st. ed. Boca Raton: CRC Press; 1996.
35. Burkhardt R, Preiss A, Joss A, Lang NP. Influence of suture tension to the tearing characteristics of the soft tissues. An in vitro experiment. Clin Oral Implants Res. 2008;19:314–9.
36. Sharp WV, Belden TA, King PH, Teague PC. Suture resistance to infection. Surgery. 1982;91:61–3.

37. Bendel LP, Trozzo LP. Tensile and bend relationships of several surgical needle materials. J Appl Biomater. 1993;3:161–7.
38. Trier WC. Considerations in the choice of surgical needles. Surg Gynecol Obstet. 1979;149:84–94.
39. Bellian KT, Thacker JG, Tribble CG, Powell DM, Becker DG, Zimmer CA, Morgan RF, Edlich RF. Biochemical performance of tapercut cardiovascular needles. Am Surg. 1991;57:591–601.
40. Pagnanelli DM, Pait TG, Rizzoli HV, Kobrine AI. Scanning electron micrographic study of vascular lesions caused by microvascular needles and suture. J Neurosurg. 1980;53:32–6.
41. Acland R. A new needle for microvascular surgery. Surgery. 1972;71(1):130–1.
42. Dujovny M, Nossovsky N, Diaz FG, Ausman JI, Berman KS. Effects of needle shape on the integrity of the vascular endothelium. Acta Neurochir. 1985;77:62–7.
43. McKernan JB, Bendel L, Freeman L, Cafferty D. Improved visibility of black surgical needles in laparoscopic surgery. Surg Endosc. 1993;7:424–6.
44. Calzetti S, Baratti M, Gresty M, Findley L. Frequency/amplitude characteristics of postural tremor of the hands in a population of patients with bilateral essential tremor: implications for the classification and mechanism of essential tremor. J Neurol Neurosurg Psychiatry. 1987;50:561–7.
45. Urban IA, Monje A. Guided bone regeneration in alveolar bone reconstruction. Oral Maxillofac Surg Clin North Am. 2019;31:331–8.
46. Elias WJ, Shah BB. Tremor. JAMA. 2014;311:948–54.
47. Elble RJ, Randall JE. Mechanistic components of normal hand tremor. Electroencephalogr Clin Neurophysiol. 1978;44:72–82.
48. Fargen KM, Turner RD, Spiotta AM. Factors that affect physiologic tremor and dexterity during surgery: a primer for neurosurgeons. World Neurosurg. 2016;86:384–9.
49. Sutton GG, Sykes K. The effect of withdrawal of visual presentations of errors upon the frequency spectrum of tremor in a manual task. J Physiol. 1967;190:281–93.
50. Argarwal GC, Gottlieb GL. Mathematical modeling and simulation of the postural and control loop. Part III. Crit Rev Biomed Eng. 1984;12:49–93.
51. Gottlieb GL, Agarwal GC. Physiologic clonus in man. Exp Neurol. 1977;54:616–21.
52. Fox JR, Randall JE. Relationship between forearm tremor and the biceps electromyograph. J Appl Physiol. 1970;29:103–8.
53. Carignan B, Daneault JF, Duval C. Quantifying the importance of high frequency components on the amplitude of physiologic tremor. Exp Brain Res. 2009;202:299–306.
54. Harwell RC, Ferguson RL. Physiologic tremor and microsurgery. Microsurgery. 1983;4:187–92.
55. Stiles RN. Frequency and displacement amplitude relations for normal hand tremor. J Appl Physiol. 1976;40:44–54.
56. Stiles RN, Randall JE. Mechanical factors in human tremor frequency. J Appl Physiol. 1967;23:324–30.
57. Safwat B, Su EL, Gassert R, Teo CL, Burdet E. The role of posture, magnification, and grip force on microscopic accuracy. Ann Biomed Eng. 2009;37:997–1006.
58. Elman MJ, Sugar J, Fiscella R, et al. The effect of propranolol versus placebo on resident surgical performance. Trans Am Opthalmol Soc. 1998;96:283–94.
59. Verrelli DI, Qian Y, Wilson MK, Wood J, Savage C. Intraoperative tremor in surgeons and trainees. Interact Cardiovasc Thorac Surg. 2016;23:410–5.
60. Thacker JG, Rodeheaver G, Moore JW, Kauzlarich JJ, Kurtz L, Edgerton MT, Edlich RF. Mechanical performance of surgical sutures. Am J Surg. 1975;130:374–80.
61. Tera H, Aberg C. Tensile strengths of twelve types of knot employed in surgery, using different suture materials. Acta Chir Scand. 1976;142:1–7.
62. Meyle J. Suture materials and suture techniques. Periodontology. 2006;3:253–68.
63. Nordström RE, Nordström RM. Absorbable versus nonabsorbable sutures to prevent postoperative stretching of wound area. Plast Reconstr Surg. 1986;78:186–90.
64. Pensalfini M, Meneghello S, Lintas V, Bircher K, Ehret AE, Mazza E. The suture retention test, revisited and revised. J Mech Behav Biomed Mater. 2018;77:711–7.

65. Abidin MR, Dunlapp JA, Towler MA, Becker DG, Thacker JG, McGregor W, Edlich RF. Metallurgically bonded needle holder jaws. A technique to enhance needle holding security without sutural damage. Am Surg. 1990;56:643–7.
66. Rubinstein C, Russell WJ. Wound closure and suturing patterns: a vector analysis of suture tension. Aust N Z J Surg. 1992;62:733–7.
67. DesCôteaux JG, Temple WJ, Huchcroft SA, Frank CB, Shrive NG. Linea alba closure: determination of ideal distance between sutures. J Investig Surg. 1993;6:201–9.
68. Varjú I, Sótonyi P, Machovich R, Szabó L, Tenekedjiev K, Silva MM, Longstaff C, Kolev K. Hindered dissolution of fibrin formed under mechanical stress. J Thromb Haemost. 2011;9:979–86.
69. Burgess LP, Morin GV, Rand M, Vossoughi J, Hollinger JO. Wound healing. Relationship of wound closing tension to scar width in rats. Arch Otolaryngol Head Neck Surg. 1990;116:798–802.
70. Pickett BP, Burgess LP, Livermore GH, Tzikas TL, Vossoughi J. Wound healing. Tensile strength vs healing time for wounds closed under tension. Arch Otolaryngol Head Neck Surg. 1996;122:565–8.
71. Pini Prato G, Pagliaro U, Baldi C, Nieri M, Saletta D, Cairo F, Cortellini P. Coronally advanced flap procedure for root coverage. Flap with tension versus flap without tension: a randomized controlled clinical study. J Periodontol. 2000;71:188–201.
72. Williams DF, Harrison ID. The variation of mechanical properties in different areas of a healing wound. J Biomech. 1977;10:633–42.
73. Hensel J, Graumont R. Encyclopedia of knots and fancy rope work. 4th ed. Cambridge: Cornell Maritime Press; 2009.
74. von Fraunhofer JA, Chu CC. Mechanical properties. In: Chu CC, von Fraunhofer JA, Greisler HP, editors. Wound closure biomaterials and devices. Boca Raton: CRC Press; 1997. p. 123.
75. Rojas-Vizcaya F. BoneModels®. 2021. http://www.bonemodels.es. Accessed 28 Mar 2021.
76. Demirseren ME, Tosa Y, Hosaka Y. Microsurgical training with surgical gauze: the first step. J Reconstr Microsurg. 2003;19:385–6.
77. Tung MA, Richards JF. Ultrastructure of the Hen's egg shell membranes by electron microscopy. J Food Sci. 1972;37:277–81.
78. Martin LB, Rose JK. There's more than one way to skin a fruit: formation and functions of fruit cuticles. J Exp Bot. 2014;65:4639–51.
79. Segado P, et al. Ultrastructure of the epidermal cell wall and cuticle of tomato fruit (solanum Lycopersicum L) during development. Plant Physiol. 2016;170:935–46.
80. Fischer MWF, Money NP. Why mushrooms form gills: efficiency of the lamellate morphology. Fungal Biol. 2010;114:57–63.
81. Ti-Sheng C, et al. Principles techniques and applications in microsurgery. Singapore: World Scientific Publishing Co.; 1986.
82. Mehdorn HM, Muller GH. Microsurgical exercises: basic techniques, anastomoses, refertilization, transplantation. New York: Theme Medical Publishers; 1989.
83. Acland R. Preconditions of microsurgical skill https://urldefense.proofpoint.com/v2/url?u=https-3A__m.youtube.com_watch-3Fv3DOXPzLAEdKhQ&d=DwICAg&c=vh6Fg FnduejNhPPD0fl_yRaSfZy8CWbWnIf4XJhSqx8&r=_aVlhOL0DwHkFpf5efnDWybFajk-TUmcdN4dz4kJ7s38o3SlqcNubAc1N_wByYPg4&m=HBmE0Tm5AOHHJzgAejo5bLRlu eKENkNfBtNFofhVq4E&s=iNrIIruTt4roW1zll2S11CZzdWoHLq-3n8qMhMP9I8M&e=. Accessed March 6, 2021.
84. Csikszentmihalyi M. Flow: The psychology of optimal experience. New York: Harper & Row New York; 1990.
85. Chu CC. Types and properties of surgical sutures. In: King MW, Gupta BS, editors. Biotextiles as medical implants. 1st ed. Oxford: Woodhead Publishing; 2013. P 234, 235, 243 and 244.

Practical Considerations in Incorporating Microsurgery to Daily Workflow

Diego Velasquez-Plata

Contents

Supplementary Information The online version contains supplementary material available at [https://doi.org/10.1007/978-3-030-96874-8_6].

D. Velasquez-Plata (✉)
Private Practice, Fenton, Michigan, USA

Adjunct Clinical Assistant Professor Periodontics and Oral Medicine Department,
The University of Michigan School of Dentistry, Ann Arbor, MI, USA
e-mail: dvelasq@umich.edu

Abstract

Adopting new technology is usually associated with change. Regardless of the connotation of this change, patterns of individual and collective work routines will most likely be altered in one way or another. The incorporation of the operating microscope into the daily periodontal and dental implant practice is a prime example of such disruption. Defining the new operational paradigm will require a total commitment from all the team members in the practice.

Early adopters (dental students and new practitioners) may have a smoother transition when compared to a well-established practitioner when considering time availability at the disposal of the microsurgeon in training. Conversely, the established practitioner will have experience that can be a catalyst for creativity and resourcefulness that will help bypass some of the challenges of the early stages of assimilation of this technology.

Regardless of the traveled path, it is important to recognize that periodontal and dental implant procedures have unique positional and interactive demands that require adaptation and customized approaches to the different procedural requirements. Adopting a healthy posture, becoming proficient with utilizing aids like indirect vision and empowering the microsurgical assisting team to be active participants in patient positioning and therapy delivery will be fundamental in the successful and fruitful transition to a microsurgical periodontal and dental implant practice.

Keywords

Ergonomics · Musculoskeletal Pain · Microscopy · Microsurgery

1 Introduction

Ergonomics has been defined as the scientific study of people and their working conditions, especially done in order to improve effectiveness [1]. Dentists, dental hygienists, and dental assistants are all exposed to risks of developing musculoskeletal disorders (MSDs). Practicing dentistry requires optimal focus and accurate execution of movements. Visualization of procedures is essential and, in an effort, to access remote targets in a dark and constrained space such as the oral cavity, unnatural positions are often forced and adopted. The physicality of this occupation requires repetitive movements, forceful exertions, exposure to vibrating objects, and uncomfortable and prolonged static postures [2]. Although recommendations have been made to lessen the occupational burden by the addition of ergonomically designed equipment, breaks between high risk tasks, instrumentation that reduces excessive force application and stretching exercises, there are still challenges that seem to perpetuate the occupational hazards in these occupations.

2   Principles of Ergonomics

2.1   Musculoskeletal Disorders Associated with Dentistry

The term work-related musculoskeletal disorders refers to MSDs to which the work environment are primary contributors, worsening and/or prolonging the symptoms associated with this condition [3]. MSDs have been acknowledged as being the primary reason for early retirement among dentists (29.5%) [4]. MSDs present in diverse forms: back problems (lower and upper back pain), hand and wrist issues (tendinitis, tenosynovitis, trigger finger, carpal tunnel syndrome, Guyon's syndrome, De Quervain's disease). Decrease in motion, loss of normal sensation, decrease grip strength, loss of normal motion range and coordination are signs of MSDs. Shoulder and neck fatigue, tingling and burning sensations in arms, wrists, hands, cramping and numbness in hands and fingers are symptoms of MSDs.

Repetitive motion and awkward postures translate into muscle fatigue and imbalance leading to tensional and compressive forces associated with micro-trauma. Muscle ischemia/necrosis develops once microtrauma incidents augment, pain arises which triggers compensatory protective muscle contraction creating joint hypomobility, nerve compression, spinal disc degeneration, herniation, and adding to a cumulative trauma disorder [5].

Data related to upper limb MSDs support a high occurrence in the dental population. Neck being the most affected segment showing a prevalence of up to 73% [6]. The presence of pain for the lower back has been reported to be as high as 67%, 40–67% for shoulder pain, and 15–20% for wrist and hands [7]. MSDs appear early in dental careers with more than 70% of dental students reporting pain by their third year [8].

Optimal posture is the result of a balanced interaction between the osseous and soft tissues supporting the spine. From a side view, the natural curves of the spine (two concave curves cervical and lumbar lordosis, and two convex, thoracic and sacral kyphosis) are all interdependent and with the exception of the limited mobility of the sacral lordosis, all of the remaining curves are highly flexible. When these curves are in a neutral position, the bony components (vertebrae) support the load with minimal muscle and ligament involvement. When off axis positions are adopted, muscle and ligament interplay increase which can lead to episodes of microtrauma as described previously. In dentistry, forward neck thrusting positions are common to gain better visual access. Under prolonged and repetitive episodes, muscles of the cervical and upper thoracic spaces must be constantly contracted to support the weight of the head in its forward posture. This can lead to muscle imbalances, predisposing to nerve impingement of the supraspinous tendon in the shoulder. Unsupported arm abduction constrains blood supply triggering trapezius myalgia. Maintaining and protecting a proper position for the cervical lordosis is essential to reduce low back pain. Tilting the seat angle by 5–15° can increase the low back curve and prevent reducing blood circulation created by underside pressure on the thighs. This downward pitch of the seat will place the hips slightly higher than the knees. Both feet must be firmly touching the floor, while sitting tall and adjusting the lumbar support of the operator's stool will help stabilize the cervical lordosis [9].

Proper selection of magnification systems is essential [10]. Maintaining working postures with greater than 20° of neck flexion have been associated with increased neck pain [11]. The use of loupes, which requires the eyes looking down while tilting the head down and forward, has been associated with ambiguous reports regarding resolution of neck pain and upper extremity MSDs [12, 13].

The operating microscope (OM) allows for optimal magnification and illumination while promoting the most neutral posture by design [14] (while using the OM the operator adopts a healthy ergonomic position by maintaining the spine erect and eyes looking straight ahead, avoiding forward/downward tilts of the head) (Fig. 1). There are accessories that facilitate adopting a healthy posture such as mechanisms to adjust the focal length over a large distance in the vertical axis without leaving the preferred working position or moving the OM or the patient's chair. Tiltable interfaces allow the operator to always maintain a comfortable upright viewing position by changing the angulation of the optical lens without moving the ocular pieces and tube extensions have been designed to meet changes in the working horizontal and vertical distance. Indirect vision is another skill of utmost importance that needs to be developed, nourished, and constantly implemented to facilitate maintaining an adequate ergonomic posture. Indirect vision could be defined as visualization afforded by use of a reflective surface. Mirrors are a common example of reflective surfaces that bounce back light rays that spawn a reverse image of the original object. Intraoral mirrors are a key component of the armamentarium for the microsurgeon. Learning to utilize indirect vision is an essential skill that facilitates work execution in a fashion consistent with healthy ergonomic principles.

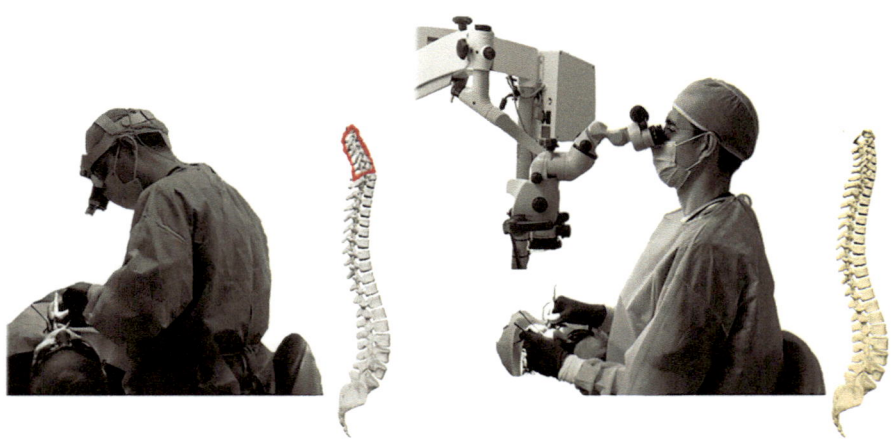

Fig. 1 Magnification systems play an important role on musculoskeletal health

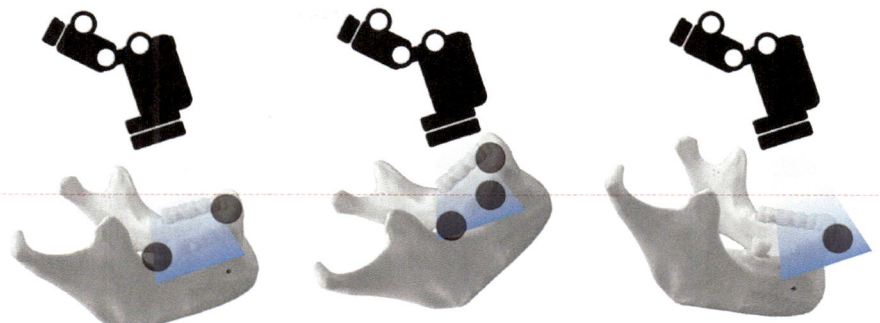

Fig. 2 Blind spots encounter when utilizing the operating microscope

When working with the operating microscope, the visual axis encounters several blind spots that can be to some extent eliminated or greatly reduced by modifying the patient and the operator's position (Fig. 2). Dental mirrors, in particular, micro-mirrors (3–5 mm in diameter) become extremely useful to achieve visual access in otherwise difficult areas to approach. Delivering precise movements under indirect vision is essential to perform incisions, clean surfaces, polish strata, flap elevation, etc.

Although the OM alone is not a complete solution for ergonomic related ailments, it is a key component, together with adequate lumbar and arm support, strong dental assisting, and adoption of a healthy and conscientious operational posture [15, 16]. The operating stool must be wide and support 2/3 of the thighs. Its back should provide adequate lumbar support and allow for vertical adjustments allocating the knees lower than the hips. Armrests must be adjustable to provide support when the arms are abducted and maintain the forearms parallel to the floor.

2.2 Working Mistakes When Using the Microscope

The utilization of an OM and ergonomically designed operator's chair does not prevent the adoption of less than ideal postural dynamics. Neck flexions, head and back inclinations, neck extensions, arm abduction, trunk rotations, and neck twists can occur and ought to be avoided. Training all the members of the microsurgical team is essential to maximize the ergonomic advantages that the OM and its support system have to offer. Unhealthy posturing needs to be constantly avoided by the microsurgeon and the microsurgical assistants, four or six handed dentistry operational protocols ought to be exercised and refined to maximize efficiency and avoid unnecessary twisting and bending movements. The operatory design for using the OM should facilitate easy access, having instruments and equipment within arms reach of the members of the operating team requiring no more than movements originating from the shoulder.

3 Implementation Stages of OM in Periodontal and Implant Procedures

Implementing the positional and ergonomic skills necessary to effectively use an OM is essential for the success of the microsurgical team. Occasional and intermittent use of the OM is only to be accepted during the learning process. Utilizing the OM from incision making to placing the last suture is the goal of the periodontal and implant microsurgical team. Sporadic, intermittent utilization of the OM disrupts the flow of treatment delivery and affects efficiency in a negative fashion. Practitioners who do not adopt a constant and uninterrupted work routine while utilizing the microscope will struggle to refine operational, visual, and ergonomic skills associated with high performance.

A word on magnification. Most periodontal and implant surgical procedures will be performed under 4×–7× magnification ranges. At times, higher magnification is warranted, for instance, when inspecting a root surface to rule out the presence of accretions, root fractures, or other irregularities that need to be dealt with when performing regenerative therapy. De-epithelializing a papilla, releasing the Schneiderian membrane, splitting epithelium from connective tissue in preparation for graft harvesting, or piecing tissue with a needle are some other examples of procedures that will benefit from performing at higher magnification (10×–15×). Performance at higher magnification is usually limited to areas where minimal or no movement is required. Narrower field of views and shallower depths of field come with the territory of higher magnification. Working under higher magnification is more demanding and with practice it will be less intrusive in the overall dynamics of surgical therapy delivery.

The following staging to implement the utilization of the OM has been suggested when introducing the incorporation of the OM to the periodontal and dental implant surgical practice (Table 1).

Table 1 Implementation stages of the operating microscope

Implementation Stages Easiest (1) Most Advanced (7)	
Stage	Activity
1	Full mouth probing
1	Prophylaxis with a rubber cup
2	Scaling and root planing (single-multiple)
2	Suture removal (anterior posterior)
3	Single anterior OSS, REG, MG
4	Single posterior OSS, REG, MG,
4	Soft tissue harvesting
5	Anterior/Posterior multiple teeth OSS, REG, MG
5	Sinus elevation
5	Anterior implant placement
6	Lingual anterior Mandible OSS, REG, MG
7	Posterior Implant Placement

OSS **resective surgery,** *REG* **regenerative surgery,** *MG* **mucogingival surgery**

First Stage: It provides an opportunity to interact with operator's and patient positioning, utilization of instruments that challenge eye-hand coordination under different magnifications and engage a dental assistant in a 4-hand assisting model.

- Full mouth probing
- Prophylaxis with a rubber cup

Second Stage: Incorporation of instruments with active/sharp surfaces that require good hand-eye coordination when handling them under the OM. Adequate patient and operator positioning is demanded in order to access different areas of the mouth (anterior and posterior areas); indirect vision is also required.

- Scaling and root planing (single teeth, multiple teeth)
- Suture removal on anterior and posterior areas of the mouth.

Third Stage: The surgical team starts interacting with a six-hand platform by treating areas that are easily accessible and require minimal indirect vision, thus freeing both hands of the microsurgeon to engage in surgical care. Work limited to a single tooth, or two contiguous teeth maximum will allow a higher range of magnification settings while executing care.

- Single anterior resective, regenerative or mucogingival therapy.

Fourth Stage: Working on posterior areas most often requires different operator, assistant, and patient positioning as well as relying on indirect vision more frequently. Starting with a single tooth or two contiguous teeth maximum requires less positional changes.

- Single posterior resective, regenerative, mucogingival therapy
- Soft tissue harvesting

Fifth Stage: Working on multiple teeth, sextans and quadrants will demand more flexibility on magnification settings which are intimately related to depth of field (the ability of the lens system to focus on objects that are near or far without having to change the OM position). Operator, patient, and dental assistant positioning may fluctuate according to the areas being treated. A more advanced eye–hand coordination is required to start performing more delicate procedures such as a manipulating the Schneiderian membrane of the maxillary antral cavity and coordination of the microscope visual axis and the alveolar plane horizontal and vertical plane when preparing an osteotomy for implant placement.

- Anterior/posterior multiple teeth undergoing resective, regenerative, and mucogingival therapy.
- Maxillary sinus elevation with both a lateral and a supracrestal approach.
- Anterior implant placement.

Sixth Stage: This stage demands proficiency with indirect vision and positioning of the patient and all team members to help deliver optimal care in areas that are more challenging to reach and require efforts to compensate discrepancies between the visual axis of the OM and the target area.

- Lingual aspects of mandibular anterior sextant undergoing resective, regenerative, and mucogingival therapy.

Seven Stage: The ultimate stage. Placing implants without a completely guided system may offer unique challenges when working on posterior areas due to the inherent discrepancies between the visual axis of the OM and the area where the implant or implants will be going. Utilizing indirect vision (mirror surfaces) or direct vision without looking through the microscope is sometimes advised to verify that distances and angulations are optimal and consistent with safe and accurate implant placement execution.

- Posterior implant placement, single or multiple units.

The above described staging approach is a recommendation that can be modified according to the skills and experience and pace of incorporation of the OM into the daily periodontal and dental implant practice of each individual microsurgeon.

4 Fundamental Aspects of Microsurgical Incorporation (Fig. 3)

4.1 Frame of Mind

Psychomotor balance and comfort are essential when performing under a surgical microscope. A clear mind, a focused mind is instrumental and has to be pursued to achieve a state that will allow for maximum concentration and performance. Basics such as good sleeping habits, avoidance of unusual amounts of stimulant beverages such as coffee, tea, or power drinks containing caffeine (i.e. if having a cup of

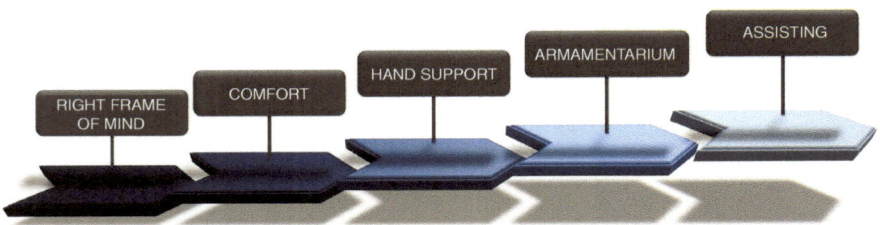

Fig. 3 Aspects to facilitate execution of microsurgical procedures

coffee every morning should not be a problem. What may turn into an issue is when the routine dosage is increased the day of using the surgical microscope). Solving pending or urgent matters is strongly advised prior to seating behind the microscope. In that way, maximum focus and attention can be procured during operating procedures.

4.2   Comfort

Seating comfortably in the operator's chair is the second most important aspect. Minimizing or avoiding fatigue during operational times is of utmost importance. Having a chair with adequate support for the hips, lower back, and arms is essential. This chair should be in solid contact with the ground, meaning, it cannot move around with ease, the seat should be positioned at such height that the thighs and knees are at a lower position when compared to that of the hips (Fig. 4).

4.3   Hand Support

Another feature is that of active support on the lower back and simultaneous two-dimensional support for the arms. These arm supports should offer mobility that allows the operator to move hands and arms accompanied by a supporting structure

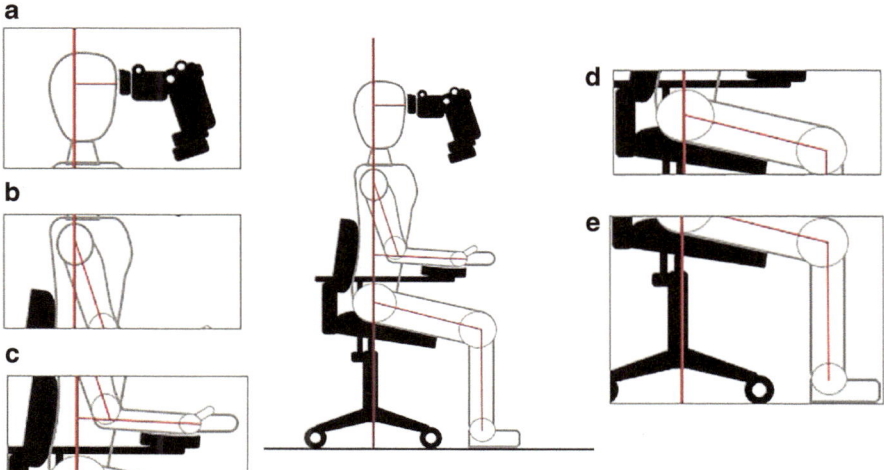

Fig. 4 Ergonomically sound posture while operating with the OM. (**a**) Head above shoulder, with a vertical tilt ranging from 0° to 20°. (**b**) Arms inclined between 0° and 25°. (**c**) Forearm parallel to the floor. (**d**) Hips at 90° to 100° with upper leg tilted downward. (**e**) Lower leg at 90° to the floor surface. Foot sole parallel to the floor in full contact

at all times. Arm support is essential to minimize muscle fatigue at the level of the shoulders, arms and wrists that can translate into deleterious tremors of different magnitudes [17].

4.4   Armamentarium

Microsurgical instruments must be available in the operating room and ready to be used as demanded. Setting up trays with specific instruments allotted by procedure to be performed or having general surgical trays that can be supplemented with specific instruments depending on the procedures being performed can be arranged as the members of the surgical assisting team see fit. Anticipating possible variants in procedural execution will save time and allow all effort to be concentrated in expeditious care delivery rather than requesting, looking for, and fetching tools and biomaterials not readily available when needed.

Having back up instruments and biomaterials in the room in case there is an unexpected need for replacement due to mechanical failure, human error (dropping an instrument/biomaterial to the ground), will be conducive to maximizing time efficiency.

4.5   Assisting

The assistant team must become proficient in reading the clinical situation at hand, anticipating movements and needs of the microsurgeon to help minimize the time in which eyes and hands are diverted away from the surgical field.

It is the experience of the author that in order to maximize efficiency of procedural execution, a six handed operational system is advantageous when compared to a four handed model. The first assistant will be occupied with immediate needs such as retraction and suction and irrigation to help get visual access to the surgical field. The second assistant can provide support to the first assistant's needs and requirements and at the same time can be preparing biomaterials, armamentarium, troubleshooting unexpected issues that arise concerning patient well-being, mechanical performance of instruments and equipment. During prolonged procedures, both assistants could switch roles to provide rest in sometimes physically and mentally demanding execution of surgical periodontal and implant care (Video 1).

A third assistant or a "roving dental assistant" has proven to be an asset to enhance workflow by assisting the two microsurgical assistants by supporting their needs and help maintain a consistent and active support to the six handed dentistry model (Video 2).

Microsurgical assistants have two ways to follow surgical procedures:

Direct Vision
Utilizing a diploscope (a microscope with two binocular viewing fields). This device allows the assistant to observe the surgical field simultaneously with the

surgeon. There are some disadvantages to this approach that can interfere with a smooth interaction and freedom of movement:

- Moving the microscope will affect the position of not only the operator but also the assistant, having to adjust not only one optical tube but two.
- It may detract from the whole field visibility to the assistant and make more difficult the interaction with the surgical field and its surroundings.

Indirect Vision
Setting up the surgical room with high-definition monitors that broadcast live the surgical field.

This approach offers flexibility as it represents the visual experience of the operator and helps identify the working surfaces, helps establish rapid communication that can quickly address needed adjustments on focus, OM position, etc., without having to coordinate the movement of multiple components and personnel, Fig. 5. As this setup is not fixated to the body of the OM, freedom of movement is higher since it does not affect any other attachments or componentry.

Part of growing and implementing an efficient microsurgical team is to distribute tasks among the microsurgical assistants. Movement economy will be maximized by a seamless integration and execution of maneuvers that lead to accurate and efficient performance. Knowing what instrument to pass and when to deliver it, anticipating the direction of the active surface that is going to be used, knowing when and when not to suction, what suction tip to use, when to irrigate, when to retract, when to blow air to clear a mirror surface when using indirect vision. These are all tasks that need to be performed harmoniously in order to reduce working

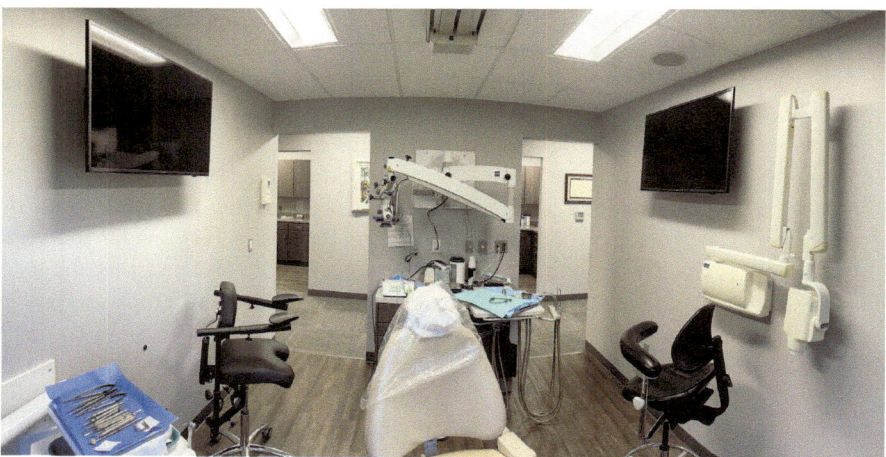

Fig. 5 Room setup to support indirect vision assistance support. High-definition monitors on opposite sides facilitate visual access by surgical assistants

times and maximize operational efficiency. Once a system such as that one is in place, working times will be reduced and improved when compared to those instances when the OM was not being utilized.

5 Economy of Movement

5.1 Assisting Models

During the initial stages of implementation of the operating microscope (OM) into periodontal and implant surgical procedures, it is very common to experience slower times in the performance of common tasks. There are factors that explain this occurrence.

First of all, visual acuity has been enhanced and with it, awareness of details increases, leading to identification of structures such as accretions, granulation tissue, bone formations, etc. that sometimes with lower magnification would be imperceptible and therefore its presence ignored altogether, requiring no further action from the operator. Instead, when working at higher magnification, the operator becomes aware of the presence of these variations and executes movements to eliminate and correct them which translates into longer operational times. This issue is corrected with practice, and it will not become a factor any longer in performance speed.

Another factor is associated with the structure and patterns of movements while operating in multiple planes and surfaces. For instance, when performing resective surgery on sextants or quadrants the field of vision and patient position needs to be adjusted in order to be able to facilitate visual access with the OM. This also applies to procedures that require accessing outer and inner surfaces of the target areas. Implementing a system that minimizes the movement of the patient's head and body position in the chair will translate into more accurate operational moves, thus maximizing the efficiency of the performance.

One last factor and perhaps the most important is the performance of the operator and the members of the microsurgical assisting team (MAT).

It is very important to maximize movement efficiency which is related to enhancing the economy of motions. When working under the microscope, the operator needs to maximize all efforts to avoid withdrawing the hands from the surgical field, performing movements within motion class I–IV under the ergonomic motion classification and avoid movements that involve twisting the torso usually involved with reaching out for instruments or materials (a motion class V) (Table 2).

Tasks like focus adjustment, minor movements of the microscope body, changing magnification levels, and so on can unnecessarily take away the hands of the operator from the surgical field and consequentially slowing down the execution of the task being performed.

Table 2 Ergonomic classification of operational movements

Motion Class	Movement
I	Moving only fingers
II	Moving only fingers and wrists
III	Movement originated from the elbow
IV	Movement originated from the shoulder
V	Movement that involves twisting or bending at the waist.

6   Positioning

Positioning refers to the interaction existing between the operating microscope, the operator, the microsurgical assisting team, and the patient. Each one of these components will be addressed separately:

6.1   Operator (Microsurgeon)

It is assumed that calibration of the OM has already been accomplished and checked. Interpupillary distance, parfocal adjustment, fine focus adjustment have already taken place. The operator will usually seat at the 11–12-o'clock position or at the 9 o'clock position depending on the working area to be approached. The seating position should be adjusted with the 90° concept in mind: hips 90° to the floor, knees are 90° to the hips, and forearms are 90° to the upper arms [18]. Arms should be resting on arm supports of the chair and feet should be completely flat against the floor. The spine should be in a neutral position, erect, and perpendicular to the floor and the eyepiece inclined so the eyes are looking at the horizon and the ears are aligned with the shoulders. The patient is moved to accommodate this position. Once the patient's head is adjusted, the hands of the operator should be at the level of the patient's mouth to facilitate the execution of fine movements. All of this is performed under low magnification. Once the target area is identified, magnification can be increased as needed. Most movements will be generated by adjusting the patient's head and moving a mirror when indirect vision is utilized. In contrast to endodontic based procedures, periodontal and implant related surgical applications require multiaxial access which demands positional changes by the operator and the assisting team. Minimization of these positional changes is to be procured by implementing surgical protocols congruent with this principle.

6.2   Assisting Team

The position of the assisting team varies depending on the target operational areas. Functions will be operated in a sitting or standing position depending on visual access and task being performed. Ideally, surgical procedures should be performed with the support of two surgical operational assistants. These two assistants should have the backing of a rover operational assistant that will be in charge of attending to their needs and requirements, for instance, reaching instruments/materials/equipment no readily available in the surgical room, preparing materials such as bone, biologics, etc., all geared towards allowing the surgical assistants to be attentive to the microsurgeons needs at all times.

The surgical assistants should have an ergonomically suited chair that will offer a solid contact with the ground surface, ease of rotational mobility to reach different surfaces and areas of the operating room, and readily allow for exiting the chair confines to adopt a standing position as needed.

When working with peripheral high-definition monitors, visual access should be readily available at all times to help monitor moves and actions occurring in the operating field.

6.3   Patient Position

Patient position will be determined by the target area (TA) which is the area being worked on. TA will also determine the position of the microsurgeon and the assisting team.

From the author's experience, this section will be divided into different subsections, each corresponding to the different TA being described.

*When describing operator (**circle**) and assistant team members (**triangle**) positions in the room, the landscape of an analog clock will be referred to, with the head support of the patient chair coinciding with the 12:00 o'clock position and consequently, the feet support of the patient chair will be aiming at the 6:00 o'clock location.*

1. Maxillary arch (Fig. 6).
    (a) Patient chair will be positioned at about 5–10° with respect to the ground line.
    (b) Operator will be at 9–12 o'clock.
    (c) Assistant 1: will be at 1–2 o'clock.
    (d) Assistant 2: will be at 10–11 o'clock.

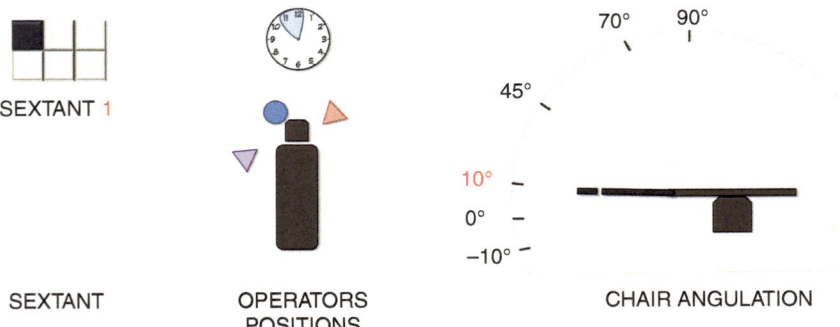

Fig. 6 Positioning maxillary arch, posterior sextants

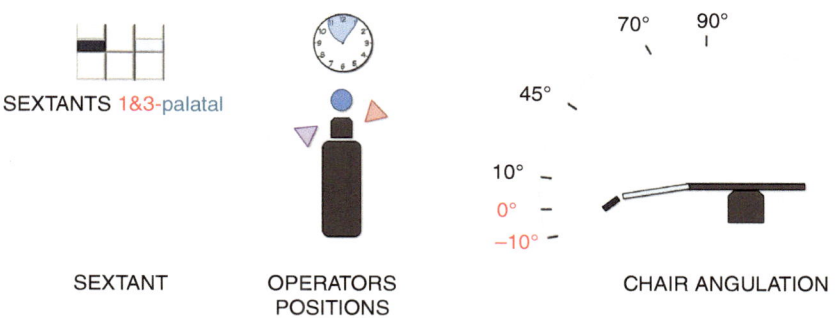

SEXTANTS 1&3-palatal

SEXTANT   OPERATORS
                 POSITIONS

CHAIR ANGULATION

Fig. 7 Maxillary arch, palatal aspects

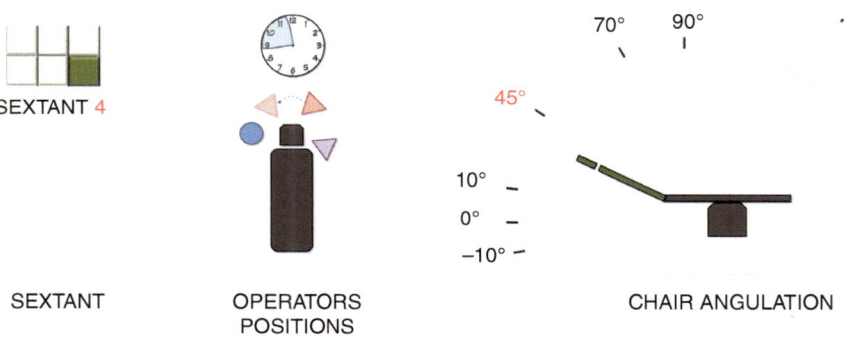

SEXTANT 4

SEXTANT   OPERATORS
                 POSITIONS

CHAIR ANGULATION

Fig. 8 Mandibular arch, posterior sextants

2. Maxillary arch, soft, and hard palate (when harvesting tissue with direct vision) (Fig. 7).
   (a) Patient chair will be positioned at about −5 to −10° with respect to the ground line.
   (b) Operator will be at 12 o'clock.
   (c) Assistant 1: will be at 1–2 o'clock.
   (d) Assistant 2: will be at 10–11 o'clock.
3. Mandibular arch posterior right and left sextants (Fig. 8).
   (a) Patient chair will be positioned at about 40–45° with respect to the ground line.
   (b) Operator will be oscillating from 9 o'clock to 12 o'clock.
   (c) Assistant 1: will be at 1–2 o'clock.
   (d) Assistant 2: will be rotating from 10 to 11 o'clock (when operator is positioned at 12 o'clock) or at 12–3 o'clock (when operator is positioned at 9 o'clock).
4. Mandibular arch, anterior sextant, buccal aspects (Fig. 9).
   (a) Patient chair will be positioned at about 40–45° with respect to the ground line.

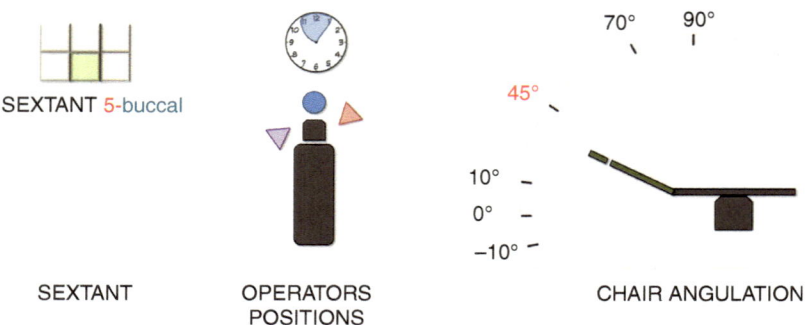

Fig. 9 Mandibular arch, anterior sextant, buccal aspects. Same positioning is valid for the maxillary arch anterior sextant, buccal aspects

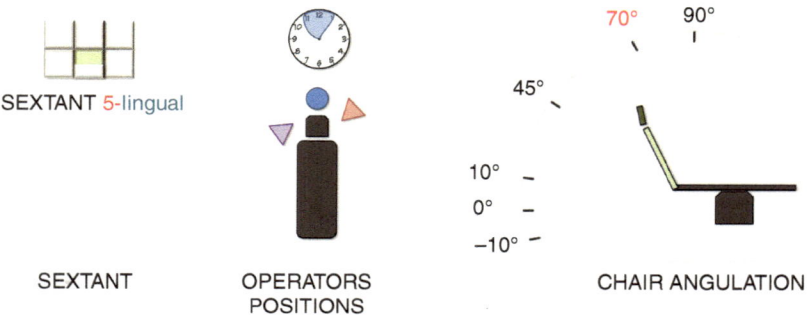

Fig. 10 Mandibular arch, anterior sextant, lingual aspects

    (b) Operator will be at 12 o'clock.
    (c) Assistant 1: will be at 1–2 o'clock.
    (d) Assistant 2: will be at 10–11 o'clock.
5. Mandibular arch, anterior sextant, lingual aspects (Fig. 10).
    (a) Patient chair will be positioned at about 70–80° with respect to the ground line.
    (b) Operator will be at 12 o'clock.
    (c) Assistant 1: will be at 1–2 o'clock.
    (d) Assistant 2: will be at 10–11 o'clock.

During these procedures, patient will be asked to actively participate with head rotations to facilitate visual access, utilizing both direct and indirect vision.

7   Infection Control

For disinfection instructions and details, the reader is advised to contact the manufacturer of the OM being utilized. The following are some general guidelines that could help discuss the best way to disinfect the OM with the respective manufacturer's technical support team.

Disinfectants are chemical solutions that can weaken or neutralize biologic agents by destroying living organisms by interfering with their metabolism or by inactivating virus particles. The utilization of these solutions prevents exposure to harmful biological agents and cross contamination.

Cleaning and disinfecting internal surfaces require delegation to technician with expertise and training on how to perform these tasks. External cleaning of the casing and mechanical external surfaces can be performed with wipes dampened with a disinfectant.

For cleaning lenses and eyepieces utilize lens paper with solutions approved by the manufacturer of the OM. Utilizing lens protectors is highly recommended to prevent splashing of bodily fluids on this delicate surface. Cleaning and replacing these protectors is much easier than dealing with an objective lens and its delicate surface. As recommended above, contact the OM manufacturer to get a list of approved disinfection solutions that are compatible with the machine being used.

Utilizing drapes and covers is highly recommended to facilitate maintenance and cleaning procedures. Some OM have asepsis sets consisting of rubber caps and handgrips that can be sterilized in autoclaves. For proper utilization of drapes, covers, and asepsis kits when available, the reader is advised to contact the manufacturer of the OM being utilized.

8 Conclusions

The incorporation of the operating microscope into a periodontal and dental implant practice is an investment in the well-being of the operator, the support surgical team, and the patient population. Being able to work in a neutral position with optimal ergonomics is health benefit that has the potential to translate into a longer professional career. The adoption of this technology requires total commitment of all stakeholders. Beyond the ultimate benefits that come along with better visualization provided by enhanced magnification paired with optimal illumination of the working field, the OM becomes a tool with a tremendous potential to improve work flow patterns, efficiency of delivery of care, and quality of therapy being provided.

When the question arises of when to start utilizing the operating microscope, the answer is always the same: now is the best time!

9 Key Points

1. Dentistry is a profession that is extremely demanding on the musculoskeletal health of the practitioner.
2. The operating microscope provides optimal magnification and illumination and promotes the most healthy ergonomic position.
3. Implementation stages can be tailored to the expertise and needs of the practitioner.

4. Microsurgery is not a solo discipline. It is a team-based effort.
5. Commitment, pursuing educational opportunities and discipline in frequent practicing will potentially translate into faster adoption of this technology into the daily periodontal and dental implant practice.

References

1. Cambridge dictionary. https://dictionary.cambridge.org/us/dictionary/english/ergonomics. Accessed 10 Feb 2021.
2. Morse T, Bruneau H, Dussetschleger J. Musculoskeletal disorders of the neck and shoulder in the dental professions. Work. 2010;35:419–29.
3. Gupta A, Bhat M, Mohammed T, Bansal N, Gupta G. Ergonomics in dentistry. Int J Clin Pediatr Dent. 2014;7:30–4.
4. Murphy DC. Ergonomics and dentistry. NY State Dent J. 1997;63:30–4.
5. Gupta A, Ankola AV, Hebbal M. Dental ergonomics to combat musculoskeletal disorders: a review. Int J Occup Saf Ergon. 2013;19:561–71.
6. Occhionero V, Korpinen L, Gobba F. Upper limb musculoskeletal disorders in healthcare personnel. Ergonomics. 2014;57:1166–91.
7. Sakzewski L, Naser-ud-Din S. Work-related musculoskeletal disorders in dentists and orthodontists: a review of the literature. Work. 2014;48:37–45.
8. Rising DW, Bennett BC, Hursh K, Plesh O. Reports of body pain in a dental student population. J Am Dent Assoc. 2005;136:81–6.
9. Plessas A, Bernardes Delgado M. The role of ergonomic saddle seats and magnification loupes in the prevention of musculoskeletal disorders. A systematic review. Int J Dent Hyg. 2018;16:430–40.
10. Chang BJ. Ergonomic benefits of surgical telescope systems: selection guidelines. J Calif Dent Assoc. 2002;30:161–9.
11. Ariens G, Bongers P, Douwes M, Miedema MC, Hoogendoorn WE, van der Wal G, Bouter LM, van Mechelen W. Are neck flexion, neck rotation, and sitting at work risk factors for neck pain? Results of a prospective cohort study. Occup Environ Med. 2001;58:200–7.
12. Hayes MJ, Osmotherly PG, Taylor JA, Smith DR, Ho A. The effect of loupes on neck pain and disability among dental hygienists. Work. 2016;53:755–62.
13. Hayes MJ, Osmotherly PG, Taylor JA, Smith DR, Ho A. The effect of wearing loupes on upper extremity musculoskeletal disorders among dental hygienists. Int J Dent Hyg. 2014;12:174–9.
14. Valachi B, Valachi K. Preventing musculoskeletal disorders in clinical dentistry: strategies to address the mechanisms leading to musculoskeletal disorders. J Am Dent Assoc. 2003;134:1604–12.
15. Niemczyk SP. Essentials of endodontic microsurgery. Dent Clin N Am. 2010;54:375–99.
16. Carr GB, Murgel CAF. The use of the operating microscope in endodontics. Dent Clin N Am. 2010;54:191–214.
17. Harwell RC, Ferguson RL. Physiologic tremor and microsurgery. Microsurgery. 1983;4:187–92.
18. Michaelides PL. Use of the operating microscope in dentistry. J Calif Dent Assoc. 1996;24:45–50.

Microscope-Assisted Periodontal and Peri-implant Plastic Surgery

Juan Carlos Duran

Contents

Supplementary Information The online version contains supplementary material available at [https://doi.org/10.1007/978-3-030-96874-8_7].

J. C. Duran (✉)

Prosthodontics Program, School of Dentistry, Faculty of Medicine, University of Desarrollo UDD, Santiago, Chile

e-mail: jcduran@udd.cl

Abstract

The use of microsurgical principles and procedures provides clinically relevant advantages over conventional macrosurgical concepts for plastic esthetic periodontal surgery. The term "periodontal microsurgery" proposed by Shanelec refers to a procedure that has advantages in periodontal surgery. The combination of an improved visual precision with the use of microsurgical tools specifically designed for this procedure allows more precise and less damaging manipulation of both soft and hard tissues and more capacity to properly debride the defect and the root surface, which increases the chances of healing by primary intention. Microsurgical procedures from incision to the final closure of the surgical wound have less extensive flap designs and enhanced vision fields that facilitate identification of defects and anatomical landmarks. Visual acuity is enhanced by both magnification and illumination when performing periodontal surgical procedures with the aid of an operating microscope (OM). Current evidence supports the benefits of OM and outcome superiority of periodontal surgical therapy with the use of OM for root coverage. It is not easy to move out of the comfort zone, especially when significant changes to the daily practice need to be implemented. This is one of the main reasons for limited use of microscopes in the periodontal field. Great determination, effort, and dedication are required to incorporate microscopy into practice; however, after it is accomplished, there is no turning back. Moreover, it takes clinical performance to a new level. The purpose of this chapter was to present the clinical experience with the use of the microscope in periodontal and peri-implant surgery.

Keywords

Periodontal microsurgery · Gingival recessions · Incisions · Sutures
Microsurgical tools

1 Introduction

Magnification and illumination translate into controlled manipulation of soft and hard tissue structures that make up the periodontium. Microsurgical procedures from incision to the final closure of the surgical wound have less extensive flap designs and enhanced vision fields that facilitate identification of defects and anatomical landmarks such as furcations, cementoenamel projections, anatomical grooves, and others (such as accretions, defective restorative margins, and caries lesions).

Mucogingival surgery has been a prevalent focus of interventions and studies looking at the advantages of utilizing the operating microscope (OM) to enhance surgical outcomes and patient experiences. This chapter will cover foundational aspects in microsurgical plastic therapy such as phenotype definitions, recession classification systems employed to enhance communication, technical applications such as incision and flap design, suture techniques, followed by therapy execution around natural teeth and dental implants.

2 Historical Background of Periodontal Microsurgery Compared with Conventional Mucogingival Interventions

Surgical procedures for correcting or eliminating anatomical, developmental, or traumatic deformities in the gingiva or alveolar mucosa benefit from the OM, which provides magnification and illumination and thus improves visual acuity and enhances precise and delicate tissue manipulation. Tissue trauma may be reduced by choosing finer suture diameters, because thinner (6–0, 7–0) sutures lead to thread breakage rather than tissue breakage [1], 7–0 sutures clearly represent a category of sutures that requires visual (OM improved visual precision) rather than tactile control in handling [1].

Therefore, it is not surprising that the field of mucogingival therapy has been an objective of various clinical studies. Burkhardt and Lang [2] conducted a 12-month randomized controlled trial to compare wound healing following mucogingival surgical interventions performed using micro- and macrosurgical approaches. According to Miller's classification, ten patients had bilateral Miller's class I and class II recession lesions [3]. In this split-mouth design, defects were randomly selected for recession coverage using either a microsurgical (test) or macrosurgical (control) approach. Fluorescent angiograms were performed to evaluate graft vascularization immediately after surgical intervention and 3 and 7 days of healing. Clinical parameters such as gingival inflammation, supragingival plaque presence, periodontal probing depth (PD), gingival recession, and clinical attachment level (CAL) were assessed prior to surgery and at 1, 3, 6, and 12 months postoperatively. All differences in vascularization and recession coverage were statistically significant. The percentage of root coverage for the test and control sites remained stable during the first 12 months at 98% and 90%, respectively. An OM (for recipient site) and prism loupes-5×− (for donor site) together with microsurgical instruments and 7–0 and 9–0 sutures were used in the test group. Conventional instruments and 4–0 sutures were used in the control group.

Francetti et al. [4]. performed a controlled clinical study and reported the treatment of 24 patients with Miller class I and II gingival recession defects (≥2 mm) were treated. Twelve patients were treated with the aid of OM (test group) and 12 patients were treated without the aid of OM (control group). Clinical parameters such as recession depth, PD, clinical attachment loss, and keratinized gingival tissue were evaluated and the measurements were recorded before surgery and after 12 months of surgery. After 12 months, the mean defect coverage in the test and control groups was 86% and 78%, respectively, and complete root coverage in the test and control groups was 58.3% and 33.4%, respectively. Qualitative esthetic assessment showed significantly less scarring and better marginal profile in the test group and no significant difference in papilla appearance between the groups.

In a case series, Andrade et al. [5] aimed to compare macro- and microsurgical techniques for root coverage using a coronally advanced flap (CAF) in combination with enamel matrix derivative (EMD). Thirty patients participated in this study. An equal number of patients were randomly assigned to the test group (TG) and the control group (CG). The microsurgical approach was used in TG, and the conventional macrosurgical approach was used in CG. Clinical parameters (gingival recession, PD, CAL, width, and thickness of keratinized tissue) were assessed before and 6 months after surgery. The discomfort level evaluation was performed 1 week after surgical intervention. At 6 months after surgery, the root coverage was 92% and 83% in TG and CG, respectively. A statistically significant increase in the width and thickness of keratinized tissue was found in TG only. All patients reported minimal postoperative discomfort. Microsurgical instruments with an OM and 5–0 and 8–0 sutures were used in TG. Conventional instruments and 5–0 sutures were used in CG.

In a randomized controlled trial, Bittencourt et al. [6] compared root coverage, postoperative morbidity, and esthetic outcomes of subepithelial connective tissue graft with and without the use of a surgical microscope for the treatment of Miller class I and II gingival recession (≥ 2 mm). Twenty-four patients were enrolled in this split-mouth study. Parameters such as depth and width of the gingival defect, width and thickness of keratinized tissue, PD, and CAL were recorded. In addition, postoperative morbidity and patient satisfaction were evaluated. At 12 months after surgery, root coverage in TG and CG was 98% and 88.3%, respectively, and complete root coverage in TG and CG was 87.5% and 58.3%, respectively. All (100%) TG patients and 79.1% CG patients were satisfied with the outcome. Patients of both the groups were treated using the same instruments and 8–0 sutures, except for the use of an OM.

It is evident that the scientific literature on the use of OM in periodontal surgical procedures mainly constitutes opinion papers, anecdotal case descriptors, and technical essays illustrating operational procedures. These types of publications are meritorious and form an important segment of the tiers of publications and clinical expertise that guide clinical care [7]. Although cohort studies and randomized controlled trials are limited (Table 1), the evidence put forth by these studies consistently suggests the outcomes of periodontal surgical procedures are superior with the use of OM. When it comes to mucogingival surgical applications and the execution of these procedures using an OM, the test groups (OM aided) consistently showed higher root coverage and superior complete root coverage compared with procedures performed without the assistance of the OM [2–4, 6]. These results are corroborated by recent meta-analysis [8], in comparison to macrosurgery, microsurgery yields an additional 6% of mean root coverage and 28% of probability for complete root coverage. Patient-reported outcomes also favored microsurgery with improved esthetics, patient's satisfaction, and reduced pain.

3 Periodontal Phenotype

The determination and classification of the periodontal phenotype [9] are essential for the planning of periodontal, restoring, implantological, and orthodontic treatments. The type of phenotype is based on anatomical characteristics such as:

- Thickness of the gingiva
- Width of the keratinized gingiva
- Osseous morphotype
- Tooth dimensions

Based on these parameters, the phenotype can be classified into the following three categories:

Thin scalloped phenotype: A phenotype characterized by a slender triangular crown, slight cervical convexity, interproximal contacts next to the incisal border, tight zone of keratinized tissue (KT) a high gingival scallop, and relatively slim alveolar bone (Fig. 1).

Table 1 Microscope-assisted periodontal surgical procedures studies

Reference	Patient group	Study type	Methods	Key results	Comments
Francetti et al. [4]	$N = 24$; single Miller's I or II	Prospective RTC	Root coverage with OM (T) and conventional (C) 12 m follow up	Defect coverage: 86% (T),78% (C) complete coverage: 58.3% (T),33.3% (C)	OM: Better results: Success and predictability
Burkhardt and Lang [2]	$N = 10$; Bilateral Miller's class I or II in maxillary canines	Prospective RTC/Split mouth	Root coverage with OM (T) and conventional (C) Fluorescent angiograms 0, 3, 7d. 12 m follow up	Vascularization: 0d 8.9 ± 1.9% (T) 7.95 ± 1.8% (C) 3d 53.3 ± 10.5% (T) 4.5 ± 5.7% (C) 7d 84.8 ± 13.5% (T) 64.0 ± 12.3% (C) Mean recession coverage 98% (T) and 90% (C)	Microsurgery improves vascularization and percentages of root coverage
Andrade et al. [5]	$N = 15$ single Miller's class I or III	Prospective RTC	Root coverage with OM (T) and conventional (C) 6 m follow up	Defect coverage: 92% (T),83% (C) complete coverage: 73% (T),46% (C)	No statistically significant differences between groups. Short duration, mix of recession (I and III) and tooth groups
Bittencourt et al. [6]	$N = 24$ single Miller's class I or II	Prospective RTC/Split mouth	With OM (T) and conventional (C) 12 m follow up	Defect coverage: 98% (T),88.3% (C) complete coverage: 87.5% (T), 58.3% (C) esthetics: 100% patients satisfied (T), 79.1% patients satisfied (C)	Although both approaches produce root coverage, OM: Yields better results

CAL clinical attachment level, *PD* probing depth, *OM* operating microscope, *T* test, *C* control, *m* month, *d* day, *RTC* randomized controlled trial

Fig. 1 Thin scalloped phenotype

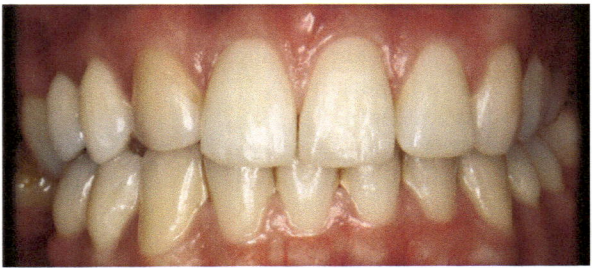

Fig. 2 Thick flat phenotype

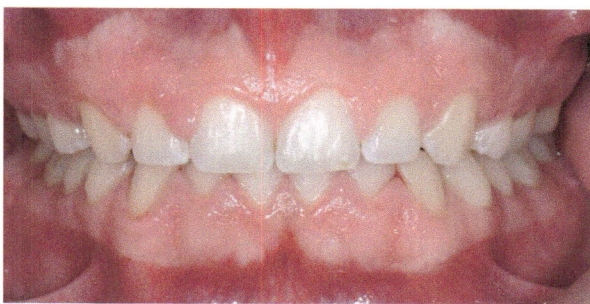

Fig. 3 Thick scalloped phenotype

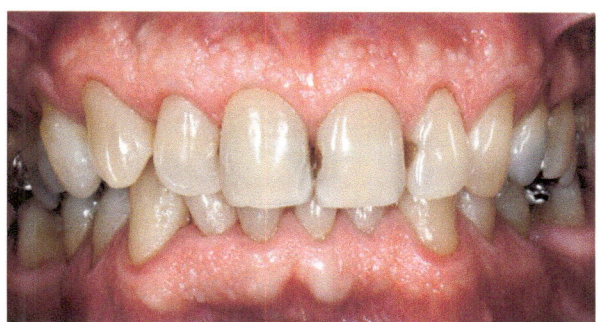

Thick flat phenotype: A phenotype characterized by more square-shaped dental crowns, pronounced cervical convexity, large interproximal contact at the apex, wide zone of KT, thick and fibrotic gingiva, and relatively thick alveolar bone (Fig. 2).

Thick scalloped phenotype: A phenotype characterized by a thick fibrotic gingiva, slim teeth, tight zone of KT, and pronounced gingival sinuation (Fig. 3).

4   Gingival Recessions

In the last few decades, the treatment of gingival recessions has gathered much interest from both surgeons and researchers, which has led to this field of periodontics to rapidly evolve, and thus, the predictability of the techniques has increased.

Generally, different approaches and techniques are available for the treatment of recessions, such as isolation or multiple, to achieve root covering. These techniques can be grouped based on the source of the donor tissue for root covering (Table 2). Thus, the techniques are grouped into pedunculated soft tissue grafting, free soft tissue grafting, and additive treatment in which biomaterials are used to replace the connective tissue.

This section will focus on the two most used techniques for the treatment of recessions: the coronal advanced flaps (CAF) and the envelope and tunneling assisted by microscope techniques. The use of a microscope allows us to perform

Table 2 Techniques based on the source of the donor tissue for root covering

Pedunculated soft tissue grafts	**Rotated** Double papilla pedicle graft **Coronal advanced** Coronal Advanced Flap (1965) Coronal advanced flap modified (De Sanctis and Zucchelli 2000, 2007) Semilunar Flap (1907)	*Treatments additives*	
			Biomaterials periodontal surgery
	Non-submerged grafts		Biological (allograft xenograft)
	Free gingival graft (1966)		Bioactive molecules (enamel matrix proteins)
Free soft tissue grafts	**Submerged grafts** Connective tissue graft subepithelial Coronal advanced flap + connective tissue graft Lateral moved coronal advanced flap + connective tissue graft Envelope Flap Raeztke (1985), Allen, Bruno (1994) Tunnel Azi Etienne (1998), Zuhr		Tissue engineering

precise and minimally invasive interventions. Shannelec [10] reported the benefits of plastic periodontal microsurgery, which are as follows:

1. Enhanced motor skills, thus perfecting surgical capabilities
2. Primary wound closure with emphasis on passive flaps
3. Use of micro-tools and micro-sutures, thus reducing tissue trauma

The microsurgical technique causes minimal trauma in the tissue, both during incision and micro-suturing. Moreover, if the first intention closure is performed, the healing time, inflammation time, and the risk of necrosis are lower compared with those after macrosurgery [11]. Two additional factors that are advantageous to the microsurgery technique are postoperative patient satisfaction and the long-term esthetic satisfaction of patients. A correlation was reported between the invasiveness and duration of the surgical technique and postoperative complications and pain [12]. Patient satisfaction and postoperative pain experience are reduced by 55% when microsurgery techniques are used [4].

Usually, the effectiveness of the root coverage procedure is measured in relation to the final position of the gingival margin with respect to the cementoenamel junction (CEJ). This provides an objective view of the result in terms of the percentage of root coverage, but not of the actual esthetic result. Macrosurgical techniques can achieve good root coverage. Cairo et al. [13] proposed the use of root coverage esthetic score (RES) that measures other clinical variables such as texture, color, and soft tissue contour in addition to the percentage of coverage achieved. The current perception of the outcomes of patients with high esthetic demand requires the

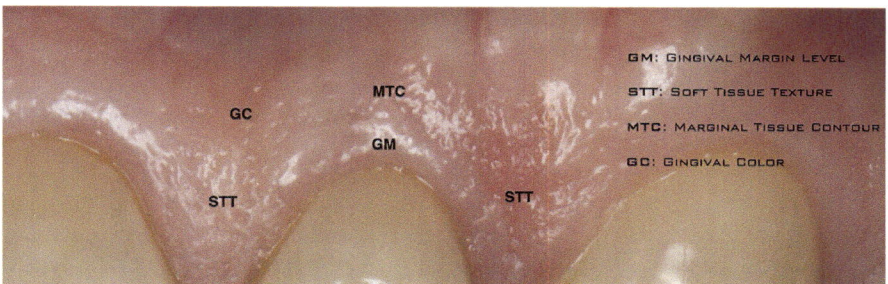

Fig. 4 Root coverage esthetic score (RES) clinical variables

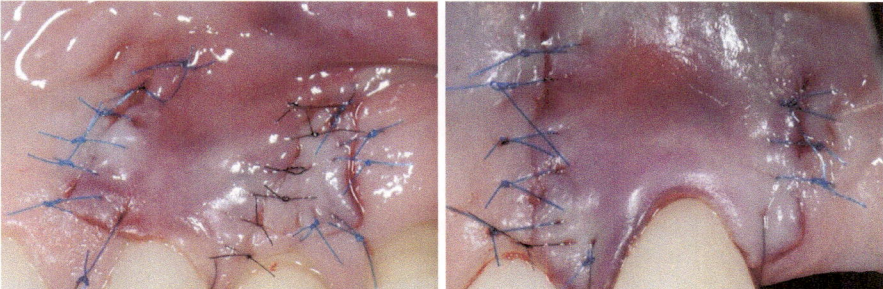

Fig. 5 Suture technique and materials in microsurgery

use of surgical techniques that do not leave scars or sequelae and are less invasive characteristics that fit perfectly with the concept of microsurgery (Fig. 4).

In mucogingival surgery, an optimal esthetic outcome can be achieved with microsurgical techniques when numerous parameters are upheld: many hours of practice for the training and mastery of the microsurgical technique of the microsurgeon, suture technique (the most important parameter), and necessary visual aids, tools, and materials [14] (Fig. 5).

Independent of the technique, various factors can affect root coverage [15], which are as follows:

• Type of recession and the risk of the interdental tissue
• Dimension, symmetry, height, and shape of the interdental papilla
• Postsurgical position of the gingival margin (ideally 1 mm in the coronal CEJ direction)
• Degree of passivity of the flap
• Tissue phenotype
• Presence of carious and non-carious cervical lesions
• Absence of the CEJ
• Flap design
• Biomodification of the root surface

- Dimension, thickness, and quality of the connective tissue graft (CTG)
- Tooth position (extrusion and buccal/lingual inclination)

5 Recession Classification

Miller [5] proposed four types of gingival recession based on the level of the gingival margin with regard to the mucogingival line and interproximal osseous tissue. The important aspect of this classification system is that it associates the type of recession with its therapeutic outcome success (Fig. 6). Most recently, Cairo et al. [16] proposed a classification system that identifies three types of gingival recession: type RT-1, does not include loss of interproximal insertion; type RT-2, the loss of interproximal insertion that is less than or equal to the buccal recession; and type RT-3, the loss of interproximal insertion is greater than that of the buccal recession (Fig. 7).

6 Incisions

The term "periodontal microsurgery" proposed by Shanelec [10, 14] refers to a procedure that has advantages in periodontal surgery. The combination of an improved visual precision with the use of microsurgical tools specifically designed for this procedure allows more precise and less damaging manipulation of both soft and hard tissues and more capacity to properly debride the defect and the root surface, which increases the chances of healing by primary intention. Based on the type of intervention, magnifications of 8× to 20× are considered ideal depending on periodontal microsurgery (Table 3). The depth of field and field of view decreases with an increase in magnification, and therefore, the maximum magnification for a

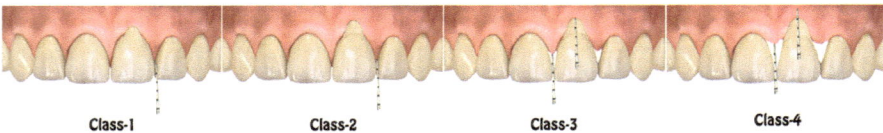

Fig. 6 Miller classification system

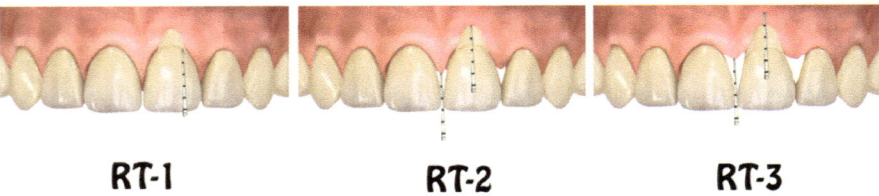

Fig. 7 Cairo classification system

Table 3 Magnification recommended for surgical periodontal procedures

Magnification recommended	Surgical interventions
6×–8×	Clinical inspections, anesthesia, entire quadrant is under operation
12×–15×	Coverage of single of a single tooth tissue recession, interdental wound closure
15×–25×	Clinical details, anatomical papillae, de-epithelized

Table 4 Field of view Vs. depth of field

Magnification (×)	Field of view (mm.)	Depth of field (cm.)
3×	64 mm	Up to 10 cm
5×	41 mm	Up to 5 cm
8×	25 mm	Up to 3.5 cm
13×	16 mm	Up to 1 cm
21×	10 mm	Up to 0.3 cm

surgical intervention is limited to approximately 12× to 20× (Video 1) for localized problems such as the coverage of a single soft tissue recession (Table 4; Figs. 8a, b, 9, and 10).

A correct incision means preservation of an adequate amount of vascularization in the flap, allowing access to the area being treated by moving the flap, preservation of the attached gingiva and making the suturing process easier. The type of incision and the angle of the blade in relation to the surface of the tissue are used to determine the thickness of the flap. Moreover, the marginal edges of the flap and its thickness should be consistent and ideally close to 1 mm [17]. The blood flow in the gingiva is mainly derived from the supraperiosteal blood vessels, which anastomize with the blood vessels of the alveolar bone and periodontal ligament in the free gingiva [18]. During incision, the blade of the scalpel should be perpendicular to the surface of the tissue regardless of any anatomic restriction that may exist. This is the only way to achieve 90° angles in the flap margins or adequate thickness on both the sides of the incision line. Bevels should be avoided, especially in thin phenotypes. Furthermore, initial incisions that cross one another should be slightly over-extended to achieve clearly defined margins and corners of consistent thickness [19].

The use of microscope greatly benefits these procedures, as it allows us to see in detail the flap thickness and incision limits, especially when dealing with fragile tissues with a limited vascular network, such as the interdental mucosa. The use of a microscope greatly improves the surgical access to the interdental or interimplant spaces. These delicate and narrow soft tissues can be sharply dissected using microblades (Keydent microblade tunnel ADSystem Munich, Germany) with the aid of clear magnified vision and preserved, thus reducing trauma and facilitating accurate wound closure (Video 2).

Based on direction, the types of incision are of two types: horizontal and vertical.

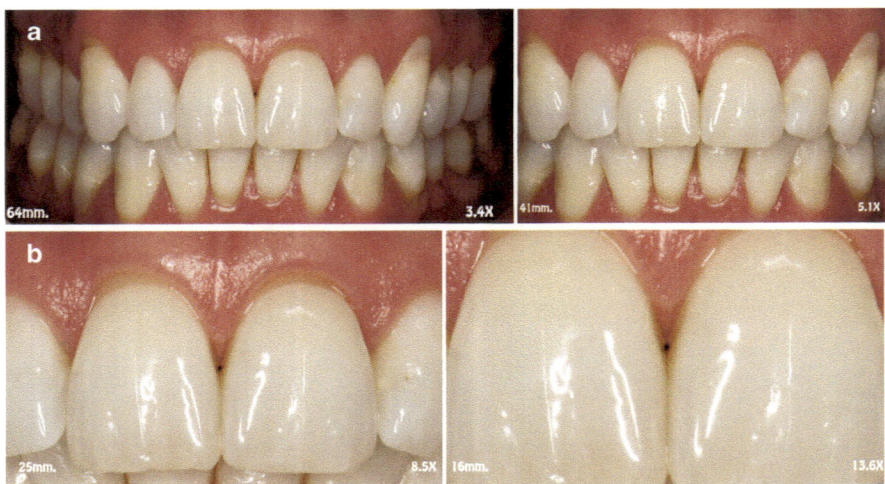

Fig. 8 (**a**) 3.4×–5.1× Magnification. (**b**) 8.5×–13.6× Magnification ideal in periodontal microsurgery

Fig. 9 21.25× Magnification in periodontal microsurgery

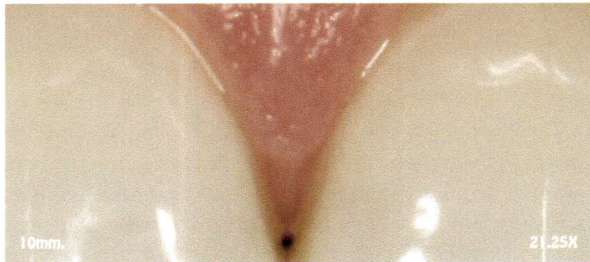

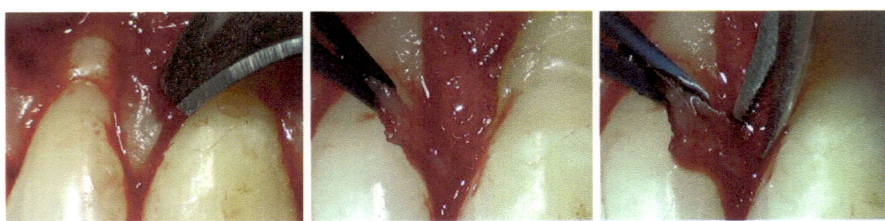

Fig. 10 Controlled manipulation of soft tissue structures that make up the periodontium

6.1   Horizontal

Sulcular incision: This type of incision maintains the marginal tissue completely intact. The blade of the scalpel is inserted through the gingival sulcus and is apically directed to the osseous tissue, maintaining contact with the dental and root surface. The whole gingival margin is incorporated into the flap and preserved in its entirety.

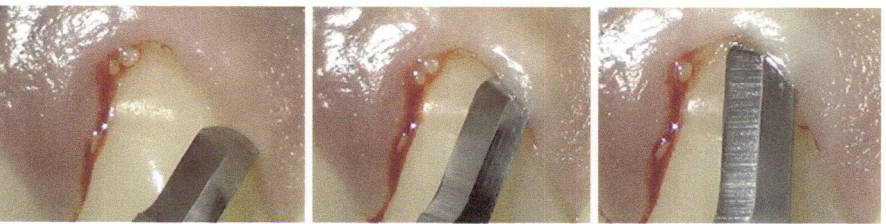

Fig. 11 Sulcular incision microblades (Swann-Morton SM67 Sheffield, England)

Fig. 12 Sulcular, marginal, and paramarginal incision

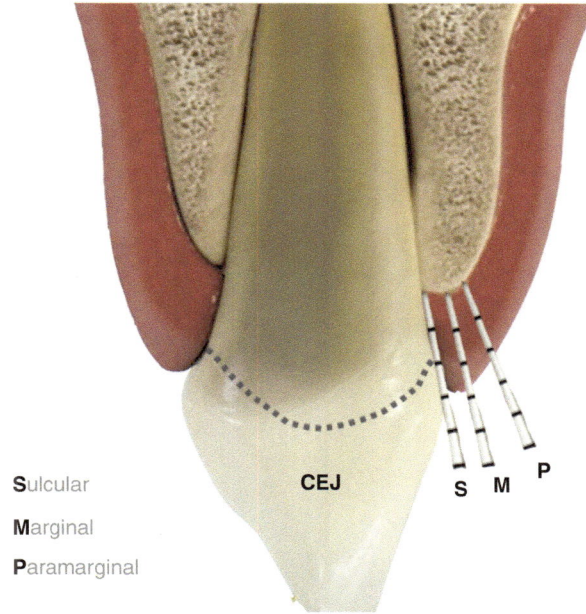

To make this process easier, the use of microblades (Swann-Morton SM67 Sheffield, England), instead of scalpel, combined with microscope for magnification provides absolute control and precision in the procedure (Fig. 11).

Paramarginal incision: This type of incision is located parallel or slightly apical to the gingival margin. The coronal tissue in the line of the paramarginal incision can be removed or de-epithelized depending on the procedure being performed [19] (Fig. 12).

6.2 Vertical

A vertical incision can be part of the design or act as a releasing incision. It is used to increase the accessibility or change the position of the flap. A vertical incision should be performed in the inter-root concavities and should have a slight

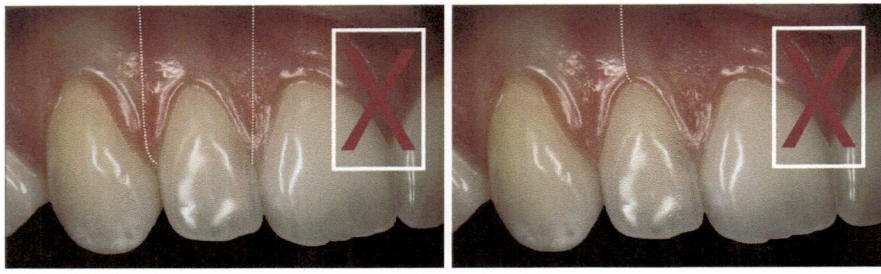

Fig. 13 Incorrect location of vertical incision

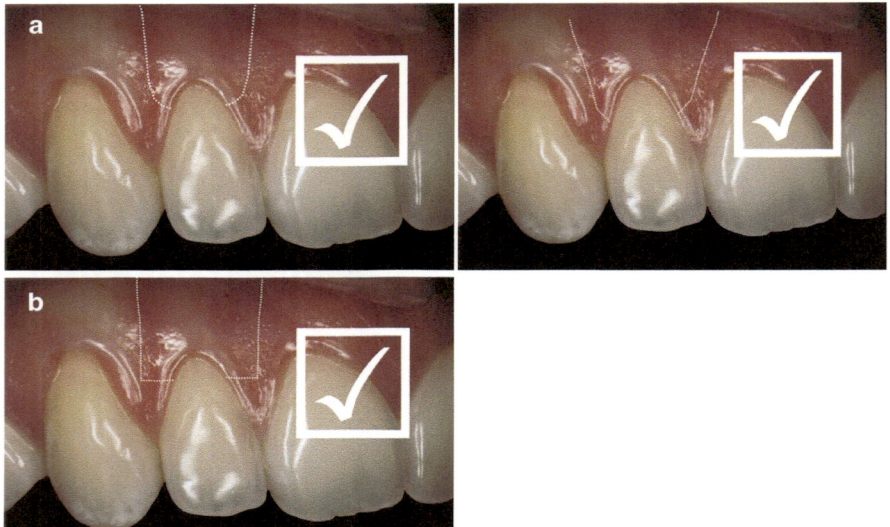

Fig. 14 (**a**) Correct location of vertical triangular incision. (**b**) Correct location of vertical trapezoidal incision

divergence (Video 3). The exact location of this incision depends on the type of procedure being performed (only coronal or apical access or displacement of the margin). The idea is to prevent flawed scarring at the interdental papilla level. Hence, an incision should be made where the papilla base meets the gingival margin and not in the middle of the papilla, dividing it into two (Fig. 13). The largest possible volume of papilla should be preserved. Therefore, the incision should not be made at the level of the gingival zenith because it increases the possibility of a future gingival recession in that area. The procedure of relocation of the gingival margin involves flap design (trapezoidal, triangular) (see treatment of gingival recession) (Fig. 14a, b).

Fig. 15 (**a**) Depending on whether the periosteum is included in the flap. (**b**) Mucoperiosteal flap (total thickness)

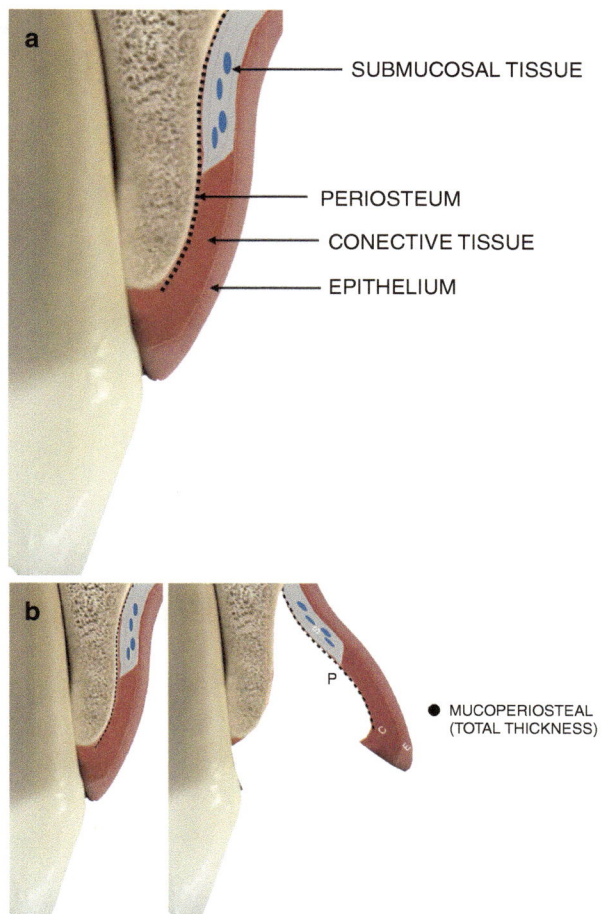

SUBMUCOSAL TISSUE

PERIOSTEUM

CONECTIVE TISSUE

EPITHELIUM

P

● MUCOPERIOSTEAL (TOTAL THICKNESS)

7 Flap Designs

Depending on whether the periosteum is included in the flap (Fig. 15a), flaps are classified as follows:

- Mucoperiosteal flap (total thickness)
- Mucosal flap (partial thickness)
- Combined flap (partial/total/partial thickness)

7.1 Mucoperiosteal Flap (Total Thickness)

This type of flap design includes the epithelium, connective tissue, and periosteum. The incision reaches the osseous tissue. This flap design has the following characteristics (Figs. 15b and 16):

Fig. 16 Mucoperiosteal
flap (total thickness)

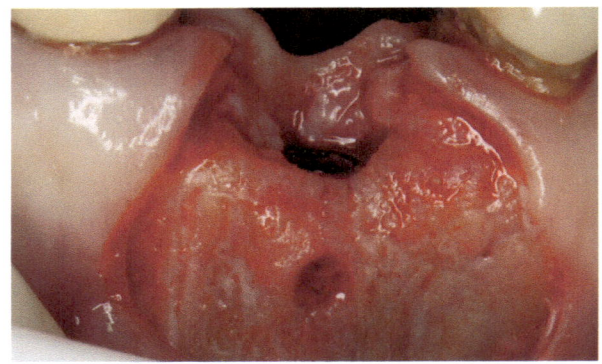

Fig. 16 Mucoperiosteal
flap (total thickness)

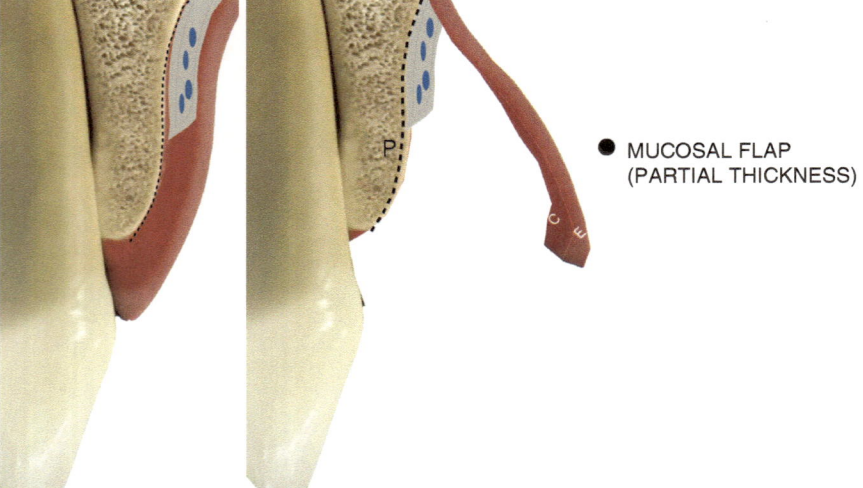

MUCOSAL FLAP
(PARTIAL THICKNESS)

Fig. 17 Mucosal flap (partial thickness)

- First intention healing
- Relatively easy to design and perform
- Adequate blood support, as the entire plexus of the periosteum is present
- Limited mobility
- Minor bleeding

7.2   Mucosal Flap (Partial Thickness)

This type of flap design includes the epithelium, subepithelial connective tissue, and periosteum layer over the osseous tissue (Fig. 17). The microsurgeon should be very attentive when performing this incision and observe the external part of the flap because the blade of the scalpel runs parallel to the mucosal tissue and a high risk

Fig. 18 Mucosal flap (partial thickness)

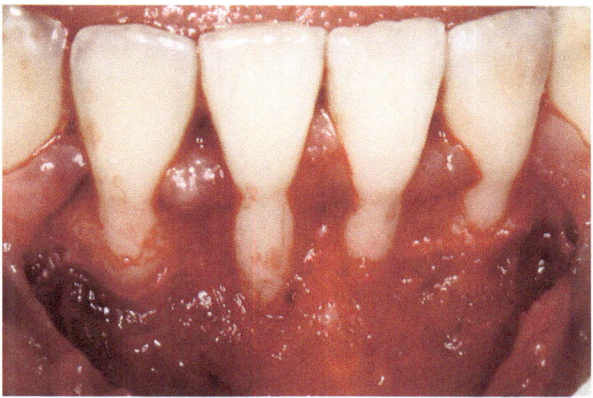

of perforation is present. The main advantage of this type of flap is its mobility, which allows its relocation in any direction without tension. This flap design has the following characteristics (Fig. 18):

- Difficult to design and carry out
- Reduced blood support due to maximized design or extension
- More bleeding
- Moderate postoperative complications such as slightly more edema

7.3 Combined Flap (Partial/Total/Partial Thickness)

This flap design was introduced by Zucchelli and De Sanctis in 2000 [20]. The concept involved moderating the flap thickness (partial/total/partial). In the most coronal part at the level of the papilla, a partial incision is made (only epithelium and connective tissue), which allows better adaptation and healing of the flap. In the middle part, complete lifting is performed, including the periosteum, with the objective of increasing the flap thickness and improving vascularization. Finally, in the most apical part, two incisions are made. One incision is made deep and parallel to the osseous tissue to release the mucosal of the periosteum and another incision is made superficial and parallel to the alveolar mucosa to release the flap from the muscular insertions and the submucosal tissue (Fig. 19). This type of flap design has been proven to be superior in the long term with regard to the stability of the percentage of root covering in the treatment of isolated maxillary recessions compared with the mucosal flap or partial thickness [21]. This flap design has the following characteristics (Fig. 20):

- Easy to perform using the proposed protocol
- Good blood flow support
- Moderate inflammation postoperatively

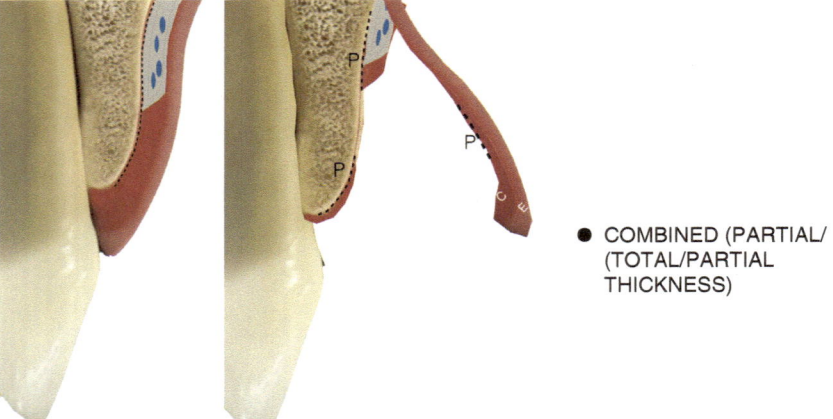

Fig. 19 Combined flap (partial/total/partial thickness)

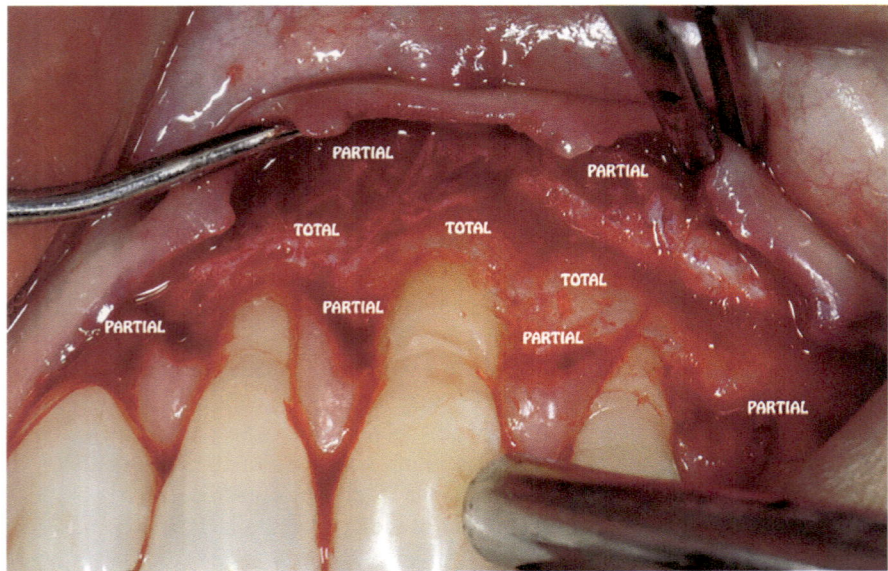

Fig. 20 Combined flap (partial/total/partial thickness)

8   Suture Techniques

The suture technique should be focused on at the surgical borders, especially in the case of a flap that has been correctly, completely, and passively executed, to avoid creating tension.

The selection of the suture material, technique, and manner of knotting plays a fundamental role in the initial stages of healing and in resistance to mechanical stress in the stages of greater inflammation [22]. As a rule, the mobile tissue should be sutured toward the immobile tissue, and to do this, it is recommended to slightly lift the immobile border with a micro-elevator (Mamadent Micro 005 papilla elevator ADS system Munich, Germany) and to permanently irrigate the tissue, which makes the manipulation and stitching of the soft tissues easier (Fig. 21a, b).

In the management of micro-sutures, the biomechanics and technique of knotting, choice of materials, and suture strength are fundamental (Fig. 22a, b).

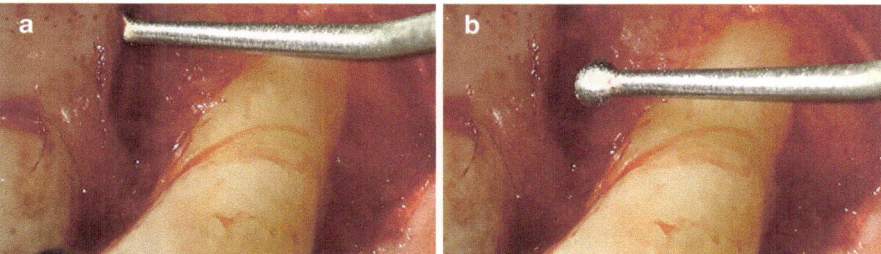

Fig. 21 (**a, b**) It is recommended to slightly lift the immobile border with a micro-elevator (Mamadent Micro 005 papilla elevator ADS system Munich, Germany)

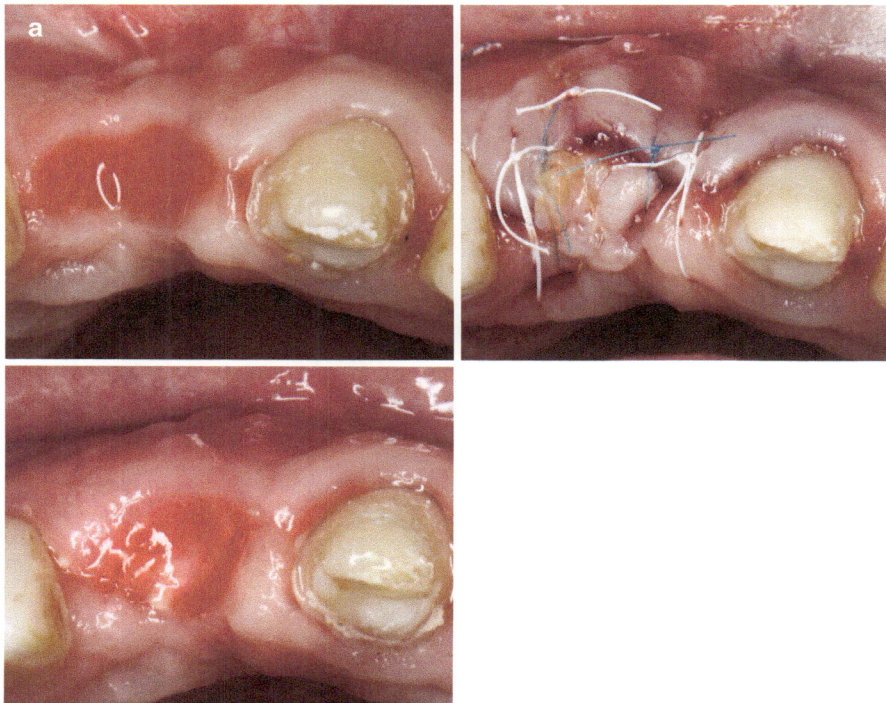

Fig. 22 (**a, b**) In the management of micro-sutures, the biomechanics and technique of knotting, choice of materials, and suture strength are fundamental

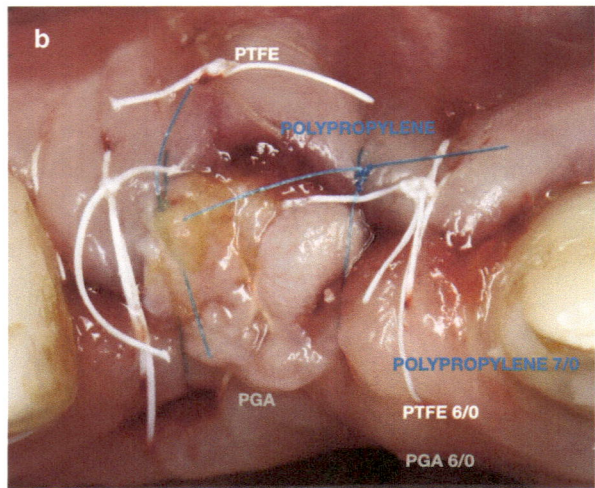

Fig. 7 (continued)

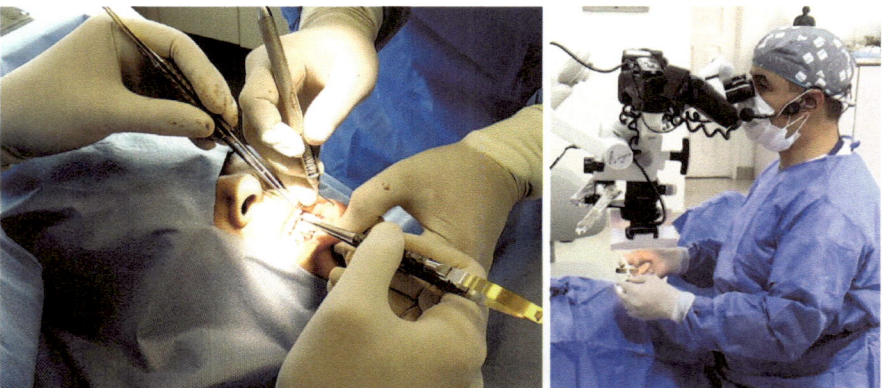

Fig. 23 The use of bimanual technique allows to work comfortably from outside the mouth in any small area, facilitating the manipulation of micro-sutures and preventing sharp injuries

The use of bimanual technique is highly recommended with instruments that are 18 cm long for suturing. This technique allows to work comfortably from outside the mouth in any small area, facilitating the manipulation of micro-sutures and preventing sharp injuries (Fig. 23). Very small needles should be inserted in the gingiva close to the area where knots will be tied (Fig. 24) (Video 4).

Table 5 Sutures and micro-sutures used in periodontal and peri-implant surgeries. Generally, based on the function, sutures are classified as follows [19]:

- *Closing sutures*
- *Tension-relieving sutures*

Fig. 24 Very small needles should be inserted in the gingiva close to the area where knots will be tied

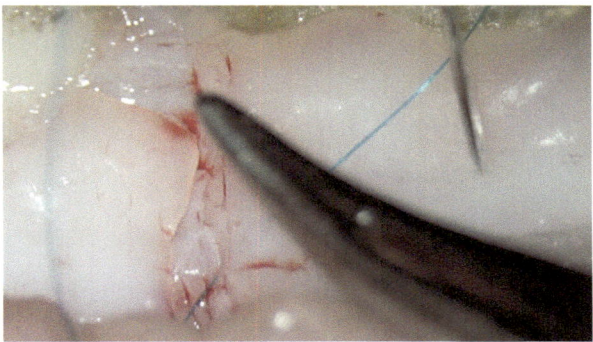

- *Combined sutures (closed and tension-relieving)*
- *Suspension sutures*
- *Fixation sutures*
- *Insertion and position sutures*

8.1   Closing Sutures

Closing sutures are used to close the gap between the surgical borders to achieve primary wound healing. It is fundamental that the manipulation of the flap is performed correctly and that no tension exists whatsoever. This ensures that the tension generated at the surgical border during the initial stages of the scarring process is minor and that the sutures do not rip the tissue or break the stitching material. The most common technique used for closure sutures is the simple interrupted suture technique. Although the simple interrupted suture technique seems to be simple, executing it in a reproducible and systematic manner with consistent and symmetrical bite size is challenging (Fig. 25) (Video 5).

Another closure suture technique is the continuous suture technique. As the name implies, sutures are not interrupted or knotted independently. The main disadvantage and the reason for limited use of the continuous suture technique are that it depends on a single knot and is generally used in large surgical borders (Fig. 26).

8.2   Tension-Relieving Sutures

The tension-relieving suture technique is used in combination with the closing suture technique to release the tension generated by postoperative inflammation and edema at the surgical border. This helps closure sutures to have better mechanical stability because closure sutures are applied after stitching and knotting tension-relieving sutures in the deeper layers of the tissue. One type of tension releasing/relieving suture technique is the mattress suture technique (vertical and horizontal variants) (Figs. 27 and 28). The mattress suture technique allows an eversion to occur at the surgical border, which should be supported by interrupted closing sutures.

Table 5 Micro-sutures

Brand name®	Material	Thread type	Suture strength	Needle	Needle	Indications	Absorbable
AD surgical	Polypropylene	Monof	6/0	12 mm	3/8	Papillary sutures anterior, periosteal sutures	No
AD surgical	Polypropylene	Monof	7/0	11 mm	3/8	Buccal releasing incision	No
Seralene	Polyvinylidene fluoride	Monof	6/0	12 mm	3/8	Standard sutures	No
Vicryl	Polyglactin 910	Braided	7/0	6.4 mm	3/8	Fixation sutures CTG	Yes
PGA	Acid polyglycolic	Monof	6/0	13 mm	3/8	Fixation sutures CTG	Yes
Monotex	Polytetrafluoroethylene	Monof	6/0	13 mm	3/8	Papillary sutures posterior	No
Prolene	Polypropylene	Monof	8/0	6.4 mm	1/2	Buccal releasing incision	No
AD surgical	Polyamide	Monof	9/0	5 mm	3/8	Buccal releasing incision, papilla base incision	No
AD surgical	Polyamide	Monof	10/0	4 mm	3/8	Buccal releasing incision, papilla base incision	No

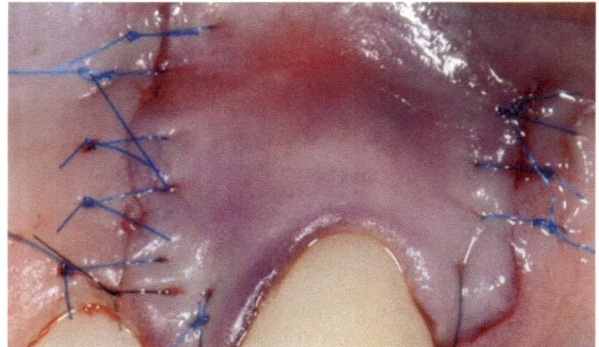

Fig. 25 Symmetrical bite size

Fig. 26 Continuous suture technique

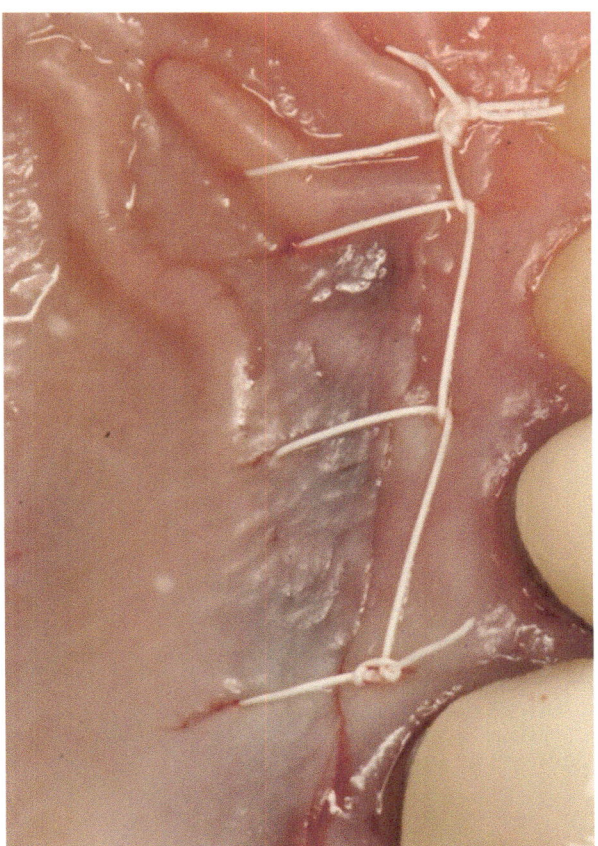

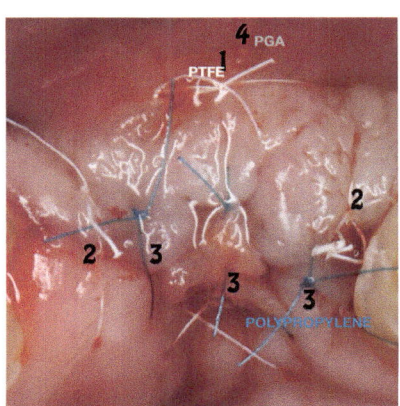

- 1-Tension-relieving sutures (PTFE 6/0)
- 2-Double Sling (Combined sutures) (PTFE 6/0)
- 3-Closing sutures (Polypropylene 7/0)
- 4-Fixation sutures (PGA 6/0)

Fig. 27 The mattress suture technique (vertical and horizontal variants)

Fig. 28 Tension-relieving sutures

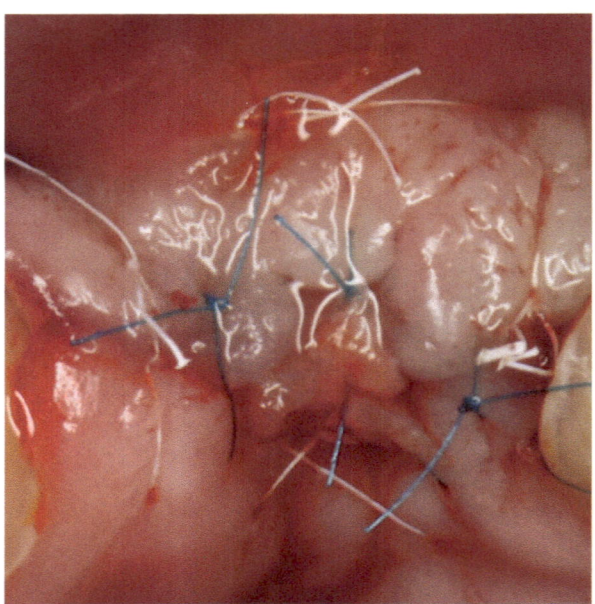

Fig. 29 The double sling technique combines two interrupted closing sutures of different bite sizes in different tissue layers

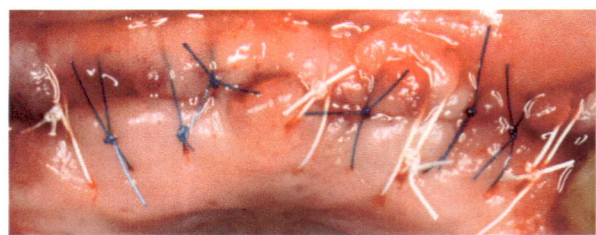

8.3   Combined Sutures (Closing and Tension-Relieving Sutures)

Combined sutures relieve tension and close the surgical border in an accurate and safe manner. The double sling technique [23] combines two interrupted closing sutures of different bite sizes in different tissue layers (Fig. 29). The suture with the largest bite size releases the tension and the suture with smaller bite size closes the surgical border and both the sutures are knotted in one place.

8.4   Suspension Sutures

Suspension sutures are used to fix the new positions of the flap, when it is moved (coronal, apical, or lateral). The anchoring zones of suspension sutures can be dental palatal zone, soft tissue palatal zone, and contact points (Fig. 30).

Fig. 30 Suspension
sutures

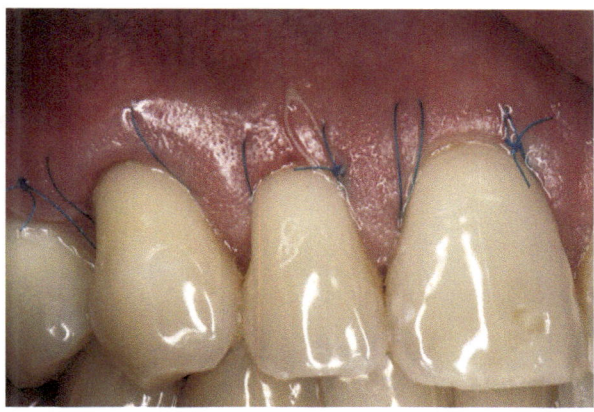

8.5   Point-of-Contact Sling Sutures

Point-of-contact sling sutures are the most commonly used sutures in plastic microsurgeries for the treatment of gingival recession with a modified tunnel [24]. They are designed to displace the flap in the coronal and palatal directions to adapt and stabilize the soft tissue toward the root surface in its new position while avoiding dead spaces and zones of greater edema and clot formation. Many variations of this technique are used to achieve the goal. These sutures are generally attached to an interdental contact point created by a composite. Based on the severity of the recession, the sutures can be horizontal, oblique, or vertical. Once the design has been selected (horizontal, oblique, or vertical), suturing is initiated by inserting the needle from the apical to coronal part depending on the degree of displacement required, which could be at the level of the papilla base or apical to the last suture, and exiting almost from the vertex of the papilla. Thereafter, the needle is passed below the contact point and the short end is used to interweave it with the long end that goes in the palatal direction. The knot is tied at the coronal end toward the buccal or palatal area, taking care that the occlusion does not touch the knot and break it postoperatively (Fig. 31a, b) (Video 6).

8.6   Fixation Sutures

Fixation sutures are used to fix a membrane or CTG to a determined position for gingival recession treatment or gingival augmentation. These sutures unite the graft by anchoring to the periosteum, papilla, or the same flap in its internal area (Fig. 32).

8.7   Insertion Sutures

Insertion sutures are used in tunnel procedures for the placement of the CTGs inside them (Fig. 33).

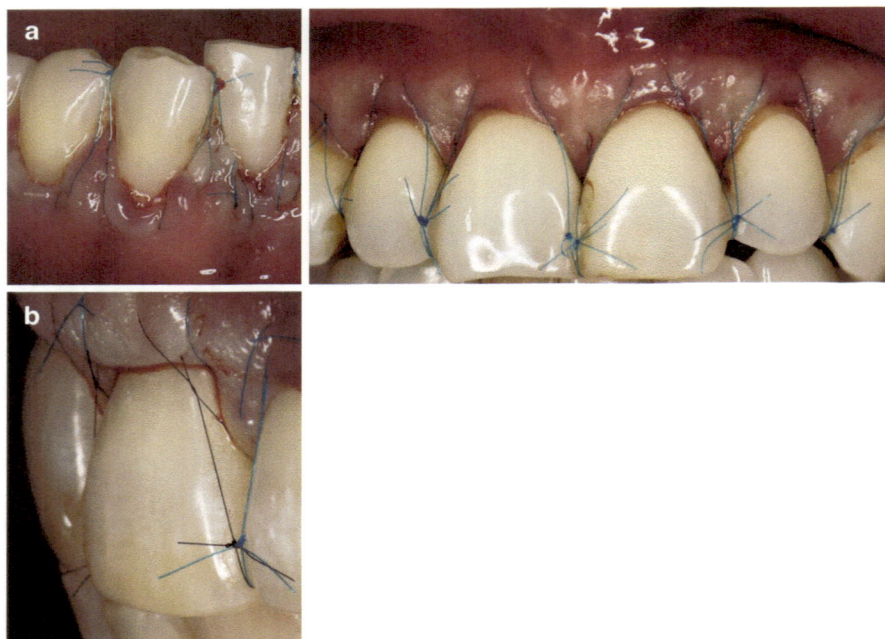

Fig. 31 (**a, b**) Point-of-contact sling sutures

Fig. 32 Fixation sutures
are used to fix CTG

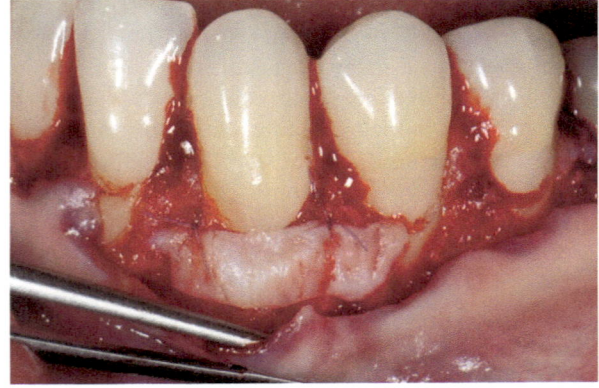

9   Treatment of Single Gingival Recessions

9.1   Trapezoidal Flap (CAF with Vertical Incisions)

The trapezoidal flap technique was described and modified by Zucchelli and De Sanctis in 2007 [25]. This design consists of two horizontal incisions of 3 mm in each papilla, and two slightly divergent vertical incisions in a trapezoidal shape (Fig. 34). An essential requirement for this technique is that the apical zone in relation to the recession should have at least 2 mm of keratinized gingiva.

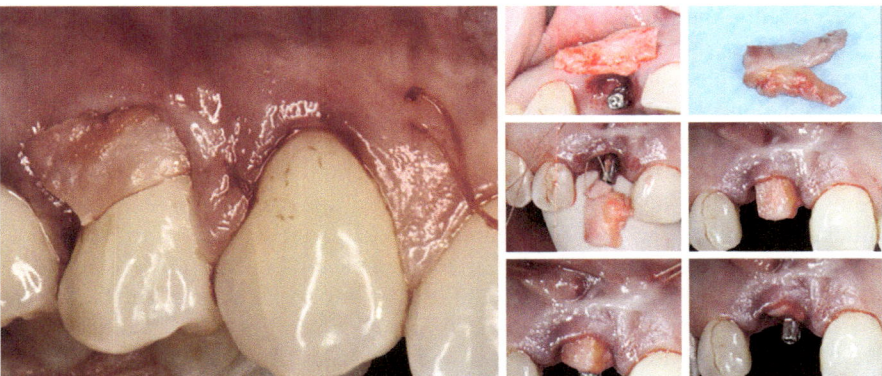

Fig. 33 Insertion sutures

Fig. 34 Trapezoidal flap (CAF with vertical incisions)

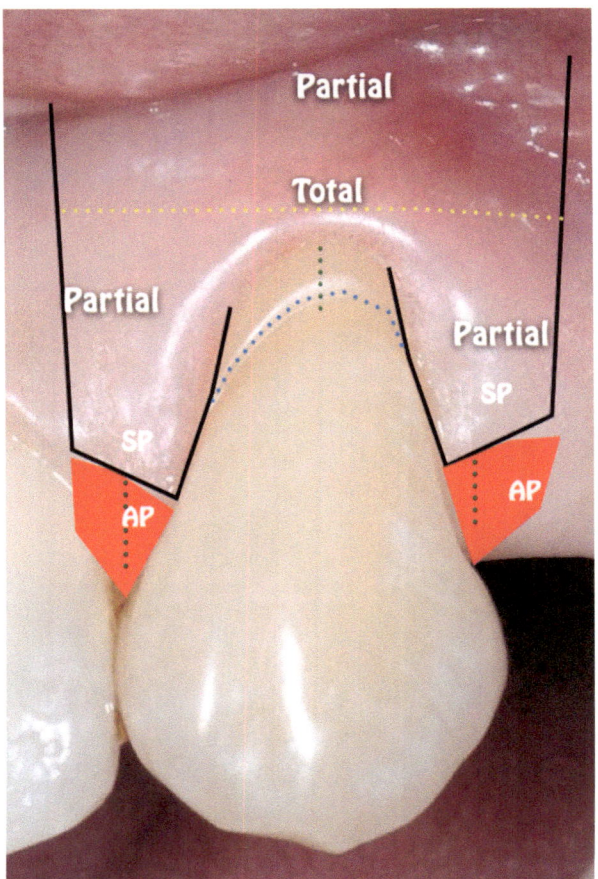

Horizontal incisions constitute the new surgical papilla (SP), and the position of these incisions depends on the degree of coronal displacement in relation to the depth of the recession being treated. The extension of coronal displacement is calculated and 1 mm is added in the coronal direction in relation to the CEJ to compensate for the postsurgical contraction of the gingival margin. Vertical incisions are made 3–4 mm along the mucogingival line. Thereafter, the SP should be removed from the underlying tissue as a partial thickness flap having consistent thickness, which is achieved by keeping the scalpel blade parallel to the osseous tissue. Once both the SP have been lifted, the apical part of the gingival margin is performed with a muco-periosteal elevator of complete thickness. The flap should be lifted approximately 3 mm apical to the residual bone crest. Thereafter, the vertical incisions are beveled toward the internal section of the flap, with the objective of leaving the periosteum on the surgical border and reducing the risk of scarring along the incision. To allow the flap to be passive and to be moved without tension, a deep incision parallel to the osseous tissue is made in the apical part of the flap to allow for the disinsertion of muscular and submucosal fibers of the periosteum. Further, a superficial incision is made parallel to the alveolar mucosa to detach the muscular insertions from the connective tissue of the alveolar mucosa (Fig. 35).

Fig. 35 Combined flap (partial/total/partial thickness)

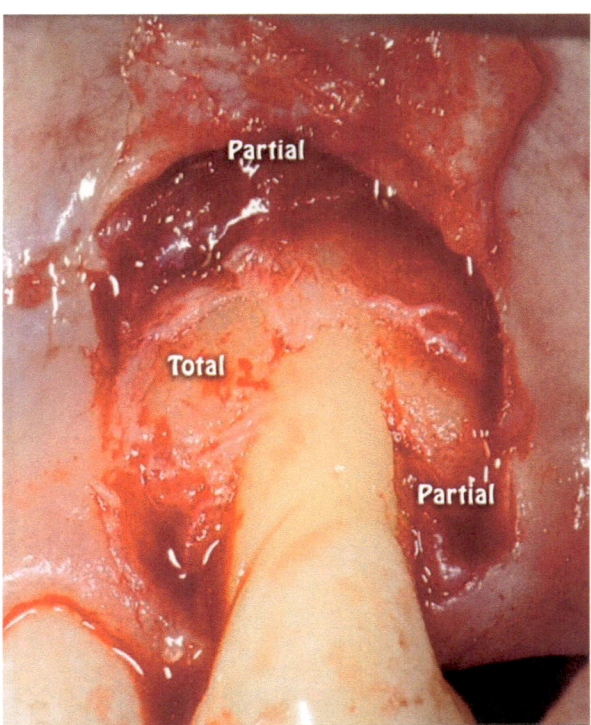

Fig. 36 Polypropylene 7/0 and 8/0 nylon sutures were used

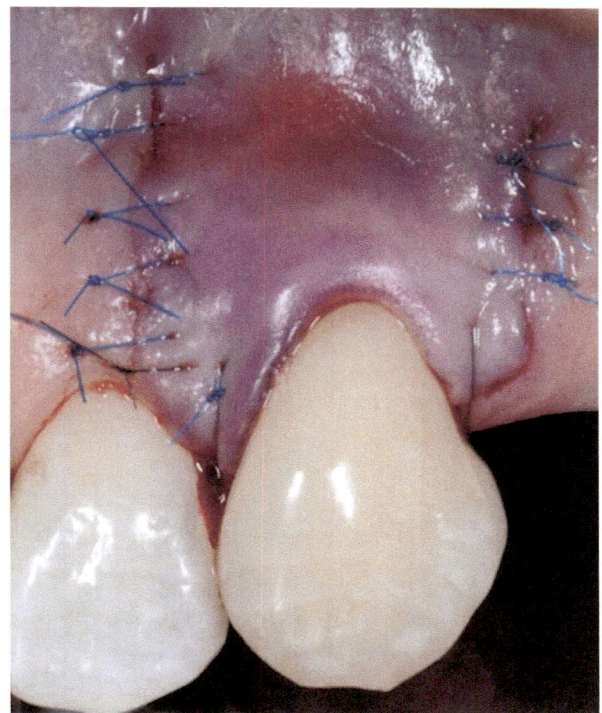

The biomodification of the root surface is performed by root planning while avoiding contact between the root surface and osseous deficiency to preserve the connective tissue fibers that are in the root cementum. Additionally, the root surface can be conditioned with the local application of ethylenediaminetetraacetic acid (EDTA, 24%) followed by irrigation with the Enamel matrix derivative (Emdogain Straumann, Basel, Switzerland), after the removal of EDTA.

The anatomical papilla (AP) is de-epithelized to expose the connective tissue that receives the internal connective tissue of the coronally displaced SP. This procedure can be made easier by using microsurgical tools such as Castroviejo scissors and microblades (Morita Micro 15c Kyoto, Japan).

First, the vertical incisions are sutured with simple closing sutures using 7/0 or 8/0 non-absorbable monofilament threads (Polypropylene, Nylon, AD Surgical Sunnyvale CA, USA) while keeping the bite size symmetrical. It is important to use needles with a length shorter than 8 mm to suture vertical incisions easily. Finally, a suspension suture is placed in the papilla base anchored to the palatine (Fig. 36) (Video 7).

The sutures are removed after 2 weeks (Fig. 37). Postsurgical evaluations are performed at 2 weeks, 4 weeks, 12 weeks, 6 months, and 12 months after the surgery (Figs. 38 and 39).

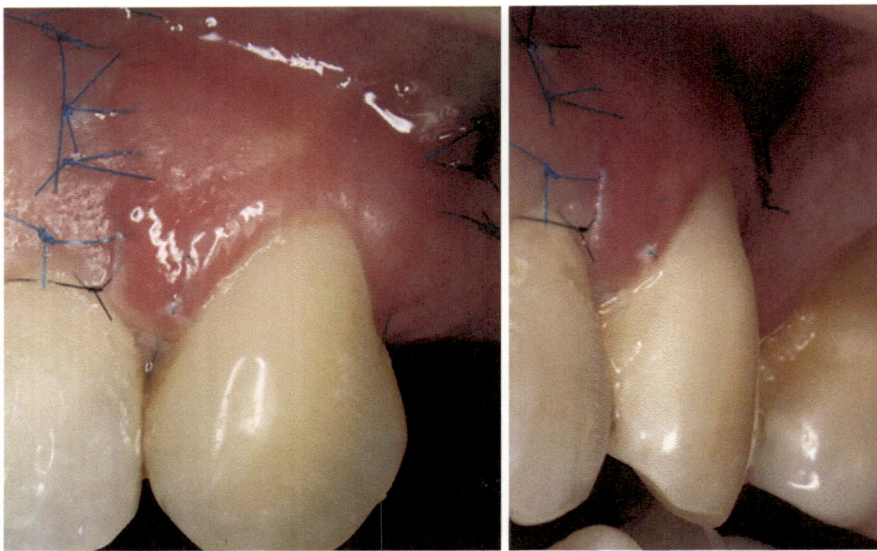

Fig. 37 The sutures are removed after 2 weeks

9.2   Laterally Moved CAF

The laterally moved CAF technique was described [26] and modified by Zucchelli and De Sanctis [27]. This flap design has many characteristics in common with the trapezoidal CAF. The main requirement of this technique is that the donor zone adjacent to the recession should have 3 mm of keratinized gingiva from the apical to coronal region and 6 mm in the meso-distal region plus the width of the recession being treated (Fig. 40). This technique is not recommended when the esthetic demands of the patient are high.

The approach to the flap is partial/total/partial. This creates the SP1 that is laterally advanced or in some cases is moved in the coronal direction. The mesial papilla AP1 is de-epithelized to expose the connective tissue and unite it with the internal area of the connective tissue of the pedicle. The suturing method is the same as in the trapezoidal flap technique, starting with the vertical incisions from apical to coronal region and ending with a suspension suture from the base of the SP1 to the base of the AP1 anchored to the palatal aspect of the tooth. Polypropylene 7/0 and 8/0 nylon sutures were used (Polypropylene, Nylon, AD Surgical Sunnyvale CA, USA) (Figs. 41, 42, 43, 44, 45, 46, 47, and 48) (Video 8).

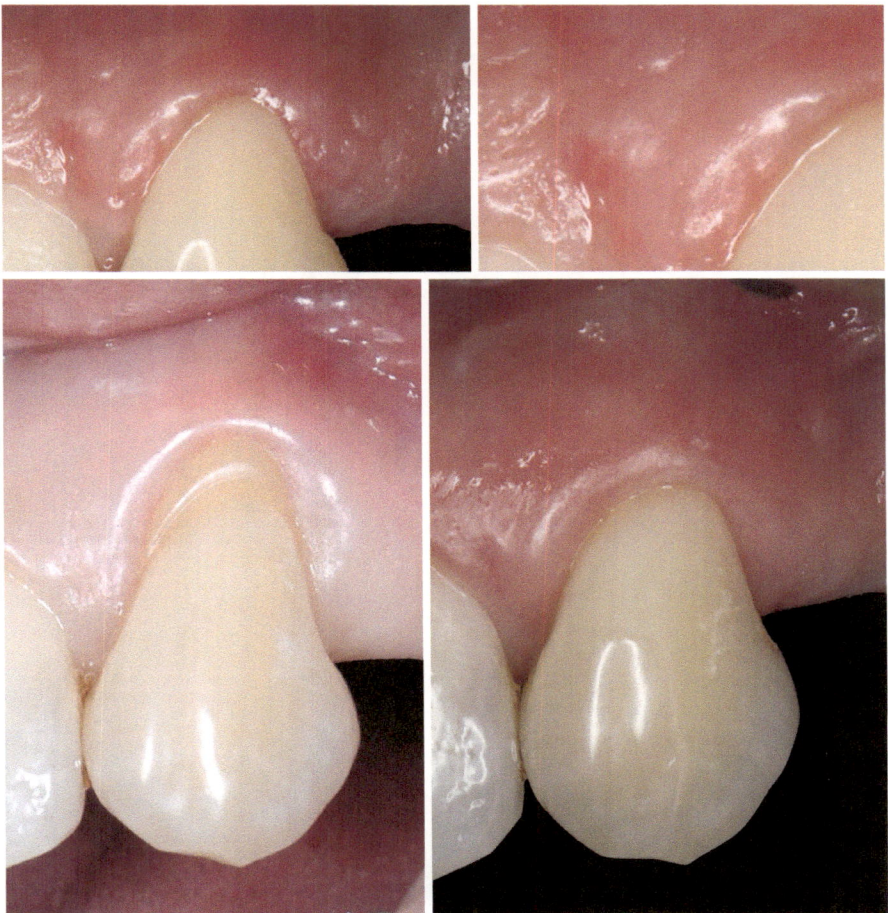

Fig. 38 Postsurgical evaluations are performed at 6 months after the surgery

9.3 CAF in Envelope Without Vertical Incision

This approach is the modification of the CAF for multiple teeth described by Zucchelli and De Sanctis in 2000 [28]. Oblique incisions are made at the papilla level to create the SP, and a partial/total/partial thickness flap is created to achieve the displacement and passivity of the flap. In this case, a bilaminar technique with CTG is used (Fig. 49). Evaluation is performed at 3 months after surgery (Fig. 50).

Fig. 39 Postsurgical evaluations are performed at 12 months after the surgery

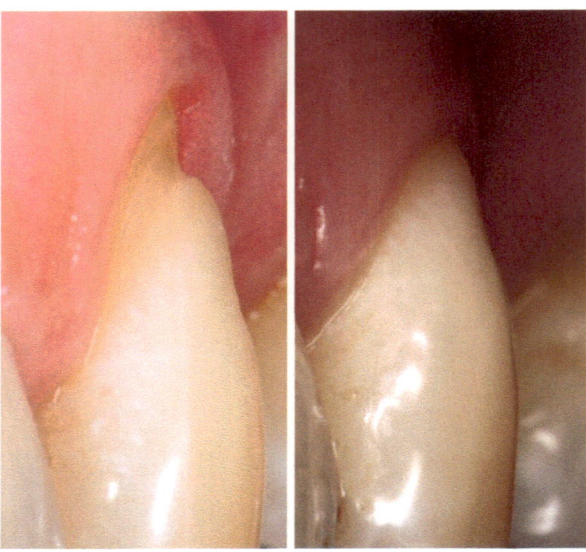

Fig. 40 Flap design laterally moved CAF

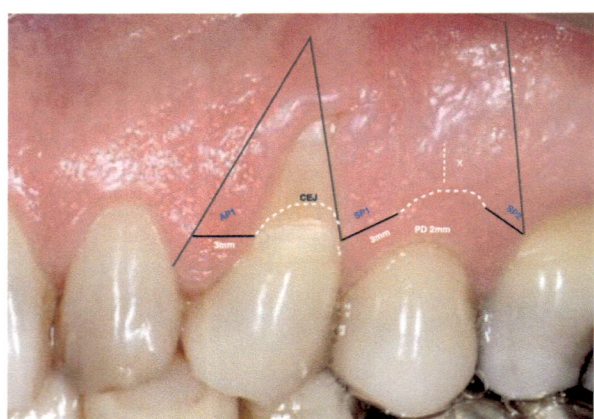

9.4   Envelope Without Incision

The envelope without incision technique was described by Raetzke in 1985 [29] and modified by Allen in 1994 [30], the first procedure without flap for root covering of single recessions. This technique was modified to increase flap mobility to displace it coronally and enhance the suture techniques at the same end. An incision-free procedure enhances the vascularization of the flap and graft and avoids scarring.

Patient after RT1 Cairo orthodontic treatment with the modified envelope technique and CTG (Fig. 51a–c) (Video 9).

Fig. 41 Polypropylene 7/0 and 8/0 nylon sutures were used

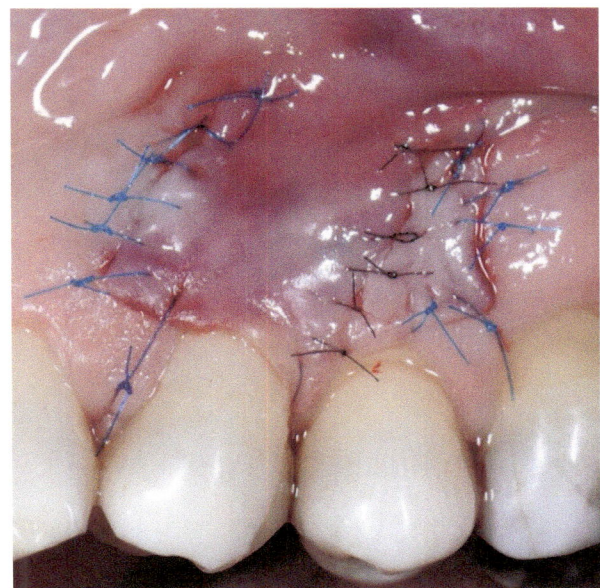

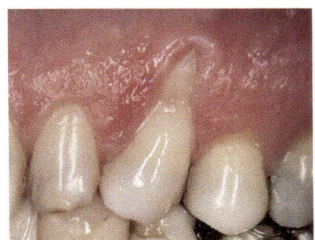
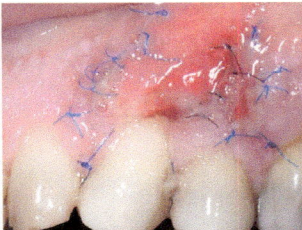
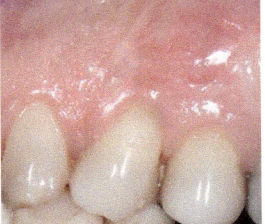

Fig. 42 Postsurgical evaluations at 7 days and 6 months after surgery

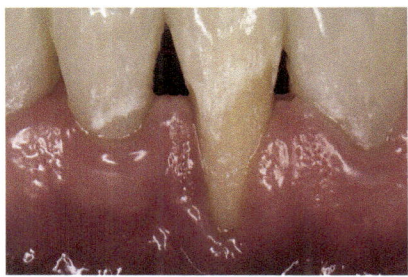
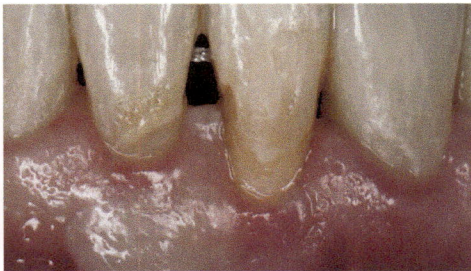

Fig. 43 Post-orthodontic treatment, type 2 Cairo recession, and a displaced lateral flap

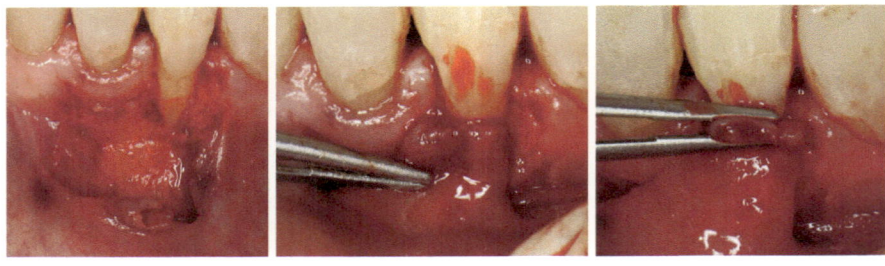

Fig. 44 De-epithelized grafting CTG with 7/0 sutures

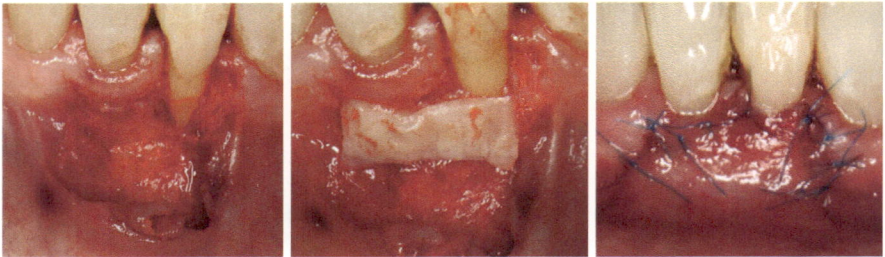

Fig. 45 7/0 polypropylene sutures

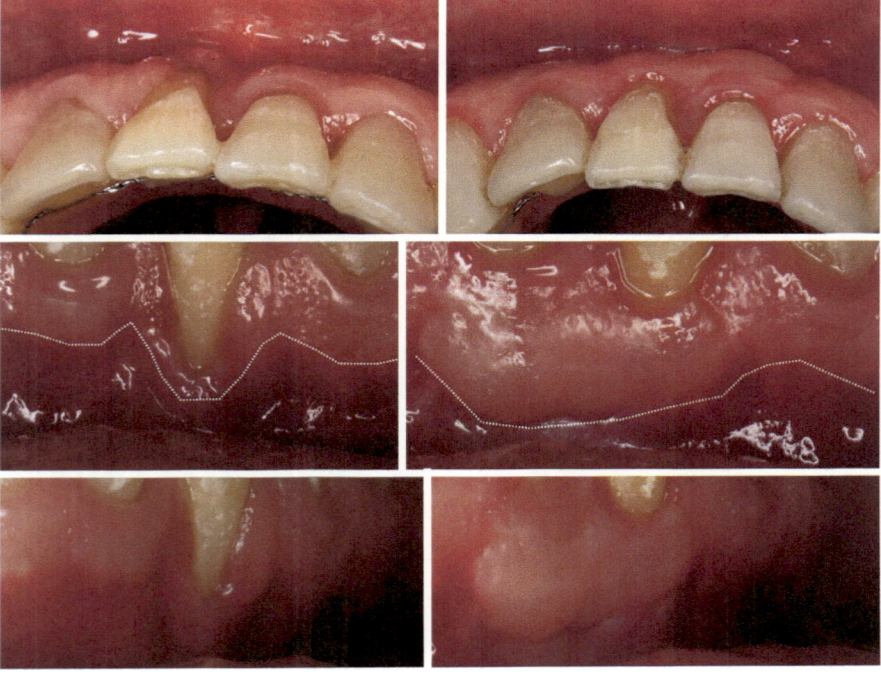

Fig. 46 Evaluation at 6 months after surgery

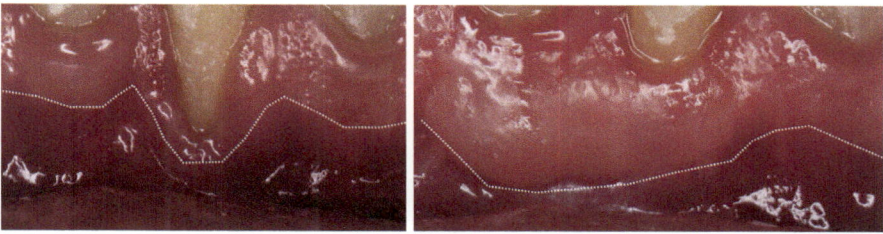

Fig. 47 Evaluation of a displaced lateral flap with a CTG at 5 years after surgery

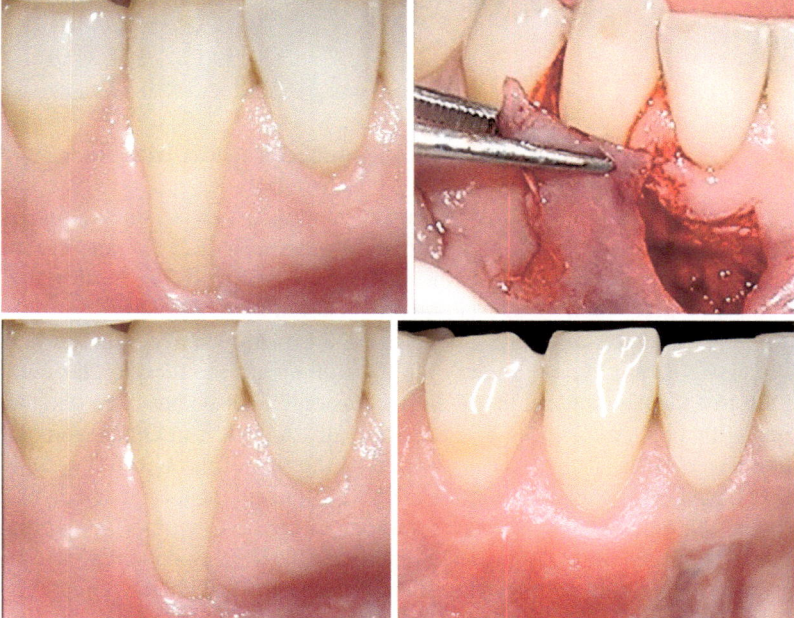

Fig. 48 Evaluation of the patient who received post-orthodontic treatment with displaced lateral flap and CTG at 5 years after surgery

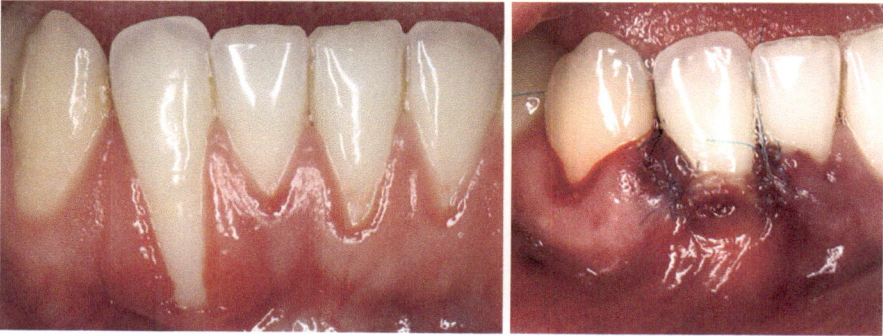

Fig. 49 In this case, a bilaminar technique with CTG is used

Fig. 50 Evaluation is
performed at 3 months
after surgery

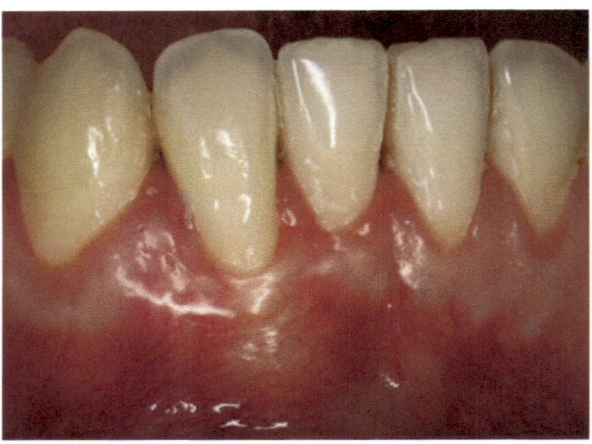

Fig. 50 Evaluation is performed at 3 months after surgery

9.5   Laterally Closed Tunnel for Isolated Mandibular Recession

The laterally closed tunnel for isolated mandibular recession technique was described by Sculean [31] and modified by Carranza [32]. It was specifically designed for deep and ideally narrow isolated recessions (RT1, 2) in mandibular incisors. It involves making of a supraperiosteal tunnel with microsurgical tools: a microscalpel microblade tunnel (Keydent ADS system Munich, Germany), micro papilla elevator, and microtunnelers. An incision parallel to the alveolar mucosa is made to free the submucosal tissue until a tensionless tissue has been obtained and the recession being treated can be closed laterally. A graft is obtained from the connective tissue of the palate and is inserted in the tunnel through 6/0 polyglycolic acid (PGA, AD Surgical Sunnyvale CA, USA) sutures in the mesial and distal directions, and the recession borders are sutured over the CTG with 7/0 polypropylene sutures (Polypropylene, AD Surgical Sunnyvale CA, USA) with simple stitches and border approximation knotting. Thus, the graft is submerged in the tunnel (Fig. 52).

10   Treatment of Multiple Gingival Recessions

There are two types of approaches for the treatment of multiple recessions: the CAF in the envelope [28] and the modified tunneling [24, 33, 34].

10.1   CAF in Envelope

The design of the displaced coronal flap is based on oblique incisions made in the papilla from the base of the papilla to the vertex, taking the point of greater recession as a reference as the axis of greater rotation of the flap. In this case, it is the lateral one. Each oblique incision created a SP [28] (Fig. 53). A partial/total/partial thickness flap was made, using the same protocol described in the trapezoidal flap, to achieve coronal displacement and passivity. Before suturing, the anatomical

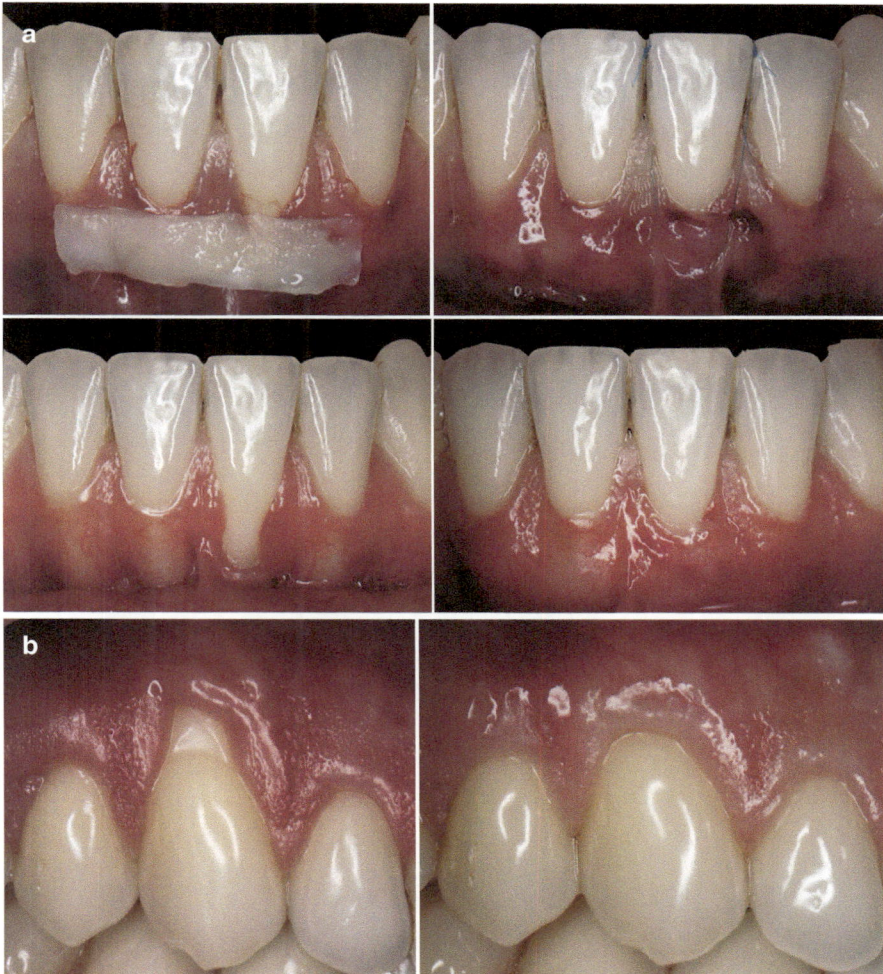

Fig. 51 (**a**) Patient after RT1 Cairo orthodontic treatment with the modified envelope technique and CTG. (**b**, **c**) Postsurgical evaluations at 5 years after surgery

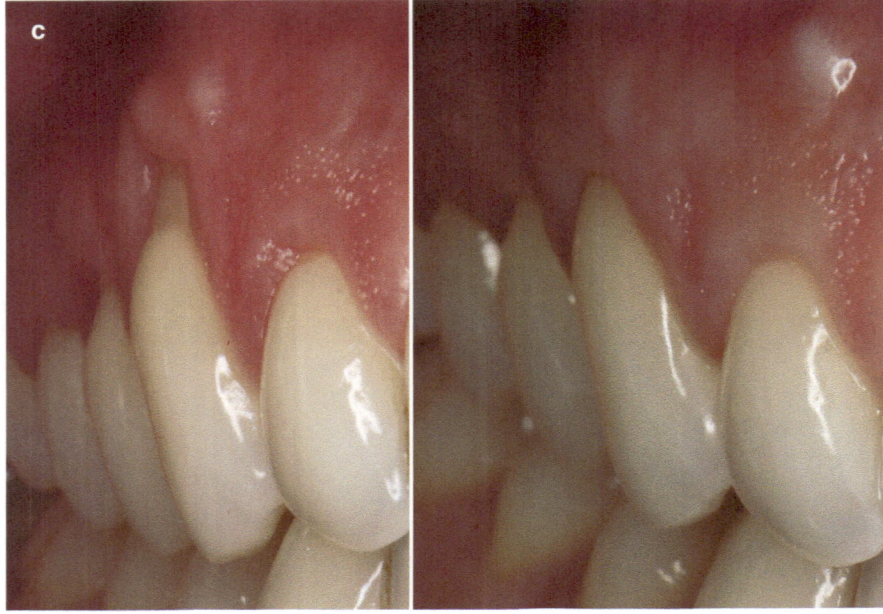

Fig. 7 (continued)

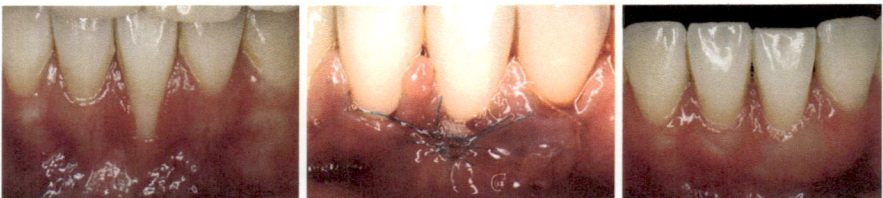

Fig. 52 Laterally closed tunnel for isolated mandibular recession

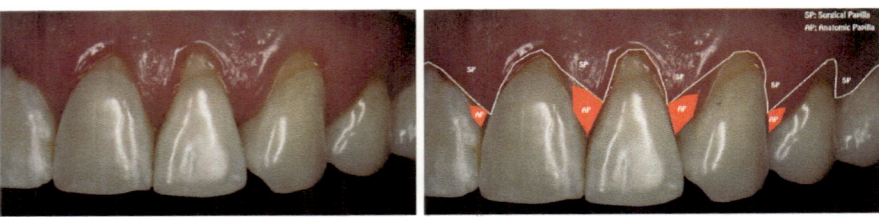

Fig. 53 Flap design CAF in envelope

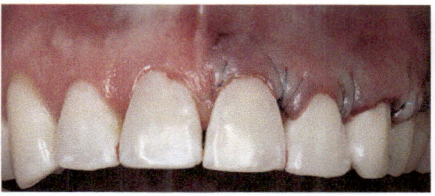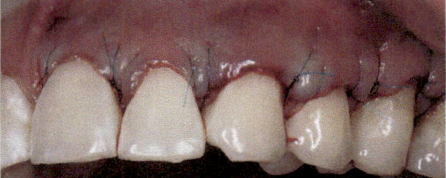

Fig. 54 Immediate postsurgical

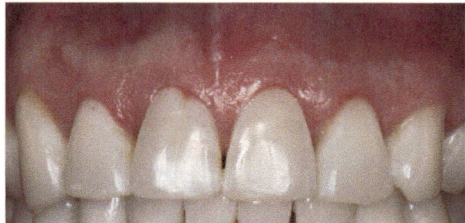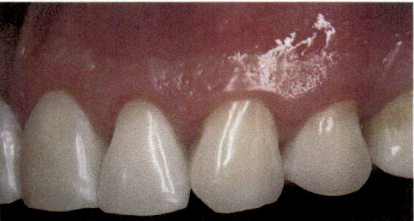

Fig. 55 Evaluation performed at 6 months after surgery

papilla was de-epithelized to receive the connective tissue of the SP and sutured with suspension sutures (7/0 polypropylene sutures) (Polypropylene, AD Surgical Sunnyvale CA, USA) to palatine from the base of the SP to the base of the anatomical papilla (Figs. 54, 55, 56, and 57; Video 10).

10.2   Modified Tunnel

Modified tunnelling technique was described by Azzi and Etienne [24] in 1998, popularized by Zabalegui [33] in 1999 and modified by Zuhr [34] in 2007. It consists of making a tunnel through intrasulcular, continuing with a mucosal partial thickness flap (supraperiosteal technique), encompassing the entire adhered gingiva. At the mucogingival line, a dissection is made to free the submucosal and muscular tissues and to achieve the necessary mobility to displace the flap in the coronal direction. Another important aspect is the freedom of the base of the papillae, which should be created in a delicate and careful manner (micro papilla elevator Mamadent Micro 005 papilla elevator ADS system Munich, Germany), without touching the tip, palatinal, or lingual part of the papilla. A greater flap mobility is achieved in this manner.

The use of micro-tools specially designed for this purpose (microtunnelers, microelevators, micro papilla elevators, and microscalpels for tunneling Mamadent ADS system Munich, Germany) is essential because they ensure a clean, minimally invasive technique with a low risk of piercing the gingiva and mucosa (Figs. 58 and 59).

The suture technique should be based on immobilization of the flap, which has been displaced several millimeters in the coronal direction from its initial position.

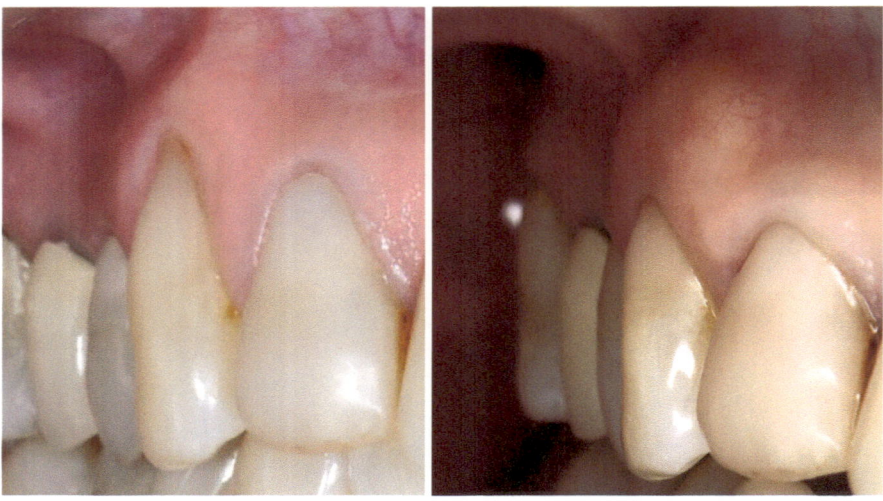

Fig. 56 Evaluation performed at 1 year after surgery

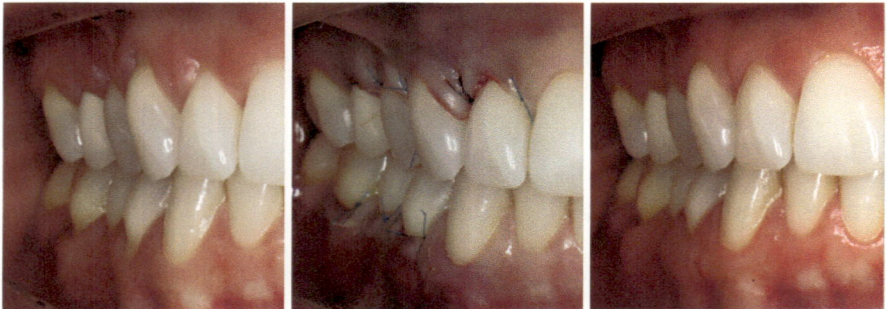

Fig. 57 Evaluation before and after 1 year of surgery with coronal advanced flap

Suspension sutures are usually anchored to the contact point (intentionally or provisionally made with a flowable composite in the most incisal section close to the contact point). This suturing technique involves introduction of the needle from the base of the recession toward the papilla as close as possible to the vertex, where the needle exits the vestibular site. Thereafter, the needle is grabbed at its base, weaved underneath the contact point, and knotted in the incisal section close to the contact point. Before knotting, it is important to ensure that the short end of the suture is underneath the long end and that the suture applies a strength vector toward the coronal and palatine zones. In addition, 7/0 polypropylene sutures are used (Polypropylene, AD Surgical Sunnyvale CA, USA) (Fig. 60).

The orientation of the suture at the level of the papilla can be vertical, horizontal, or oblique depending on the depth of the recession (Fig. 61). Oblique orientation is recommended for deeper recessions, whereas vertical and horizontal orientations

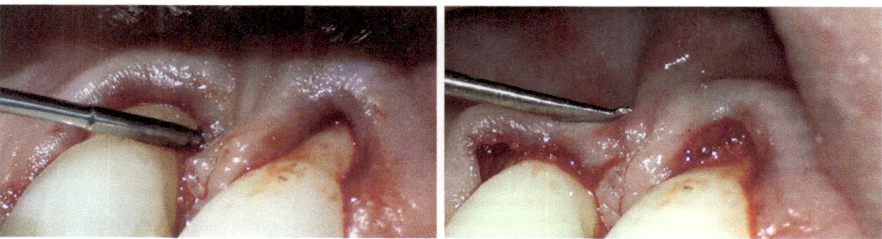

Fig. 58 Microtunnelers, micro papilla elevators, Mamadent Micro 005 papilla elevator ADS system Munich, Germany for tunneling

Fig. 59 Microtunnelers, micro papilla elevators, Mamadent Micro 005 papilla elevator ADS system Munich, Germany for tunneling

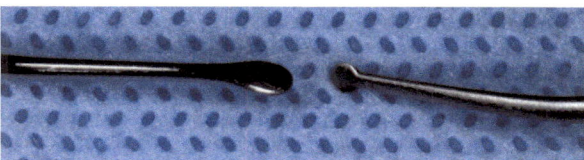

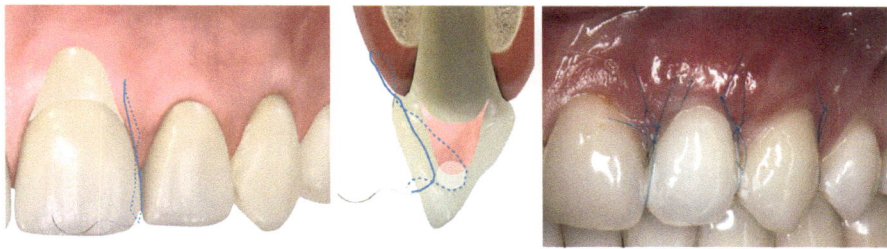

Fig. 60 Point-of-contact sling sutures, 7/0 polypropylene sutures are used

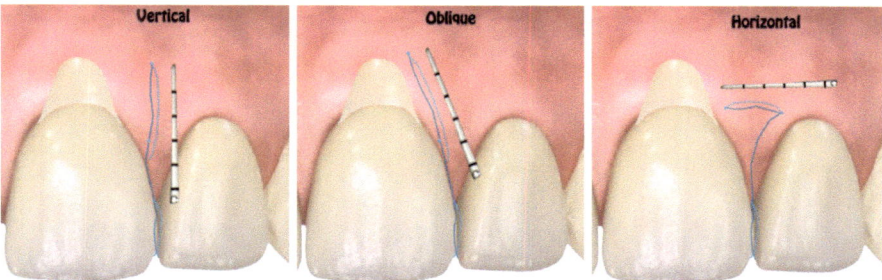

Fig. 61 The orientation of the suture at the level of the papilla can be vertical, horizontal, or oblique depending on the depth of the recession

are recommended for not so deep recessions. (Figs. 62, 63, 64, 65, 66, 67, 68, 69, 70, 71, 72, 73, 74, and 75; Videos 11 and 12).

Fig. 62 Female patient with multiple type I recessions and darkening of the central 2.1

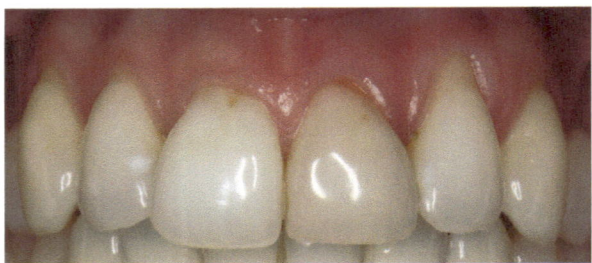

Fig. 63 Tunneling with connective tissue grafting in the lateral zone 2.2

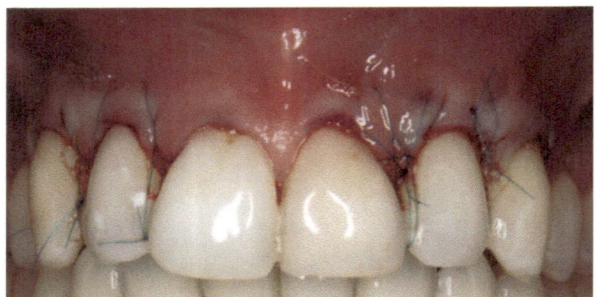

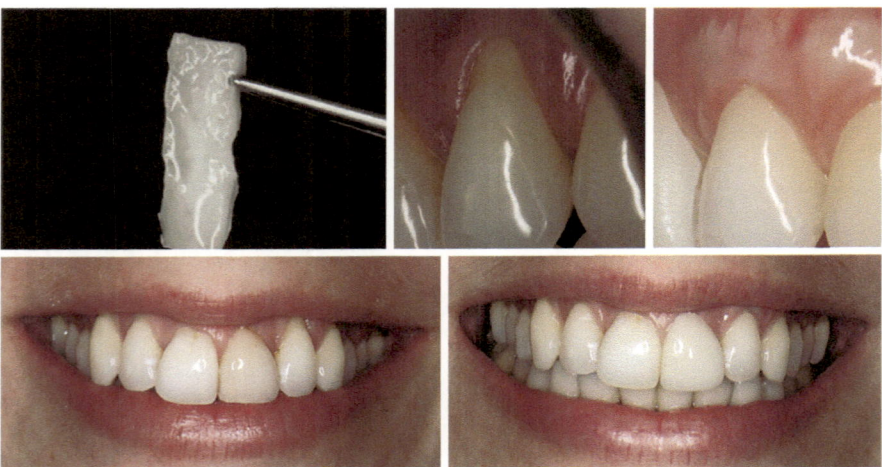

Fig. 64 Evaluation performed at 1 year after surgery

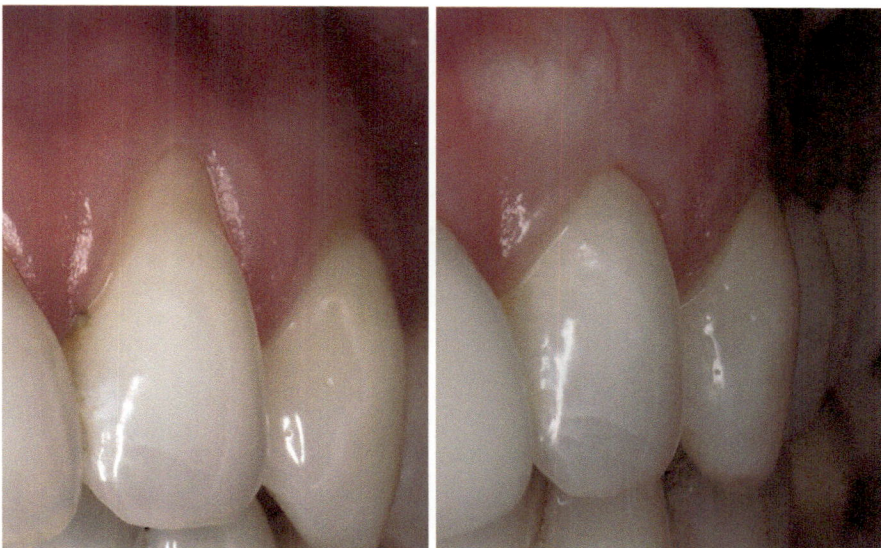

Fig. 65 Lateral view at 1 year after surgery

Fig. 66 Female patient
with multiple type I
recessions and non-carious
cervical lesions treated
with a displaced coronal
flap and ceramic veneers.
Evaluation after 5 years of
treatment

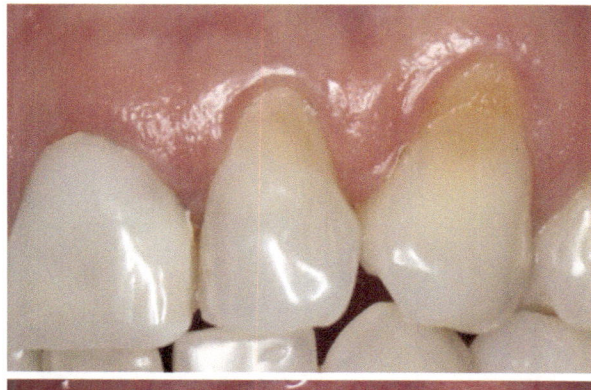

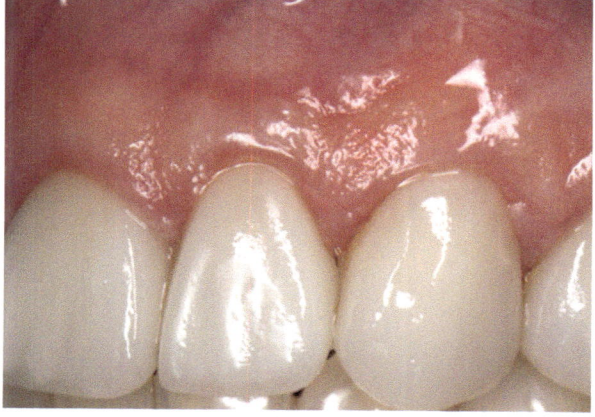

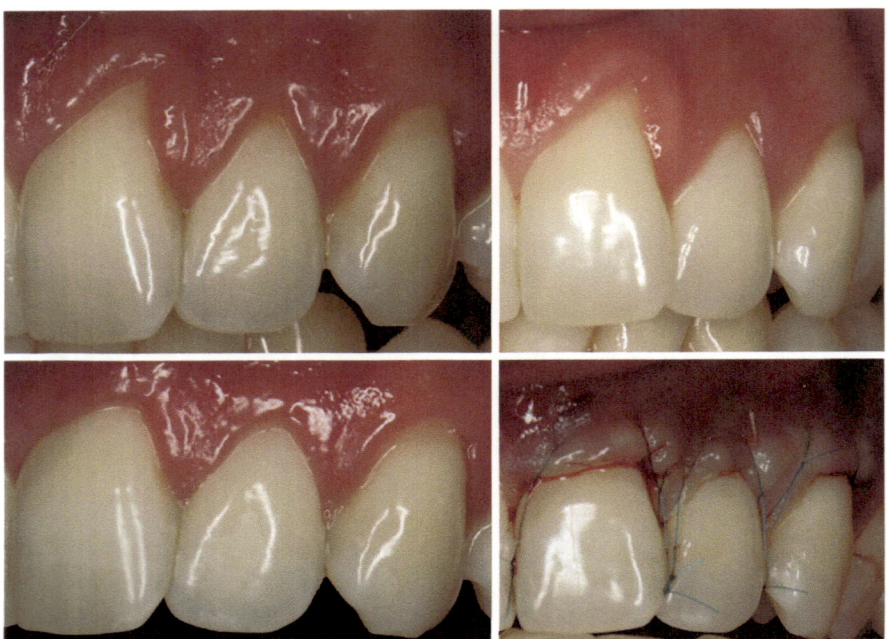

Fig. 67 Male patient with multiple type I recessions treated with tunneling and connective tissue graft post-orthodontic treatment. Evaluation after 1 year of treatment

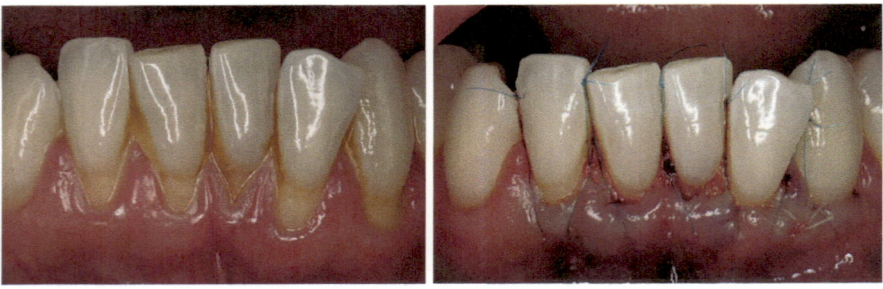

Fig. 68 Female patient with multiple type I recession treated with tunneling and connective tissue graft

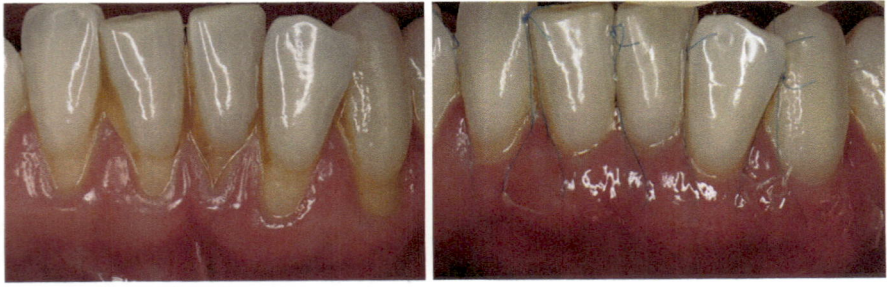

Fig. 69 Evaluation at 6 months after treatment

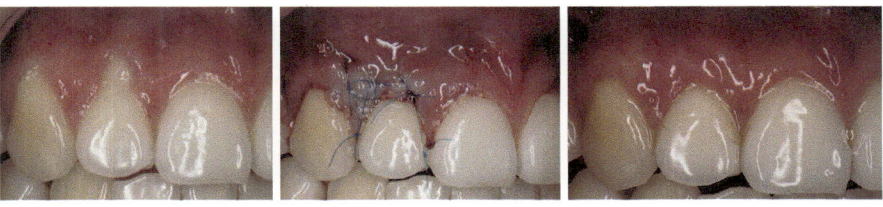

Fig. 70 Female patients with multiple type I recessions treated with tunneling and connective tissue graft

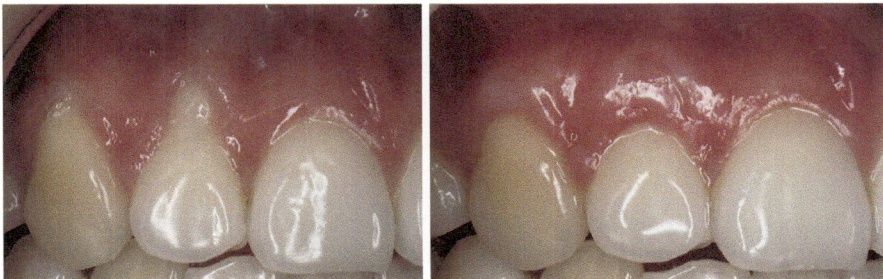

Fig. 71 Evaluation after 6 months of treatment

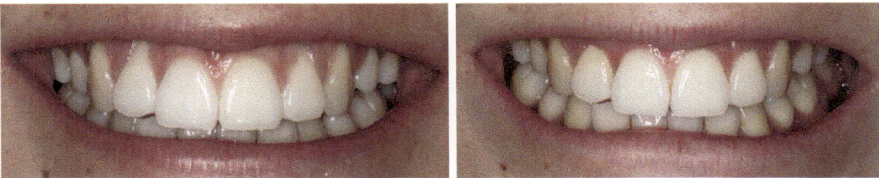

Fig. 72 Evaluation after 6 months of treatment

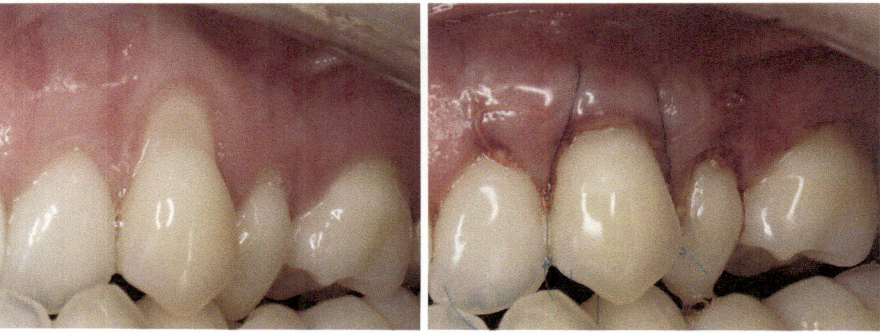

Fig. 73 Female patient with multiple type I recessions treated with tunneling and connective tissue graft

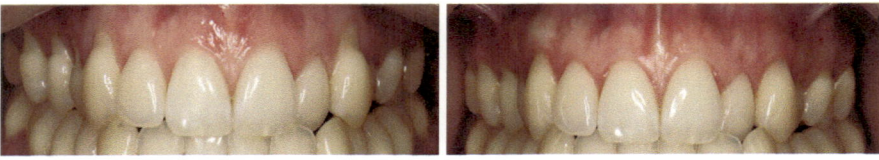

Fig. 74 Evaluation after 6 months of treatment

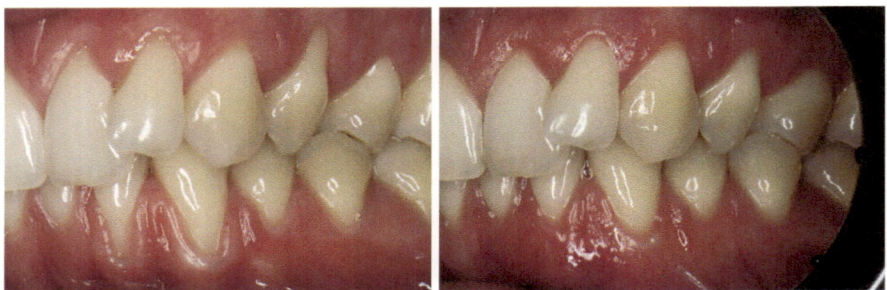

Fig. 75 Male patient with multiple type I recessions treated with tunneling and connective tissue graft. Evaluation after 1 year of treatment

11   Microscope-Assisted Autograft Harvesting

Autologous connective tissue is the ideal tissue to reconstruct soft tissue defects such as root and peri-implant covering, increased toothless ridge, and prosthetic gingival thickening among others [35, 36]. The grip on the graft with the use of magnification and illumination provided by a surgical microscope aids in the identification of the type of intervened tissue and to create a more symmetrical graft in thickness and size, which is an essential requirement for its survival. Although working in the palatine area with a microscope is not very comfortable for the operator, it is recommended to have and use pivotal objectives and slanted optics. This allows the microsurgeon to maintain an upright comfortable position at all times, independent of the angle in the oral cavity, which makes the position and access to the palate easier.

There are mainly three techniques to obtain a graft of palate connective tissue:

11.1   Trapdoor Technique

This technique was described by Edel et al. [35] in the year 1974. It involves the creation of a partial thickness flap with a horizontal incision (same size as that of the graft in a meso-distal sense) and two vertical incisions (at least 2 mm away from the gingival margin and apically extending 1 mm beyond the graft in the apico-coronal direction). All of the initial incisions should be perpendicular, and the thickness of the graft should be determined by the horizontal incision (approx. 1 mm). At that point, the angle of the scalpel blade is changed and is made parallel to the tissue, while ensuring that the thickness is consistent throughout the whole graft, horizontal incisions meet vertical incisions, and connective tissue is removed. Finally, the access flap is sutured with simple interrupted 7/0 polypropylene sutures (Polypropylene, AD Surgical Sunnyvale CA, USA).

11.2   Envelope Technique

The envelope technique was first described by Hurzeler et al. [36] and modified by Lorenzana et al. [37]. This technique involves a single horizontal incision, through which a flap of partial thickness is created to access the subepithelial connective tissue. In this technique, the thickness of the soft tissue of the palate should not be less than 3 mm (Fig. 76).

The horizontal incision should be 4 mm greater than the meso-distal width of the graft and the envelope should be at least 2 or 3 mm apical to the apico-coronal limit of the graft. A horizontal incision is made 2 mm away from the gingival margin (Fig. 77). Thereafter, a second incision is made parallel to the tissue by changing the direction of the scalpel to create an envelope. After the envelope has been created, the deep surface is accessed and through three incisions (horizontal, coronal, and apical) that meet the vertical incision, the connective tissue graft is obtained (Fig. 78).

The donating area is sutured with suspension sutures with crossed teeth or horizontal mattress sutures as reported by Borguetti [24] (Fig. 79).

11.3   Connective Tissue Graft (De-epithelialized Epithelium)

This technique is a modification of the free epithelial graft [38], is recommended when the palate thickness is not sufficient (<3 mm) to obtain connective tissue using other techniques. A free epithelized graft was dissected through a horizontal

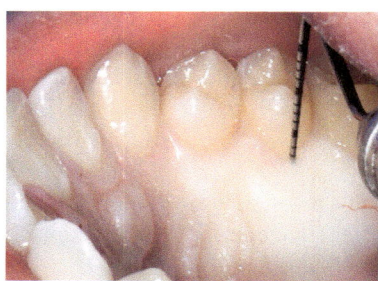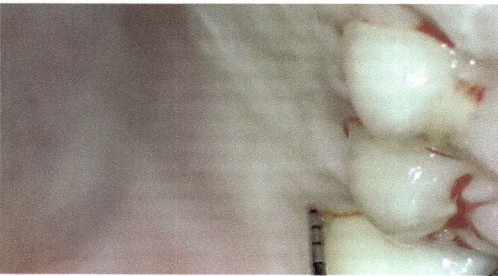

Fig. 76 The thickness of the soft tissue of the palate should not be less than 3 mm

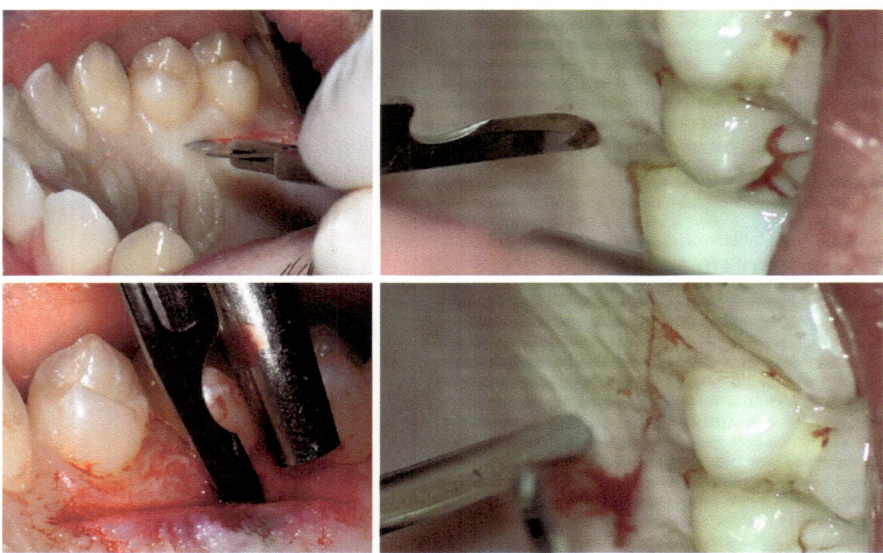

Fig. 77 The horizontal incision

incision 2 mm away from the gingival margin. The angle of the scalpel blade should be perpendicular to the osseous tissue and the depth should be according to the thickness of the required tissue (1–1.5 mm). The length of the meso-distal part of the incision depends on the size of the desired graft, which depends on the wound being treated. Thus, vertical incisions (mesial and distal) are made according to the size of the desired graft. Thereafter, the blade is rotated within the horizontal incision and made parallel to the osseous tissue. The graft is excised from the meso-coronal corner and through the length of the horizontal coronal incision to the meso-apical corner (Fig. 80). It is important to ensure that the graft is of the same thickness and size. Lastly, the apical horizontal incision is made by bringing together the apical part of the vertical incisions to release the graft.

The epithelial layer of the graft is removed under a magnification of more than 6× to be able to differentiate between the epithelium (appears shining when illuminated) and the connective tissue (appears dull when illuminated). The epithelium is removed using a new blade placed parallelly to the external surface of the graft. The epithelial (rough) tissue and connective (soft) tissue can be differentiated based on the appearance (Fig. 81; Video 13).

The donating area is sutured with suspension sutures with crossed teeth or horizontal mattress sutures (Fig. 82).

The exposed area of the palate is protected with a resorbable collagen membrane and is sutured to immobilize it for greater postoperative comfort. An acrylic stent can be used to protect the palate for 7 days (Fig. 83).

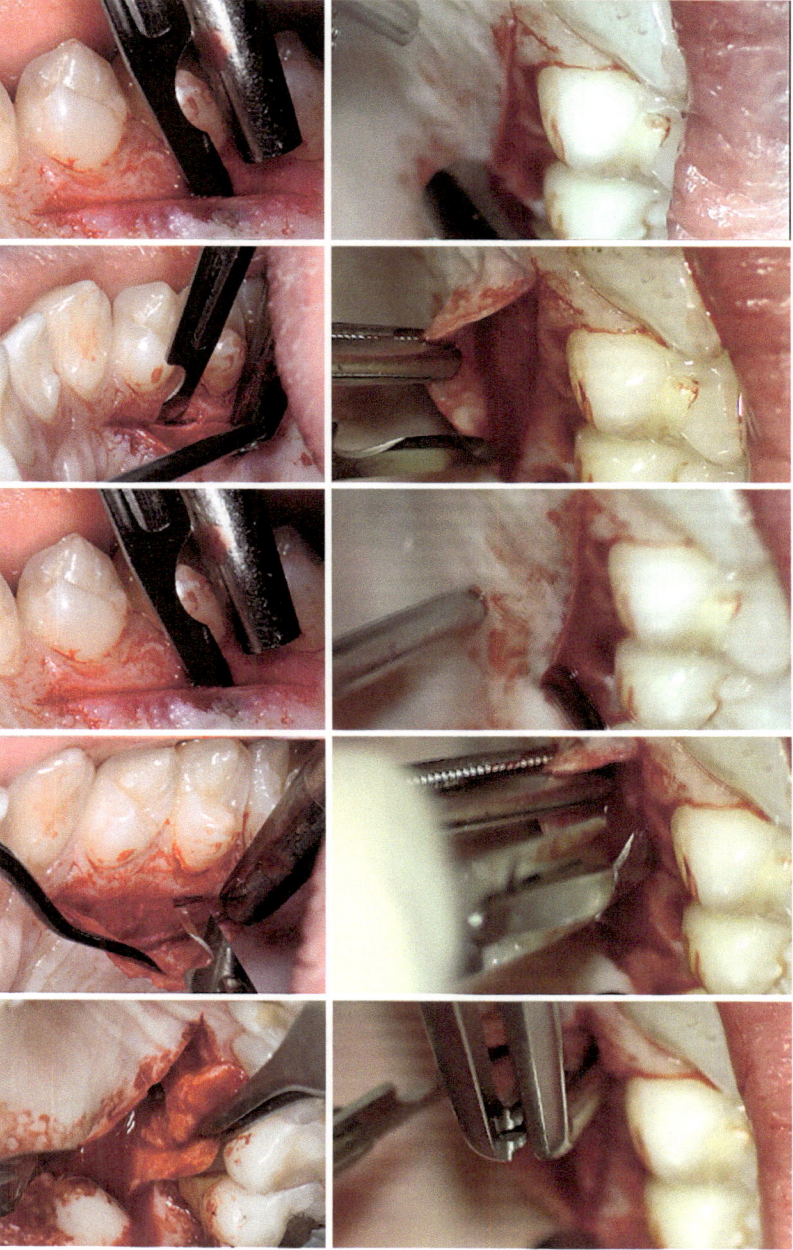

Fig. 78 Thereafter, a second incision is made parallel to the tissue by changing the direction of the scalpel to create an envelope. After the envelope has been created, the deep surface is accessed and through three incisions (horizontal, coronal, and apical) that meet the vertical incision, the connective tissue graft is obtained

Fig. 79 The donating area is sutured with suspension sutures with crossed teeth or horizontal mattress sutures as reported by Borguetti

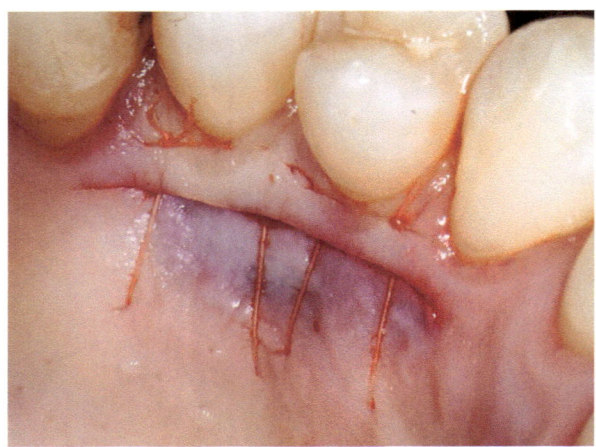

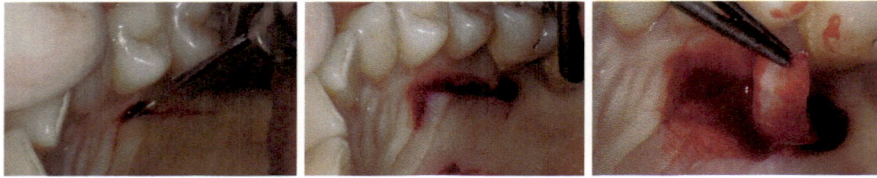

Fig. 80 The graft is excised from the meso-coronal corner and through the length of the horizontal coronal incision to the meso-apical corner

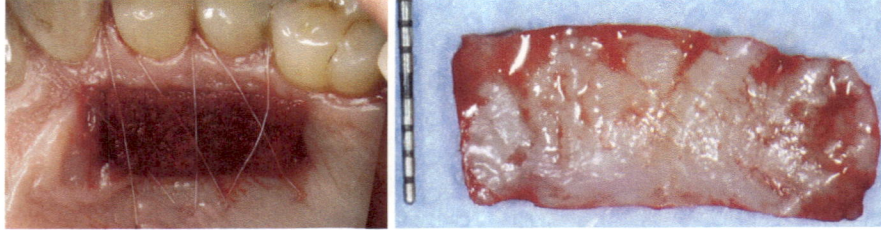

Fig. 81 The epithelial (rough) tissue and connective (soft) tissue can be differentiated based on the appearance

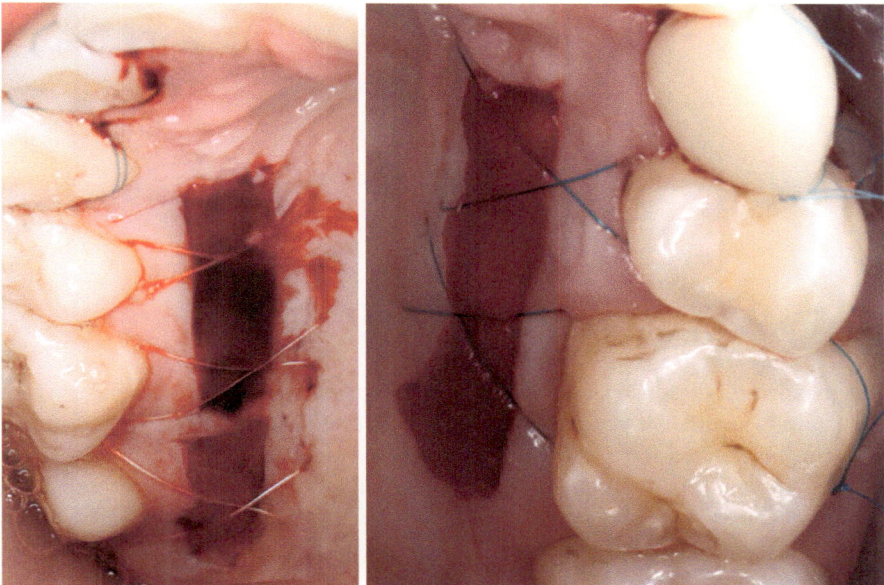

Fig. 82 The donating area is sutured with suspension sutures with crossed teeth or horizontal mattress sutures

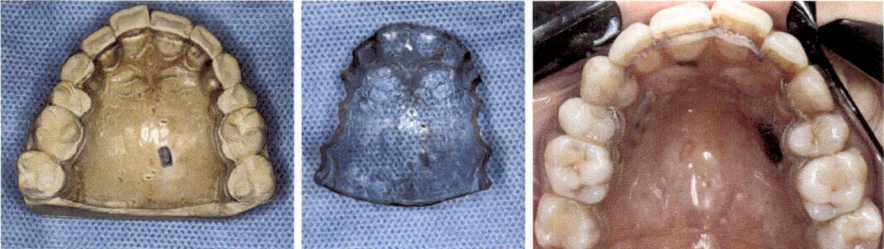

Fig. 83 An acrylic stent can be used to protect the palate for 7 days

12   Treating Non-carious Cervical Lesions Associated with Gingival Recessions Defects

12.1   Classification of Root Defects

The effects of the tooth surface or CEJ are described in the literature as non-carious cervical lesions (NCCLs) [39]. In many cases, the CEJ cannot be recognized when NCCLs occur. This is a clinical problem given that the CEJ acts as a reference point for the diagnosis and treatment of gingival recessions [40]. The absence of an identifiable CEJ can be because of erosion, abrasion, and abfraction, resulting in

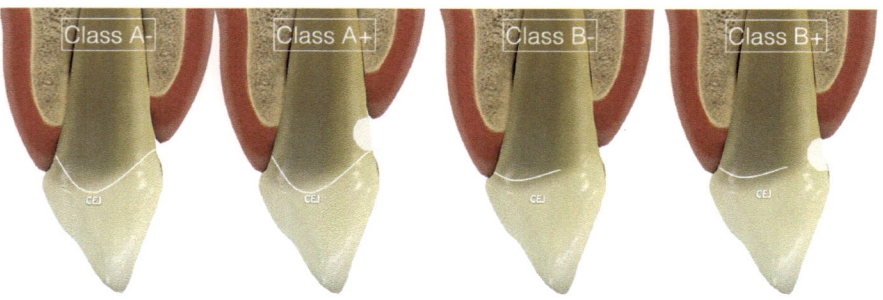

Fig. 84 Classification of root defects

diagnostic problems as well as serious surgical challenges when the root surface is structurally significantly affected [41]. Piniprato et al. [42] described a classification system for affected tooth surface in the areas of gingival recession. Based on the visual presence (A) or absence (B) of the CEJ and the presence (+) or absence (−) of a tooth surface discrepancy caused by the loss of tissue, there are four possible classes (A+, A−, B+, and B−) (Fig. 84).

12.2 Digitally Guided Root Coverage Predetermination: A Multidisciplinary Approach

The absence of an identifiable CEJ can be because of erosion, abrasion, and abfraction, resulting in diagnostic problems as well as serious surgical challenges when the root surface is structurally significantly affected [43]. The ideal treatment for crown-radicular NCCL should be a combination of restorative and periodontal treatments. Different approaches have been presented in terms of the sequence of clinical actions that should be performed to achieve a successful outcome. However, completing the restorative therapy before mucogingival surgery has been found to have several clinical advantages for both procedures: restorations can be easily performed and finished in an isolated field with no interference of the soft tissues. In addition, root coverage surgery is facilitated by the reconstruction of the emergence profile of the clinical crown, which provides a stable, smooth, and convex anatomy for surgical flap repositioning [44, 45]. The main objective of a periodontal surgical procedure for esthetic root coverage is to adequately reposition soft tissues to reproduce an ideal and natural emergence profile and thereby protect the underlying structures. Although different authors have proposed different techniques to treat this type of defect, there is no consensus on treatment protocols for a deep cavity (≥3 mm) beyond the CEJ (Fig. 85a). Zucchelli et al. [45] defined topographically the maximum root coverage after a mucogingival surgical correction (Fig. 85b). This maximum line of root covering substitutes the CEJ when it is not clinically detectable or the conditions for a complete covering are absent (e.g., complete height of the papilla). Although factors such as the partial loss of the height of the papilla, dental rotation, extrusion, and occlusal abrasion should be considered for pre-surgical analysis. The most common mistake is not being able to establish the location of the CEJ in the recession zone and mistaking it for abrasion. Hence, the use of a 20× high magnification microscope is essential because it allows us to clearly differentiate between tissues, enamel and dentin, root surface, presence of cervical lesions, cavities, and restorations (Video 14). Generally, the CEJ is a curved and convex line, unlike abrasion lines that are flat and concave. In the absence of the CEJ, it is recommended to reconstruct it using one of the various methods available [45, 46].

A chart illustrating the decision-making process for treating NCCLs associated with gingival recessions is presented (modified Zucchelli [43]) (Fig. 85c).

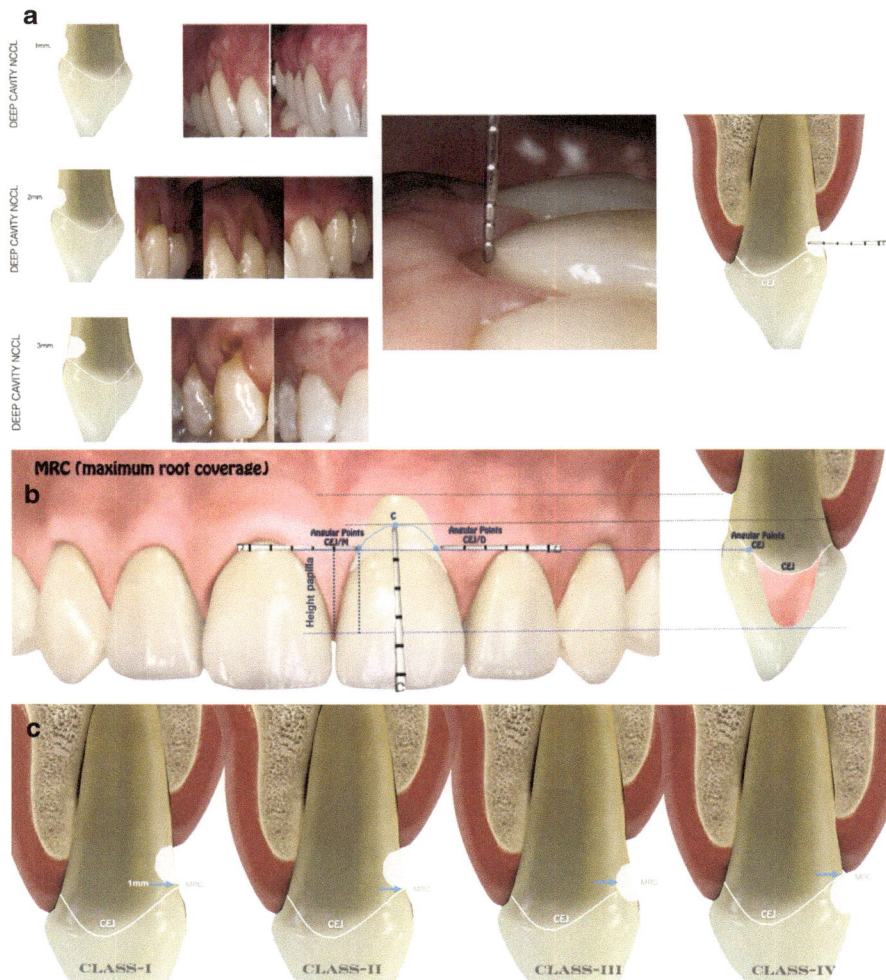

Fig. 85 (**a**) Deep cavity NCCL. (**b**) The maximum root coverage. (**c**) A chart illustrating the decision-making process for treating NCCLs associated with gingival recessions

12.3   Treatment Options

12.3.1 Class 1
A CAF or tunnel is indicated when the maximum line of coverage is 1 mm coronal to the NCCLs and the defect is less than 1 mm deep (Fig. 86).

12.3.2 Class 2
A CAF or tunnel is indicated when the maximum line of coverage is on the coronal border of NCCLs and the defect is less than 2 mm deep. Connective tissue graft is indicated for a patient with a fine phenotype (Fig. 87).

12.3.3 Class 3 (Option 1)
A coronal displaced flap or tunnel is indicated when the maximum line of coverage is in the middle of the NCCLs and the defect is greater than 2 mm (Fig. 88).

12.3.4 Class 3 (Option 2)
A coronal displaced flap or tunnel is indicated when the maximum line of coverage is in the middle of the NCCLs and the defect is greater than 2 mm. A connective tissue graft is indicated for patients with a fine phenotype (Fig. 89).

12.3.5 Class 4
Only restorative treatment is indicated when the maximum line of coverage is apical to the NCCLs (Fig. 90).

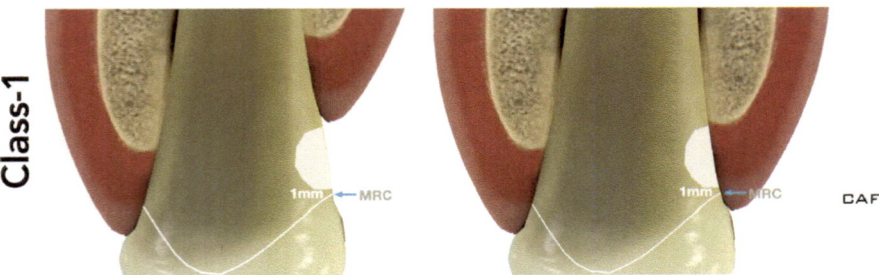

Fig. 86   Class-1

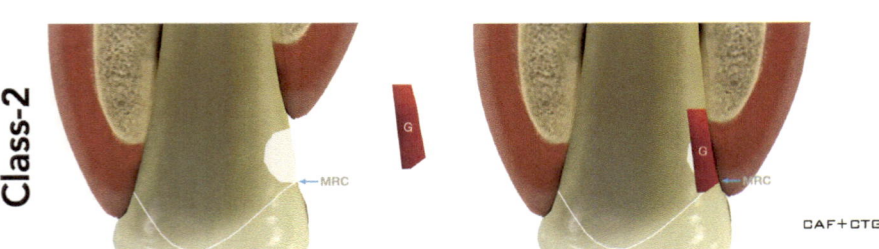

Fig. 87   Class-2

Class-3 (option 1)

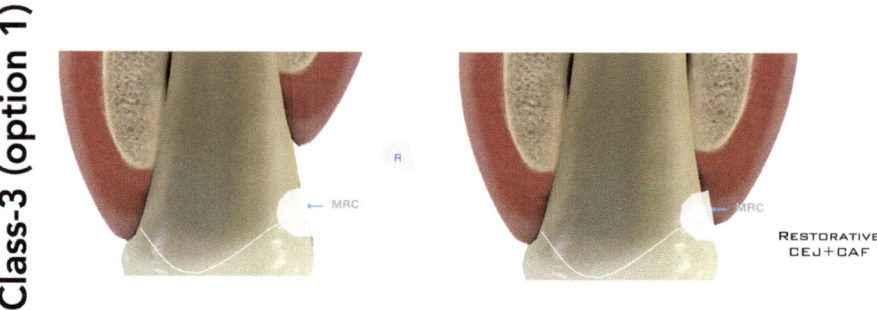

Fig. 88 Class-3 option-1

Class-3 (option 2)

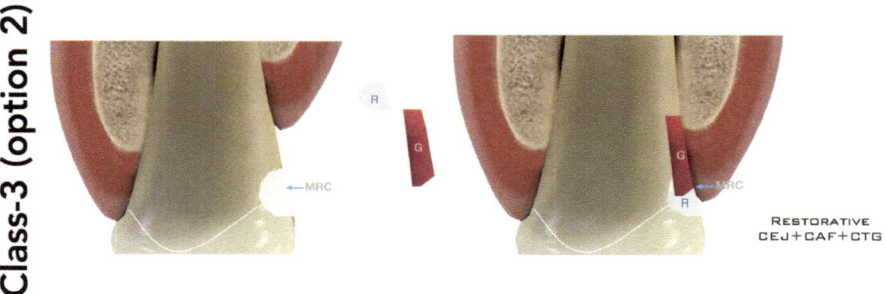

Fig. 89 Class-3 option −2

Class-4

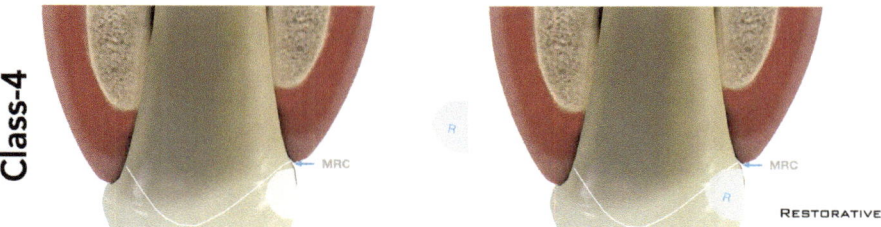

Fig. 90 Class-4

The incorporation of computer-aided design/computer-aided manufacturing CAD/CAM technology into the profession opens the door for new and innovative possibilities for dental treatment. Currently, the method to determine the CEJ and maximum line of root covering is through digital means. This protocol has been adopted from previous reports [45, 46].

Clinical Case A female patient with multiple inferior recession type I (RT-I) Cairo, NCCL B (+), and a thick phenotype (Fig. 91a). Treatment protocol (Class 3 Option 2): hygienic phase, treatment of the NCCL and reconstruction of the CEJ (Fig. 91b), and surgery (Fig. 91c). Tunneling in zones 3.3 and 4.3 was performed using connective tissue grafts.

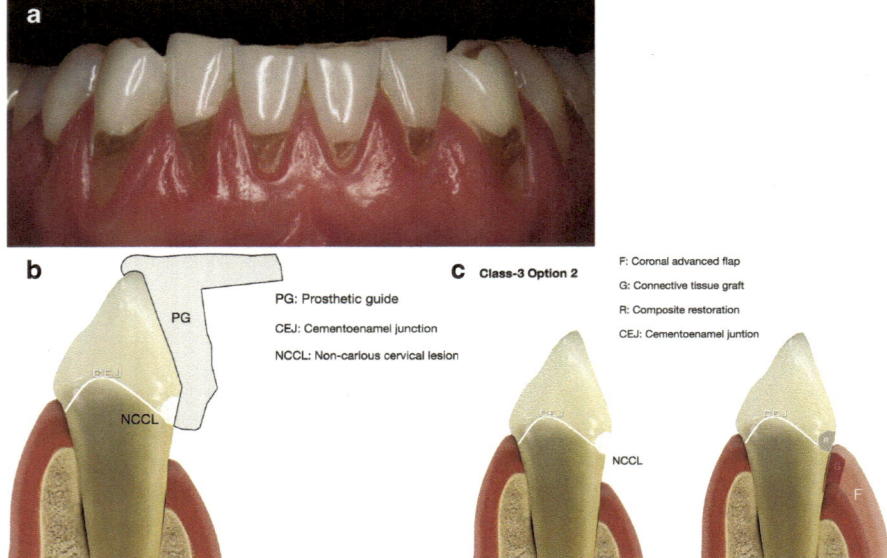

Fig. 91 (**a**) A female patient with multiple inferior recession type I (RT-I) Cairo, NCCL B (+), and a thick phenotype. (**b**) A prosthetic guide was designed for the reconstruction of the CEJ and projected on a digital model. (**c**) Treatment protocol (Class 3, Option 2)

Fig. 92 A digital impression

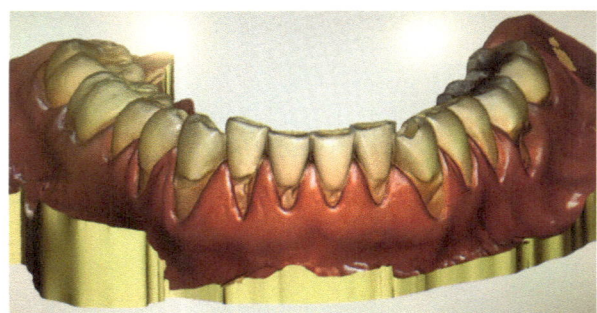

12.4   Restorative Treatment

1. A digital impression and intraoral photographs of the maxilla or jaw to be treated were captured (Fig. 92).
2. Stereolithography models were exported to the Meshmixer (Autodesk trademarks) software (Fig. 93).
3. The location of the angular points of the CEJ was clinically established to transfer the data to the digital model (Fig. 94).
4. Projection to the CEJ location was performed by measuring the height of the papilla, the vertical distance between the horizontal line of angular points of both

Fig. 93 Stereolithography models

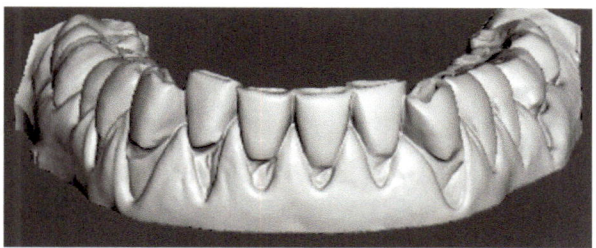

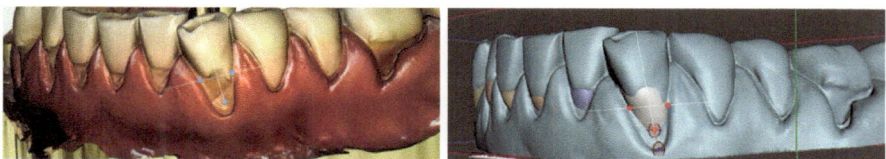

Fig. 94 The location of the angular points of the CEJ

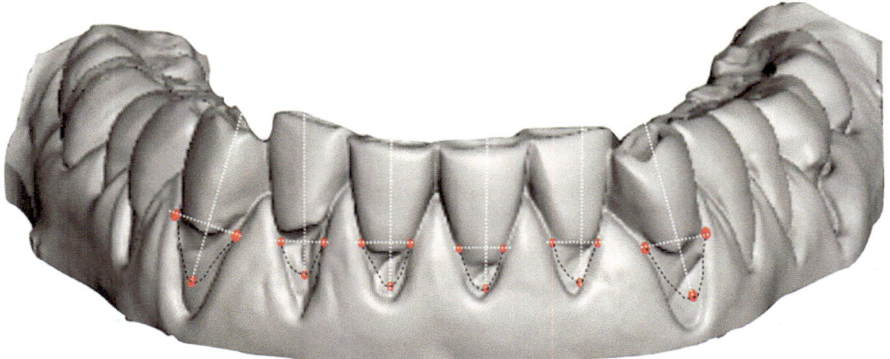

Fig. 95 Projection to the CEJ location

adjacent teeth, and the peak of the papilla using a digital model (Fig. 95). After obtaining the mesial and distal points, they were brought together by a curve-sinuated line that depended on the scalloping associated with patient's phenotype (Fig. 96).

5. A prosthetic guide was designed for the reconstruction of the CEJ and projected on a digital model (Fig. 97).
6. The CEJ reconstruction prosthetic guide was printed (Fig. 98).
7. After testing the adaptation of prothesis to the mouth (Fig. 99) (Video 15), the area was completely isolated for the CEJ and NCCL reconstruction with composite resin (Fig. 100).
8. The restoration was completed after grinding heads to polish (Figs. 101 and 102).

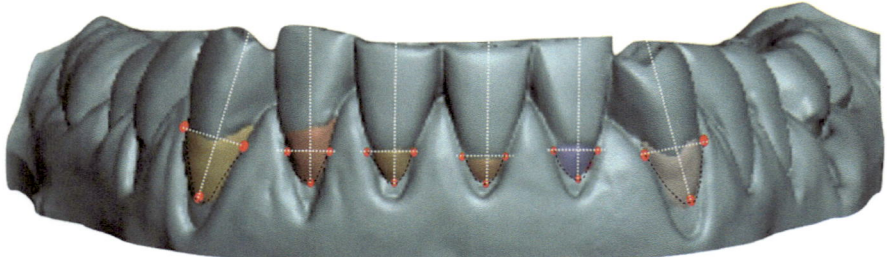

Fig. 96 After obtaining the mesial and distal points, they were brought together by a curve-sinuated line that depended on the scalloping associated with patient's phenotype

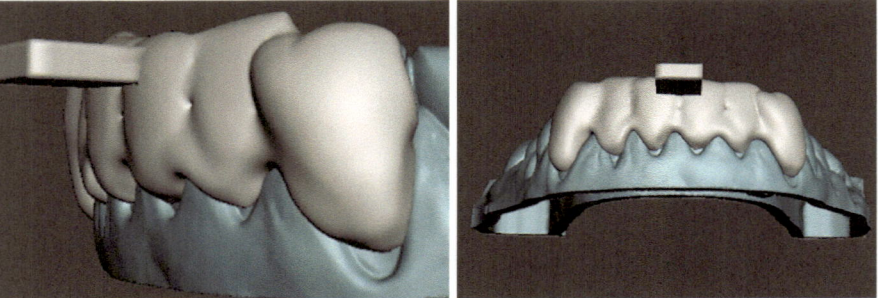

Fig. 97 A prosthetic guide was designed for the reconstruction of the CEJ

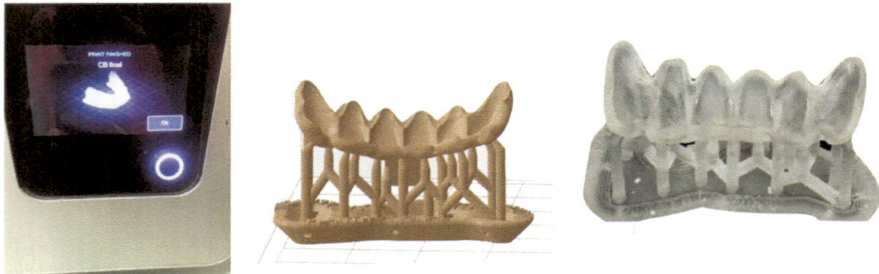

Fig. 98 Prosthetic guide was printed

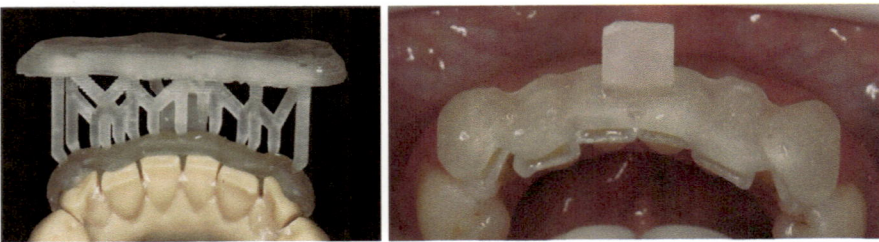

Fig. 99 After testing the adaptation of prothesis to the mouth

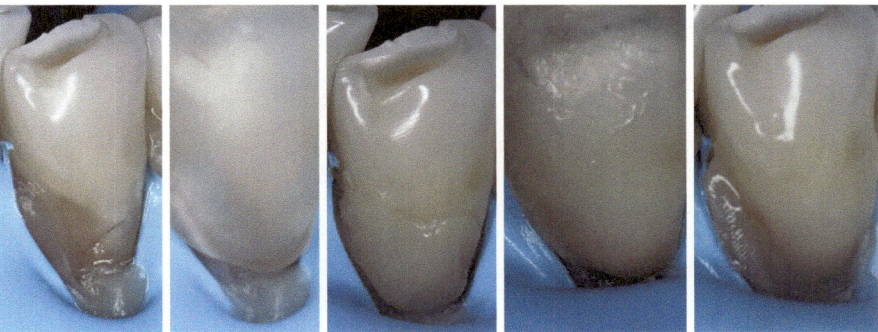

Fig. 100 The area was completely isolated for the CEJ and NCCL reconstruction with composite resin

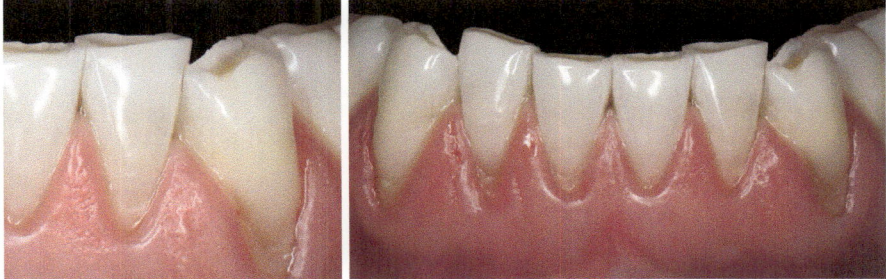

Fig. 101 The restoration was completed after grinding heads to polish

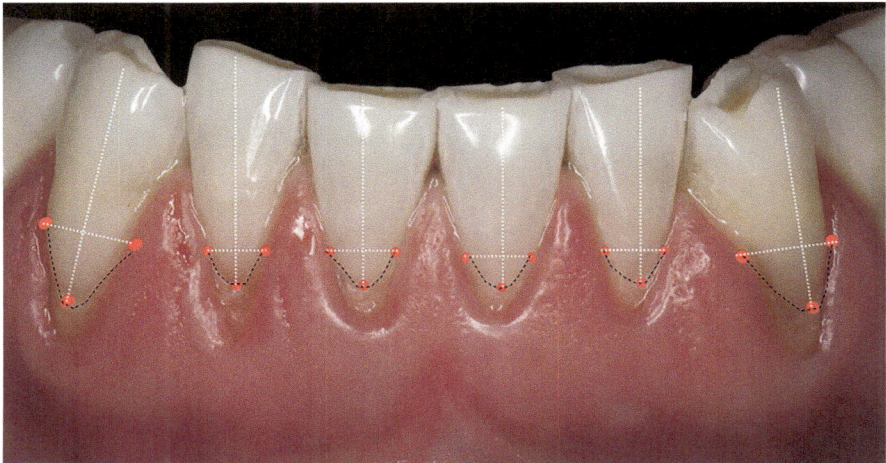

Fig. 102 Projection digital to the CEJ reconstruction

12.5   Surgical Treatment

9. The modified tunnel plus connective tissue graft (MTT + CTG) technique was selected (Fig. 103).
10. Point-of-contact sling 7/0 polypropylene sutures (Polypropylene, AD Surgical Sunnyvale CA, USA) (Figs. 104, 105, and 106). Evaluation at 2 weeks post-treatment and suture removal (Fig. 107).
11. The incisal borders are reconstructed (Fig. 108).
12. Evaluation at 6 months post-treatment (Fig. 109).

Clinical Case A non-smoker, female patient without any relevant medical conditions complained of poor esthetics and tooth sensitivity. The patient had RT-I Cairo, multiple recession defects in the maxillary and mandibular zones. The teeth had deep abrasion caused by an acidic diet and hard brushing was observed (Fig. 110).

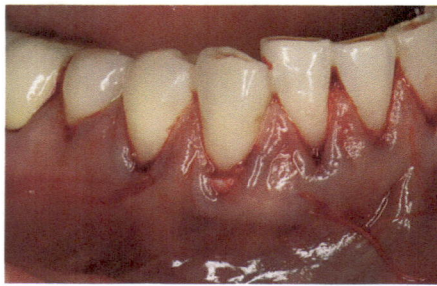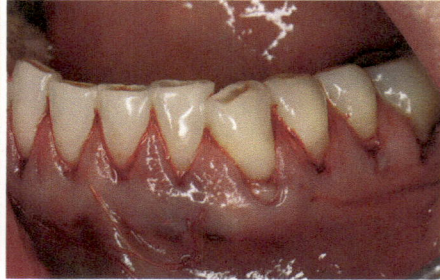

Fig. 103 The modified tunnel plus connective tissue graft

Fig. 104 Point-of-contact sling 7/0 polypropylene sutures

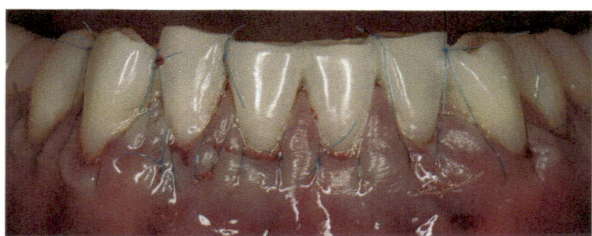

Fig. 105 Point-of-contact sling 7/0 polypropylene sutures

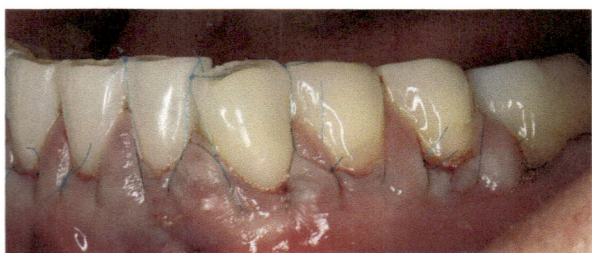

Fig. 106 Point-of-contact sling 7/0 polypropylene sutures

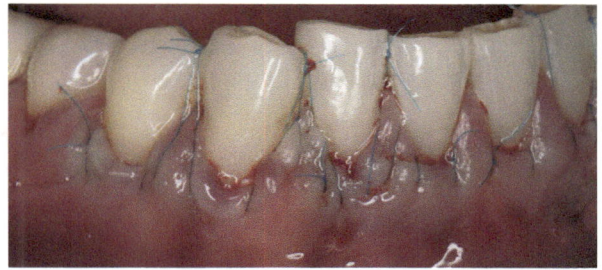

Fig. 107 Evaluation at 2 weeks post-treatment and suture removal

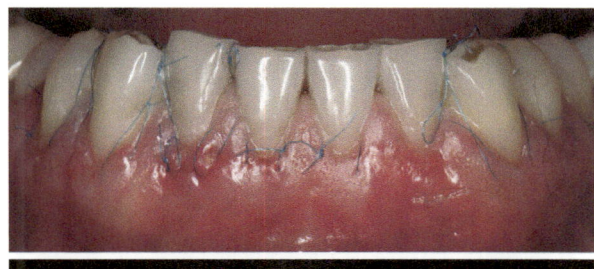

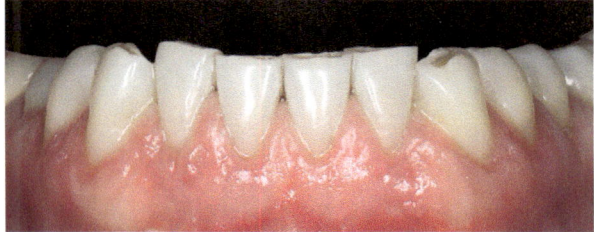

Fig. 108 The incisal borders are reconstructed

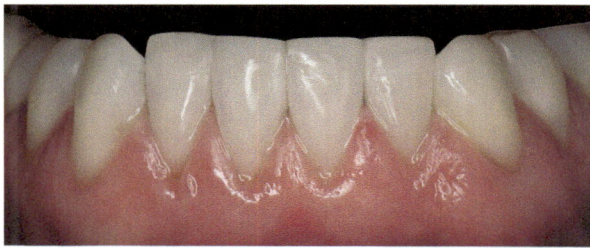

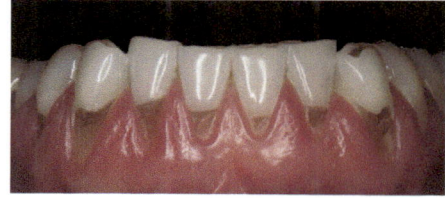
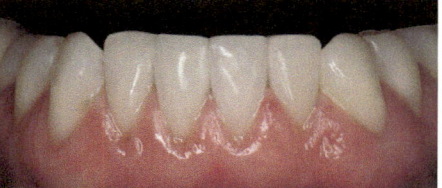

Fig. 109 Evaluation at 6 months post-treatment

Before starting the treatment, the occlusion of the patient was stabilized with a mouth guard. The patient was instructed to reduce the acidity of the diet, change the toothbrush, and modify the brushing technique. The CEJ level was identified using the Pini Prato's technique (Fig. 111).

The cervical defect had a depth of 2.5 mm, no decay, and a positive vitality. According to Pini Prato's classification [42], the lesion was Type B+ (Fig. 112).

12.6 Restorative Treatment

In teeth 2.1, 2.2, 2.3, 2.4, 2.5, 3.3, 3.4, and 3.5, the therapeutic CEJ and lost enamel were restored with composite resin, sandblasting, adhesive technique, and thorough polishing of the surface (Fig. 113).

12.7 Surgical Treatment Plan (Right Side)

In teeth 1.1, 1.2, 1.3, 1.4, 1.5, 1.6, 4.1, 4.2, 4.3, 4.4, 4.5, and 4.6, the modified tunnel technique described by Azzi and Etienne with connective tissue graft (MTT + CTG) was performed [24].

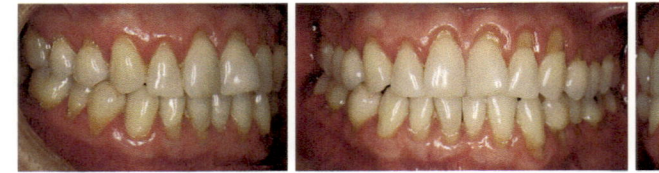

Fig. 110 The patient had RT-I Cairo, multiple recession defects in the maxillary and mandibular zones

Fig. 111 The CEJ level was identified using the Pini Prato's technique

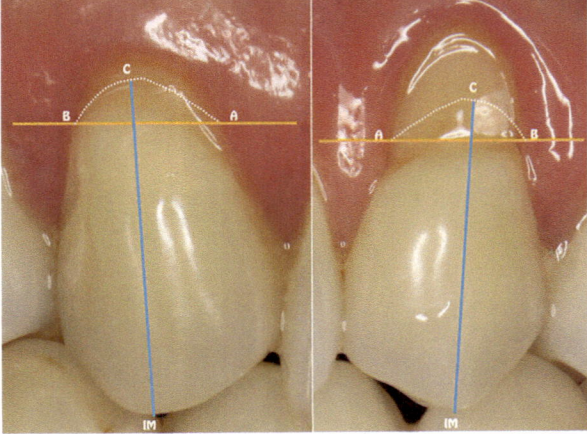

Identification of CEJ level

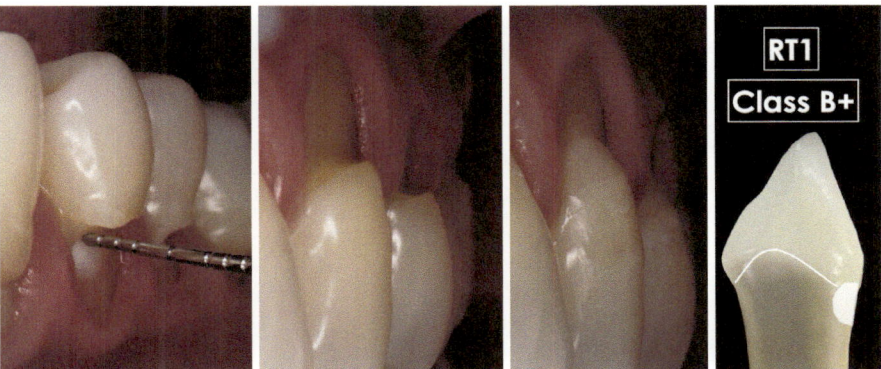

Fig. 112 The cervical defect had a depth of 2.5 mm, no decay, and a positive vitality. The lesion was Type B+

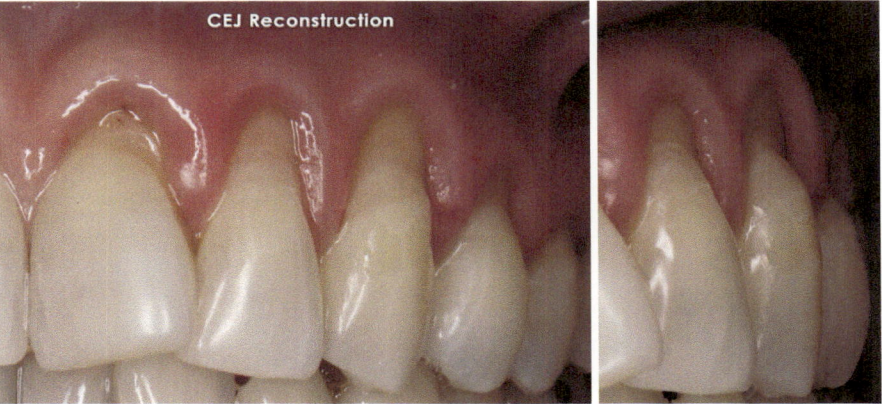

Fig. 113 In teeth 2.1, 2.2, 2.3, 2.4, 2.5, 3.3, 3.4, and 3.5, the therapeutic CEJ and lost enamel were restored with composite resin

12.8 Surgical Treatment Plan (Left Side)

In teeth 2.1, 2.2, 2.3, 2.4, 2.5, and 2.6, the CAF technique was performed, as described by De Sanctis and Zucchelli [28] (Figs. 114a, b, 115, and 116).

12.9 Mandibular Surgical Plan (Left Side)

Root polishing was performed under infiltrative anesthesia. Subsequently, submarginal incisions were made (Fig. 117). To increase the thickness of the soft tissue to improve long-term stability, the CAF technique with a connective tissue graft (CAF + CTG) was used in teeth 3.2, 3.3, 3.4, 3.5, and 3.6 (Fig. 118a, b; Video 16).

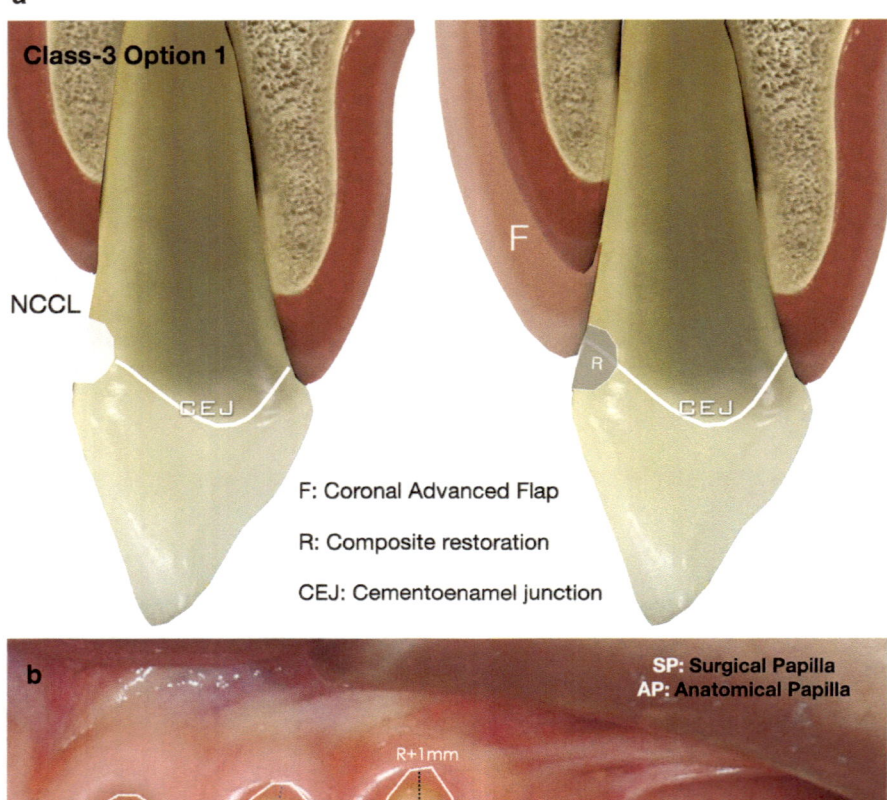

Fig. 114 (**a**) Treatment protocol (Class 3 Option 1). (**b**) In teeth 2.1, 2.2, 2.3, 2.4, 2.5, and 2.6, the CAF technique

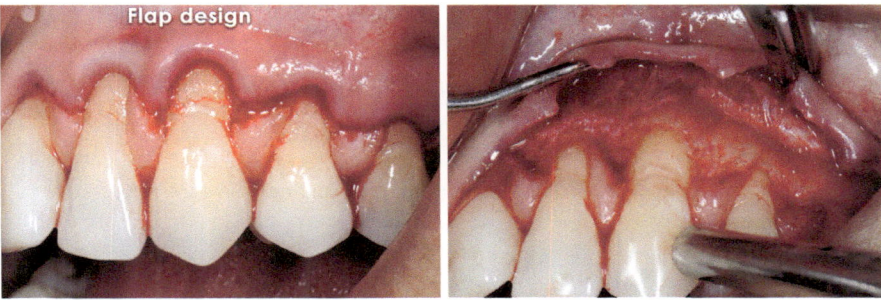

Fig. 115 Flap design

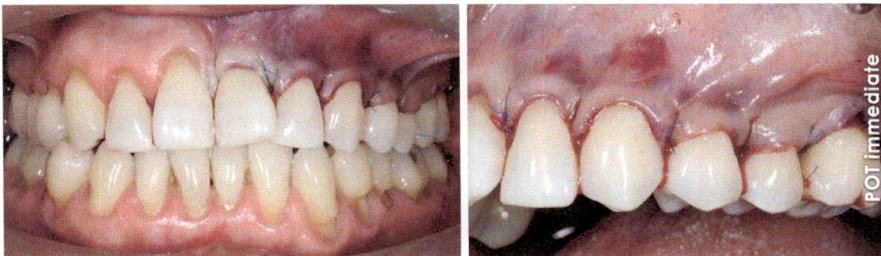

Fig. 116 Postsurgical immediate

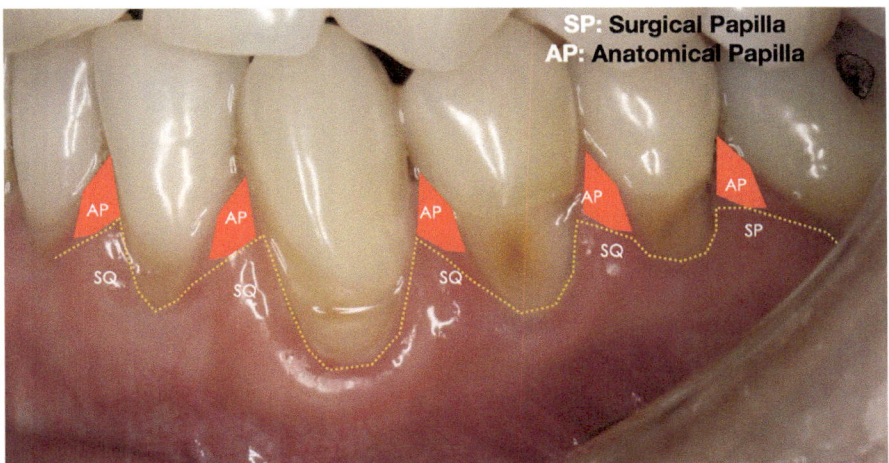

Fig. 117 Submarginal incisions were made

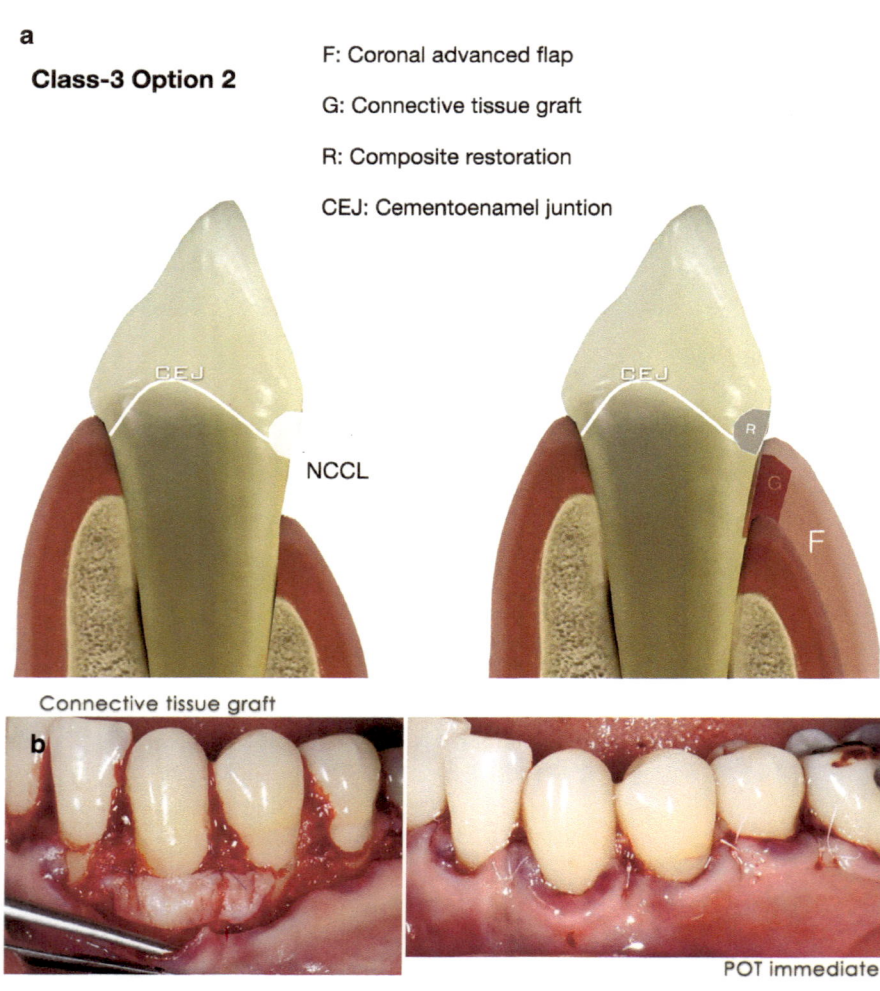

a

Class-3 Option 2

F: Coronal advanced flap

G: Connective tissue graft

R: Composite restoration

CEJ: Cementoenamel juntion

Connective tissue graft

b

POT immediate

Fig. 118 (**a**) Treatment protocol (Class 3, Option 2). (**b**) Technique with a connective tissue graft (CAF + CTG) was used in teeth 3.2, 3.3, 3.4, 3.5, and 3.6

12.10 Clinical Outcomes

Esthetic outcome and root coverage in the four quadrants were achieved with the MTT + CTG, CAF, and CAF + CTG techniques. The stability of the gingival tissues was maintained after 3 years in all quadrants, regardless of the surgical technique used. The mucogingival line did not migrate to a position other than that obtained after surgery (Fig. 119a–c).

Clinical Case A non-smoker, female patient without any relevant medical conditions presented with an RT-I Cairo recession in teeth 5 and 6 with a thin gingival

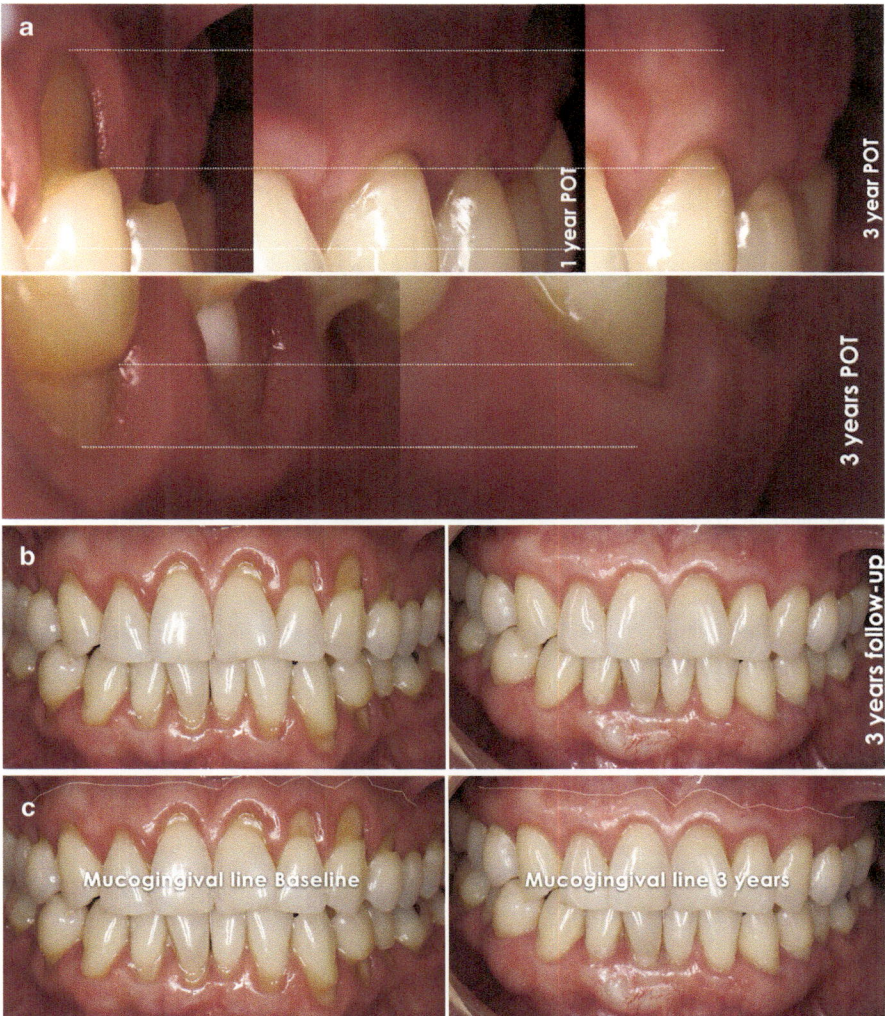

Fig. 119 (**a**) Lateral view evaluation at 1 and 3 year post-treatment. (**b**) Frontal view 3 years follow-up. (**c**) Frontal view mucogingival line 3 years follow-up

phenotype [47] (Fig. 120). NCCLs were present in both teeth. The canine and premolar recessions were described as Type A+ according to the Pini Prato classification, meaning that the CEJ was identifiable and a step was present between the CEJ and abrasion lesion. The cervical lesion depths in teeth 6 and 5 were 2.5 and 1 mm. Scheme of the periodontal and restorative approach for the treatment of the NCCL is shown in Fig. 121.

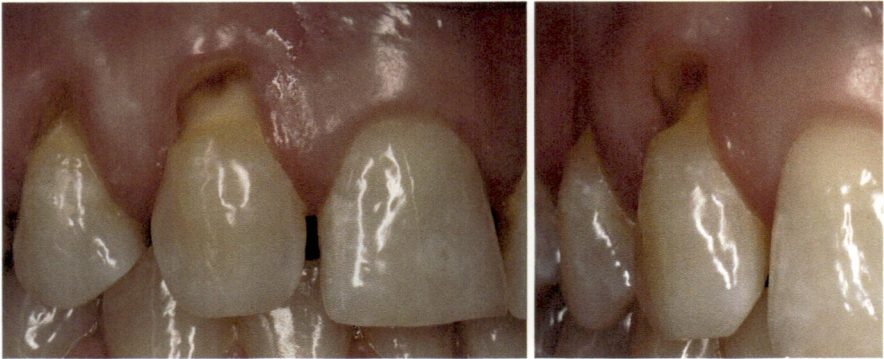

Fig. 120 A non-smoker, female patient without any relevant medical conditions presented with an RT-I Cairo recession in teeth 5 and 6 with a thin gingival phenotype

Fig. 121 Scheme of the periodontal and restorative approach for the treatment of the NCCL

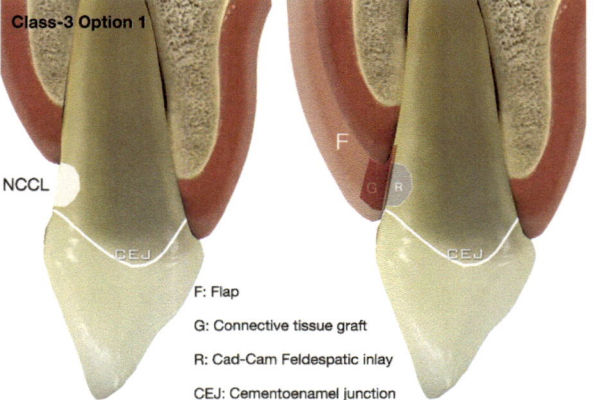

F: Flap
G: Connective tissue graft
R: Cad-Cam Feldespatic inlay
CEJ: Cementoenamel junction

12.11   Restorative Treatment

After local anesthesia, cervical lesions in teeth 1.4 and 1.3 were cleaned and flattened using rotary instruments at high speed. Digital optical impressions of teeth 1.4 and 1.3 were obtained (Fig. 122). An indirect restoration was designed for tooth 1.3 using specialized software. A cervical feldspathic ceramic inlay was milled using a milling unit. After milling, the restoration was confirmed intraorally and absolute isolation was performed. The adhesive cementation process was performed according to the manufacturer's instructions. The cervical lesion in tooth 1.4 was shallower and smaller than that in tooth 1.3; hence, cervical lesion in tooth 1.4 was restored with direct composite (Fig. 123).

Fig. 122 Digital optical impressions

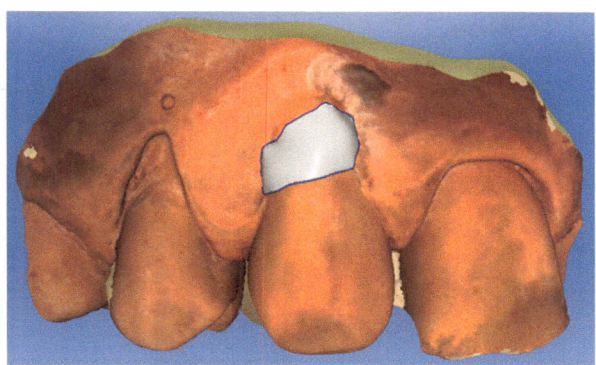

Fig. 123 Cervical lesion in tooth 1.4 was restored with direct composite

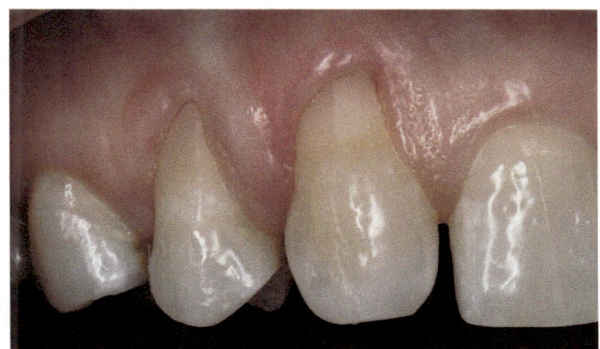

12.12   Surgical Treatment

A microblade was used to create a mucogingival tunnel from teeth 1.6–1.2. All muscle insertions were released to facilitate coronal soft tissue advancement. CTG was harvested from the palate using the one-incision approach. The graft was 12 mm long, 5 mm wide, and 2 mm thick. The subepithelial CTG was inserted into the mucogingival tunnel and its coronal limit was fixed at the CEJ level of teeth 1.4 and 1.3 with vertical mattress and sling sutures. Final flap anchoring to the palatal aspect of both teeth was performed with a 7/0 sling suture (Polypropylene, AD Surgical Sunnyvale CA, USA) (Fig. 124). This procedure allowed intimate adaptation of the buccal flap over the underlying CTG.

12.13   Clinical Outcomes

Complete root coverage was achieved. Parameters showed that bleeding on probing BOP maintained negative, PD remained stable, and relative gingival recession RGR and CAL decreased by 2.3 mm showing a favorable integration of the restoration and a predictable response of soft tissues during the entire follow-up period

(Figs. 125 and 126). Clinical measurements of teeth 1.4 and 1.3 are presented in (Table 6). At 60 month follow-up, cone beam computed tomography of tooth 1.3 was requested for imaging analysis (Fig. 127) and final photographs were captured. Treatment outcomes and their evolution were compared schematically (Figs. 128, 129, and 130).

Fig. 124 Final flap anchoring to the palatal aspect of both teeth was performed with a 7/0 sling suture

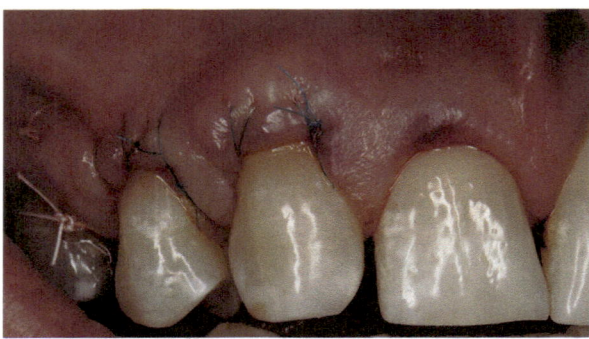

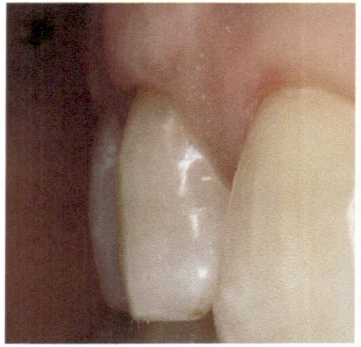 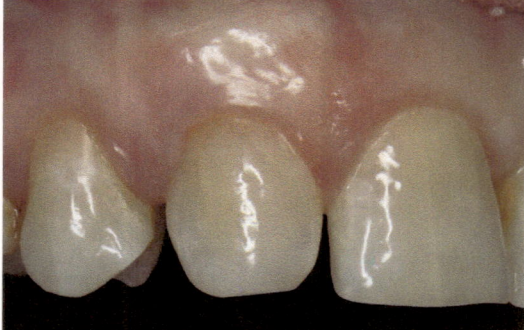

Fig. 125 Complete root coverage was achieved

Fig. 126 Parameters showed that bleeding on probing BOP maintained negative, PD remained stable

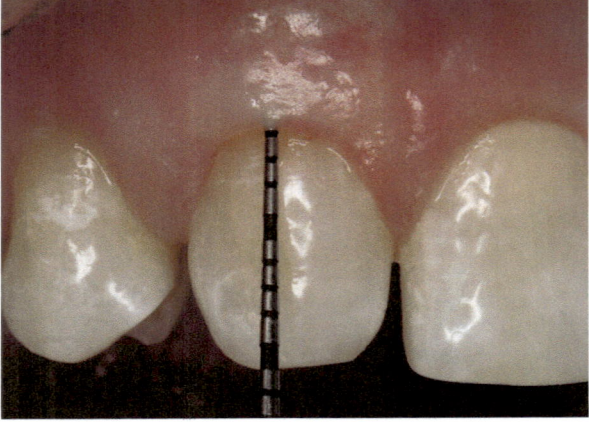

Table 6 Recorded parameters measurements

Tooth 1.3	Baseline	12 Months	24 Months	36 Months	60 months
BOP	(–)	(–)	(–)	(–)	(–)
PD	2 mm	2 mm	2 mm	2 mm	2 mm
RGR	(–) 2.3 mm	0 mm	0 mm	0 mm	0 mm
CAL	4.3 mm	2 mm	2 mm	2 mm	2 mm
Tooth 1.4	Baseline	12 months	24 months	36 months	60 months
BOP	(–)	(–)	(–)	(–)	(–)
PD	2 mm	2 mm	2 mm	2 mm	2 mm
RGR	(–) 1.5 mm	0 mm	0 mm	0 mm	0 mm
CAL	3.5 mm	2 mm	2 mm	2 mm	2 mm

BOP bleeding on probing, *PD* probing depth, *RGR* relative gingival recession, *CAL* relative clinical attachment level determined by PD + RGR

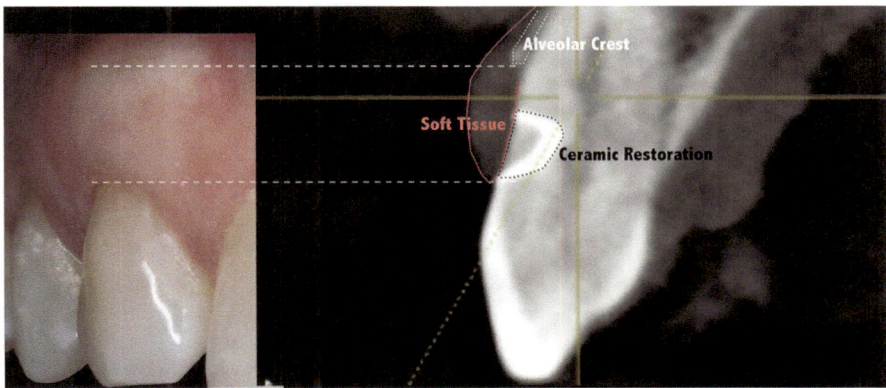

Fig. 127 At 60 month follow-up, cone beam computed tomography of tooth 1.3 was requested for imaging analysis

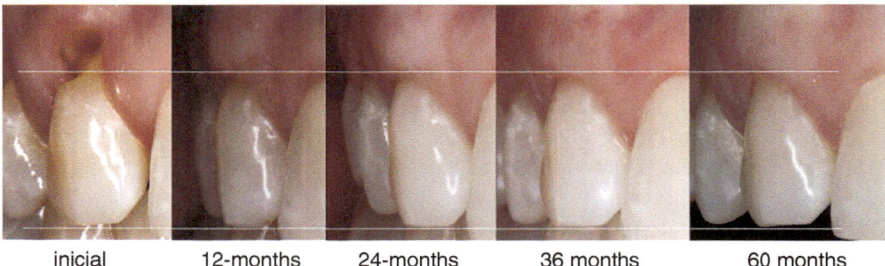

inicial   12-months   24-months   36 months   60 months

Fig. 128 Treatment outcomes and their evolution were compared schematically

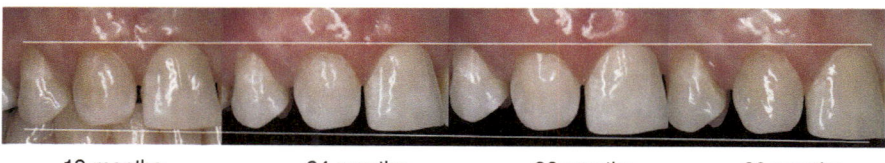

12-months   24-months   36 months   60 months

Fig. 129 12, 24, 36, 60 months follow-up

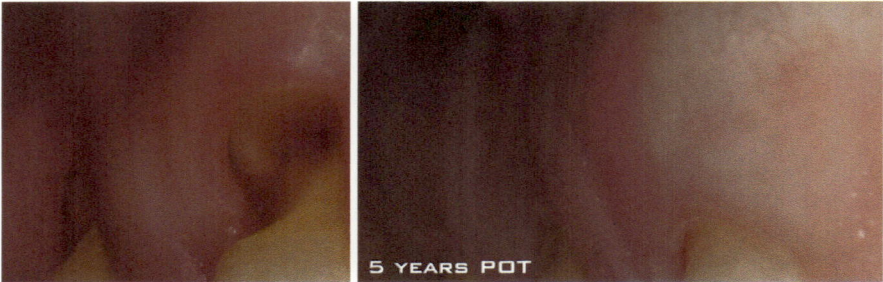

Fig. 130 12, 24, 36, 60 months follow-up

13 Treatment of Peri-implant Soft Tissues Dehiscences/ Deficiencies in the Esthetic Zone

The final goal of an implant-supported restoration in the esthetic zone is to achieve long-term esthetic and functional performance. From the surgical point-of-view, achieving a harmonious gingival margin without sudden changes in tissue height while keeping the papilla undamaged and preserving the convexity of the outline of the alveolar crest is a desirable result. This depends on the following four anatomical and surgical parameters [48] (Fig. 131a–c):

1. The submucous position of the implant platform
2. The precise 3D position of the implant
3. The long-term stability of the peri-implant soft tissue outline
4. The volumetric symmetry of clinical crown between the implant zone and contralateral teeth.

Since Furhauser [49] proposed the Pink Esthetic Score in 2005 to evaluate the peri-implant soft tissue, the results and treatment of soft tissue in implant therapy are evaluated using seven clinical variables (Fig. 132).

The preparation and development of the zone implant prior to implant placement have been emphasized as one of the most effective methods of preventing possible defects and complications in soft tissues. Apical displacement of the peri-implant facial tissue can be defined as a recession of the peri-implant margin, mucous recession or dehiscence, deficiency, or dehiscence of the soft tissue or soft tissue defect. The term peri-implant soft tissue dehiscence/deficiency (PSTD) may be the most appropiate [50].

The management of the peri-implant tissue can be based on the management time point:

1. Immediate management during the placement of implants
2. Later management on rehabilitated implants

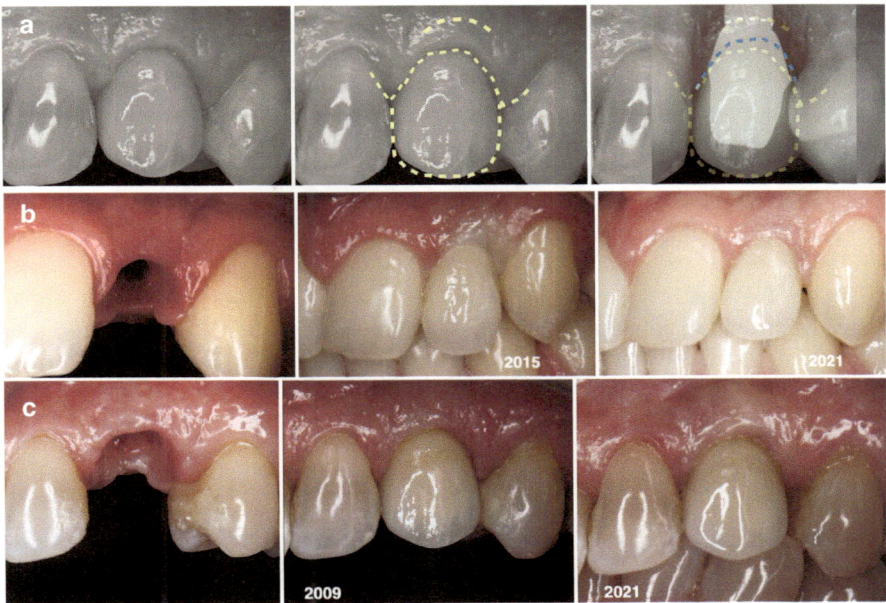

Fig. 131 (**a**) The final goal of an implant-supported restoration in the esthetic zone is to achieve long-term esthetic and functional performance. (**b**) Implant-supported restoration 6 years follow-up. (**c**) Implant-supported restoration 11 years follow-up

P.E.S.

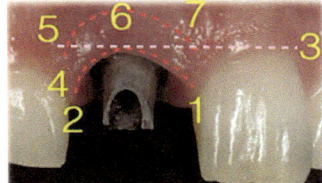

Variables	0	1	2
Mesial Papilla	Missing	Incomplete	Complete
Distal Papilla	Missing	Incomplete	Complete
Soft Tissue Level	> a2 mm.	1 – 2 mm.	< a 1 mm.
Soft Tissue Counter	Unnatural	Virtually Natural	Natural
Alveolar Process deficiency	Clearly Resorbed	Slightly Resorbed	No difference
Soft Tissue Color	Clear Difference	Slightly Difference	No difference
Soft Tissue Texture	Clear Difference	Slightly Difference	No difference

Fig. 132 Pink esthetic score [49]

13.1   Immediate Management During the Placement of Implants

The management of peri-implant soft tissues during implant placement should be complemented with precise prosthetic management of the provisional restorations [51] to ensure the correct development of the emergent esthetic profile. It has been suggested that a connective tissue graft should be placed to enhance the phenotype and compensate the dimensional changes in the alveoli after extraction [52].

Clinical Case A 35-year-old male patient was referred from orthodontics, in his cone beam analysis horizontal bone loss is observed (Figs. 133, 134, 135, 136, 137, 138, 139, 140, and 141).

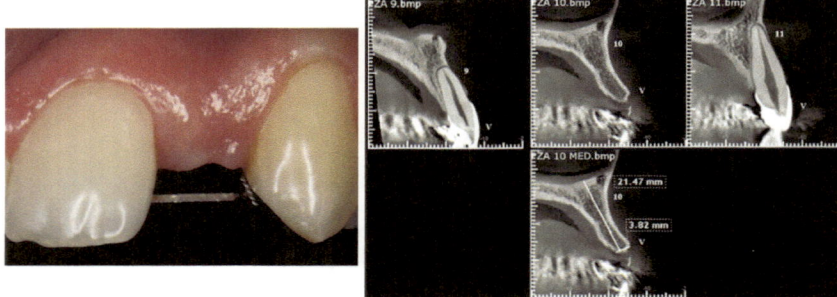

Fig. 133 A 35-year-old male patient was referred from orthodontics

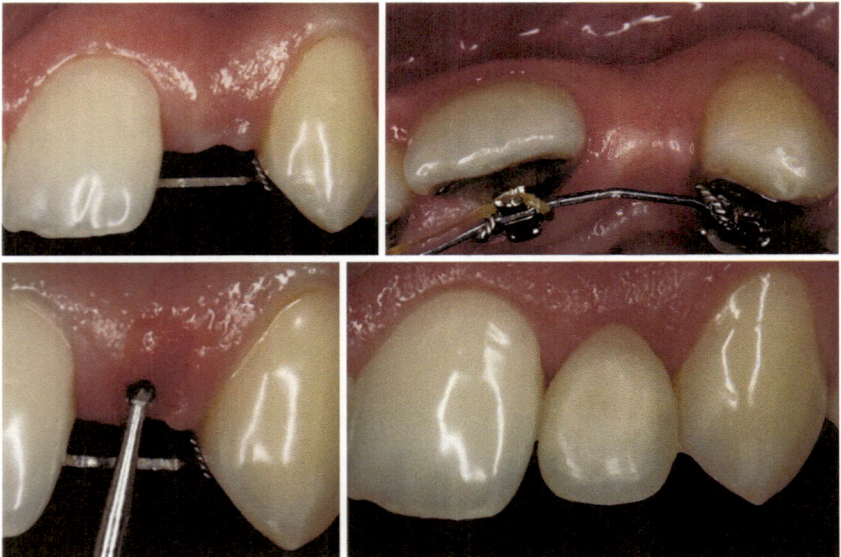

Fig. 134 Slight sculpting of gingival tissue was performed to prepare for adhesive provisional restoration

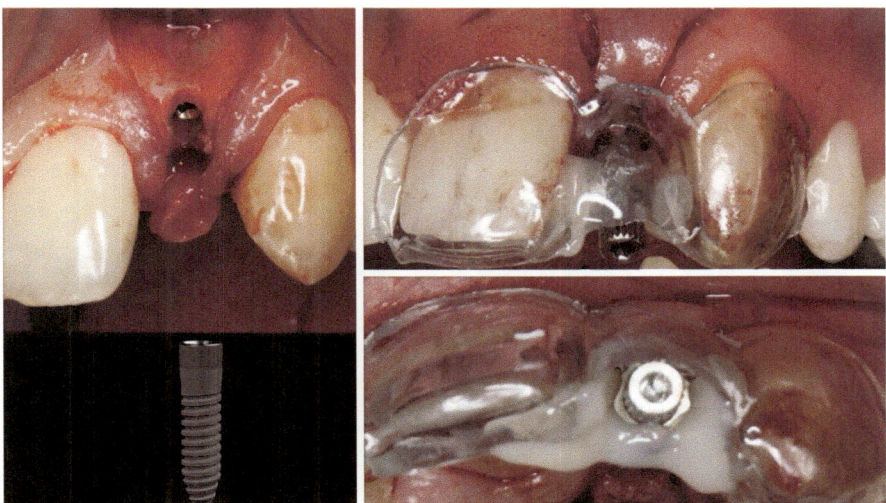

Fig. 135 A 3.0 diameter implant installation and indexing of implant position to perform provisional restoration

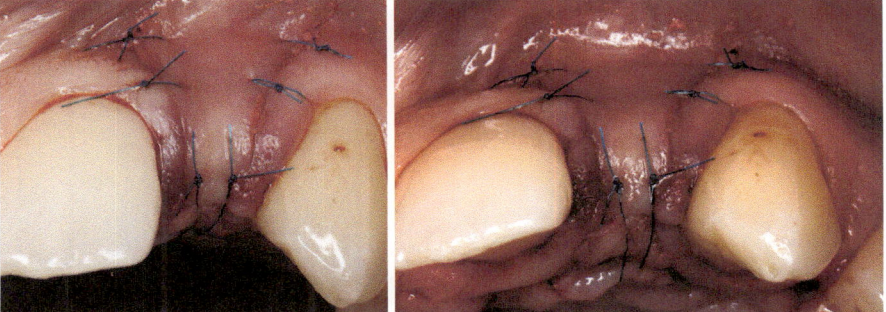

Fig. 136 Bone graft placement and primary wound closure with 7/0 polypropylene sutures

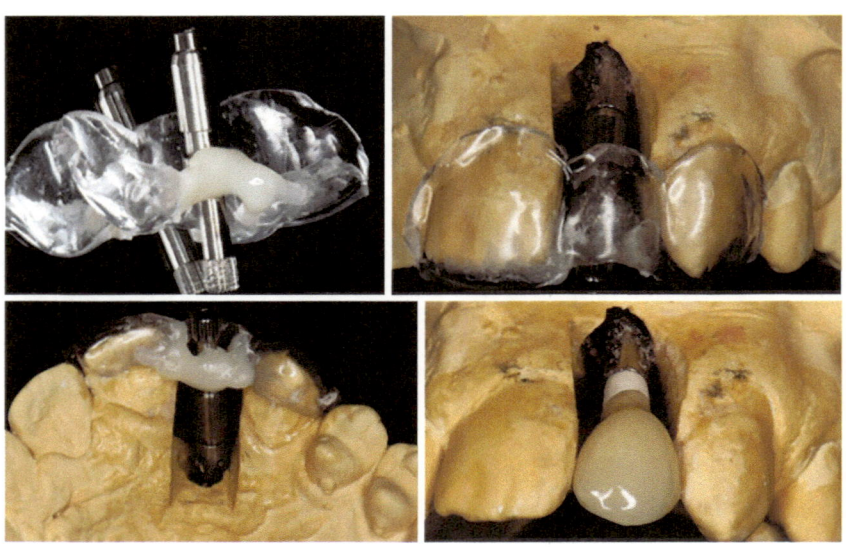

Fig. 137 Fabrication of the implant-supported fixed interim restoration (ISFIR) in the laboratory

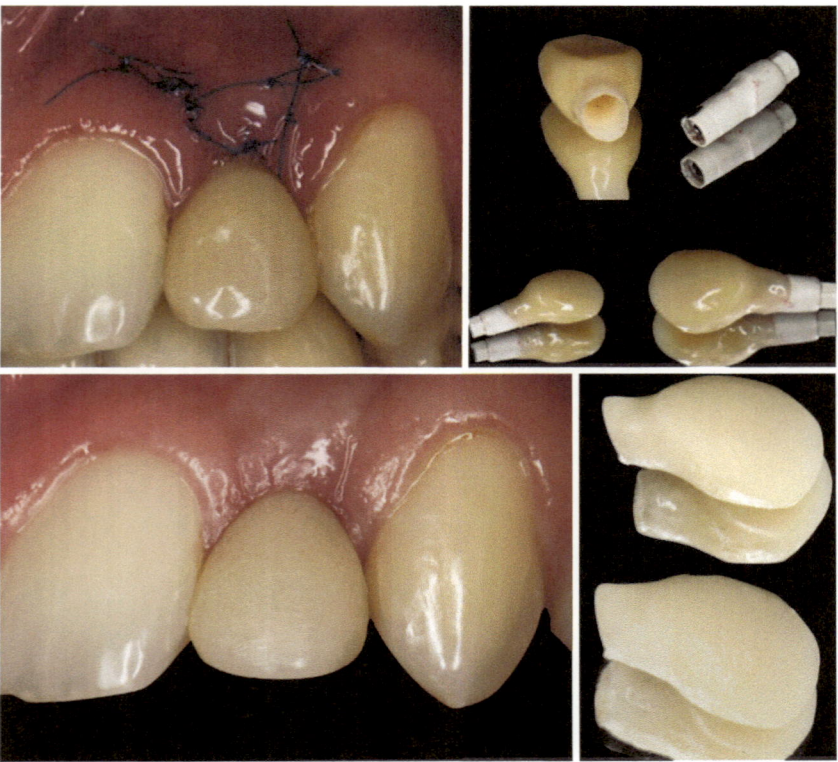

Fig. 138 Implant connection and provisional installation

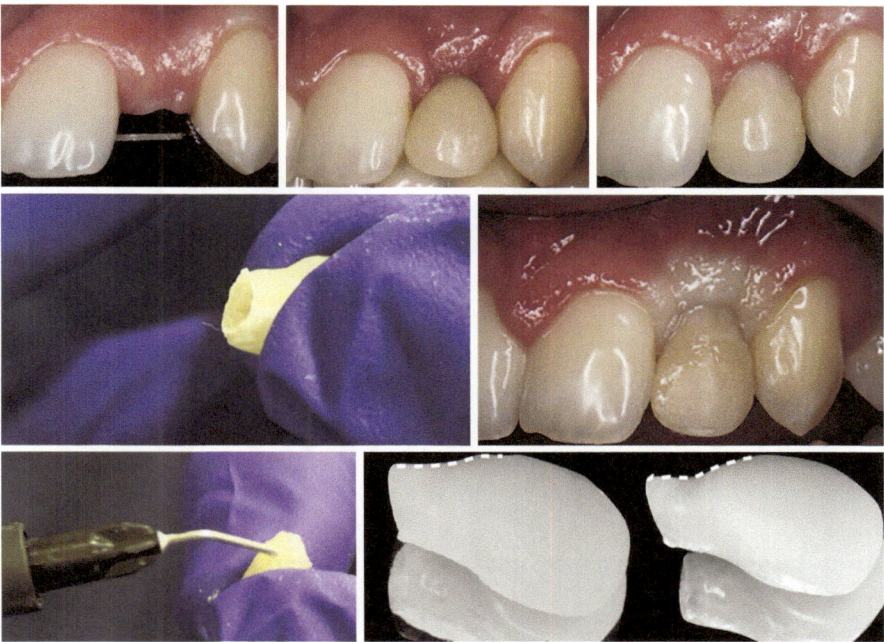

Fig. 139 Critical and subcritical contour management in the ISFIR for apical zenith displacement

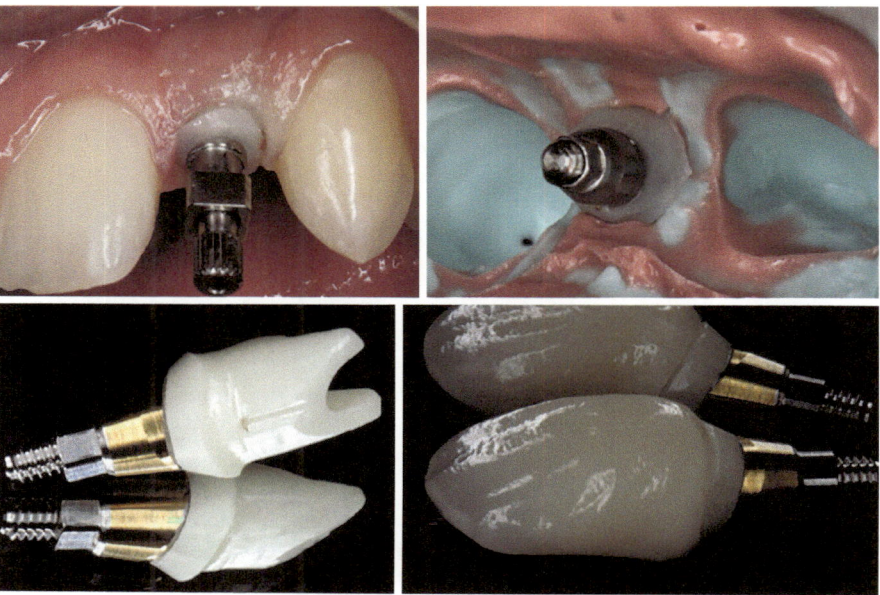

Fig. 140 Custom abutment for capturing and transferring the emergence profile, impression, CAD/CAM abutment and ceramic crown

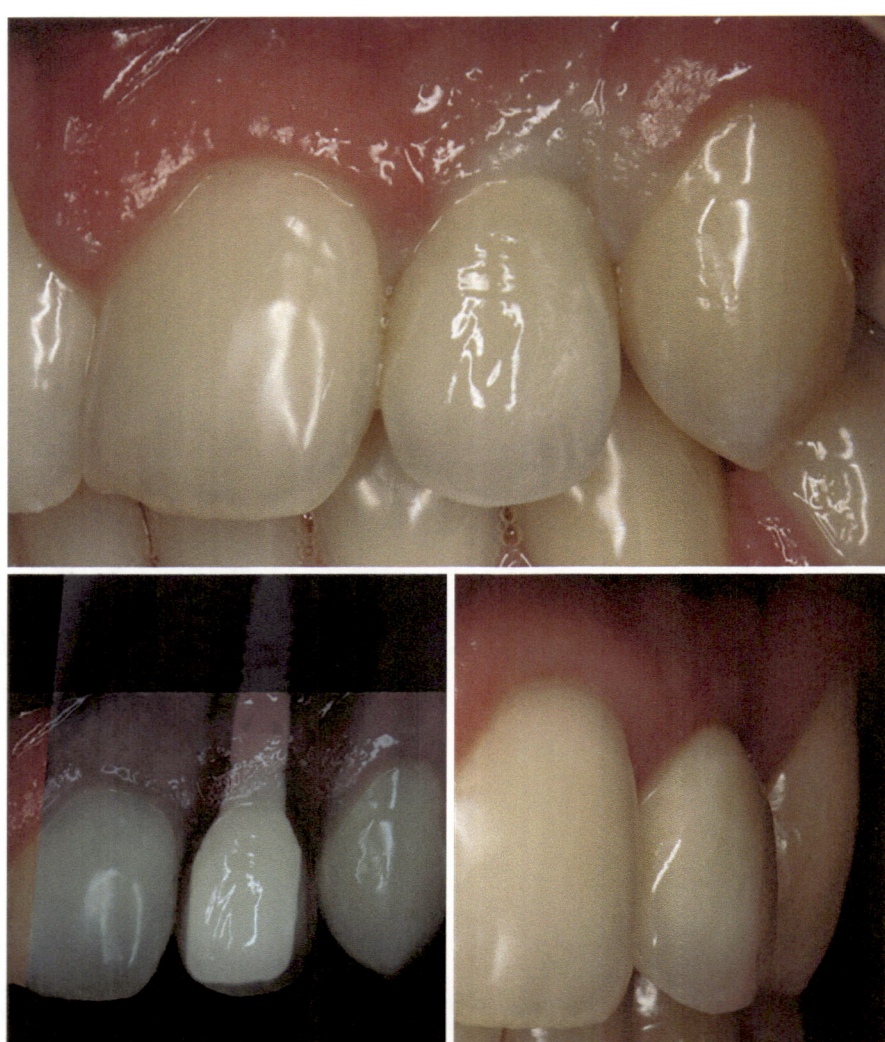

Fig. 141 Installation of custom abutment and crown. Radiographic control

Clinical Case A 60-year-old female patient with a lost canine tooth in 1.3, total plate loss, and horizontal defect in soft and hard tissues (Figs. 142, 143, 144, 145, 146, and 147).

Clinical Case A 53-year-old male patient with poor periodontal prognosis in the central tooth 1.1, total plate loss, and horizontal defect in soft and hard tissues (Figs. 148, 149, 150, 151, 152, 153, and 154).

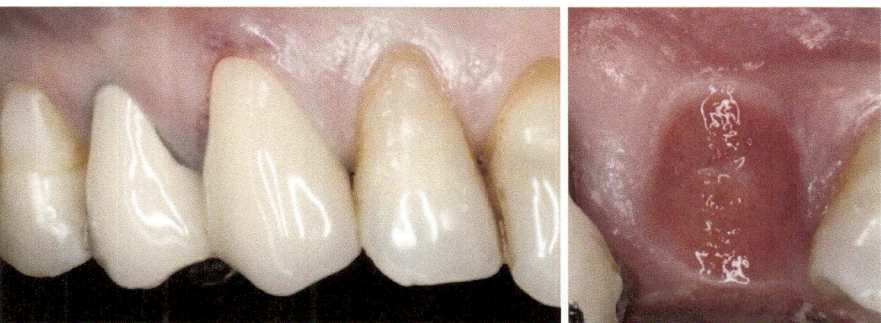

Fig. 142 A 60-year-old female patient with a lost canine tooth in 1.3, total plate loss, and horizontal defect in soft and hard tissues

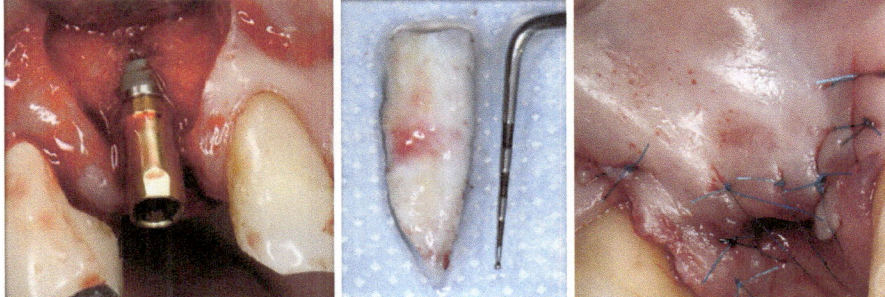

Fig. 143 Implant installation with connective tissue graft (7/0 polypropylene sutures)

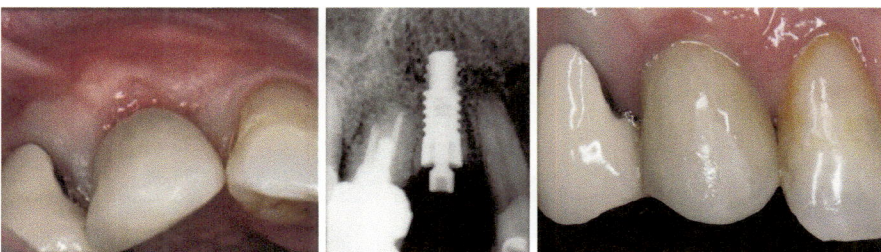

Fig. 144 Evaluation at 8 weeks after ISFIR

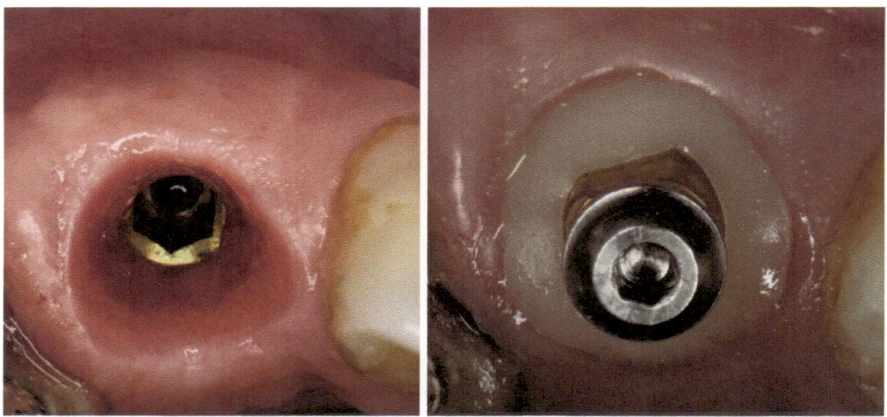

Fig. 145 Evaluation at 6 months

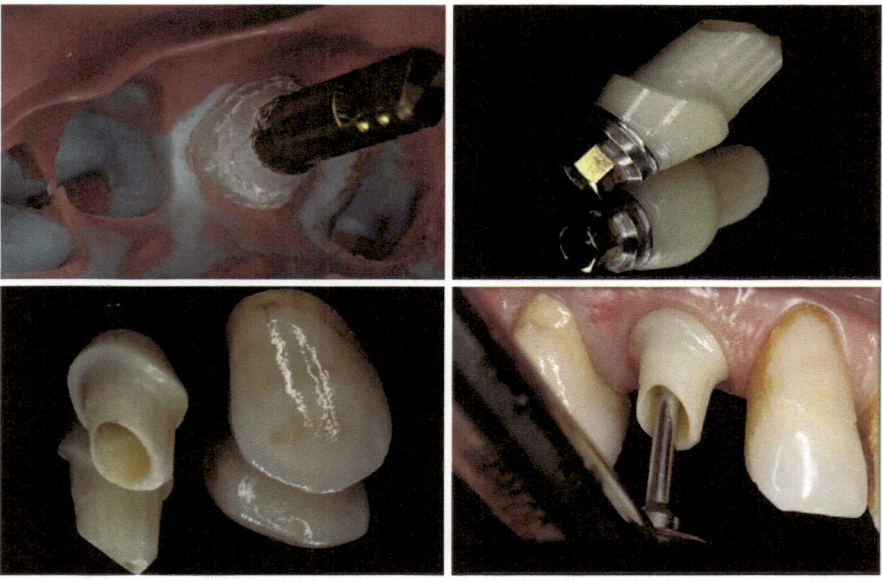

Fig. 146 Custom abutment to copy emergence profile, impression, CAD/CAM abutment, and ceramic crown

13.2   Later Management on Rehabilitated Implants

The incidence and prevalence of PSTD are high, which can be attributed to the following factors: the amount of post-implant keratinized gingiva, protocol for implant installation (immediate or mediate), phenotype, surgical experience of the microsurgeon, and 3D position of the implant [53]. The decision-making process for the

Fig. 147 Lateral and frontal intraoral view at 24 months after treatment

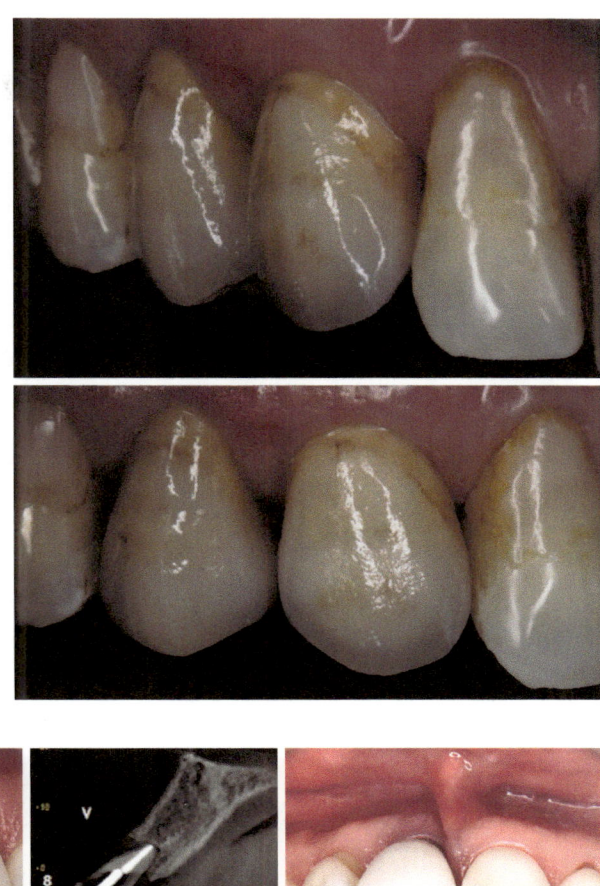

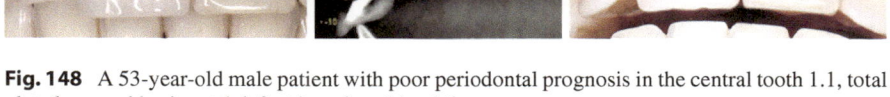

Fig. 148 A 53-year-old male patient with poor periodontal prognosis in the central tooth 1.1, total plate loss, and horizontal defect in soft and hard tissues

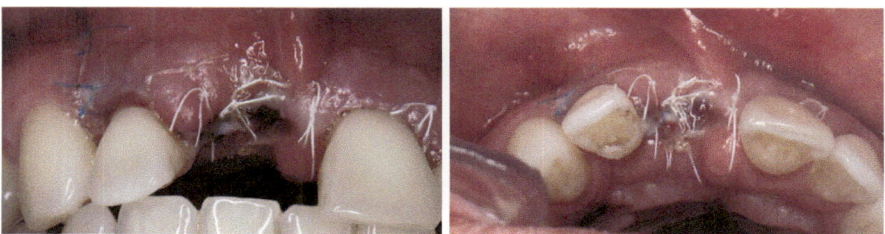

Fig. 149 Implant installation with connective tissue graft and bone graft substitutes (7/0 polypropylene sutures and 6/0 polytetrafluorethylene sutures)

Fig. 150 Evaluation at
6 months

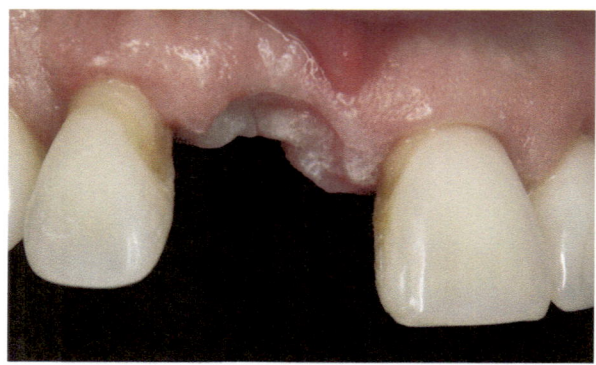

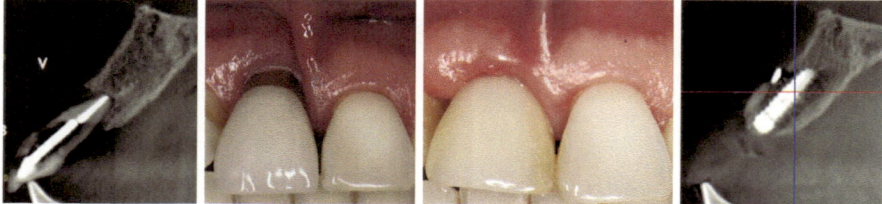

Fig. 151 Implant connection and implant-supported fixed interim restoration

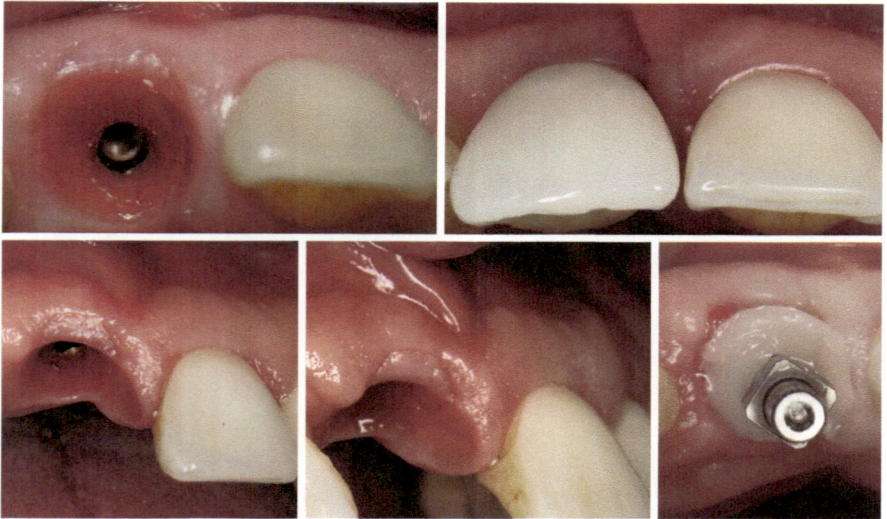

Fig. 152 Custom abutment transfer to copy emergence profile

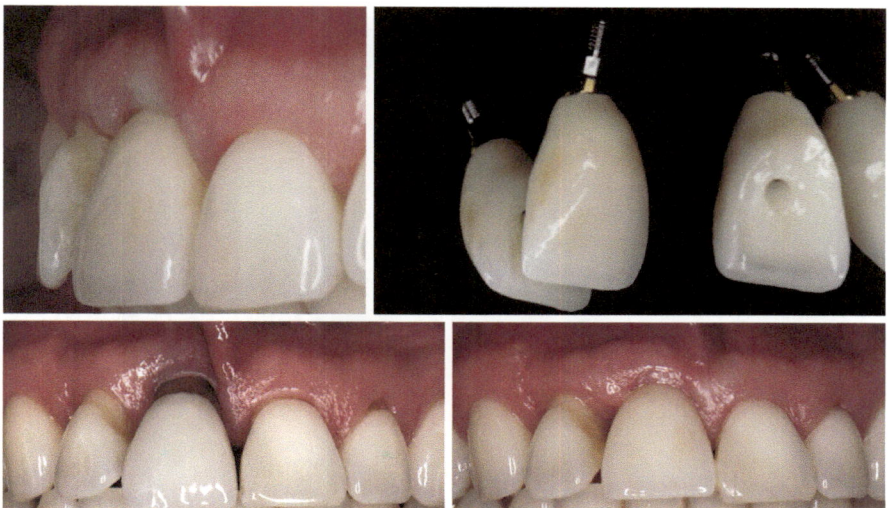

Fig. 153 Lateral and frontal intraoral view at 12 months after treatment

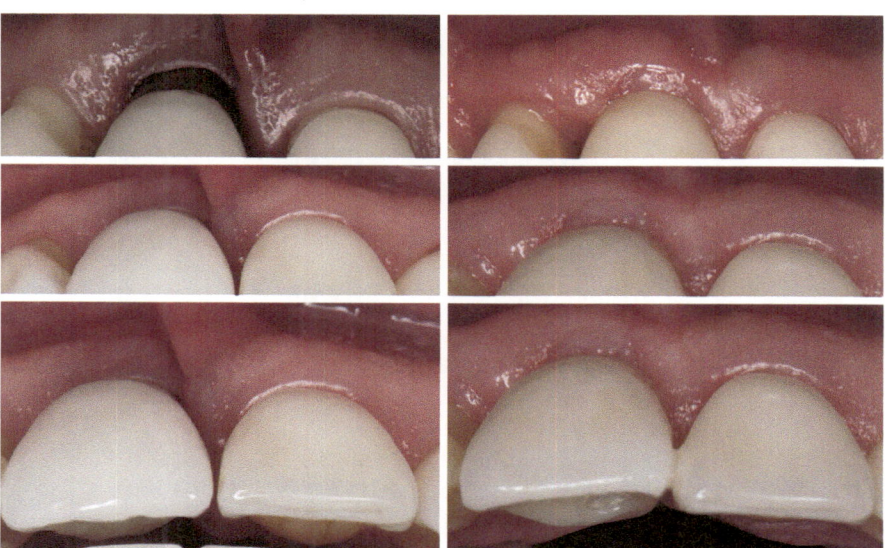

Fig. 154 Before and after peri-implant contour

treatment of PSTD is complex and requires a thorough study of the current condition and the possible causes of PSTD. Zucchelli et al. [54] (Table 7) proposed a new classification system and recommendations to support the decision-making process in the treatment of PSTDs.

Table 7 Peri-implant soft tissue dehiscence/deficiency

Class	PSDT	Recommended surgical/prosthetic treatment
I	Soft Tissue Margin is located same level of the gingival margin homologous tooth	CAf or TUNNEL+ CTG Combined prosthetic-surgical approach
II	Soft Tissue Margin is located apical level of the gingival margin homologous tooth, implant-supported crown profile is located palatal to the profile of adjacent teeth	No crown removal, CAf + TUNNEL + CTG Combined prosthetic-surgical
III	Soft Tissue Margin is located apical level of the gingival margin homologous tooth, implant-supported crown profile is located facially to the profile of adjacent teeth. The head of the implant, evaluated after crown removal, is inside the straight imaginary line that connects the profile of the adjacent teeth at the level of the gingival margin	Crown removal, CAf + TUNNEL + CTG Combined prosthetic-surgical approach Soft tissue augmentation with
IV	Soft Tissue Margin is located apical level of the gingival margin homologous tooth, implant-supported crown profile is located facially to the profile of adjacent teeth. The head of the implant, evaluated after crown removal, is inside the straight imaginary line that connects the profile of the adjacent teeth at the level of the gingival margin	Combined prosthetic-surgical approach Soft tissue augmentation with submerged healing Implant Removal
Subclass		
A	The tip of both papilla is ≥3 mm coronal to the ideal position of soft tissue margin of the implant-supported crown	
B	The tip of at least one papilla is ≥1 mm but <3 mm coronal to the ideal position of the soft tissue margin of the implant supported crow	
C	The height of at least one papilla is <1 mm coronal to the ideal position of the soft tissue margin of the implant-supported crown	Does not apply for class I PSTD

13.3   Classification of Peri-implant Soft Tissues Defects

13.3.1 Multidisciplinary Approach

Clinical Case A 40-year-old female patient with class III, subclass B PSTD, vestibular deficiency, volume loss (Figs. 155, 156, 157, 158, 159, and 160).

Clinical Case A 47-year-old male patient with class I, subclass A PSTD, vestibular deficiency, and volume loss had active fistula at the middle 1/3 vestibular level.

Combined treatment: Removal of the crown CAF and CTG, implant-supported fixed interim restoration for creating a new emergent profile and new rehabilitation over the implant (Figs. 161, 162, 163, 164, 165, and 166).

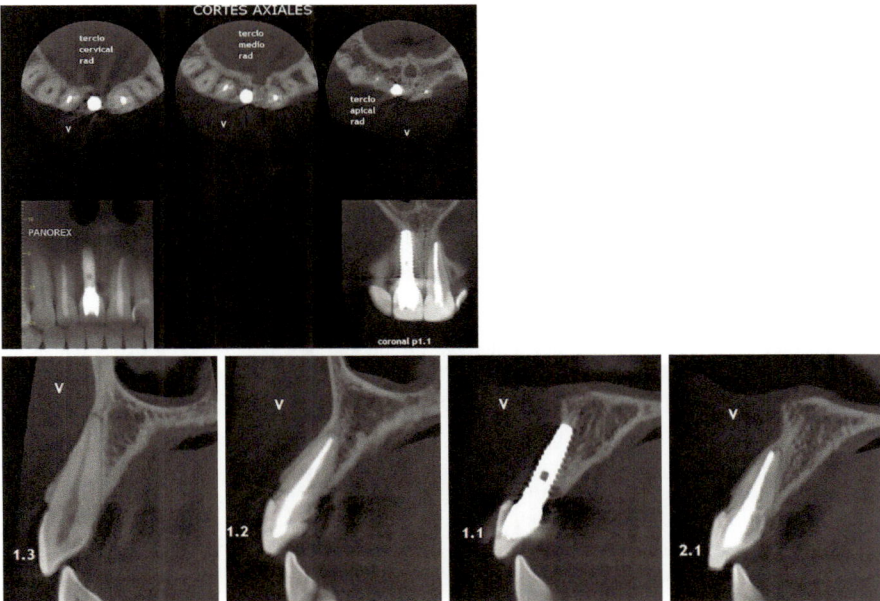

Fig. 155 A 40-year-old female patient with class III, subclass B PSTD

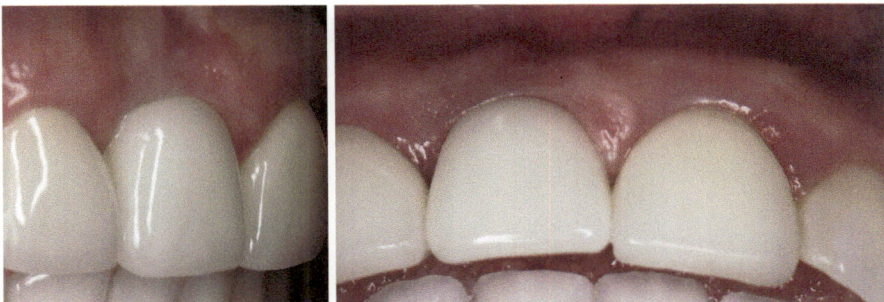

Fig. 156 Vestibular deficiency, volume loss, and loss of the distal papilla (1.5 mm). Profile of the crown over the implant within the imaginary line between the crowns of adjacent teeth

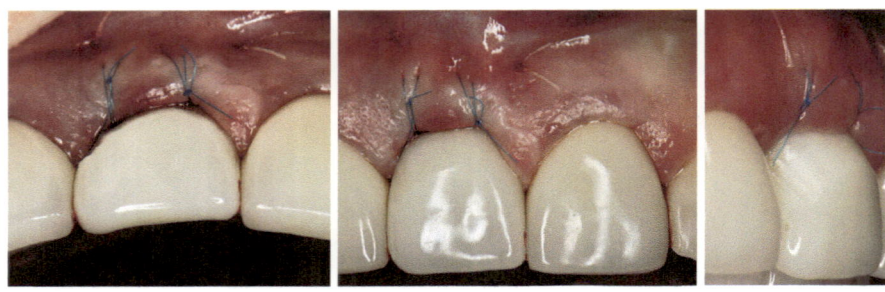

Fig. 157 Combined treatment: removal of the crown tunneling and CTG, implant-supported fixed interim restoration for creating a new emergent profile and new rehabilitation over implant and change in adjacent teeth crowns. Removal of crowns over the implant, critical and subcritical outlines were modified through over-contour elimination

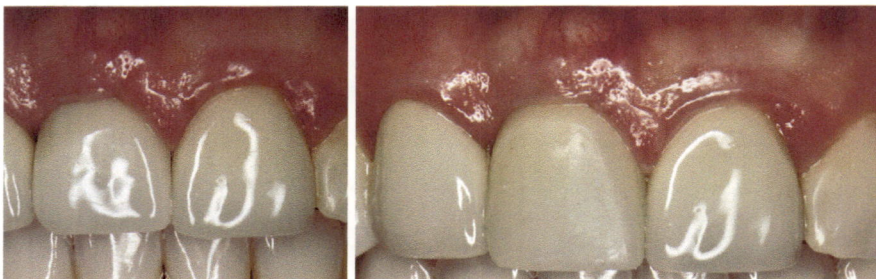

Fig. 158 Evaluation of new implant-supported fixed interim restoration over implant to modify the height zenith and develop a new emergence profile after 4 weeks of treatment

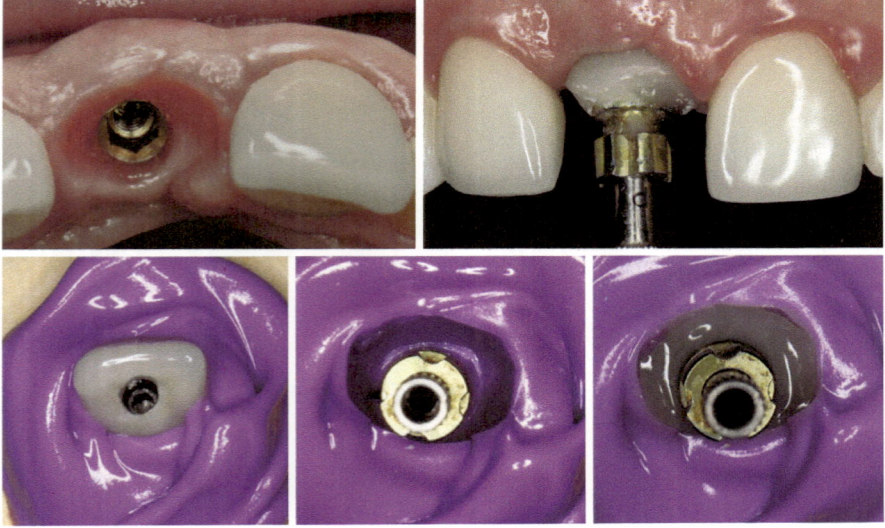

Fig. 159 Custom abutment transfer to copy emergence profile

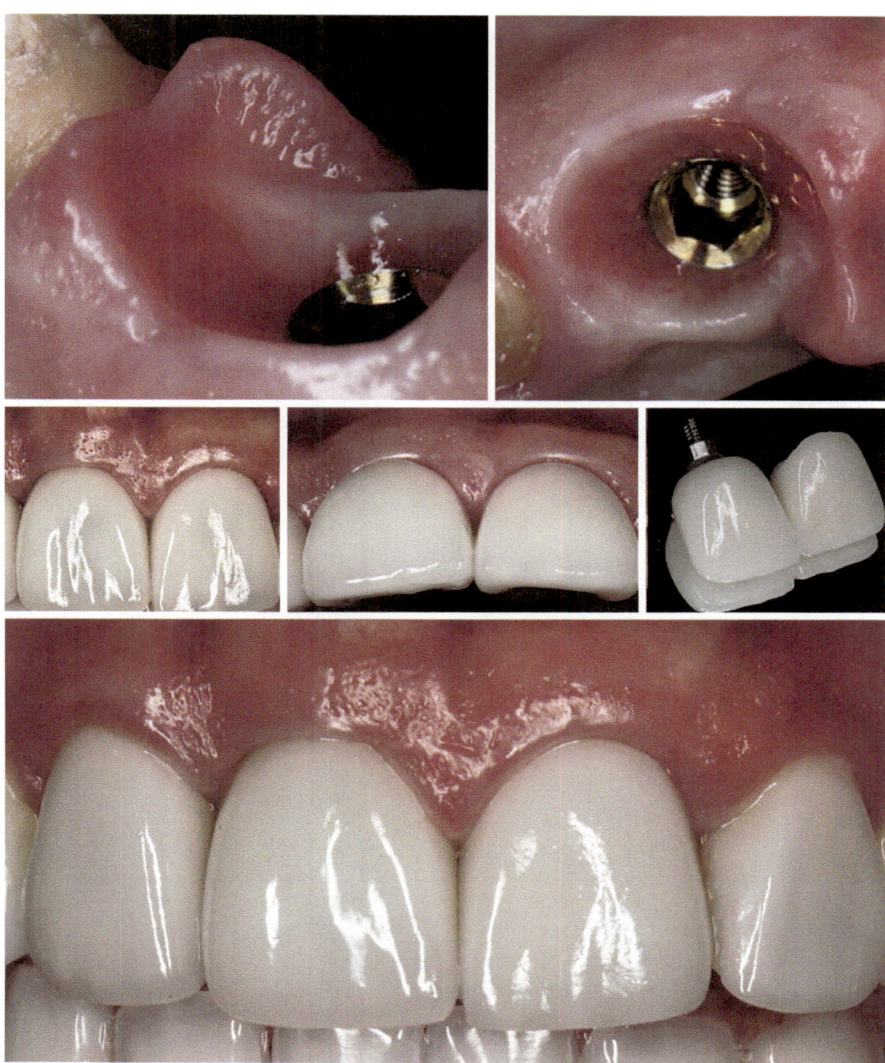

Fig. 160 Definitive restorations resulting in marked increase in peri-implant vestibular volume

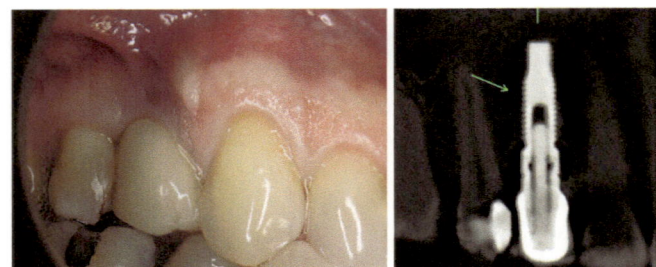
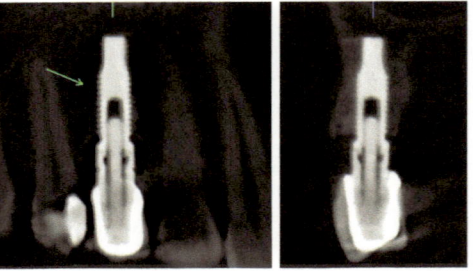

Figs. 161 A 47-year-old male patient with class I, subclass A PSTD, vestibular deficiency, and volume loss had active fistula at the middle 1/3 vestibular level

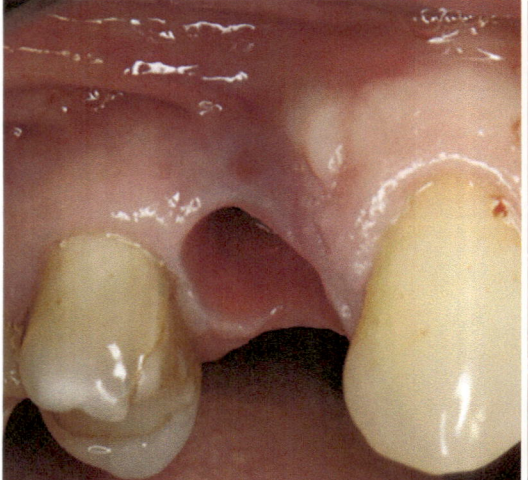
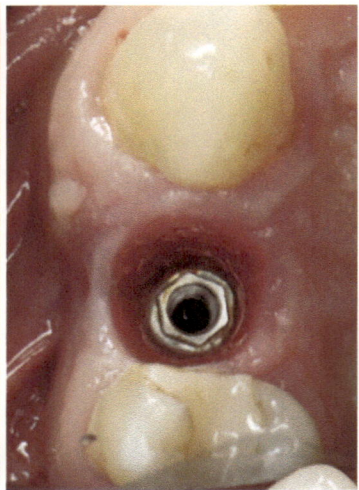

Fig. 162 Lateral and occlusal view

Fig. 163 Combined treatment: removal of the crown CAF and CTG, implant-supported fixed interim restoration for creating a new emergent profile and new rehabilitation over the implant

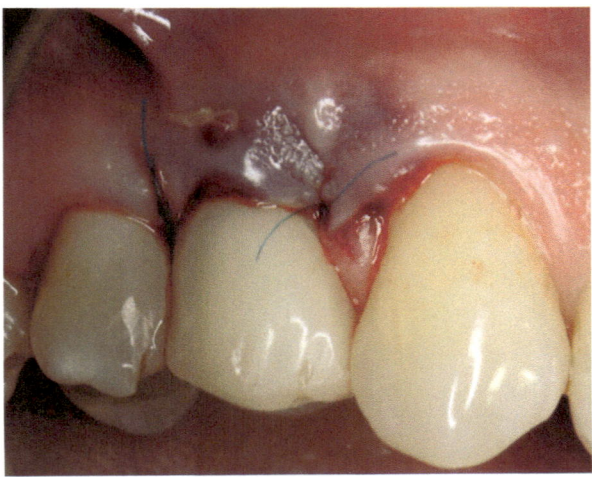

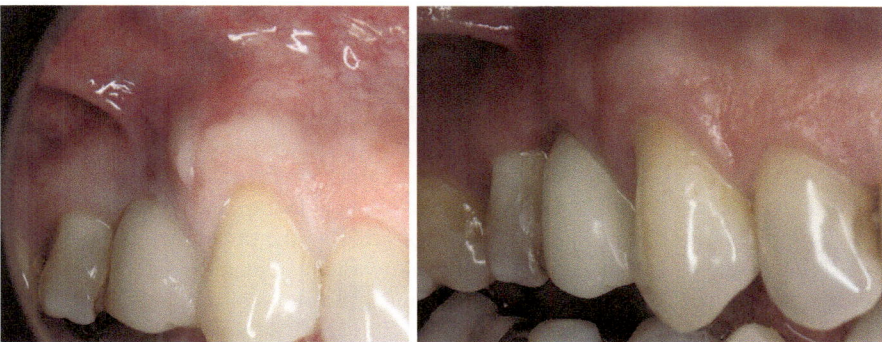

Fig. 164 Before and after surgery 6 months follow-up

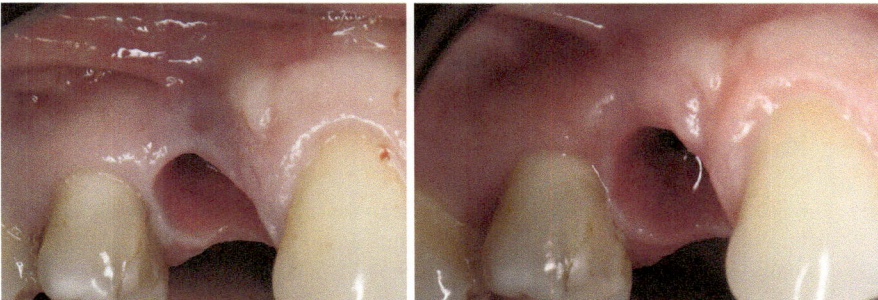

Fig. 165 Lateral view 6 months follow-up

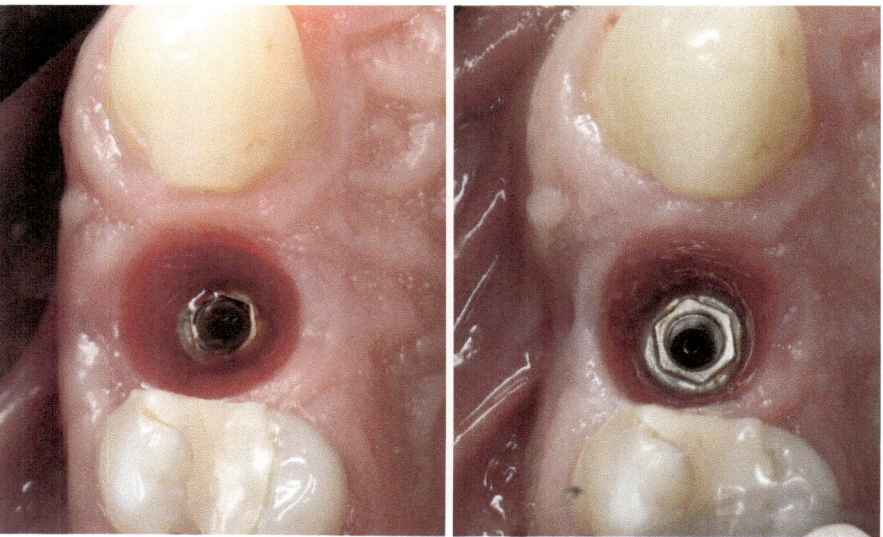

Fig. 166 Occlusal view 6 months follow-up

14 Conclusions

Microsurgical procedures usually require less extensive flap designs and offer enhanced vision fields that facilitate identification of defects and anatomical landmarks. The use of microsurgical principles and procedures provides clinically relevant advantages over conventional macrosurgical concepts and applications for plastic esthetic periodontal and peri-implant surgical therapy.

Current evidence supports the benefits of utilizing the operating microscope for periodontal and peri-implant plastic surgical treatment. Outcome superiority of root coverage surgical therapy with the use of magnification enhancing tools has been documented in the literature. This is validating clinical experience based reports that constitute the bulk of the evidence supporting this treatment approach. It is evident that the operating microscope is a superior magnification tool that has the potential to enhance esthetic outcomes in periodontal and peri-implant plastic therapy. Needless to say, the microsurgeon and the microsurgical team has to develop the necessary skills to take full advantage of what this technology has to offer.

15 Key Points

1. The use of micro-instruments and micro-sutures allows finer procedures that are difficult to achieve using macro-instruments and macro-sutures.
2. Visual acuity is enhanced by both magnification and illumination when performing periodontal surgical procedures with the aid of an OM. This translates into the controlled manipulation of soft and hard tissue structures that make up the periodontium.
3. A detailed exhaustive diagnosis and meticulous evaluation of the association of NCCls with gingival resection using a microscope is the key to decision-making in multidisciplinary treatment.
4. It is not easy to move out of the comfort zone, especially when significant changes to the daily practice need to be implemented. This is one of the main reasons for limited use of microscopes in the periodontal field. Great determination, effort, and dedication are required to incorporate microscopy into practice; however, after it is accomplished, there is no turning back. Moreover, it takes clinical performance to a new level.

References

1. Burkhardt R, Preiss A, Joss A, Lang NP. Influence of suture tension to the tearing characteristics of the soft tissues: an in vitro experiment. Clin Oral Impl Res. 2008;19:314–9.
2. Burkhardt R, Lang NP. Coverage of localized gingival recessions: comparison of micro and macrosurgical techniques. J Clin Periodontol. 2005;32:287–93.
3. Miller PD. A classification of marginal tissue recession. Int J Periodontics Restorative Dent. 1985;5:9–13.

4. Francetti L, Del Fabbro M, Calace S, et al. Microsurgical treatment of gingival recession: a controlled clinical study. Int J Periodontics Restorative Dent. 2005;25:181–8.
5. Andrade PF, Grisi MFM, Marcaccini AM, et al. Comparison between micro and macrosurgical techniques for the treatment of localized gingival recession using coronally positioned flaps and enamel matrix derivative. J Periodontol. 2010;81:1572–9.
6. Bittencourt S, Ribeiro EDP, Sallum EA, et al. Surgical microscope may enhance root coverage with subepithelial connective tissue graft: a randomized-controlled clinical trial. J Periodontol. 2012;83:721–30.
7. Nevins M. Editorial: limitations of evidence-based dentistry. Int J Periodontics Restorative Dent. 2017;37:779.
8. Di Gianfilippo R, Wang IC, Steigmann L, et al. Efficacy of microsurgery and comparison to macrosurgery for gingival recession treatment: a systematic review with meta-analysis. Clin Oral Invest. 2021; https://doi.org/10.1007/s00784-021-03954-0.
9. Zweers J, Thomas RZ, Slot DE, Weisgold AS, Van der Weijden GA. Characteristics of periodontal biotype, its dimensions, associations and prevalence: a systematic review. J Clin Periodontol. 2014;41:958–71.
10. Shanelec DA, Tibbetts L. A perspective on the future of periodontal microsurgery. Periodontol. 2000;1996(11):58–64.
11. Van Hattam A, James J. A model for the study of epithelial migration in wound healing. Virchows Arch B Cell Pathol Incl Mol Pathol. 1979;30:221–30.
12. Curtis JW Jr, McLain JB, Hutchinson RA. The incidence and severity of complications and pain following periodontal surgery. J Periodontol. 1985;56:597–601.
13. Cairo F, Rotundo R, Miller PD, Pini Prato GP. Root coverage esthetic score: a system to evaluate the esthetic outcome of the treatment of gingival recession through evaluation of clinical cases. J Periodontol. 2009;80:705–10. https://doi.org/10.1902/jop.2010.100278.
14. Tibbetts L, Shanelec DA. An overview of periodontal microsurgery. Curr Opin Periodontol. 1994:187–93.
15. Rasperini G, Acunzo R, Limiroli E. Decision making in gingival recession treatment scientific evidence and clinical experience. Clin Adv Periodont. 2011;1(1):41–52.
16. Cairo F, Nieri M, Cincinelli S, Mervelt J, Pagliaro U. The interproximal clinical attachment level to classify gingival recessions and predict root coverage outcomes: an explorative and reliability study. J Clin Periodontol. 2011;38:661–6.
17. Baldi C, et al. Coronally advanced flap procedure for root coverage. Is flap thickness a relevant predictor to achieve root coverage? A 19-case series. J Periodontol. 1999;70:1077–84.
18. Lindhe J, Karring T. Anatomy of the periodontium. In: Lindhe J, Karring T, Lang NP, editors. Clinical periodontology and implant dentistry. 3rd ed. Copenhagen: Munksgaard; 1997. p. 19–68.
19. Otto Z. Plastic-esthetic periodontal and implant surgery: a microsurgical approach. Quintessence Publishing Co, Ltd; 2012. p. 51–4.
20. Zucchelli G, De Santis M. Treatment of multiple recessions-type defects in patients with esthetic demands. J Periodontol. 2000;71:1506–14.
21. Clementini M, Discepoli N, Danesi C, de Sanctis M. Biologically guided flap stability: the role of flap thickness including periosteum retention on the performance of the coronally advanced flap–a double-blind randomized clinical trial. J Clin Periodontol. 2018;45:1238–46. https://doi.org/10.1111/jcpe.12998.
22. Griffin TJ, Hur Y, Bu J. Basic suture techniques for oral mucosa. Clin Adv Periodont. 2011;2011(1):221–32.
23. Wachtel H, Fickl S, Zuhr O, Hurezeler M. The double sling suture. A modified technique for primary wound closure. Eur J Esthet Dent. 2006;1:314–24.
24. Azzi R, Etienne D. Recouvrement radiculaire et reconstruction papillaire par greffon conjonctif enfoui sous un lambeau vestibulaire tunnelisé et tracté coronairement. Journal de Parodontologie et d'Implantologie Orale. 1998;17:71–7.
25. Zucchelli G, De Sanctis M. Coronally advanced flap: a modified surgical approach for isolated recessions-type defects. J Clin Periodontol. 2007;34(3):262–8.

26. Grupe J, Warren R. Repair of gingival defects by a sliding flap operation. J Periodontol. 1956;27:290–5.
27. Zucchelli G, De Sanctis M. Laterally moved, coronally advanced flap: a modified surgical approach for isolated recession type defects. J Periodontol. 2004;75:1734–41.
28. Zucchelli G, De Sanctis M. Treatment of multiple recession-type defects in patients with esthetic demands. J Periodontol. 2000;71:1506–14.
29. Raetzke PB. Covering localized areas of root exposure employing the "envelope" technique. J Periodontol. 1985;56:397–402.
30. Allen AL. Use of the supraperiosteal envelope in soft tissue grafting for root coverage. I. Rationale and technique. Int J Periodontics Restorative Dent. 1994;14:216–27.
31. Sculean A, Allen E. The laterally closed tunnel for the treatment of deep isolated mandibular recessions: surgical technique and a report of 24 cases. Int J Periodontics Restorative Dent. 2018;38:479–87. https://doi.org/10.11607/prd.3680.
32. Carranza N, Pontaloro C. Laterally stretched flap with connective tissue graft to treat single narrow deep recession defects on lower incisors. Clin Adv Periodont. 2019;9:29–33.
33. Zabalegui I, Sicilia A, Cambra J, Gil J, Sanz M. Treatment of múltiple adjacent gingival recessions with the tunnel subepithelial connective tissue graft: a clinical report. Int J Periodont Restorat Dentist. 1999;1999(19):199–206.
34. Zurh O, Flick S, Wachtoll H, Bolz W, Hurzeler MB. Covering of gingival recessions with a modified microsurgical tunnel technique- a case report. Int Periodont Restorat Dent. 2007;27:456–63.
35. Edel A. Clinical evaluation of free connective tissue grafts used to increase the width of keratinised gingival. J Clin Periodontol. 1974;1:185–96.
36. Hurzeler M, Weng O. A single incision technique harvest subepithelial contective tissue graft from the palate. Int J Periodontics Restorative Dent. 1999;19:279–87.
37. Lorenzana ER, Allen EP. The single-incision palatal harvest technique: a strategy for aesthetics and patient comfort. Int J Periodont Restorat Dent. 2000;2:297–305.
38. Zucchelli G, Mele M, Stefanini M, Mazzotti C, Marzadori M, Montebugnoli L, de Sanctis M. Patient morbidity and root coverage outcome after subepithelial connective tissue and de-epithelialized grafts: a comparative randomized-controlled clinical trial. J Clin Periodontol. 2010;37:728–38. https://doi.org/10.1111/j.1600-051X.2010.01550.x.
39. Pedrine M, Bovi G, Zaffalon M, Nociti F Jr, et al. The influence of local anatomy on the outcome of treatment of gingival recession associated with non-carious cervical lesions. J Periodontol. 2010;81:1027–34.
40. Deliberador T, Bosco A, Martins T, Nagata M. Treatment of gingival recessions associated to cervical abrasion lesions with subepithelial connective tissue graft. A case Report. Eur J Dent. 2009;3:318–23.
41. Cortellini P, Bissada NF. Mucogingival conditions in the natural dentition: Nar- rative review, case definitions, and diagnostic considerations. J Periodontol. 2018;89(Suppl 1):S204–13. https://doi.org/10.1002/JPER.16-0671.
42. Pini-Prato G, Franceschi D, Cairo F, Nieri M, et al. Classification of dental surface defects in areas of gingival recession. J Periodontol. 2010;81:885–90.
43. Zucchelli G, Gori G, Mele M, Stefanini M, et al. Non carious cervical lesions associated with gingival recessions. A decisión-making process. J Periodontol. 2011;82:1713–24.
44. Zucchelli G, Testori T, De Sanctis M. Clinical and anatomical factors limiting treatment outcomes of gingival recession: a new method to predetermine the line of root coverage. J Periodontol. 2006;77:714–21.
45. Zucchelli G, Mele M, Stefanini M, Mazzotti C. Predetermination of root coverage. J Periodontol. 2010;81:1019–26.
46. Pini Prato GP, Cario F. A technique to identify and reconstruct the cementoenamel junction level using combined periodontal and restorative treatment of gingival recession. A prospective study. Int J Periodontics Restorative Dent. 2010;30:573–81.
47. Durán JC, Alarcón C, De la Jara D, Pino R, Lanis A. Multidisciplinary treatment of deep non-carious cervical lesion with a CAD/CAM chairside restoration in combination with periodontal

surgery: a 60-month follow-up technique report. Clin Adv Periodontics. 2021;11:8792. https://doi.org/10.1002/cap.10152.

48. Belser UC, Bernard JP, Buser D. Implant-supported restorations in the anterior region: prosthetic considerations. Pract Periodontics Aesthet Dent. 1996;8:875–83.

49. Furhauser R, et al. Evaluation of soft tissue around single-tooth implant crowns: the pink esthetics score. Clin Oral Implants Res. 2005;16:639–44.

50. Mazzotti C, Stefanini M, Felice P, Bentivogli V, Mounssif I, Zucchelli G. Soft-tissue dehiscence coverage at peri-implant sites. Periodontol. 2000;2018(77):256–72.

51. Lemongello G. Customized provisional abutment and provisional restauration for an immediately-placed implant. PPAD. 2007;19(7):419–24.

52. Tsuda H, et al. Peri-implant tissue response following connective tissue and bone grafting in conjunction with immediate single- tooth replacement in the esthetic zone: a case series. Int J Oral Maxillofac Implants. 2011;26:427–36.

53. De Bruyn H, Raes S, Matthys C, Cosyn J. The current use of patient-centered/reported outcomes in implant dentistry: a systematic review. Clin Oral Implants Res. 2015;26(Suppl 11):45–56.

54. Zucchelli G, Tavelli L, Stefanini M, et al. Classification of facial peri-implant soft tissue dehiscences/deficiencies at single implant sites in the esthetic zone. J Periodontol. 2019:1–9. https://doi.org/10.1002/JPER.18-0616.

Microscope-Assisted Laser Ablation of Gingival Pigmentation

Akira Aoki, Koji Mizutani, and Risako Mikami

Contents

Supplementary Information The online version contains supplementary material available at [https://doi.org/10.1007/978-3-030-96874-8_8].

A. Aoki (✉) · K. Mizutani · R. Mikami
Department of Periodontology, Graduate School of Medical and Dental Sciences, Tokyo Medical and Dental University (TMDU), Tokyo, Japan
e-mail: aoperi@tmd.ac.jp

Abstract

Unsightly gingival pigmentations can markedly detract from a patient's esthetic appearance. Oral melanin deposition is the most frequently observed physiological pigmentation in the gingiva. Conversely, as iatrogenic pigmentations, metal or amalgam tattoos are occasionally observed following unintentional tissue contamination during dental treatment. Previously, mechanical and surgical treatments have been the primary means of removing such pigmentations; however, those removal procedures were relatively invasive and not necessarily effective, in particular, for metal tattoo removal. Patient demand is increasing for the removal of gingival pigmentation and the recovery of esthetic appearance, especially in the anterior labial gingiva. Thus, other more useful tools or methods have been sought. Recently, laser soft tissue surgery has attracted attention, and less invasive depigmentation procedures have been implemented using different types of dental lasers. Among those lasers, Er:YAG laser has notably advantageous properties for soft tissue surgery with its minimal thermal influence and precise ablation under water spray. Furthermore, the combination of Er:YAG laser with microscopy facilitates safe and effective pigmentation removal, uneventful and favorable wound healing, as well as successful outcomes in improving discoloration. In this chapter, the characteristics of Er:YAG laser, the details regarding minimally invasive procedures for microscope-assisted laser ablation of gingival melanin and metal tattoo pigmentations, and exemplary clinical cases are presented.

Keywords

Melanin · Metal tattoos · Pigmentation · Esthetic · Laser · Minimally invasive Microsurgery

1   Introduction: Gingival Pigmentation

Healthy gingival color is an essential component of a charming smile, especially in patients with a high smile line [1]. Normal physiologic gingival color is coral or salmon pink depending on physiological variations of periodontal tissue, such as degree of vascularization, epithelial thickness, and the amount of melanin pigment [2]. According to the spectrophotometric CIELAB color system ($L^*a^*b^*$) defined by the International Commission on Illumination (abbreviated CIE), which expresses color as three values: L^* for perceptual lightness, and a^* and b^* for the four unique colors of human vision (red, green, blue, and yellow), the averaged coordinates of gingival tissue around the upper central incisor are reportedly approximately 43–50 for L^*, 15–24 for a^*, and 10–23 for b^* [3–5].

The etiology of oral pigmentation may be physiological or pathological. As a physiological pigmentation, visible oral melanin pigmentation of intraoral tissue is most frequently observed in the gingiva tissue [6]. Melanin is pigment synthesized

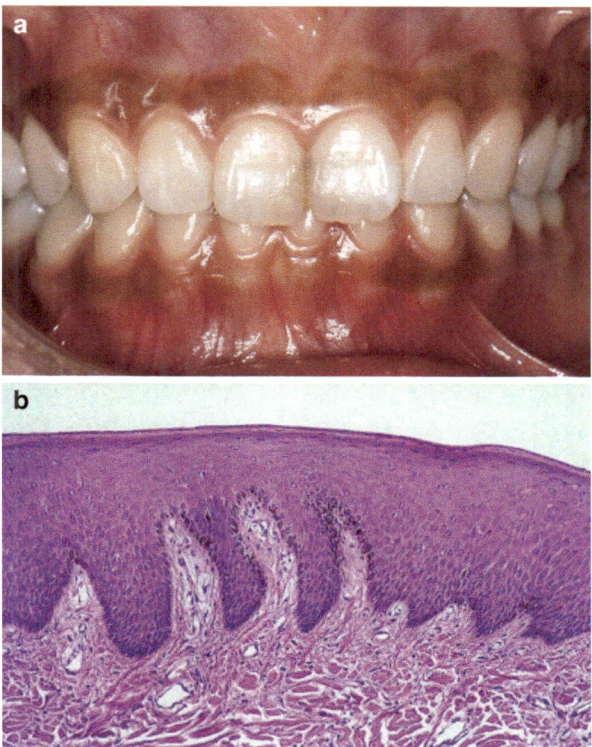

Fig. 1 Melanin hyperpigmentation. A 19-year-old female, non-smoker. Generalized moderate to severe melanin hyperpigmentation observed in the attached gingiva of the upper and lower arches (**a**). Histology of melanin pigmentation in a dog (**b**). Melanocytes in the basal cell layer of the gingival epithelium produce melanin that deposits in the epithelium and occasionally in the underlying connective tissue, which causes discoloration of gingiva, resulting in an unesthetic appearance. [Picture from Ishii S et al. Application of an Er:YAG laser to remove gingival melanin hyperpigmentation. *J Jpn Soc Laser Dent.* 2002;13:89–96; with permission. © copyright (2002) J Jpn Soc Laser Dent] [8]

and stored in melanosomes that are produced by melanocytes [7]. Melanocytes are located in the epithelial basal cell layer and can cause dark-colored changes in the gingiva, known as melanin hyperpigmentation (MH) (Fig. 1) [9]. MH occurs in all human races [6]. According to Suzuki et al. [3], the averaged $L^*a^*b^*$ of melanin pigmented oral tissue is reportedly approximately 42 (50: value of normal gingival tissue in their study) for L^*, 16 (23) for a^*, and 15 (23) for b^*. Pathological oral pigmentations can be caused by drugs, smoking, genetics, inflammation, exposure to UV rays, endocrine disturbances (Addison's disease, Albright and Nelson's syndrome, acromegaly), malignant melanoma, and other systemic diseases [10]. Therefore, a detailed medical history of the patient and further histopathological examination is crucial in determining whether the pigmentation is physiological or pathological [2].

Fig. 2 Metal tattoo pigmentation. A 52-year-old female. Severe black-colored gingival discoloration, namely metal tattoos, observed at marginal area of upper central incisors. [Picture from Ishikawa I, Aoki A, Takasaki A. Potential applications of erbium:YAG laser in periodontics. *J Periodont Res*. 2004;39:275–85; with permission. © copyright (2015) Blackwell Munksgaard Ltd] [11]

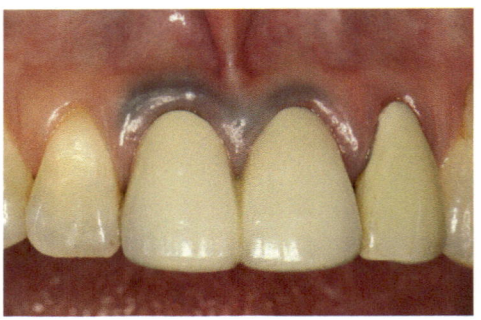

Conversely, as an iatrogenic pigmentation, a metal or an amalgam tattoo is occasionally observed following its unintentionally induction during dental treatment (Fig. 2). The metal/amalgam tattoo is the blue-gray pigmentation caused by the inadvertent deposition of metallic materials (as microdebris or microfragments derived from dental prostheses) into the gingiva adjacent to the teeth undergoing dental treatment. Reportedly, 3.3% of adults in the USA have metal/amalgam tattoos [12] and the presence of metals (Ag, Hg, Cu, Fe, Zn, S, Se, Ca, P, and Si) used in dental alloys were found in the metal tattoos within gingival tissue [13, 14]. The pigmented areas vary from very small spots to large areas that can be present in gingiva involving multiple teeth and causing serious esthetic problems.

Even though MH and amalgam tattoos are not medical problems, patient demands are increasing for their removal in order to recover an esthetic appearance, especially in the anterior labial gingiva. The techniques used to manage gingival color have become more important in order to meet patients' expectations of esthetically pleasing results following dental procedures.

2   Application of Lasers in Gingival Depigmentation

The basic concept of gingival depigmentation is the physical removal of gingival tissue surrounding discolored areas. That should be efficiently achieved by precisely detecting and accessing the layers where melanin or metal associated pigments are deposited. Special attention should be given not to cause residuum and/or pigmentation recurrence.

Various therapeutic methods for MH removal have been developed, such as bur abrasion, electrosurgery, chemical surgery, cryosurgery, laser surgery, gingivectomy, flap surgery, gingival grafting, and combinations thereof [1, 9]. One of the proposed modalities, laser surgery, is proven to reduce treatment invasiveness and is widely acknowledged [2]. Different lasers have been applied to remove MH, such as CO_2 [15], diode [16], Nd:YAG [17], and Er:YAG [2, 8, 18–21] lasers.

As for metal tattoo removal, the effective methods have never been established due to difficulties in surgical procedures and the lack of adequate instrumentation. Previously, some case reports have reported techniques using soft tissue grafts [connective tissue grafts (CTG) [22], free gingival grafts (FGG) [23] to remove metal tattoos. However, while the esthetics improved, these surgical procedures were reported to be highly invasive, complicated to use, and having results that were not always effective. In particular, surgical procedures such as flap elevation, graft harvesting, and suturing (required at both graft donor and pigmented recipient sites) prolonged treatment time, increased postoperative pain, and heightened risks of gingival recession, deformity, and defects. Recently, the advantageous effects of laser application have attracted attention, and less invasive metal tattoo removal has been implemented using different types of lasers, such as diode [24], Q-switched alexandrite [25], Er:YAG [11, 26, 27], and Er,Cr:YSGG [28] lasers, and successful outcomes have been reported.

Laser ablation for gingival depigmentation is recognized as an effective, safe, comfortable, and reliable technique which does not employ incisions and suturing, as compared to conventional methods [1]. However, in areas of thin and delicate gingiva, the CO_2, diode, and Nd:YAG lasers risk producing gingival ulceration and recession, due to their relatively strong thermal and/or deeply penetrating effects [17] (Fig. 3).

In recent years, the use of Er:YAG lasers for gingival depigmentation has gained increasing recognition for its ability for efficient soft tissue ablation with extremely low thermal damage to lased tissues. From 2002 to 2004, for the first time, our group reported several cases of successful gingival MH [8, 18] and metal tattoo removal [11] using an Er:YAG laser in combination with a microscope, demonstrating excellent esthetic improvements.

In this chapter, as a novel minimally invasive method for gingival depigmentation, we will introduce microscope-assisted gingival depigmentation using an Er:YAG laser.

3 Er:YAG Laser-Assisted Gingival Depigmentation

3.1 Indication for Depigmentation of Gingiva

Before performing gingival pigmentation removal, a differential diagnosis must be determined since melanomas occasionally resemble melanin pigmentations or metal tattoos. Proper diagnosis should be established after obtaining the patient's medical history and conducting a careful clinical examination. If there is any suspicion of melanoma considering the patient's clinical appearance and medical history, a preliminary incisional biopsy may be indicated to confirm a diagnosis of melanin or metal tattoo pigmentation [30]. Also, patients with chronic periodontitis should undergo periodontal therapy prior to depigmentation treatment.

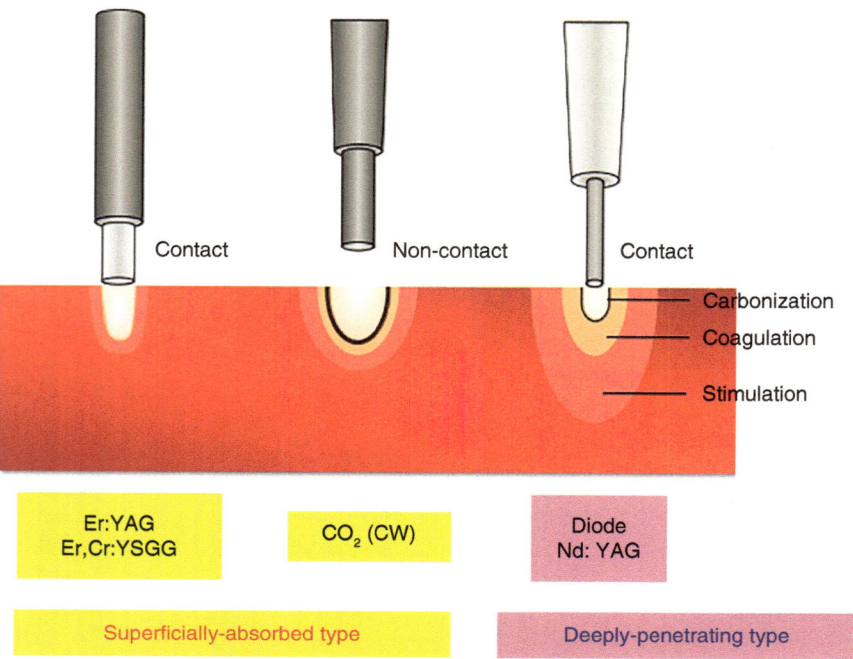

Fig. 3 Classification of lasers according to their penetration depth. One is a superficially absorbed type (shallowly penetrating type), in which the laser light does not penetrate or scatter deeply, and the other is a deeply penetrating type. CO_2, carbon dioxide; CW, continuous wave; Er,Cr:YSGG-erbium, chromium-doped yttrium-scandium-gallium-garnet; Er:YAG, erbium-doped yttrium-aluminum-garnet; Nd:YAG, neodymium-doped yttrium-aluminum-garnet. [Picture and legend from Aoki A et al. Periodontal and peri-implant wound healing following laser therapy. *Periodontol 2000.* 2015;68(1): 217–269; with permission. © copyright (2015) John Wiley & Sons A/S] [29]

3.2   Characteristics of Er:YAG Laser

Due to its high absorption by water (Fig. 4) [31, 32], the pulsed Er:YAG laser (2,940 nm) has an excellent capacity for ablating both soft and hard biological tissues with minimal thermal side effects. Thus, the Er:YAG laser can be applied not only for oral soft tissue surgery but also for hard tissue treatments such as caries removal, root surface debridement, and bone ablation [33]. Currently, the Er:YAG laser has the broadest range of periodontal applications and remains one of the most suitable lasers for periodontal therapy [29, 33, 34]. This laser employs fiberoptic or articulated mirror arm systems with various delicate contact tips for different treatment purposes. We have been using the following Er:YAG laser apparatuses: DELight® Dental Laser (Hoya ConBio, Fremont, CA, USA); Erwin AdvErL® or Erwin AdvErL Evo® (J. Morita Mfg. Corp., Tokyo, Japan); Light walker® (Photona, Slovenia) (Figs. 5, 6, and 7). As another laser in the erbium laser family, the Er,Cr:YSGG laser (2,780 nm) shows performance similar to the Er:YAG. Unlike the

Fig. 4 Laser absorption spectrum for water. Data were calculated from Hale and Querry [31]. Ar (488 nm), Diode (810 nm), Nd:YAG (1,064 nm), Er,Cr:YSGG (2,780 nm), Er:YAG (2,940 nm), and CO_2 (10,600 nm) are indicated in the figure

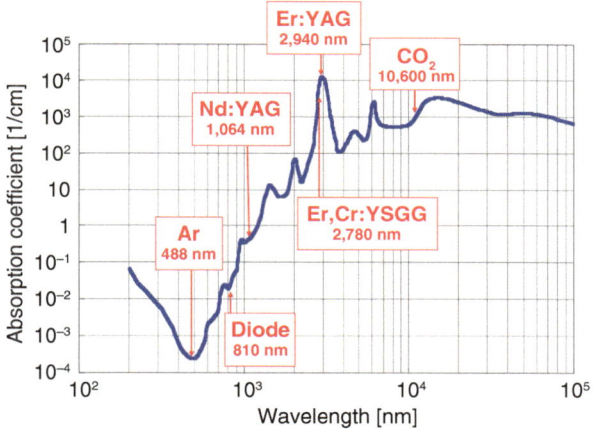

Er:YAG laser, the Er,Cr:YSGG laser's energy is absorbed more by hydroxyl (OH-) ions than by water molecules [35].

3.3 Ablation Mechanism and Thermal Effects

Among dental lasers, the Er:YAG laser has the highest absorption by water [31, 32] (Fig. 4) and thus efficiently ablates soft tissues with no visible thermal effects on the surrounding tissues during irradiation, particularly when it is used in combination with a water spray (Fig. 8) [33].

In vivo studies reported that the width of the thermally changed layer following Er:YAG laser incision was only 10–50 µm (porcine skin in non-contact mode) [36] or approximately 20 µm following Er:YAG laser contact ablation of gingival tissue in rats [37]. An ex vivo study demonstrated that the width of the coagulation layer on porcine gingival tissue following Er:YAG laser ablation was minimal compared to other dental lasers and electrosurgery: approximately 18 µm with water spray and 38 µm with no water spray (Fig. 9) [38]. Between the two types of erbium lasers, the effect of soft tissue ablation seems to be greater in the Er:YAG laser than in the Er,Cr:YSGG laser with less thermal side effects [38, 39].

3.4 Soft Tissue Ablation and Wound Healing Following Er:YAG Laser Surgery

Conventionally, scalpels have been mainly employed in soft tissue surgery. In the case where hemostasis is required following elimination of marginal gingival tissue in restorative or prosthetic therapy, electrosurgery has been frequently employed.

Fig. 5 Er:YAG laser
apparatus. Erwin
AdvErL™ Evo, J. Morita
Mfg. Corp., Kyoto, Japan

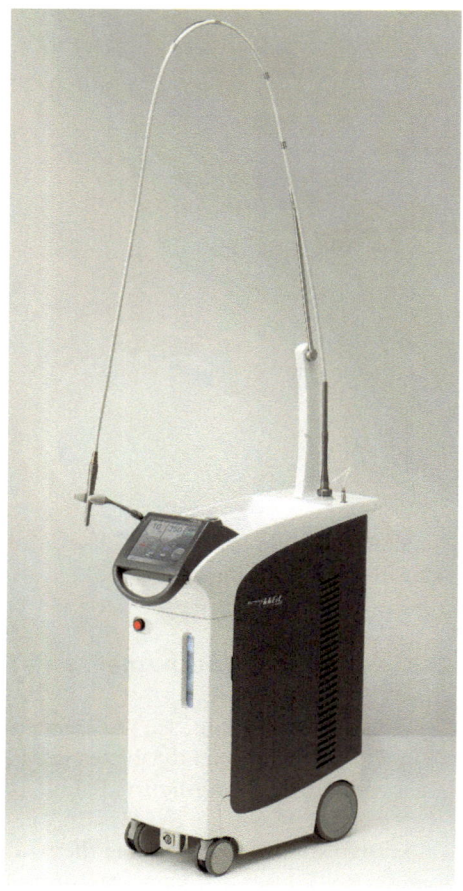

Fig. 6 Er:YAG laser handpiece with a
contact tip

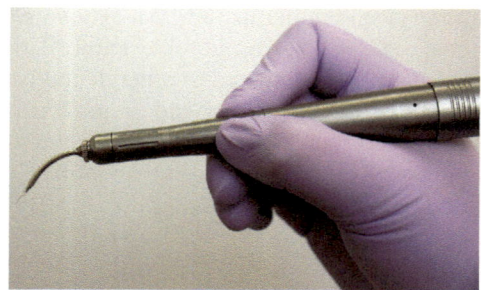

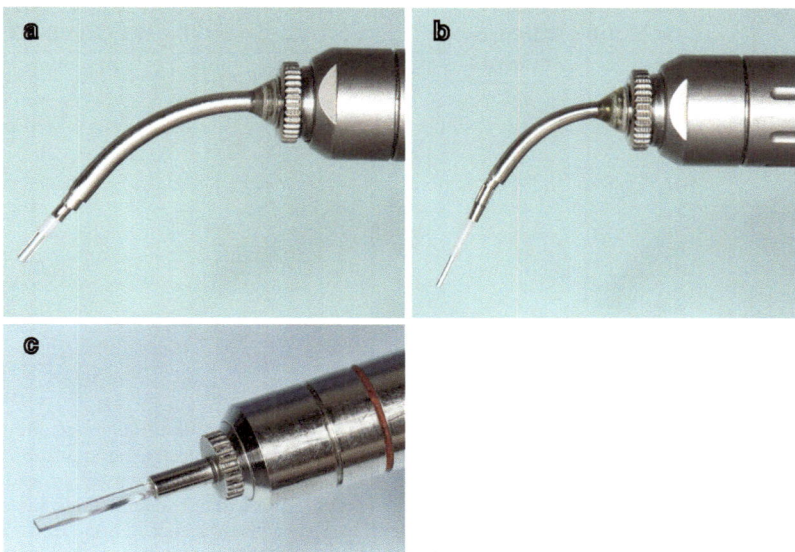

Fig. 7 Contact tips for Er:YAG laser irradiation. (**a**) Conventional cylindrical contact tip made of quartz glass, with curvature of 80°, a round end with a diameter of 600 μm and approximately 65% laser transmission (C600F; Erwin AdvErL™ Evo, J. Morita Mfg. Corp., Kyoto, Japan). (**b**) Cylindrical contact tip made of quartz glass with a diameter of 400 μm (C400F; J. Morita Mfg. Corp.). (**c**) Chisel tip made of sapphire glass, with a rectangular pointed head of 1.40 × 0.45 mm dimension and approximately 82% laser transmission (P/N 625-8746; DELight™, HOYA Conbio, Fremont, CA, USA)

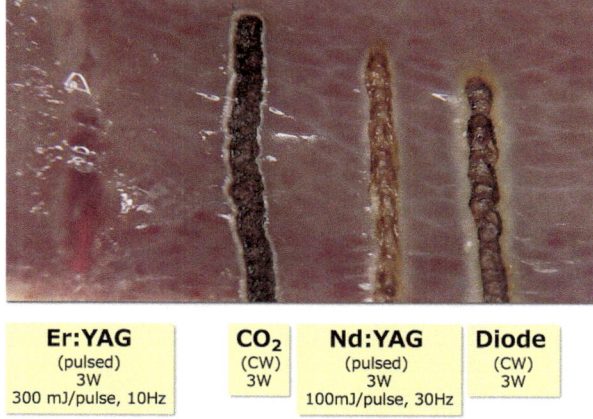

Er:YAG	CO$_2$	Nd:YAG	Diode
(pulsed)	(CW)	(pulsed)	(CW)
3W	3W	3W	3W
300 mJ/pulse, 10Hz		100mJ/pulse, 30Hz	

Fig. 8 Effects of four different types of lasers on soft tissue. Following photothermal ablation caused by lasers, various degrees of thermal denaturation were observed on the irradiated site (chicken liver). The pulsed Er:YAG laser effectively ablates soft tissue, with minimal coagulation and no carbonization. The continuous wave CO$_2$ laser also easily ablated soft tissue, but severe carbonization was evident with relatively thin coagulation. The pulsed Nd:YAG laser produced relatively thick coagulation with moderate carbonization. The CW diode laser produced the greatest coagulation, as well as moderate carbonization (Courtesy of Dr. Junji Kato). [Modified pictures and legend from Aoki A et al. Periodontal and peri-implant wound healing following laser therapy. *Periodontol 2000.* 2015;68(1): 217–269; with permission. © copyright (2015) John Wiley & Sons A/S] [29]

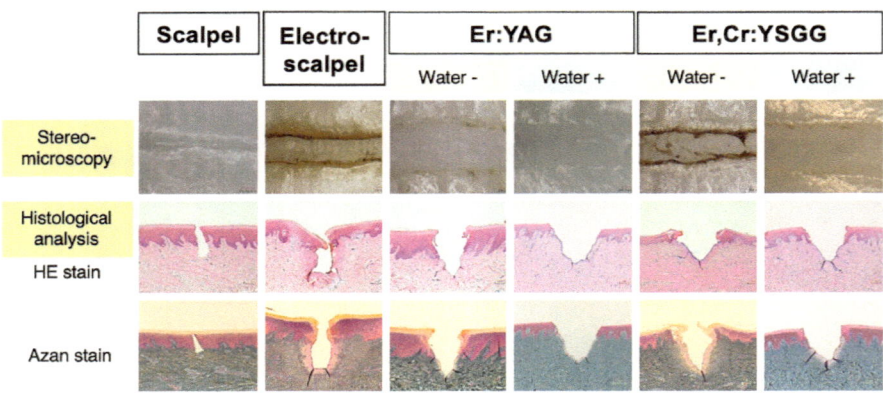

Fig. 9 Stereomicroscopy and histological analysis following gingival tissue ablation/cutting with Er:YAG laser, Er,Cr:YSGG laser, and electroscalpel. Stereomicroscopically, carbonization of the groove edge and bottom was negligible after Er:YAG with/without water spray and after Er,Cr:YSGG with water spray, and moderate after Er,Cr:YSGG without water and electroscalpel. The epithelial wound edges were smooth for scalpel, Er:YAG with/without water, and Er,Cr:YSGG with water, while epithelial collapse was observed with Er,Cr:YSGG without water and electroscalpel. Thickness of coagulated layer was minimal for Er:YAG (37.7 ± 9.6 μm) followed by Er,Cr:YSGG (50.6 ± 5.7 μm) and electroscalpel (82.0 ± 26.2 μm). Thermally affected layer around the coagulation was not detected for Er:YAG and the layer was minimally observed in Er,Cr:YSGG (65.7 ± 27.6 μm), followed by electroscalpel (94.2 ± 30.1 μm). The total width of coagulated and thermally affected layer was minimal (37.7 ± 9.6 μm) for Er:YAG and was significantly thinner as compared to Er,Cr:YSGG (116.4 ± 31.7 μm) and electroscalpel (176.2 ± 55.2 μm). With the use of water spray, coagulation was significantly reduced for Er:YAG (17.9 ± 2.1 μm) and for Er,Cr:YSGG (33.1 ± 1.4 μm), and thermally affected layer was none for both lasers. The total width was also reduced for Er:YAG (17.9 ± 2.1 μm) and Er,Cr:YSGG (33.1 ± 1.4 μm), with water spray. [Modified pictures and legend from Kawamura R, et al.: Ex vivo evaluation of gingival ablation with various laser systems and electroscalpel. *Photobiomodul Photomed Laser Surg*, 38:364–373, 2020; with permission. © copyright (2020) Mary Ann Liebert A/S] [38]

Electrosurgery is capable of readily incising soft tissues with good hemostasis [40]. However, delayed wound healing following such gingival tissue management, with a potential risk of thermal damage [37] and necrosis of the underlying periosteum and alveolar bone, can be a complication [41–43]. Compared to electrosurgery, laser treatment offers some advantages, such as greater patient comfort and safety with less postoperative pain and fewer complications. The Er:YAG laser-treated sites show faster and more favorable gingival wound healing compared to electrosurgery sites, suggesting that the Er:YAG laser is a suitable tool for periodontal soft tissue management (Fig. 10) [37].

Erbium lasers reveal precise ablation with minimal thermal effects among available dental lasers [36, 38, 44], resulting in the speediest and most uneventful wound healing. Wound healing following Er:YAG laser gingivectomy in dogs is relatively fast and clinically and histologically comparable to that of scalpel surgery [45]. In particular, sufficient bleeding and blood clot formation in the ablated defects are assured by the minimal hemostasis seen during erbium laser surgery, resulting in secure wound healing [37].

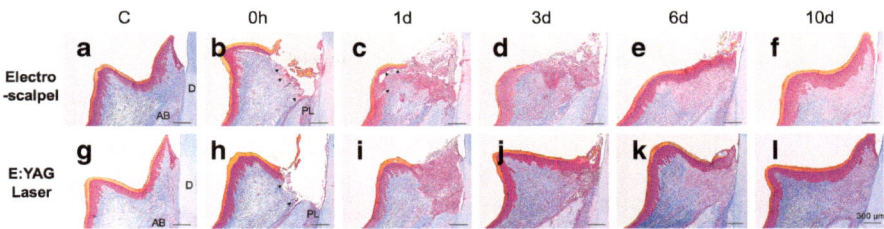

Fig. 10 Histological photomicrographs of the gingival defect following ablation with electroscalpel treatment (electrosurgery) (**a–f**) or Er:YAG laser irradiation (**g–l**). Before treatment (nontreated control: C), there was no inflammation in the gingiva (**a, g**). At 0 h (immediately after), compared to the electrosurgery (**b**), much less changed (coagulated) layer was observed on the treated connective tissue surface of the gingival defect in the Er:YAG laser (**h**) (arrowheads). At day 1, faster and more mature fibrin clot formation was observed in the Er:YAG laser (**i**) than in the electrosurgery (**c**). In the Er:YAG laser, re-epithelialization was almost completed at day 3 (**j**), while in the electrosurgery, collapse of the epithelial (arrowheads) and connective tissue layer progressed up to day 3 (**b, c, d**), and re-epithelialization was delayed and completed by day 6 (**e**). Inflammation of gingiva was scarce at both sites at day 10 (**f, l**), but connective tissue maturation was delayed in the electrosurgery (**f**). AB: alveolar bone, D: root dentin, PL: periodontal ligament. (Azan stain) [Pictures and legend from Sawabe M et al.: Gingival tissue healing following Er:YAG laser ablation compared to electrosurgery in rats. *Lasers Med Sci.* 2015;30 [2]:875–83; with permission. © copyright (2013) Springer-Verlag London 2013] [37]

In addition, lasers possess the interesting and characteristic property of biological effects (photobiomodulation: PBM) induced by low-level laser therapy (LLLT) [46, 47]. Briefly, during high-level laser irradiation (HLLT) a certain amount of energy simultaneously scatters or penetrates into the surrounding or underlying tissues, stimulating biological response, which in turn helps the promotion of wound healing/regeneration [48–50]. These effects are believed to be related to photochemical reactions within cells. PBM causes various biological effects, such as activation of wound healing [46, 51, 52], reduction of inflammation [53], as well as pain relief [51, 54].

PBM with Er:YAG laser is reported to cause promotion of cell proliferation [55–58], through phosphorylation of extracellular signal-regulated protein kinase (MAPK/ERK) [56], upregulation of galectin 7 expression [58], and the activation of temperature-sensitive transient receptor potential (TRP) channels [57].

Regarding pain perception, Zeredo et al. [59] performed oral soft tissue incisions in rats and examined the amplitude of the jaw-opening reflex measured by the digastric muscle electromyogram, in order to quantify the nociceptive response evoked by the surgical incisions. Consequently, mean reflex amplitudes evoked by laser were significantly smaller than those by scalpel, thus demonstrating that Er:YAG laser incision was less painful than scalpel incision. A systematic review of Mikami et al. [60] showed that soft tissue treatment associated with periodontal therapy using erbium lasers (Er:YAG and Er,Cr:YSGG) more effectively suppresses pain as compared to conventional treatment methods.

3.5   Advantages of Er:YAG Laser Microsurgery in Esthetic Gingival Procedures

Esthetic procedures such as recontouring or reshaping of gingiva and crown lengthening can be successfully performed with lasers [61]. Compared to other available lasers, the erbium lasers can be safely utilized for esthetic procedures due to its minimal thermal side effects [38, 44]. The additional use of water cooling further minimizes thermal effects while providing a clear surgical view. Also, use of delicate contact tips can control the amount of soft tissue ablation more precisely than with the other lasers. With no obvious indicators of thermal damage, e.g., carbonization and coagulation of the irradiated surface, wound healing can be more rapid and uneventful [11, 33, 62, 63].

In recent case reports, the excellent ability of Er:YAG laser in gingival MH and tattoo removal, followed by significant improvement in esthetics, has been reported [8, 18–21]. The pigmented gingival tissue can be accurately, less invasively, and easily ablated by Er:YAG laser under clear view. Following Er:YAG laser melanin depigmentation in dogs, the width of the thermally affected layer in gingival connective tissue is reported to be approximately 5–20 μm [64]. The minimal thermal effects of Er:YAG lasers are advantageous for viewing lased surfaces, subsequent wound healing, and pain control.

Furthermore, the application of the Er:YAG laser in combination with a surgical microscope enables the procedure to be more precise, safe, and complete (Fig. 11). The clear magnified view under water spray enables accurate and careful laser irradiation using fine contact tips, avoiding excessive irradiation and subsequent undesirable postsurgical adverse events, including gingival recession and deformities. This is facilitated by the surrounding delicate area of marginal gingiva and papillae, and the tissue attachments to the root surfaces, being securely preserved. These technical advantages of Er:YAG laser microsurgery lead to improved wound healing with less postoperative pain and facilitates delicate and complicated procedures which cannot be achieved by conventional treatments.

In our clinic, the following surgical microscopes have been used for periodontal microsurgery: Wild Heerbrugg MS-C; Leica Geosystems, Heerbrugg, Switzerland; or OPMI PROergo; Carl Zeiss Meditec AG, Oberkochen, Germany. Usually, a 10–20× low magnification setting is used for the initial rough ablation and then a 20–40× high magnification setting is employed for refinement of the treated area.

3.6   Er:YAG Laser Irradiation Safety

The most important thing to note in the safety of laser clinical applications is prevention of accidental irradiation to the eyes. The eye has the lowest maximum permissible exposure (MPE) threshold in the body. Since the wavelength of the Er:YAG laser is absorbed by the surface layer of the eyeball, accidental irradiation may

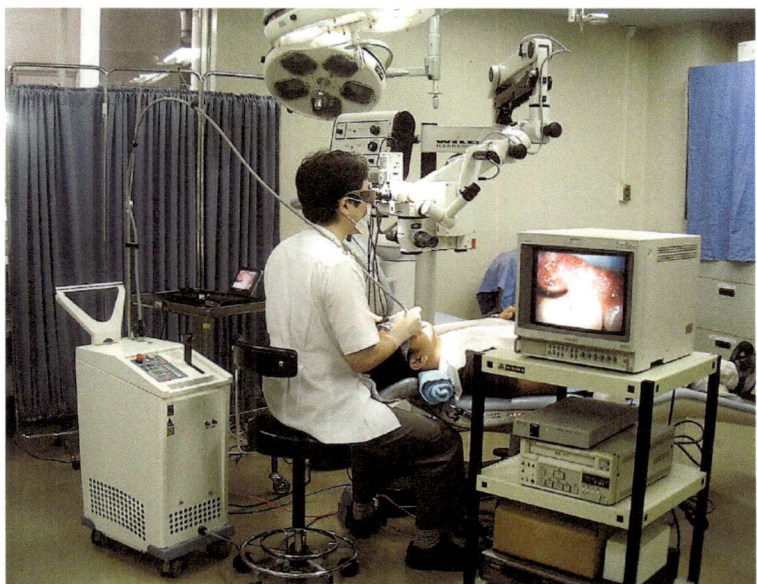

Fig. 11 Er:YAG laser microsurgery. Er:YAG laser, microscope, and monitor are employed for melanin depigmentation. [Picture from Ishii S et al. Application of an Er:YAG laser to remove gingival melanin hyperpigmentation. *J Jpn Soc Laser Dent.* 2002;13:89–96; with permission. © copyright (2002) J Jpn Soc Laser Dent] [8]

cause thermal damage to the cornea. Therefore, prior to laser treatment, the patient, assistant, and operator must be equipped with protective eyewear (goggles) in order to safeguard the eyes against reflections and scattering of laser light during treatment. The goggles must be selected according to the specific wavelength of the laser. The goggles we are using have an optical density (OD) of 4.5, which means the Er:YAG laser energy is reduced to $1/10^{4.5}$ (Transmission 0.003%) through the goggle (YL250S-Er:YAG, Yamamoto Kogaku Co., Ltd., Higashi-Osaka-city, Japan) (Fig. 12). Disinfection, sterilization, and maintenance of protective eyewear are performed according to the product manufacturer's manual. The goggles' lenses, corresponding to Er:YAG laser wavelength, are colorless and transparent and do little to reduce the coaxial light intensity of the microscope. It is known that the Er:YAG laser light is absorbed by the microscope's internal lens while being transmitted through the microscope, and that its energy is significantly attenuated [65]. However, in order to ensure safety, it is desirable to attach a specific protective filter (Prototype for Er:YAG, Yamamoto Kogaku Co., Ltd., Higashi-Osaka, Japan; OD 8.0), which efficiently absorbs the Er:YAG laser light but does not absorb coaxial light, to the objective lens (Fig. 13). The filter can be attached by using a special attachment and is sterilized by plasma gas.

Fig. 12 Protective eyewear (goggles) for Er:YAG laser irradiation (YL250S-Er:YAG, Yamamoto Kogaku Co., Ltd., Higashi-Osaka-city, Japan). Optical density (OD) 4.5, Transmission 0.003%

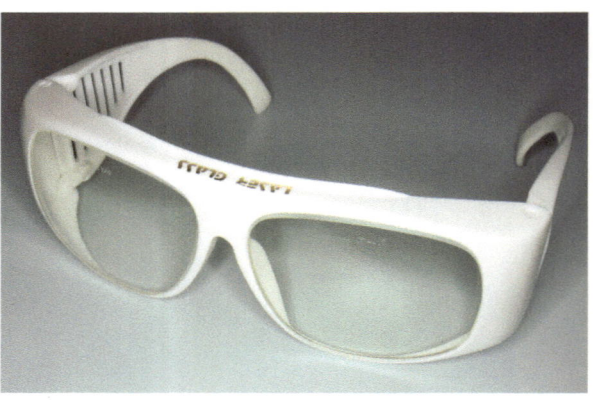

4 Removal of Melanin Pigmentation

4.1 Procedures of Melanin Depigmentation Under Microscope

Melanin depigmentation with Er:YAG laser is performed under local/topical anesthesia or no anesthesia, depending on the severity and extent of the pigmentation, as well as patients' preference. Slight and localized pigmentation can be treated with topical or no anesthesia.

Laser irradiation is performed at an energy level of 50 to 80 mJ/pulse on the panel setting (actual energy output 25–40 mJ/pulse; energy density 8.8–14.2 J/cm^2 per pulse for 600 μm diameter contact tip) and repetition rate of 10–30 Hz under water spray in an oblique contact mode with 20–30° angulation to the surface.

The initial ablation of pigmented tissue in the broad area is usually performed at 10–20 times magnification under microscopic monitoring, with the papillary edges and the free gingival margins initially left untreated. For right-handed operators, the treatment is initially directed from the right to the left side, scraping the pigmented epithelial tissue. The laser beam is applied using a "brush technique" or "sweeping motion technique," i.e., continuous and slow movement of the beam with overlapping of the laser spots. Basically, the brownish dark-colored epithelial tissue is softer compared to the underlying white-colored connective tissue, and thus excessive ablation of the connective tissue does not usually occur with oblique contact irradiation under a clear surgical field created by water spray (Movie 1).

The recommended contact tips are a curved-type round-ended tip (C600F, 600 μm diameter, Morita) or a chisel type square-ended tip (P/N 625–8746, 1.40 × 0.45 mm, HOYA) (Fig. 7). The chisel tip is appropriate for the broad area of treatment, enabling rapid treatment and leaving a smooth ablated surface (Movie 2).

After the first entire ablation of the treated area, the slight remaining pigmentation (including slightly dotted or occasionally multiple linear pigmentations, such as the bottom of rete pegs of epithelium) is carefully removed at 20–30 times higher magnification with delicate adjustment of focus. Also, if necessary, the papillary edges and the free gingival margin surfaces are ablated (Movie 3). Thus, the use of

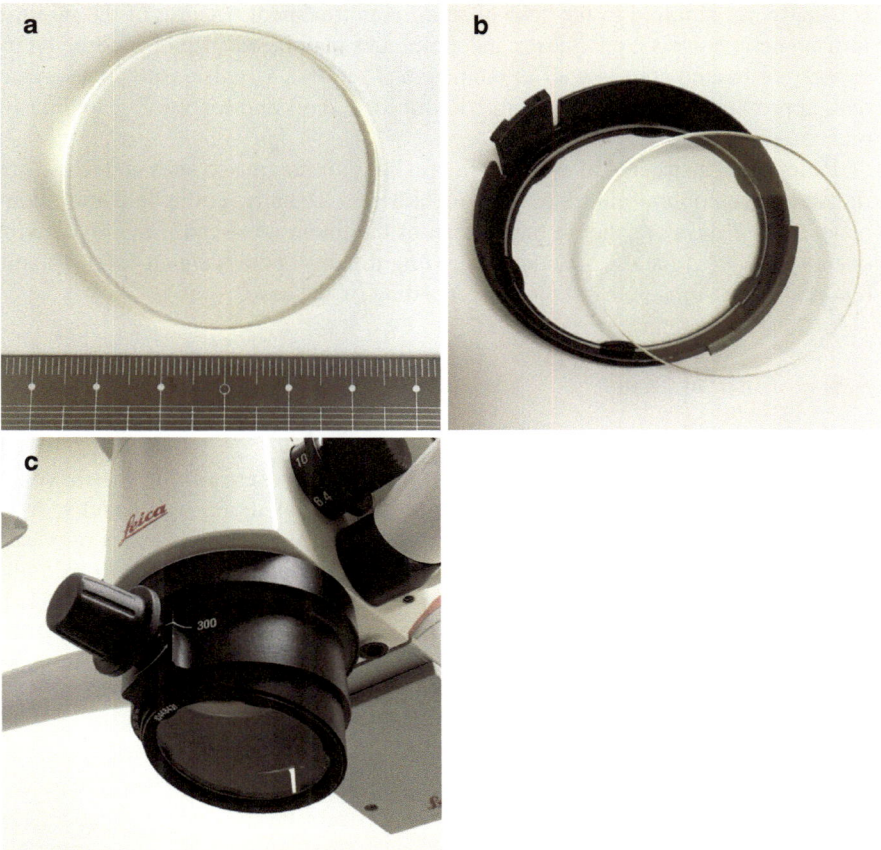

Fig. 13 Attachment of a specific filter to the objective lens of the microscope. In order to ensure safety to the eyes, it is desirable to attach a specific protective filter which efficiently absorbs the Er:YAG laser light (Prototype for Er:YAG, Yamamoto Kogaku Co. Ltd.; diameter 50 mm, thickness 2 mm, Optical density [OD] = 8.0) (**a**). The filter can be installed by stacking it inside the objective lens protection cover (**b**, **c**)

a surgical microscope facilitates the thorough detection and near-complete elimination of slightly remaining pigmentation, as well as careful irradiation of the delicate areas of the gingival margin and papilla.

4.2   Wound Healing and Pain Perception

Immediately after the procedure, white-colored gingival connective tissue is exposed with slight bleeding; however, spontaneous hemostasis is achieved in a few minutes and no suturing is required. Periodontal dressings are generally not required, but may be applied depending on the patients' preference. Postoperative medication is usually not required in the case of small area treatment because of the minimal invasiveness; however, analgesics and antibiotics may be advised depending on the severity of treated area as well as the patients' request. Usually, with areas greater than approximately 5×5 mm^2, amoxicillin for 2 days and loxoprofen sodium for pain are prescribed.

Patients are instructed to avoid tooth brushing for the treated sites and to use oral rinses (benzethonium chloride, etc.) for 1 week. Usually, epithelialization completes in 4–7 days depending on the size of treatment area, and tissue maturation occurs in approximately 2 weeks. Regarding the postoperative pain level, patients report slight-to-moderate pain level, depending on the case.

4.3 Clinical Cases

4.3.1 Case 1

A 28-year-old male patient requested the removal of severe MH in the maxillary anterior area [2] (Fig. 14a). The patient's periodontal tissue was healthy. After administration of local anesthesia (0.9 ml of 2% lidocaine), Er:YAG laser microsurgery was performed under water spray at a panel energy setting of 70 mJ/pulse (actual energy output ~35 mJ/pulse, energy density ~12.4 J/cm^2/pulse) and 30 Hz in oblique contact mode using a curved contact tip with a 600 μm diameter (Fig. 14b). The pigmented epithelial tissue was carefully and efficiently ablated without major thermal changes in the irradiated connective tissue (magnification, 10–20×) (Fig. 15) (Movie 1). After major removal of the pigmented attached gingival tissue, slightly remaining pigmented tissue was carefully ablated including the outer surface of the gingival margin and papilla (magnification, 20–30×) (Movie 3). It was possible to avoid leaving melanin-deposited tissue and perform the procedure efficiently by flushing the debris with the Er:YAG laser water spray under microscopic monitoring (Fig. 14c).

Slight bleeding was observed immediately after ablation, but spontaneous hemostasis was achieved within a few minutes and no visible thermal changes such as carbonization and severe coagulation of the gingival tissue were observed. No periodontal pack or postoperative medication were applied. The patient felt low to moderate pain according to a visual analogue scale (VAS) score of 18 (max 100), reported the night after treatment, with no pain reported 1 day following ablation. 1 week postoperatively, ablated gingiva showed almost complete epithelialization with a healthy appearance (Fig. 14d) and 2 weeks postoperatively, gingival thickness recovered. Complete healing was observed 1 month postoperatively (Fig. 14e). Three months postoperatively, the treated site was stable and the patient was very satisfied with the gingival color improvement (Fig. 14f).

4.3.2 Case 2

A 28-year-old female patient, with no smoking history requested a full-mouth gingival depigmentation of moderate MH (Fig. 16a, b). In this case, the full-mouth buccal gingival treatment was performed per quadrant. All four 30-min sessions

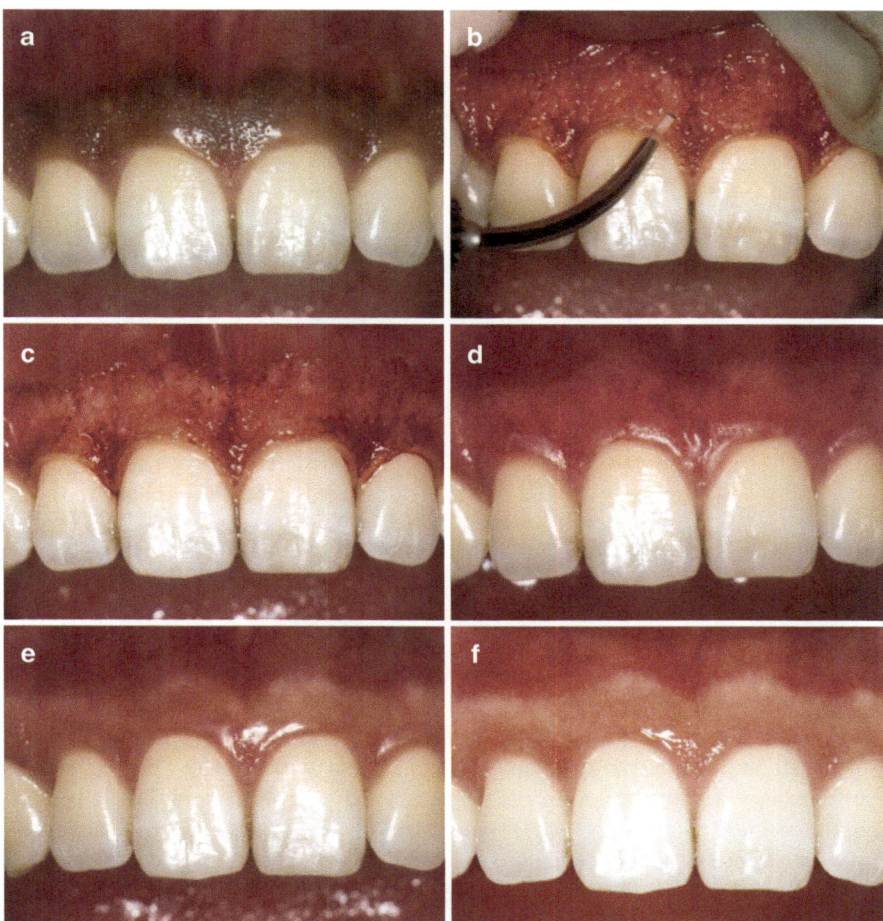

Fig. 14 Er:YAG laser microsurgery for melanin depigmentation: Case 1 presentation. A 28-year-old male. Generalized severe melanin hyperpigmentation in the upper arch, on the first visit (**a**). Er:YAG laser microsurgery was performed for melanin depigmentation. The use of surgical microscope facilitates the thorough detection and near-complete elimination of small areas of remaining pigmentation, as well as careful irradiation of the delicate area of the gingival margin and papilla (**c**). Under a modest amount of local anesthesia, Er:YAG laser irradiation (panel energy setting 70 mJ/pulse, 30 Hz, with water spray) was performed in oblique contact mode using an 80° curved tip with a 600 μm diameter (**b**). Immediately after Er:YAG laser melanin depigmentation, there are no severe thermal injuries such as carbonization and severe coagulation of the gingival tissue (**c**). 1 week postoperatively, ablated gingiva showed rapid epithelialization with a healthy appearance (**d**). 4 weeks postoperatively, complete healing was observed without recurrences, gingival recessions, or deformities (**e**). 3 months postoperatively, the gingival color is excellently improved (**f**). [Pictures and legend from Pavlic V et al. Gingival melanin depigmentation by Er:YAG laser: A literature review. *J Cosmet Laser Ther* 20:85–90, 2018; with permission. © copyright (2017) Taylor & Francis Group, LLC.] (Case details provided by Akira Aoki) [2]

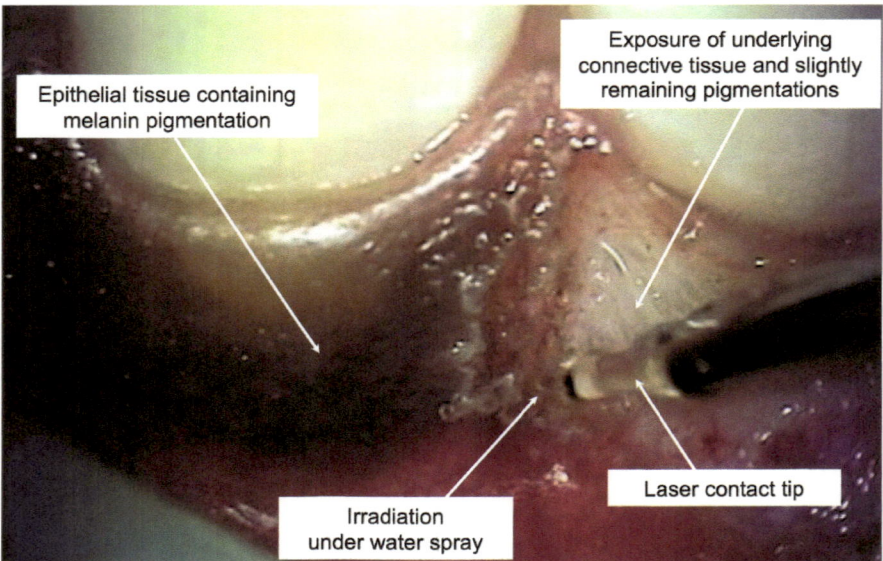

Epithelial tissue containing
melanin pigmentation

Exposure of underlying
connective tissue and slightly
remaining pigmentations

Laser contact tip

Irradiation
under water spray

Fig. 15 Magnified view while performing microsurgery for melanin depigmentation

were conducted under local anesthesia (0.6 ml of 2% lidocaine) and under the microscope (magnification, 6–20×).

For efficient removal, the entire surface layer was first ablated with a chisel-shaped tip at a panel energy setting of 80 mJ/pulse (actual energy output ~40 mJ/pulse, energy density 10.2 J/cm^2/pulse) and 20 Hz with water spray while preserving the cervical gingiva (Fig. 16c). Then, the spotty areas of residual melanin deposits were selectively removed using a fine contact tip with 400 μm in diameter at a panel energy setting of 40–60 mJ/pulse (actual energy output ~20–30 mJ/pulse, energy density ~15.9–23.9 J/cm^2/pulse) and 10 Hz. Although Er:YAG laser has a low hemostatic effect, bleeding spontaneously stopped within a few minutes postoperatively (Fig. 16d).

A realization of virtually no postoperative pain was achieved by a minimally invasive procedure that carefully removed only epithelium and colored connective tissue. Nonetheless, mild irritation by spicy and salty food was reported. 2 days after surgery, a white-colored pseudomembranous appearance was evident on the treated surface (Fig. 16e). One week after the operation, the epithelium was completely healed, and connective tissue thickness was partially recovered (Fig. 16f). One month after the operation, the thickness of the gingiva completely recovered without signs of recurrence and/or gingival recession (Fig. 16g). The location of the cervical gingiva has not changed. Six months after final treatment, the desired esthetic improvement was achieved (Fig. 16h). The improved gingival color has been maintained for 1 year (Fig. 16i).

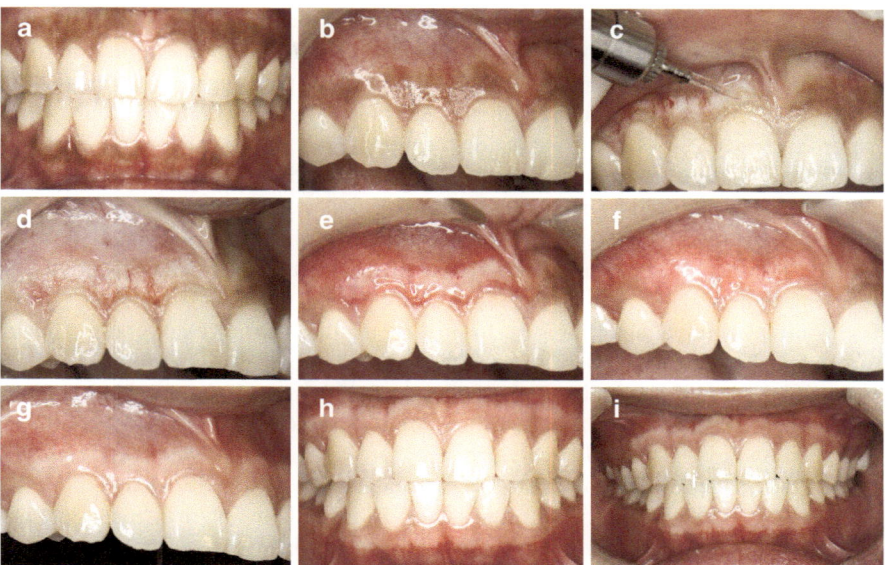

Fig. 16 Er:YAG laser microsurgery for melanin depigmentation: Case 2 presentation. Removal of gingival melanin hyperpigmentation using an Er:YAG laser. A 28-year-old never smoker female. Before treatment (**a, b**). Er:YAG laser irradiation was performed with water spray in oblique contact mode using a chisel tip (panel energy setting 80 mJ/pulse, 20 Hz) and a 400 µm diameter tip (40–60 mJ/pulse, 10 Hz) under local anesthesia. The gingival epithelium containing pigmentation was easily and effectively removed by Er:YAG laser irradiation (**c**). Immediately after surgery. No major thermal damage, such as carbonization, was observed (**d**). Two days after surgery (**e**). Seven days after the procedure, ablated area was covered with migrated epithelium. The patient reported no discomfort except for slight pain on the day of treatment (**f**). One month after the procedure, favorable wound healing was maintained without any gingival tissue defects or recession (**g**). Six months after final treatment, desired esthetic improvement was achieved (**h**). 1 year after treatment. The gingival color maintains a natural esthetic appearance (**i**). (Case details provided by Koji Mizutani)

5 Removal of Metal Tattoo Pigmentation

5.1 Procedures of Metal Tattoo Depigmentation Under Microscope

With the combination of Er:YAG laser and microscope, minimally invasive and safe therapy is possible. Most of the treated sites are in the maxillary anterior region, followed by the mandibular anterior and premolar areas. Generally, a small amount of local anesthesia (0.2–0.45 ml) is sufficient for this procedure, and occasionally, procedures involving slight to mild pigmentation can be performed with topical or no anesthesia at all, depending on the severity and area of pigmentations.

Laser irradiation is performed at a panel energy setting of 50–80 mJ/pulse (actual energy output ~25–40 mJ/pulse; energy density ~8.8–14.2 J/cm^2 per pulse for 600 μm diameter contact tip) and repetition rates of 10–30 Hz under a water spray in a vertical or oblique contact mode with 30–90° angulation to the surface. The recommended contact tips are curved-type round-ended tips (C400F or C600F, 400 or 600 μm in diameter, Morita) (Fig. 7). The total chair time is approximately 20–40 min per session, of which 2–10 min are spent on laser irradiation, and the remaining time is used for observation of the irradiated site, visualizing metal debris by focusing the microscope, and changing the angulation of the objective lens to visualize irradiation of the other sides within one ablation defect. Laser irradiation is performed intermittently and repeatedly for short time periods.

Minimal gingival ablation is performed on the black or gray-colored pigmented areas to expose the metal debris deposited in the connective tissue. The visual field, magnified approximately 10–30×, facilitates the accurate and safe ablation of the gingival tissue and minimizes the wound areas. Subsequently, the metal debris and the surrounding discolored connective tissue are carefully removed. Due to limited wound access space, the microscope's orientation is occasionally changed in order to see every wall of the wound from inside. To limit their fine invasion of the gingiva, the micro-metal fragments within connective tissue must be identified and selectively removed. In order to precisely accomplish that, a surgical microscope is significantly more advantageous, by virtue of its high magnification and coaxial light source, than low-magnification loupes.

The papillary edges, free gingival margins, and, in particular, periodontal tissue attachment to the root surface are preserved in order not to cause tissue detachment and subsequent gingival recession by excessive and inadvertent irradiation. In the case of severe or widespread pigmentations, such as those involving ≥5 mm², the area to be treated is divided into separate sections in order to secure the blood supply within the remaining marginal gingival tissue, and treatment is performed in multiple sessions on different days with intervals of approximately 1 month.

The minimal hemostatic effect of the Er:YAG laser is advantageous for wound healing, because postoperative bleeding secures blood clot formation and subsequent granulation in the ablation defect, resulting in favorable wound healing without unexpected gingival defects. Importantly, injury should be minimized to further secure blood clot formation and retention within the ablated defect, thereby further contributing to the prevention of postoperative tissue defects.

Recently, as a least invasive surgery, a novel technique called "Er:YAG laser micro-keyhole laser surgery (EL-MIKS)" was introduced [27]. In the EL-MIKS procedure, the micro-keyholes are prepared as small as possible under microsurgery (Fig. 17a).

Firstly, a keyhole with a diameter of 1–2 mm is prepared by Er:YAG laser (with a contact tip 400 or 600 μm in diameter) in the center of the pigmentation area (Fig. 17b). The laser is irradiated vertically at the energy level of 60–80 mJ/pulse on the panel (actual energy output approximately 30–40 mJ/pulse; energy density 23.9–31.2 J/cm² per pulse for 400 μm diameter contact tip) and 20–30 Hz. The deposited metal microfragments as well as surrounding discolored connective tissue are eliminated.

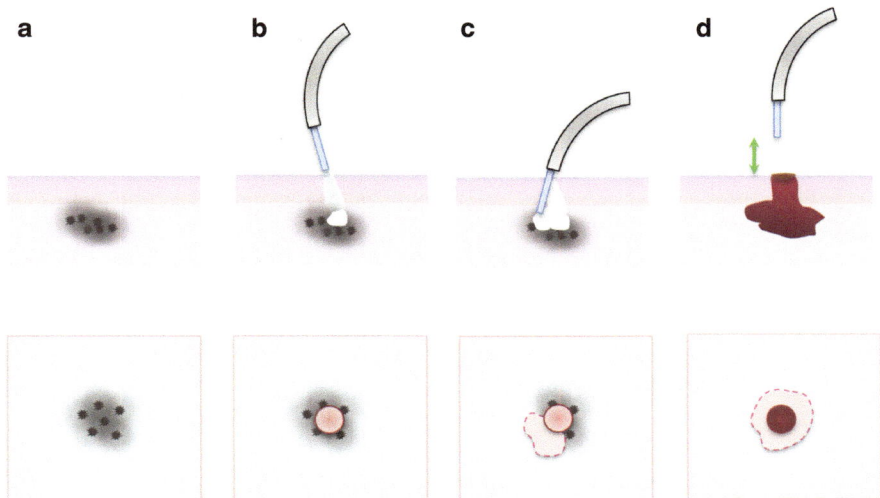

Fig. 17 Er:YAG laser micro-keyhole laser surgery (EL-MIKS). Step-by-step procedure of EL-MIKS for removing metal tattoos (**a**). Making a small keyhole with a diameter of 1–2 mm to access the pigmented gingival connective tissue for ablation of metal fragments and the surrounding discolored connective tissue using an Er:YAG laser (**b**). Shifting the laser direction to ablate the metal and surrounding tissue. Carefully preserving intact the overlaying epithelium of the discolored tissue (**c**). Eliminate micro-metal fragments as much as possible through the keyhole so as not to expand the size of the keyhole. After tissue evaporation, the ablated space fills with blood. Defocused irradiation (without water spray) of the micro-keyhole entrance is performed at a distance of more than 5 mm between the laser tip and gingiva. The blood clot is stabilized within the evaporated space (**d**). (Illustration by Koji Mizutani)

Secondly, the lateral walls of the pigmentations, within the keyhole, are evaporated by irradiation at an inclined angle, preserving the epithelium and not expanding the keyhole entrance (Fig. 17c). Then, the accessible metal pieces and surrounding pigmented connective tissue are carefully evaporated in the undercut areas. Occasionally, in order to observe the inside clearly, a laser tip or periodontal probe is employed to retract the marginal gingiva of the keyhole. A coaxial water spray, accompanying the Er:YAG laser irradiation, is able to flush out the debris of metal microfragments and tissue from the keyhole.

Thirdly, the irradiation angle should be repeatedly changed in various directions within the micro-keyhole to evaporate the pigmented tissue as much as possible, within the limits of accessibility. After blood has filled the tissue defect, the blood surface at the entrance of keyhole is coagulated by defocused irradiation at 60–80 mJ/pulse on the panel setting (400 or 600 μm diameter contact tip) and 10–20 Hz without water spray, in order to make the blood clot stable and stimulate its wound healing (Fig. 17d).

In the case of widespread pigmentation, additional micro-keyholes are prepared at a distance of 3 mm or more from each other. The area accessible through one micro-keyhole is 3–5 mm². Therefore, if a planned depigmentation area approximates 10–15 mm^2, a few micro-keyholes can be additionally prepared to allow treatment in one session. During the preoperative examination, it is recommended to consider how many micro-keyholes will be required in one session and how many sessions will be required in total, based on the total area and number of sites of the tattoos. In general, multiple sessions are recommended for widespread or severe cases larger than 5 mm^2, as well as for cases with multiple pigmentation areas. If multiple sessions are required, they should be performed at one-month intervals.

According to this protocol for EL-MIKS, generally, antibiotics and analgesics may not be indicated. However, depending on the severity of treated area as well as the patient's felt need, amoxicillin for 2 days and loxoprofen sodium may be prescribed. Patients are instructed to avoid tooth brushing for the treated sites and to use oral rinses such as benzethonium chloride for 1 week.

5.2 Wound Healing and Pain Perception

Slight-to-moderate bleeding observed during laser surgery can be dispersed by the water spray, and hemostasis is spontaneously achieved immediately after treatment. Postoperative wound healing is usually favorable with almost no postoperative pain reported [26]. One week postoperatively, the treated sites are epithelialized or epithelializing, with slight tissue depressions occasionally evident. By 2–4 weeks, wound healing is almost complete. In general, adverse events, including side effects or complications, are rarely observed. In our clinical experience, there was only one occurrence (approximately 1% incidence rate) which involved bleeding 3 days postsurgical as a result of the patient scratching the area while sleeping.

In most cases, pigmentation can be removed completely, resulting in subsequent satisfactory esthetic improvements without impaired gingival morphology, although slight discoloration remains in some cases after treatment. In the case of severe pigmentation, remaining slight discoloration derived from ionized metal components usually disappears gradually over about 6 months after treatment, if the metal microfragments have been completely removed. This gradual disappearance occurs because the discolored connective tissues may gradually excrete the bound ionized metal components following removal of metal deposits. Basically, patients are satisfied with the stable esthetic improvements [26].

5.3 Clinical Cases

5.3.1 Case 1

A 42-year-old female patient presented with widespread severe metal tattoo pigmentation around multiple teeth including the marginal area of thin gingiva in the maxillary anterior region (Fig. 18a, b) [26]. Porcelain-fused metal crowns were evident on her maxillary central and lateral incisors and right canine. After removal of these original crowns, and provisionalization, the referring prosthodontist requested removal of the metal tattoos before crown refabrication. Periodontal disease was not detected around the teeth and the probing pocket depths were ≤3 mm.

The treatment was divided into three sessions at 1-month intervals to minimize the area treated during each session and to secure the blood supply in the remaining marginal gingiva. After confirming the successful outcomes of the first treatment session (Fig. 18c), the second and third treatment sessions were conducted. During each microsurgery session, Er:YAG laser irradiation was very carefully performed under water spray at a panel energy setting of 50 mJ/pulse (actual energy output ~25 mJ/pulse, energy density ~8.8 J/cm^2/pulse) and 30 Hz with a small amount of local anesthesia. The discolored gingiva was penetrated and the pigmented site with the metal debris deposition was reached under microscope. Then, the exposed metal deposits were carefully removed and the surrounding discolored connective tissue was vaporized (Fig. 18d). The magnification settings were mainly 10–20× for the large areas of ablation and 20–40× for refinement of specific sites. The thin marginal gingiva and associated root surface attachments were carefully preserved by avoiding inadvertent or excessive irradiation that could cause gingival recession (Fig. 18e). Total chair time was 40 min per session, of which, approximately 5–8 min comprised laser irradiation. Spontaneous hemostasis was achieved with almost no postoperative bleeding (Fig. 18f).

One week after treatment, the treated areas were epithelialized, or epithelializing, and a slight gingival depression was observed (Fig. 18g); this depression healed, and the gingiva reverted to its original form at approximately 2 weeks (Fig. 18h). No postoperative pain was reported; the VAS scores were zero at all time points. Three months after treatment, new porcelain-fused metal crowns were fabricated. The patient's gingival discoloration improved considerably without impairing gingival contour, such as gingival recession or deformity. Unfortunately, horizontal scar tissue remained in the attached gingiva, subsequent to an apicoectomy performed by the patient's endodontist to address a periapical lesion (Fig. 18i, j). While the scar tissue could be removed by Er:YAG laser ablation, the patient did not pursue treatment because the scar was not evident while smiling.

5.3.2 Case 2

A representative case of EL-MIKS is shown in Fig. 19. An extensively widespread metal tattoo with total area of over 15 mm^2 was found in the maxillary right lateral incisor gingiva of a 61-year-old female [27] (Fig. 19a, b). During the preoperative examination and consultation, the patient was informed of a treatment plan requiring multiple sessions.

After administration of a small amount local anesthesia, Er:YAG laser irradiation was very carefully performed under water spray at a panel energy setting of 60–80 mJ/pulse (actual energy output ~30–40 mJ/pulse, energy density ~23.9–31.8 J/cm^2/pulse) and 30 Hz with a 400 μm diameter contact tip.

The first session was limited to the distal pigmentation of the apical area with treatment performed through one micro-keyhole (Fig. 19c, d). During the second session, the mesial, midbuccal, and distal pigmentation of the coronal area were treated using five new micro-keyholes (Fig. 19e). During the third session, any

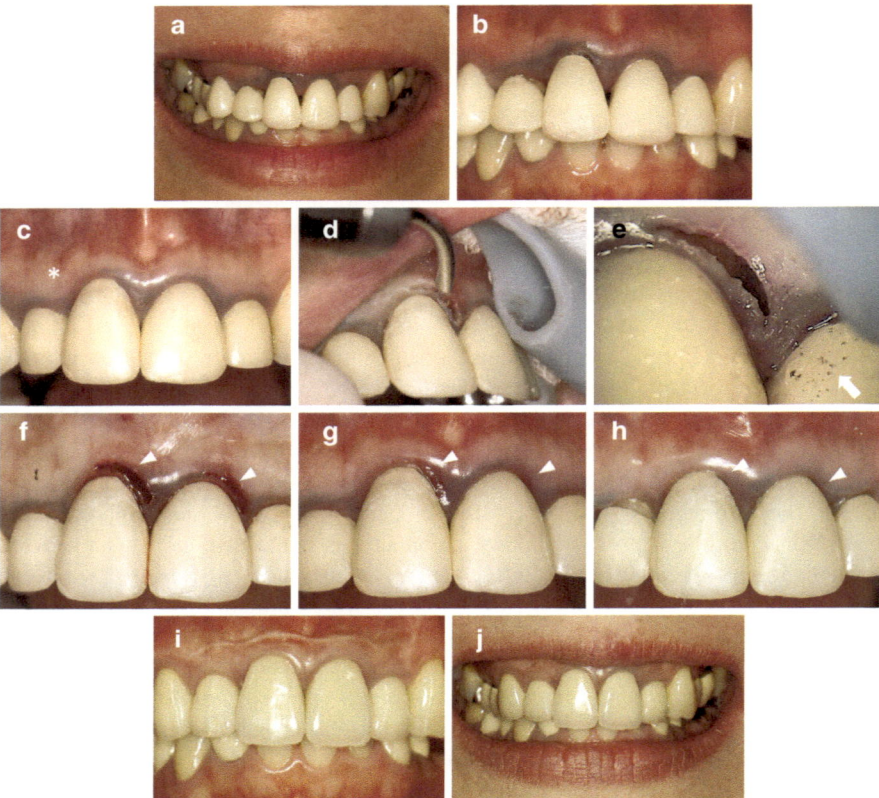

Fig. 18 Er:YAG laser microsurgery for metal tattoo removal: Case 1 presentation. A 42-year-old female. She had severe planar pigmentation in the thin gingiva of the maxillary anterior region, which disrupted the appearance of her smile (**a, b**). After confirming the successful outcomes of the first treatment session (* indicates the site of the first session) (**c**) the second treatment session using an Er:YAG laser (panel energy setting 50 mJ/pulse, 30 Hz, with water spray) was conducted under local anesthesia at the mesial site of the maxillary right central incisor (**d**). Temporary crowns were fabricated before the laser treatment (**c**). Minimal linear gingival ablation to remove metal debris was performed with care to preserve the marginal gingiva and interdental papillae (**e**). The white arrow indicates the metal debris removed from the gingiva. Immediate postoperative view (**f**). The white arrowheads indicate the two treatment sites. One week after treatment (**g**). Postoperatively, a slight linear gingival depression is present at the mesial site of the right central incisor. At 1 month after treatment, the gingiva had healed completely, and the irradiated area was decolorized (**h**). Facial views following final prosthodontic treatment and a total of five Er:YAG laser microsurgical sessions (**i, j**). Esthetic gingival appearance was achieved. The prosthodontic treatment was conducted by Dr. Masayuki Morizawa, Tokyo Medical and Dental University. The horizontal scar occurred subsequent to surgical endodontic treatment. [Pictures and legend from Mikami R, et al. A novel minimally invasive approach for metal tattoo removal with Er:YAG laser. *J Esthet Restor Dent.* 2021;33(4):550–9; with permission. © copyright (2021) Wiley Periodicals LLC.] (Case details provided by Akira Aoki) [26]

remaining pigment and metal that could not be completely removed previously were mostly eliminated through four new micro-keyholes (Fig. 19f). One week after the third session, the ablated area was covered with migrated epithelium (Fig. 19g). The remaining slight gingival discoloration spontaneously disappeared during gingival turnover following the surgery.

The patient reported almost no postoperative pain at any stage of the treatment and was very satisfied with the esthetic improvement of the gingival appearance and color. Three months after the EL-MIKS procedures, the prosthetic was replaced with an all-ceramic crown (Fig. 19g). The improved gingival color has been maintained for 2 years (Fig. 19h).

6 Closing Remarks

The Er:YAG laser can treat gingival tissue accurately and ablate gingival tissue easily using fine contact tips. Its minimal thermal effects are advantageous for inspecting treated surfaces, pain control, and subsequent wound healing during and after soft tissue surgery. The use of water spray during irradiation improves the view of the surgical field and further minimizes the thermal influence. Thus, Er:YAG laser is a most suitable choice for esthetic soft tissue management.

Furthermore, microscope-assisted Er:YAG laser irradiation enables the gingival pigmentations to be carefully and precisely removed while minimizing tissue invasion, which reduces treatment difficulties, minimizes postoperative pain, and postoperatively induces favorable and uneventful wound healing. In particular, the novel minimally invasive procedure for metal tattoo removal using an Er:YAG under microscopic monitoring is much simpler, easier, and less invasive than conventional periodontal surgical approaches. Therefore, Er:YAG laser microsurgery may be more reliable and could offer significant benefits to patients by alleviating physical and mental stresses via reduced chair time and the absence of nearly all postoperative pain.

Although loupes are an option for obtaining a magnified field of view, it is difficult to achieve the same result with loupes. Indeed, performance using a surgical microscope at low magnification is same as that of loupes. But, in gingival depigmentation procedures, in particular for tatto removal, much higer magnifications such as 20–40× with sufficient coaxial light are required for identifying and selectively removing pigmentations, controlling ablation, and refining pigmentation removal. In thse delicate situations, surgical microscopes are more advantageous, compared to loupes, and highly recommended.

Melanin and metal tattoo depigmentation of gingiva can be performed safely and effectively by Er:YAG laser microsurgery, resulting in favorable wound healing and considerable esthetic improvements of gingival discoloration with negligible side effects or complications and notably less operative pain [26].

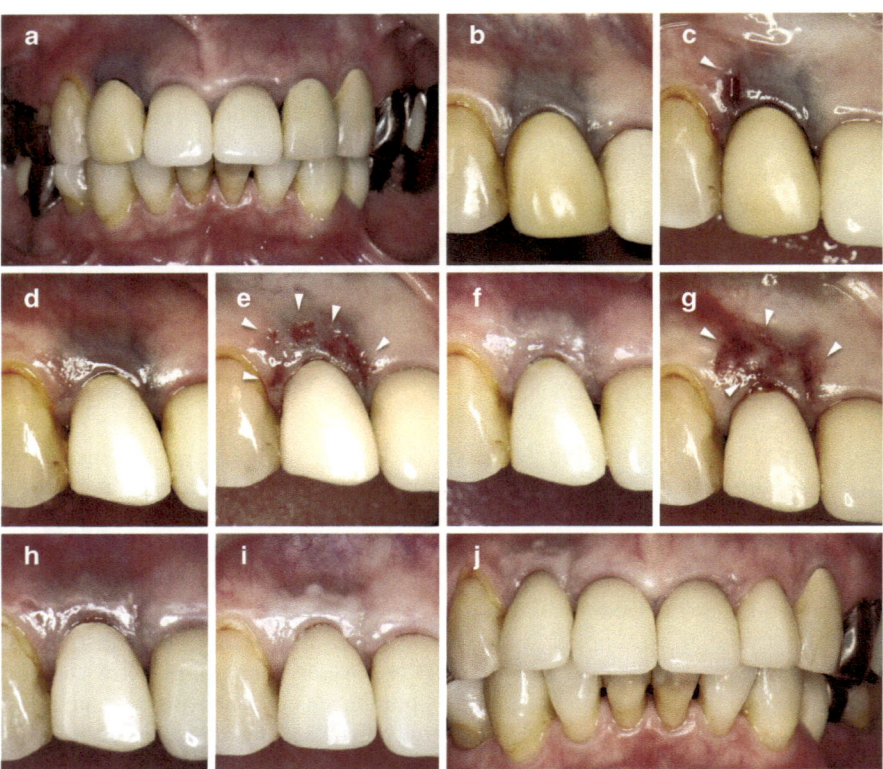

Fig. 19 Er:YAG laser microsurgery for metal tattoo removal: Case 2 presentation. A representative case of Er:YAG laser micro-keyhole laser surgery (EL-MIKS) on an extensively widespread metal tattoo. A 61-year-old female with a prominent metal tattoo in the gingiva of maxillary right lateral incisor (**a**). All procedures were performed with a microscope and Er:YAG laser (panel energy setting 60–80 mJ/pulse, 20 Hz, with water spray) under local anesthesia. A cylinder-shaped curved contact tip with a diameter of 400 μm (C400F, Morita Inc., Japan) was used. In addition, a microscope (M320, Leica) at a magnification of 20× was used to make the micro-keyholes as small as possible (**b**). Immediately after the first session. Only the apical part of the distal pigmentation was treated through one micro-keyhole (**c**). Second session was performed 1 month after the first surgery. The area treated in the first session was completely epithelized (**d**). The mesial, midbuccal, and distal pigmentation of the coronal area were treated using five new micro-keyholes (**e**). Third session was performed 1 month after the second session (**f**). The deposited pigments in the deep mesial region were removed through four micro-keyholes (**g**). One week after the third session, the ablated area was covered with migrated epithelium (**h**). Three months after the third session, the gingival pigmentation had completely disappeared. Since the metal fragments causing the pigmentation had been removed, the slightly remained discoloration spontaneously disappeared with the gingival turnover. Recession of the marginal gingiva was generally prevented. Note the crown was replaced (**i**). Two years after the procedures. The improved gingival color has been maintained and the patient was esthetically satisfied with the treatment (**j**). [Pictures and legend from Mizutani K, et al. Novel flapless esthetic procedure for the elimination of extended gingival metal tattoos adjacent to prosthetic teeth: Er:YAG laser micro-keyhole surgery. *J Prosthodont Res.* 2022;66(2):346–52; with permission. © copyright (2021) Japan Prosthodontic Society. Published by Elsevier Ireland] (Case details provided by Koji Mizutani) [27]

7 Key Points

1. Gingival melanin or metal tattoo pigmentation is occasionally observed and produces esthetic problems for patients while smiling.
2. When treating gingival pigmentations, the operator needs to pay attention to the risk of melanoma as a contraindication.
3. Among dental lasers, the Er:YAG laser effectively and precisely ablates soft tissues with extremely minimal thermal influences.
4. Er:YAG laser using water spray minimizes thermal changes to the irradiated soft tissue, making it a safe and effective choice for depigmentation procedures.
5. Microscope use during depigmentation procedures allows clear detection of melanin pigmentation and metal debris embedded in the connective tissue.
6. Microscope-assisted Er:YAG laser surgery can precisely and safely remove pigmentation with minimal wounds. In particular, Er:YAG laser micro-keyhole laser surgery (EL-MIKS) provides the least invasive procedure.
7. Microscope-assisted Er:YAG laser irradiation can delicately ablate pigmentation and prevent excessive and inadvertent ablation of surrounding tissues, resulting in no postoperative gingival recession and deformity.
8. Water spray during irradiation rinses away bleeding as well as ablated tissues and keep the operative field clear under microscopic view.
9. Microscope-assisted Er:YAG laser irradiation can promote wound healing by providing minimally invasive surgery as well as the photobiomodulation (PBM) effects of the laser.
10. When using a laser device, it is necessary to pay attention to safety. Wearing protective goggles is essential to protect against reflections and scattered light during irradiation. Also, during microsurgery, it is desirable to attach a specific protective filter to efficiently absorb the laser light to the objective lens.

Acknowledgements The authors appreciate Professor Verica Pavlic, University of Banja Luka, Bosnia and Herzegovina, and Dr. Walter Meinzer, Tokyo Medical and Dental University, Japan for their kind support in manuscript preparation.

References

1. Lin YH, Tu YK, Lu CT, Chung WC, Huang CF, Huang MS, et al. Systematic review of treatment modalities for gingival depigmentation: a random-effects poisson regression analysis. J Esthet Restor Dent. 2014;26:162–78. https://doi.org/10.1111/jerd.12087.
2. Pavlic V, Brkic Z, Marin S, Cicmil S, Gojkov-Vukelic M, Aoki A. Gingival melanin depigmentation by Er:YAG laser: a literature review. J Cosmet Laser Ther. 2018;20:85–90. https://doi.org/10.1080/14764172.2017.1376092.
3. Suzuki M. A colorimetric study of pigmented lesions on oral mucos. J Stomatol Soc Jpn. 2010;77:35–41. (in Japanse, English abstract)
4. Huang JW, Chen WC, Huang TK, Fu PS, Lai PL, Tsai CF, et al. Using a spectrophotometric study of human gingival colour distribution to develop a shade guide. J Dent. 2011;39(Suppl 3):e11–6. https://doi.org/10.1016/j.jdent.2011.10.001.

5. Gomez-Polo C, Montero J, Gomez-Polo M, Martin Casado AM. Clinical study on natural gingival color. Odontology. 2019;107:80–9. https://doi.org/10.1007/s10266-018-0365-2.
6. Dummett CO, Barens G. Pigmentation of the oral tissues: a review of the literature. J Periodontol. 1967;38:369–78. https://doi.org/10.1902/jop.1967.38.5.369.
7. Raposo G, Marks MS. Melanosomes--dark organelles enlighten endosomal membrane transport. Nat Rev Mol Cell Biol. 2007;8:786–97. https://doi.org/10.1038/nrm2258.
8. Ishii S, Aoki A, Kawashima Y, Watanabe H, Ishikawa I. Application of an Er:YAG laser to remove gingival melanin hyperpigmentation. J Jpn Soc Laser Dent. 2002;13:89–96. (in Japanse, English abstract)
9. Bakhshi M, Rahmani S, Rahmani A. Lasers in esthetic treatment of gingival melanin hyperpigmentation: a review article. Lasers Med Sci. 2015;30:2195–203. https://doi.org/10.1007/s10103-015-1797-3.
10. Kauzman A, Pavone M, Blanas N, Bradley G. Pigmented lesions of the oral cavity: review, differential diagnosis, and case presentations. J Can Dent Assoc. 2004;70:682–3.
11. Ishikawa I, Aoki A, Takasaki A. Potential applications of erbium:YAG laser in periodontics. J Periodontal Res. 2004;39:275–85. https://doi.org/10.1111/j.1600-0765.2004.00738.x.
12. Shulman JD, Beach MM, Rivera-Hidalgo F. The prevalence of oral mucosal lesions in U.S. adults: data from the Third National Health and Nutrition Examination Survey, 1988–1994. J Am Dent Assoc. 2004;135:1279–86. https://doi.org/10.14219/jada.archive.2004.0403.
13. Aoyagi H, Katagiri M. Long-term effects of Ag-containing alloys on mucous tissue present in biopsy samples. Dent Mater J. 2004;23:340–7. https://doi.org/10.4012/dmj.23.340.
14. Joska L, Venclikova Z, Poddana M, Benada O. The mechanism of gingiva metallic pigmentations formation. Clin Oral Investig. 2009;13:1–7. https://doi.org/10.1007/s00784-008-0206-8.
15. Nakamura Y, Hossain M, Hirayama K, Matsumoto K. A clinical study on the removal of gingival melanin pigmentation with the CO2 laser. Lasers Surg Med. 1999;25:140–7. https://doi.org/10.1002/(sici)1096-9101(1999)25:2<140::aid-lsm7>3.0.co;2-7.
16. Yousuf A, Hossain M, Nakamura Y, Yamada Y, Kinoshita J, Matsumoto K. Removal of gingival melanin pigmentation with the semiconductor diode laser: a case report. J Clin Laser Med Surg. 2000;18:263–6. https://doi.org/10.1089/clm.2000.18.263.
17. Atsawasuwan P, Greethong K, Nimmanon V. Treatment of gingival hyperpigmentation for esthetic purposes by Nd:YAG laser: report of 4 cases. J Periodontol. 2000;71:315–21. https://doi.org/10.1902/jop.2000.71.2.315.
18. Kawashima Y, Aoki A, Ishii S, Watanabe H, Ishikawa I. Er:YAG laser treatment of gingival melanin pigmentation. In: Ishikawa I, Frame JW, Aoki A, editors. Lasers in dentistry - revolution of dental treatment in the new millennium. Amsterdam: Elsevier Science. https://doi.org/10.1016/S0531-5131(02)01298-0.
19. Tal H, Oegiesser D, Tal M. Gingival depigmentation by erbium:YAG laser: clinical observations and patient responses. J Periodontol. 2003;74:1660–7. https://doi.org/10.1902/jop.2003.74.11.1660.
20. Azzeh MM. Treatment of gingival hyperpigmentation by erbium-doped:yttrium, aluminum, and garnet laser for esthetic purposes. J Periodontol. 2007;78:177–84. https://doi.org/10.1902/jop.2007.060167.
21. Rosa DS, Aranha AC, Eduardo Cde P, Aoki A. Esthetic treatment of gingival melanin hyperpigmentation with Er:YAG laser: short-term clinical observations and patient follow-up. J Periodontol. 2007;78:2018–25. https://doi.org/10.1902/jop.2007.070041.
22. Campbell CM, Deas DE. Removal of an amalgam tattoo using a subepithelial connective tissue graft and laser deepithelialization. J Periodontol. 2009;80:860–4. https://doi.org/10.1902/jop.2009.080613.
23. Dello Russo NM. Esthetic use of a free gingival autograft to cover an amalgam tattoo: report of case. J Am Dent Assoc. 1981;102:334–5. https://doi.org/10.14219/jada.archive.1981.0036.
24. Gojkov-Vukelic M, Hadzic S, Pasic E. Laser treatment of oral mucosa tattoo. Acta Inform Med. 2011;19:244–6.
25. Shah G, Alster TS. Treatment of an amalgam tattoo with a Q-switched alexandrite (755 nm) laser. Dermatol Surg. 2002;28:1180–1. https://doi.org/10.1046/j.1524-4725.2002.02121.x.

26. Mikami R, Mizutani K, Nagai S, Pavlic V, Iwata T, Aoki A. A novel minimally-invasive approach for metal tattoo removal with er:YAG laser. J Esthet Restor Dent. 2021;33(4):550–9. https://doi.org/10.1111/jerd.12721.
27. Mizutani K, Mikami R, Tsukui A, Nagai S, Iwata T, Aoki A. Novel flapless esthetic procedure for the elimination of extended gingival metal tattoos adjacent to prosthetic teeth: Er:YAG laser micro-keyhole surgery. J Prosthet Dent 2022;66(2):346–52. https://www.jstage.jst.go.jp/article/jpr/66/2/66_JPR_D_21_00045/_pdf.
28. Yilmaz HG, Bayindir H, Kusakci-Seker B, Tasar S, Kurtulmus-Yilmaz S. Treatment of amalgam tattoo with an er,Cr:YSGG laser. J Investig Clin Dent. 2010;1:50–4. https://doi.org/10.1111/j.2041-1626.2010.00011.x.
29. Aoki A, Mizutani K, Schwarz F, Sculean A, Yukna RA, Takasaki AA, et al. Periodontal and peri-implant wound healing following laser therapy. Periodontol. 2000;2015(68):217–69. https://doi.org/10.1111/prd.12080.
30. Lambertini M, Patrizi A, Fanti PA, Melotti B, Caliceti U, Magnoni C, et al. Oral melanoma and other pigmentations: when to biopsy? J Eur Acad Dermatol Venereol. 2018;32:209–14. https://doi.org/10.1111/jdv.14574.
31. Hale GM, Querry MR. Optical constants of water in the 200-nm to 200-μm wavelength region. Appl Opt. 1973;12:555–63. https://doi.org/10.1364/AO.12.000555.
32. Niemz MH. Laser-tissue interaction. In: Fundamentals and applications. Berlin: Springer; 1996.
33. Aoki A, Sasaki K, Watanabe H, Ishikawa I. Lasers in non-surgical periodontal therapy. Periodontology. 2000;2004(36):59–97. https://doi.org/10.1111/j.1600-0757.2004.03679.x.
34. Aoki A, Mizutani K, Takasaki AA, Sasaki KM, Nagai S, Schwarz F, et al. Current status of clinical laser applications in periodontal therapy. Gen Dent. 2008;56:674–87. Erratum in: Gen Dent 57(1):94
35. Featherstone JDB. Caries detection and prevention with laser energy. Dent Clin N Am. 2000;44:955–69.
36. Walsh JT Jr, Flotte TJ, Deutsch TF. Er:YAG laser ablation of tissue: effect of pulse duration and tissue type on thermal damage. Lasers Surg Med. 1989;9:314–26. https://doi.org/10.1002/lsm.1900090403.
37. Sawabe M, Aoki A, Komaki M, Iwasaki K, Ogita M, Izumi Y. Gingival tissue healing following Er:YAG laser ablation compared to electrosurgery in rats. Lasers Med Sci. 2015;30:875–83. https://doi.org/10.1007/s10103-013-1478-z.
38. Kawamura R, Mizutani K, Lin T, Kakizaki S, Mimata A, Watanabe K, et al. Ex vivo evaluation of gingival ablation with various laser systems and electroscalpel. Photobiomodul Photomed Laser Surg. 2020;38:364–73. https://doi.org/10.1089/photob.2019.4713.
39. Walsh JT Jr, Cummings JP. Effect of the dynamic optical properties of water on midinfrared laser ablation. Lasers Surg Med. 1994;15:295–305. https://doi.org/10.1002/lsm.1900150310.
40. Klokkevold PR, Takei HH, Carranza FA. General principles of periodontal surgery. In: Newman MG, Takei HH, Klokkevold PR, Carranza FA, editors. Carranza's clinical periodontology. 11th ed. St. Louis: Elsevier; 2012. p. 533.
41. Azzi R, Kenney EB, Tsao TF, Carranza FA Jr. The effect of electrosurgery on alveolar bone. J Periodontol. 1983;54:96–100. https://doi.org/10.1902/jop.1983.54.2.96.
42. Simon BI, Schuback P, Deasy MJ, Kelner RM. The destructive potential of electrosurgery on the periodontium. J Periodontol. 1976;47:342–7. https://doi.org/10.1902/jop.1976.47.6.342.
43. Sinha UK, Gallagher LA. Effects of steel scalpel, ultrasonic scalpel, CO_2 laser, and monopolar and bipolar electrosurgery on wound healing in Guinea pig oral mucosa. Laryngoscope. 2003;113:228–36. https://doi.org/10.1097/00005537-200302000-00007.
44. Merigo E, Clini F, Fornaini C, Oppici A, Paties C, Zangrandi A, et al. Laser-assisted surgery with different wavelengths: a preliminary ex vivo study on thermal increase and histological evaluation. Lasers Med Sci. 2013;28:497–504. https://doi.org/10.1007/s10103-012-1081-8.
45. Aoki A, Miura M, Akiyama F, Sasaki K, Matsuyama T, Eguchi T, et al. Soft tissue treatment with the Er:YAG laser at a high pulse repetition rate: gingivectomy and melanin removal in beagle dogs. In: 7th international congress on lasers in dentistry, Brussel, Belgium, abstract handbook. 2000. p. 1.

46. Mester E, Spiry T, Szende B, Tota JG. Effect of laser rays on wound healing. Am J Surg. 1971;122:532–5. https://doi.org/10.1016/0002-9610(71)90482-x.
47. Mester E, Mester AF, Mester A. The biomedical effects of laser application. Lasers Surg Med. 1985;5:31–9. https://doi.org/10.1002/lsm.1900050105.
48. Gholami L, Asefi S, Hooshyarfard A, Sculean A, Romanos GE, Aoki A, et al. Photobiomodulation in periodontology and implant dentistry: part 1. Photobiomodul Photomed Laser Surg. 2019;37:739–65. https://doi.org/10.1089/photob.2019.4710.
49. Gholami L, Asefi S, Hooshyarfard A, Sculean A, Romanos GE, Aoki A, et al. Photobiomodulation in periodontology and implant dentistry: part 2. Photobiomodul Photomed Laser Surg. 2019;37:766–83. https://doi.org/10.1089/photob.2019.4731.
50. Ohsugi Y, Niimi H, Shimohira T, Hatasa M, Katagiri S, Aoki A, et al. In vitro cytological responses against laser photobiomodulation for periodontal regeneration. Int J Mol Sci. 2020;21:9002. https://doi.org/10.3390/ijms21239002.
51. Enwemeka CS, Parker JC, Dowdy DS, Harkness EE, Sanford LE, Woodruff LD. The efficacy of low-power lasers in tissue repair and pain control: a meta-analysis study. Photomed Laser Surg. 2004;22:323–9. https://doi.org/10.1089/1549541041797841.
52. Woodruff LD, Bounkeo JM, Brannon WM, Dawes KS, Barham CD, Waddell DL, et al. The efficacy of laser therapy in wound repair: a meta-analysis of the literature. Photomed Laser Surg. 2004;22:241–7. https://doi.org/10.1089/1549541041438623.
53. Albertini R, Aimbire FS, Correa FI, Ribeiro W, Cogo JC, Antunes E, et al. Effects of different protocol doses of low power gallium-aluminum-arsenate (Ga-Al-As) laser radiation (650 nm) on carrageenan induced rat paw ooedema. J Photochem Photobiol B. 2004;74:101–7. https://doi.org/10.1016/j.jphotobiol.2004.03.002.
54. Bjordal JM, Johnson MI, Iversen V, Aimbire F, Lopes-Martins RA. Low-level laser therapy in acute pain: a systematic review of possible mechanisms of action and clinical effects in randomized placebo-controlled trials. Photomed Laser Surg. 2006;24:158–68. https://doi.org/10.1089/pho.2006.24.158.
55. Pourzarandian A, Watanabe H, Ruwanpura SM, Aoki A, Ishikawa I. Effect of low-level Er:YAG laser irradiation on cultured human gingival fibroblasts. J Periodontol. 2005;76:187–93. https://doi.org/10.1902/jop.2005.76.2.187.
56. Aleksic V, Aoki A, Iwasaki K, Takasaki AA, Wang CY, Abiko Y, et al. Low-level Er:YAG laser irradiation enhances osteoblast proliferation through activation of MAPK/ERK. Lasers Med Sci. 2010;25:559–69. https://doi.org/10.1007/s10103-010-0761-5.
57. Kong S, Aoki A, Iwasaki K, Mizutani K, Katagiri S, Suda T, et al. Biological effects of Er:YAG laser irradiation on the proliferation of primary human gingival fibroblasts. J Biophotonics. 2018;11:e201700157. https://doi.org/10.1002/jbio.201700157.
58. Ogita M, Tsuchida S, Aoki A, Satoh M, Kado S, Sawabe M, et al. Increased cell proliferation and differential protein expression induced by low-level Er:YAG laser irradiation in human gingival fibroblasts: proteomic analysis. Lasers Med Sci. 2015;30:1855–66. https://doi.org/10.1007/s10103-014-1691-4.
59. Zeredo JL, Sasaki KM, Yozgatian JH, Okada Y, Toda K. Comparison of jaw-opening reflexes evoked by Er:YAG laser versus scalpel incisions in rats. Oral Surg Oral Med Oral Pathol Oral Radiol Endod. 2005;100:31–5. https://doi.org/10.1016/j.tripleo.2004.11.012.
60. Mikami R, Mizutani K, Sasaki Y, Iwata T, Aoki A. Patient-reported outcomes of laser-assisted pain control following non-surgical and surgical periodontal therapy: a systematic review and meta-analysis. PLoS One. 2020;15:e0238659. https://doi.org/10.1371/journal.pone.0238659.
61. Coluzzi DJ, Convissar RA. Esthetic laser dentistry. In: Atlas of laser applications in dentistry. Hanover Park, IL: Quintessence Publishing Co, Inc; 2007. p. 133–51.
62. Ishikawa I, Aoki A, Takasaki AA, Mizutani K, Sasaki KM, Izumi Y. Application of lasers in periodontics: true innovation or myth? Periodontol. 2000;2009(50):90–126. https://doi.org/10.1111/j.1600-0757.2008.00283.x.
63. Watanabe H, Ishikawa I, Suzuki M, Hasegawa K. Clinical assessments of the erbium:YAG laser for soft tissue surgery and scaling. J Clin Laser Med Surg. 1996;14:67–75. https://doi.org/10.1089/clm.1996.14.67.

64. Aoki A, Ishikawa I. Application of the Er:YAG laser for esthetic management of periodontal soft tissues. In: Brugnera Junioir A, Pinheiro A, Pecora JD, editors. The 9th international congress on laser in dentistry, Sao Paulo (Brazil), July 21–24, 2004. Bologna: Medimond; 2005. p. 1–6.
65. Saegusa H, Watanabe S, Anjo T, Ebihara A, Suda H. Safety of dental lasers to the eye - irradiation under a microscope with/without eye protectors. Jpn J Conserv Dent. 2007;50:432–9. (in Japanse, English abstract)

Microscope-Assisted Periodontal Regenerative Therapy

Pierpaolo Cortellini and Diego Velasquez-Plata

Contents

Supplementary Information The online version contains supplementary material available at [https://doi.org/10.1007/978-3-030-96874-8_9].

P. Cortellini
Private Practice, Florence, Italy

Accademia Toscana di Ricerca Odontostomatologica (ATRO), Florence, Italy

European Research Group on Periodontology, ERGOPerio, Genova, Italy

Department of Oral Health Sciences, KU Leuven and Dentistry (Periodontology), University Hospitals Leuven, Leuven, Belgium
e-mail: sandro@cortellini.org

D. Velasquez-Plata (✉)
Private Practice, Fenton, MI, USA

Adjunct Clinical Assistant Professor, Periodontics and Oral Medicine Department, The University of Michigan School of Dentistry, Ann Arbor, MI, USA
e-mail: dvelasq@umich.edu

© The Author(s), under exclusive license to Springer Nature Switzerland AG 2022
H.-L. (A.) Chan, D. Velasquez-Plata (eds.), *Microsurgery in Periodontal and Implant Dentistry*, https://doi.org/10.1007/978-3-030-96874-8_9

Abstract

Performing minimally invasive periodontal regenerative surgical procedures utilizing the operating microscope demands a unique approach encompassing specialized armamentarium, knowledge of handling properties of biomaterials, specific flap designs and suturing techniques.

    This chapter reviews historical landmarks in periodontal regeneration treating infrabony and furcation defects. Principles behind biologically driven flap design are described and recommendations are made to achieve optimal soft and hard tissue handling, maintaining adequate flap perfusion and wound stability, all in the pursuit of healing through primary intention.

    Workflow during periodontal regenerative therapy utilizing the operating microscope is presented, emphasizing technical tips on flap design, defect debridement, biomaterial application and tissue approximation. Errors most frequently committed and actions to avoid are discussed, as well as recommendations for the post-operative and maintenance phases of patient care.

Keywords

Minimally invasive surgery · Infraosseous defect · Regeneration · Guided tissue regeneration · Biocompatible materials

1 Introduction

1.1 Definition of Terms

Microscope-assisted periodontal regenerative therapy is par excellence the model of minimally invasive therapy executed with the help of surgical tools that allow visual and hand access into constrained spaces. Magnification and coaxial illumination are key elements that facilitate delivery of care associated with regenerative therapy. When describing microscope-assisted periodontal regenerative therapy (PRT), there are several terms that ought to be defined prior to delving into this topic.

Regeneration: Reproduction or reconstitution of a lost or injured part in a manner similar or identical to its original form [1].

Periodontal Regeneration: The formation of new bone, new cementum, and periodontal ligament about a tooth root surface previously exposed to bacterial plaque [2].

Microsurgery: Surgical procedure performed under a microscope [3].

Periodontal Microsurgery: Refinement of basic surgical techniques made possible by the improvement in visual acuity gained with the use of the surgical microscope [4].

Periodontal Minimally Invasive Surgery: This concept consists of the use of much smaller incisions than those traditionally used for periodontal regeneration, the maintenance of as much of the blood supply as possible to aid in wound healing, primary closure of the surgical incision, and minimize patient discomfort.

1.2 Role of the OM and Microsurgical Instruments and Materials in Periodontal Regenerative Therapy (PRT)

The introduction of the operating microscope (OM) in periodontics has led to a natural adoption of the principles that guide minimally invasive procedures. PRT results and predictability have been enhanced to levels not reported prior to the incorporation of the OM into this discipline [5]. Enhanced magnification and powerful coaxial sources of illumination allow the operator to get visual and tactile access to the operating field, designing flaps by the topographic configuration of the osseous lesions to be treated, exploring root surfaces and identifying etiologic factors, mapping extension of the intraosseous defects, treating root surfaces with manual and mechanically driven instrumentation, delivering regenerative materials (membranes, bone grafts, and biologic modifiers alone or combined) as needed, and approximating wound edges to achieve primary closure under passive suture-guided tissue approximation, thus optimizing wound stability.

Microsurgical instruments have been designed to manipulate delicate tissues (microtissue forceps), to perform accurate and small incisions in equally small interproximal spaces (microsurgical blades, ophthalmic knives), elevate tissue in a controlled and delicate fashion (microsurgical soft tissue elevators), debride inflammatory tissue and remove accretions from root surfaces (micro-curettes, microsurgical scissors, mechanical instruments endowed with diamond-coated tips), visually assess root surfaces, furcation fornix areas (micromirrors), and procure primary closure under passive wound edge approximation (microtissue forceps, microneedle holders, microsurgical sutures and needles). These components of the microsurgical armamentarium allow the execution of fine psychomotor movements both visually and tactile driven with the ultimate goal of providing an ideal environment for biologically driven periodontal regenerative therapy.

2 Historical Background

2.1 Landmark Events in Periodontal Regenerative Therapy of Intrabony Defects

Implementation of PRT is most valuable around teeth that show bone loss characterized by the presence of intraosseous defects. Preservation of gingival architecture and improving the health and prognosis of the natural dentition are desired treatment outcomes. Prichard in 1957 reported the predictable formation of new attachment in intrabony periodontal lesions [6]. Prichard's technique was efficient when treating three-wall intraosseous defects, however, when dealing with two- and one-wall intraosseous defects, the results were not as predictable. This observation was confirmed in clinical and histological studies [7, 8]. To enhance regenerative outcomes, the placement of bone grafts in the intraosseous defects was advocated [9]. Intraoral autogenous grafts obtained from edentulous ridges, retromolar mandibular zones, maxillary tuberosities and extraction sockets were utilized as sources [10, 11]. Utilization of extraoral autogenous graft material was also reported, although this modality was not embraced as a routine procedure in part due to the morbidity associated with the procurement of the graft material itself and observed side effects on the recipient site such as root resorption and ankylosis [12–14]. In view of the inherent limitations associated with autogenous intraoral and extraoral techniques, allografts were scrutinized and adopted as grafting materials. Ample histologic human evidence of utilizing decalcified freeze-dried bone allografts (DFDBA) for periodontal regeneration was provided in 1989 by Bowers et al. [15, 16], and the efficacy of freeze-dried bone allografts (FDBA) was demonstrated by Mellonig in 1991 [17].

Xenografts have also been utilized safely in humans [18]. Radiographic and clinical evaluation showed equal results in clinical attachment gain when compared to autogenous bone grafts in a total of 92 intrabony defects in humans [19].

Alloplasts come in different presentations: hydroxyapatite (crystalline, dense, porous), plaster of paris, polymers, calcium carbonates, tricalcium phosphate, and bioglass. Histologically, areas treated with these biomaterials show fibrous encapsulation and lead to a healing by repair, rather than regeneration of the periodontal structures [20].

Guided tissue regeneration was first reported by Nyman, proving that the placement of a physical barrier to regulate cell migration from gingival epithelium favors periodontal ligament-sourced healing and its subsequent regenerative outcomes [21].

Biologically active regenerative materials promote the healing process, enhancing predictability of results. Regeneration utilizing enamel matrix derivatives (EMDs) has been amply supported in the literature since its introduction in 1997 [22]. Documentation of utilizing EMDs in minimally invasive procedures shows successful outcomes and confirms the versatility of this biomaterials when flap design is of minimal extension enhancing the biologic stability necessary for regenerative therapy [23–25].

Application of growth factors for regenerative purposes have been showcased by Nevins [26] whose group worked with recombinant human platelet-derived growth factor (rh-PDGF) and Kitamura [27] whose team worked with fibroblast growth factor (FGF)-2. These biomaterials have shown a significant therapeutic result in terms of linear bone growth when treating intraosseous defects around natural teeth.

2.2 Landmark Events in Minimally Invasive Surgery of Intrabony Defects

The concept of minimally invasive surgery can be traced back to an editorial published in the *British Journal of Surgery* by Fitzpatrick and Wickham in 1990 [28].

These authors observed the changes occurring in the operating theatres across surgical specialties that had one common denominator: ensuring that trauma of surgical access was reduced to a minimum while still achieving the intended therapeutic aims. The field of regenerative periodontal therapy was not excluded of these revolutionary surgical changes. Since Harrell and Rees illustrated the concept of minimally invasive surgical procedures for periodontal regeneration in 1995 [29], different flap designs and suture techniques have been introduced with the purpose of minimizing surgical access, diminishing tissue trauma, enhancing wound closure, providing stability and protection to the blood clot, and avoiding soft tissue recession while facilitating visual and mechanical access to intrabony defects. The MIS technique was subsequently illustrated in several other publications [30–32].

Flap design has played an important role in the development and application of MIS principles. Takei et al. [33] introduced a papilla preservation technique to protect the interproximal space hosting the intraosseous defect by avoiding incisions directly on the col area, thus facilitating primary closure. The palatal approach proposed by this technique was modified 10 years later when Cortellini et al. [34] described both the modified papilla preservation technique and, a few years later, the simplified papilla preservation flap [35]. These novel techniques provided surgical access from the buccal aspect instead. This surgical modality required a well-defined protocol on incision extension and location, soft tissue manipulation, suturing, and closure. It is important to recall that nonabsorbable and resorbable barriers were being utilized, and due to their size and nature, incision and flap extension had to be more extensive.

Flap design continued its evolution defined by increased knowledge and experience pertaining to biologic guiding principles such as wound stability, blood clot protection, and introduction of biomaterials that were more compatible with minimally invasive procedures. The incorporation of magnification tools such as the OM allowed for optimal visual access and illumination, two fundamental requirements when executing surgical therapy in narrow, deep, and constrained spaces.

The advantages of the utilization of the OM in regenerative therapy has been reported by Cortellini and Tonetti in a prospective cohort study published in 2001 [36]. The purpose of that study was to evaluate the outcomes of a microsurgical approach in regenerative therapy of deep intrabony defects. Twenty-six patients with one deep interdental intrabony defect each (clinical attachment level loss of at least 6 mm and radiographic evidence of a deep intrabony defect) were enrolled. These patients were treated with guided tissue regeneration utilizing either nonresorbable or absorbable membranes depending on the configuration of the intraosseous defect. These defects were accessed via papilla preservation flap techniques aided by an OM and microsurgical instruments. The authors observed that primary closure of the interdental space accessed was obtained in 92.3% of cases for the entire healing period (1 year). Gains in clinical attachment levels (CAL) were 5.4 ± 1.2 mm on average which corresponded to 82.8 ± 14.7% of the initial intrabony component of the defect. Average probing depth (PD) reduction was 5.8 ± 1.4 mm and was associated with minimal increase of gingival recession (0.4 ± 0.7 mm). It is worth noting that primary closure was obtained in 100% of the cases after the first week of surgery. Only two sites were found opened: the first one at 2 weeks and the second one at 4 weeks.

The understanding of the architectural topography of intraosseous defects has played an important role in defining flap design and wound management. The evolution of the MIS approach has witnessed the incorporation of the minimally invasive surgical technique (MIST) which limits the mesio-distal flap extension and coronal-apical reflection while minimizing trauma and maximizing tissue stability [37]. In an effort to further maximize wound stability and blood clot protection, a modified MIST (M-MIST) technique was described and illustrated with clinical cases followed up for 12 months [38]. It is important to note that all of the above work with MIST and M-MIST was performed utilizing an OM and microsurgical instruments.

In the pursuit of adhering to minimally invasive techniques, Harrel developed and later reported 36 months results utilizing a videoscope (VMIS) while treating interproximal intraosseous defects in humans [39, 40]. The described technology allows for visualization and elimination of root accretions through small surgical access incisions, a key component to make regenerative therapy more predictable.

2.3 Landmark Events in Regeneration of Furcation Defects

Flap design for buccal and lingual mandibular and buccal maxillary class II furcations, the so-called key hole, was described over 20 years ago and has not been substantially modified since [41–44].

2.4 Landmark Events in Regeneration of Combined Intrabony and Furcation Defects

Aslan et al. proposed the application of papilla preservation flaps (PPF) to get access to the intrabony component and a buccal/lingual extension to get access to the furcation area [45].

3 Principles Behind the Biologically Driven Paradigm

3.1 Setting the Ideal Condition for Periodontal Regenerative Microsurgery

Periodontal regeneration is applied to improve clinical conditions of periodontally compromised teeth presenting with deep pockets associated with clinical attachment and bone loss. Clinical objectives of periodontal regeneration are pocket reduction, attachment and bone gain, and minimal or no recession. The possibility to gain consistent amounts of periodontal support makes regeneration an approach able to change the prognosis of compromised teeth. This might occur even with minimal or no hamper to the aesthetic appearance of the treated units. Ample evidence shows that regeneration is highly predictable in the treatment of pockets associated with deep and shallow intrabony defects [46] and Class II mandibular and buccal maxillary furcations [47]. In these periodontal defects, periodontal regeneration is recommended, while the application of regeneration in Class II maxillary mesial and distal furcations is strongly suggested [48]. There is no solid evidence supporting the application of periodontal regeneration to pockets associated with Class III furcations and horizontal bone destruction.

A consistent variability of clinical outcomes, however, is evident among the different studies on periodontal regeneration [47, 49]. The observed clinical variability may depend upon differences among the enrolled patients in terms of socioeconomic background, form of periodontal disease, response to therapy, and persistence of specific pathogens; factors like clinical experience, surgical skills, and clinical organization might help to explain different outcomes reported by different clinicians. A series of prognostic factors associated with the clinical outcomes have been identified using multivariate approaches. The main sources of clinical variability are patient, defect, and surgery-associated factors [49].

Periodontal regeneration in intrabony defects and furcations has been so far tested with a variety of surgical procedures aiming at soft tissue preservation, flap elevation, defect debridement, and primary closure of the wound in the absence of tension; these efforts have been enhanced with the adoption of the concept of microscope-assisted periodontal regenerative therapy. Various materials have been proven to favor regeneration, as illustrated in a previous paragraph of this chapter. These materials are incorporated into the defect after debridement and before suturing. It is apparent that none of the tested approaches are clearly superior to the others and applicable to all the possible clinical presentations. The existing ample evidence, however, can be used to develop a "personalized" regenerative strategy [50].

In this chapter, a step-by-step decisional process will be discussed and enriched with flowcharts to guide clinicians to build a personalized regenerative strategy laying out alternatives to choose from among the most effective procedures, the fastest, the easiest, the less burdened by side effects, and the best tolerated by patients [49, 51].

Two determining factors for periodontal regeneration will be discussed: patient preparation and site preparation.

3.1.1 Patient Preparation: Patient-Related Factors

The first step of periodontal therapy is a cause-related therapy, aimed at obtaining patient compliance, reduction of oral bacterial load, and control of gingival infection.

At completion of nonsurgical cause-related therapy, patients are re-evaluated (Flowchart 1). A full periodontal examination should be registered to evaluate:

1. The compliance of the patient in terms of plaque control: a very low load of bacterial plaque is a major goal of cause-related therapy and key to periodontal regeneration. Optimal regenerative outcomes have been reported in patients maintaining full mouth plaque score lower than 15% [49].
2. The control of periodontal infection: low level of bleeding on probing is another major goal of cause-related therapy and again extremely important for the regenerative outcomes. Optimal outcomes have been reported in patients presenting with full mouth bleeding score lower than 15% [49].

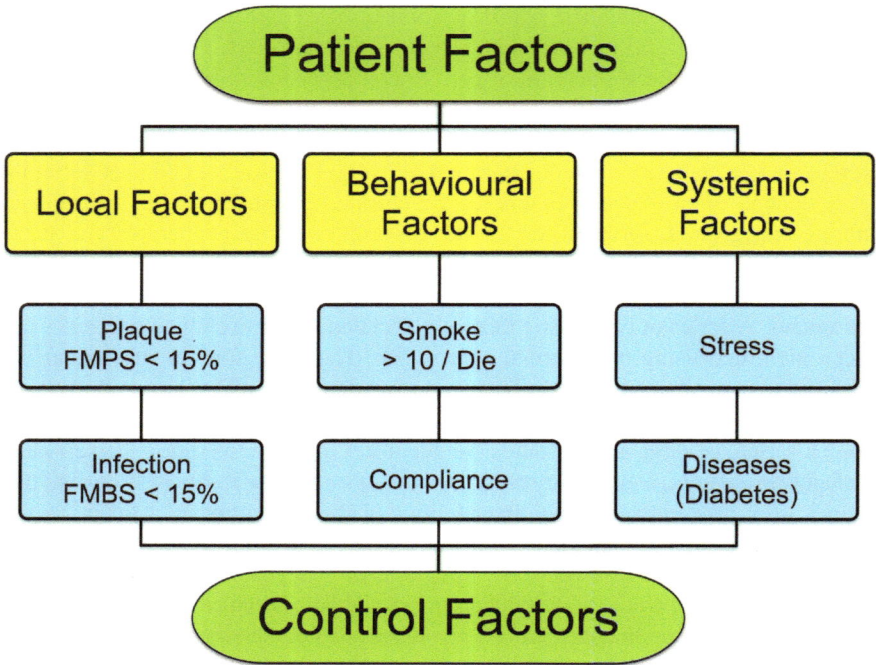

Flowchart 1 Patient associated characteristics to be controlled prior to surgery. Full mouth plaque score (FMPS), full mouth bleeding score (FMBS)

3. The presence of residual pockets or furcation defects that might indicate the need for additional periodontal surgery. Some of the residual pockets might meet the indications for periodontal regeneration, others for different surgical approaches. Ideally, regenerative procedures should be applied after the surgical treatment of pockets not amenable for regeneration, to create the ideal mouth environment for the delicate biologic regenerative process.
4. Additional goals of cause-related therapy are control of behavioral and systemic conditions, like smoking habits, stress and systemic diseases, diabetes in particular.

3.1.2 Site Preparation: Site-Related Factors

The second step aims at the control of three conditions before surgery: (1) the end-odontic status; (2) the local contamination; and (3) mobility of the involved tooth (Flowchart 2). Endodontic diagnosis and treatment, when necessary, should be performed well in advance of the regenerative surgery [52].

Vital teeth should preferably be kept vital, the only exception being periodontal breakdown involvement of the apex of the tooth. Nonvital teeth have to be successfully treated with root canal therapy. Existing root canal therapies should be evaluated, and inadequate treatments should be re-done. Local contamination of the defect-associated pocket should be as low as possible at the time of regenerative surgery. The presence of bleeding on probing (i.e., bacteria) in the defect-associated

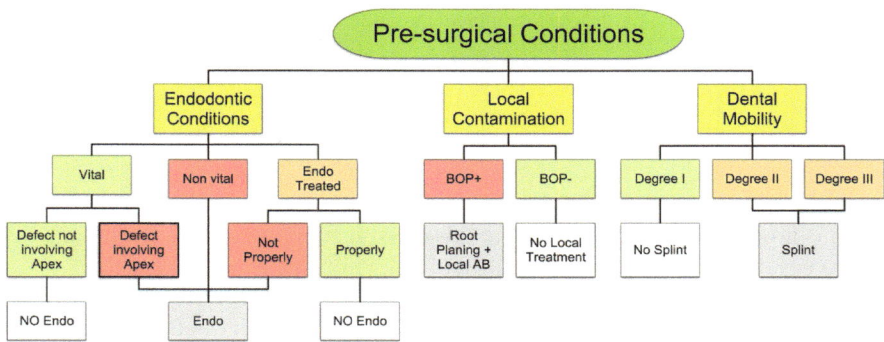

Flowchart 2 Patient conditions to be controlled prior to surgery. Antibiotics (AB); Bleeding on probing (BOP); endodontic treatment (Endo)

pocket indicates the application of gentle root planning and local antimicrobials 2–3 weeks before regeneration. Teeth with a mobility of degree II or III should be splinted prior to or immediately after the surgical procedure. Tooth mobility should be re-evaluated during the early healing phase: any increase in mobility should be detected and immediately controlled.

3.2   Biologically Driven Flap Design and Selection of the Regenerative Strategy

Clinicians are challenged with a decisional process in order to select flap design and regenerative strategy. The unique presentation of each clinical condition requires a careful preoperative evaluation of soft and hard tissue morphology and the knowledge of the biologic requirement for the regenerative event to occur.

3.2.1   Soft Tissue Architecture

Periodontal tissues are characterized by ample differences in morphology and volume in different patients and within the mouth of the same patient [53]. The term "periodontal phenotype" indicates a dimension, genetically determined, that may change through time upon environmental factors and clinical interventions and can be site-specific [54]. The assessment of periodontal phenotype is considered relevant for outcome assessment of therapy (Table 1). Overall, the distinction among different phenotypes is based upon anatomic characteristics of components of the masticatory complex, including (1) gingival phenotype, which includes in its definition gingival thickness (GT) and keratinized tissue width (KTW); and (2) bone phenotype (BP). The phenotype is generally classified as:

- *Thin scalloped* phenotype characterized by narrow zone of KT (<3mm), thin gingiva (<1 mm), and a relatively thin alveolar bone.
- *Thick flat* phenotype characterized by a broad zone of KT (≥3 mm), thick gingiva (≥1 mm), and a comparatively thick alveolar bone.

Table 1 Diagnostic tool for the classification of the soft tissue morphology

Single tooth	KT width	Gingival thickness	Gingival recession	Papilla width
Mesial				
Buccal				
Distal				
Palatal				

It is however to be underlined that this classification cannot be representative of the very ample variability among subjects and within the same subject.

It is a matter of fact that a thin phenotype has a greater tendency to retract when challenged with a pathosis or a disease or with a surgical event. A thorough analysis of gingival thickness and width is thereby mandatory before surgery. Gingival thickness can be determined observing the probe transparency when inserted into the sulcus: when the probe is visible, gingival thickness is ≤1 mm. Gingival width is measured as the distance between the gingival margin and the mucogingival junction. Another key parameter is the amount of the gingival recession at the four aspects of the tooth. Presence of ample recessions will increase the surgical difficulties and limit the regenerative potential. Measurement of the papilla width will guide the type of interproximal incision when applying a papilla preservation approach.

3.2.2 Hard Tissue Architecture

Intrabony defects have been classified according to their morphology in terms of residual bony walls, width of the defect (or radiographic angle), and in terms of their topographic extension around the tooth [55]. Three-wall, two-wall, and one-wall interproximal defects have been defined on the basis of the number of residual alveolar bone walls. Frequently, intrabony defects present a complex morphology consisting of a three-wall component in the most apical portion of the defect, and two- and/or one-wall components in the more superficial portions. Such defects are frequently referred to as combination defects. The defect morphology can be relatively simple when the intrabony defect is allocated on one aspect of the tooth. Whenever the defect is extending around the tooth, the defect morphology becomes more complex and can be different on the different aspects of the tooth. Additional expressions of bone destruction are (1) bone dehiscence at the buccal and/or the lingual aspect of the tooth and (2) the involvement of the furcation area in multirooted teeth. A recent systematic review concluded that deeper defects with narrower angles and increased number of walls exhibit improved CAL and radiographic bone gain at 12 months post-regenerative surgery [46]. However, the authors underlined that more data are needed about other aspects of defect morphology such as extension to buccal/lingual surfaces. In addition, periodontal breakdown can involve neighboring teeth creating many different morphologic conditions. There is a need to develop a more comprehensive, treatment-oriented classification that could guide clinicians in the selection of the regenerative strategy (Table 2).

Table 2 Diagnostic tool for the classification of osseous defect morphology

	Depth 1 wall	Depth 2 wall	Depth 3 wall	X-ray width	Depth dehiscence	Depth suprabony (horizontal)	Depth crater	Furcation H (degree I, II, III)	Furcation V (subclass a, b, c)
Mesial									
Buccal									
Distal									
Palatal									

3.2.3 Presurgical Assessment of the Hard and Soft Tissue Morphology

Defect morphology should be forecasted before surgery and confirmed during surgery. The presurgical assessment is based on periodontal probing and observation of periapical radiographs. The presence of an interproximal intrabony defect is guessed when a difference in the interproximal attachment level between two neighboring teeth is detected: this difference represents the depth of the intrabony defect (Fig. 1a–d). The diagnosis has to be confirmed with a periapical radiograph that provides additional information about the morphology of both the defect and the root. Radiographically, the interproximal intrabony component is normally well visible even if the depth of the defect is frequently underestimated, and the mesio-distal width of the defect can be measured. Additional information is about the root length, the amount of residual bone support, the relation with neighboring roots and information on the endodontic and root-related conditions.

When the presence of an intrabony defect is confirmed at one or both the interproximal aspects of a tooth, the extension at the buccal/lingual aspects should be carefully inspected to assess the presence of an associated bone dehiscence and/or an intrabony component (Figs. 2a–d and 3a–d). Measurement of attachment levels and bone sounding are the diagnostic tools to get solid information on the extension of periodontal/bone destruction but provide limited information about morphology of the destruction. Morphology can be guessed by combining data points about the extension of periodontal destruction, radiographic appearance, thickness of the alveolar process, size and position of the tooth, amount of gingival recession, and proximity with neighboring teeth.

The presence of osseous defects at neighboring teeth should be carefully evaluated. When multiple neighboring defects are present, the surgical approach becomes more demanding (Fig. 4a–d).

Additional information about the involvement of the furcation should be collected when dealing with a multirooted tooth. Depth of the horizontal involvement (Class I–III) and amount of vertical destruction around each single root (subclass A–C) should be assessed. A furcation involvement can be associated with horizontal or vertical bone destruction and/or with buccal/lingual bone dehiscence (Fig. 5a–d).

The analysis of *soft tissue morphology* will indicate potential, difficulties, and limits of the regenerative surgery. Examples of the most frequent scenarios are as follows:

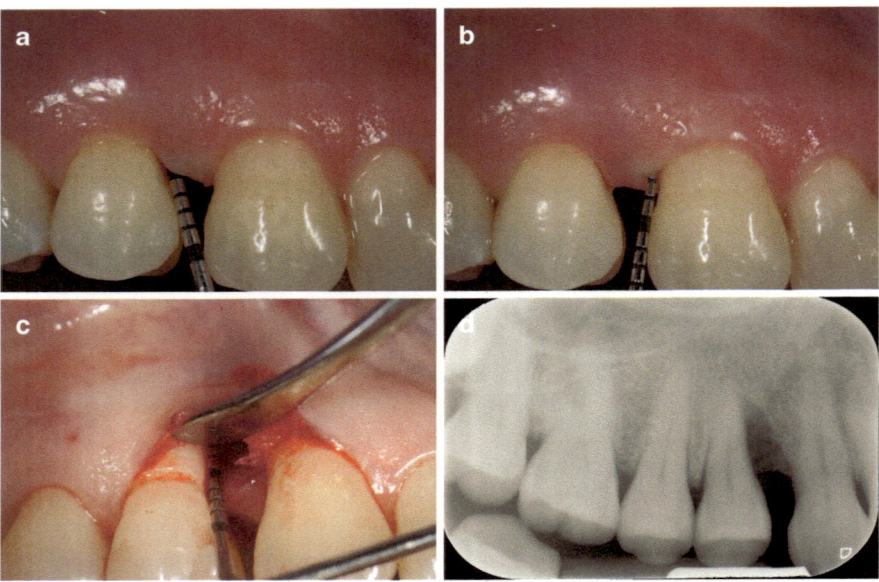

Fig. 1 Clinical detection of an intrabony defect. (**a**) 10 mm clinical attachment level at the defect-associated tooth. (**b**) 2 mm clinical attachment level at the crest-associated tooth: the difference between the two measurements forecasts an intrabony component depth of 8 mm. (**c**) Intrasurgical measurement of the intrabony depth, confirming the clinical measurement of 8 mm. (**d**) Radiographic image of the defect

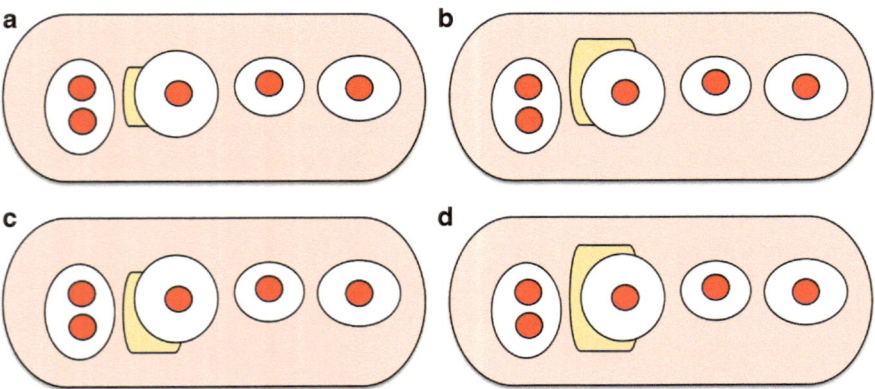

Fig. 2 (**a–d**) Schematic drawings of the involvement of a single interproximal aspect (**a**) and associated buccal (**b**) and/or palatal (**c, d**) extension of the defect

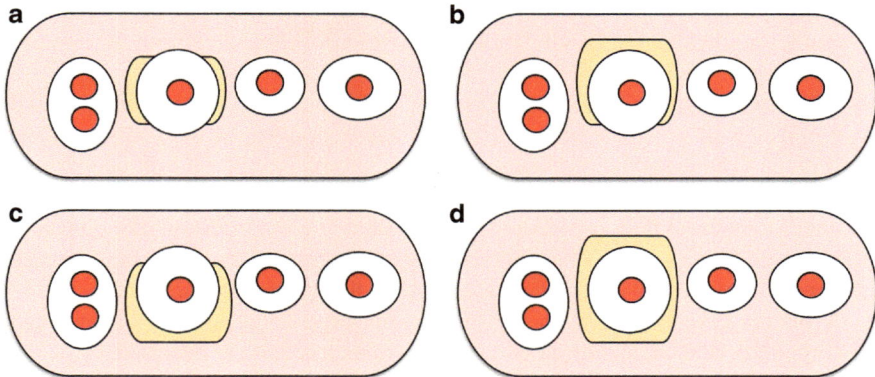

Fig. 3 (**a–d**) Schematic drawings of the involvement of both the interproximal aspects (**a**) and associated buccal (**b**) and/or palatal (**c, d**) extension of the defect

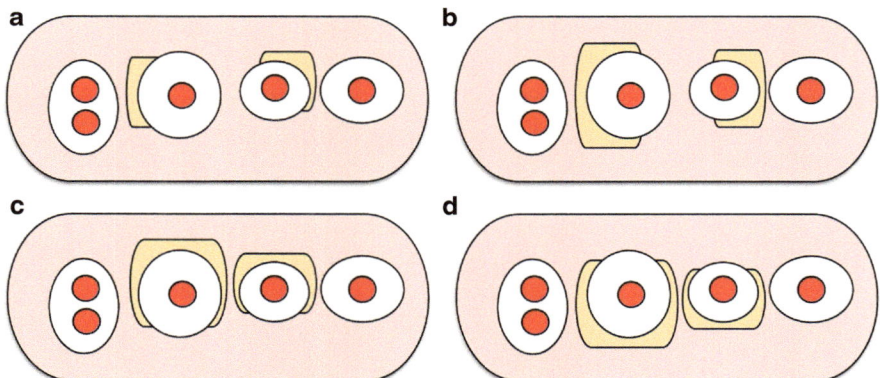

Fig. 4 (**a–d**) Schematic drawings of the involvement of multiple teeth. The interproximal defects are associated with buccal and/or palatal extension of the defect (**a–d**)

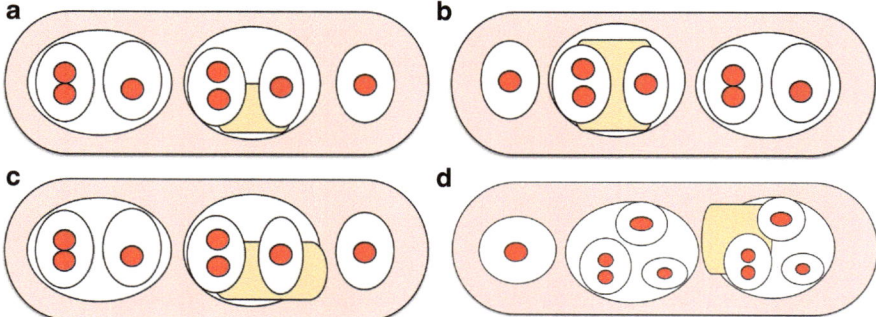

Fig. 5 (**a–d**) Schematic drawings of mandibular class II (**a**) and III (**b**) key-hole furcation involvement and mandibular (**c**) and maxillary (**d**) class II furcation involvement combined with interproximal defects

- Thick phenotype with no or minimal gingival recession and a well-preserved convex and wide interdental papilla is the most desirable condition for regenerative surgery (Fig. 6).
- A thin phenotype will increase the risk for potential intrasurgical damages to the gingival wall and potential soft tissue contraction in the postsurgical period (Fig. 7). The odds for the latter will become greater when a thin phenotype is associated with a buccal bone dehiscence and when a biomaterial is positioned under the buccal flap. A potential solution could be the insertion of a connective tissue graft to modify the phenotype either 3 months before or during regenerative surgery. The latter will increase the complexity of the procedure.
- A buccal gingival recession will determine the coronal limit for regeneration (Fig. 8). A potential solution is coronal advancement of the buccal flap.
- A palatal/lingual recession will determine the coronal limit for regeneration with very limited possibilities to overcome the problem (Fig. 9a, b).
- A very thin papilla will increase the risk for failure of the primary closure, especially in the molar area (Fig. 10). Presence of biomaterials and especially an overfill will increase the odds for this side effects.

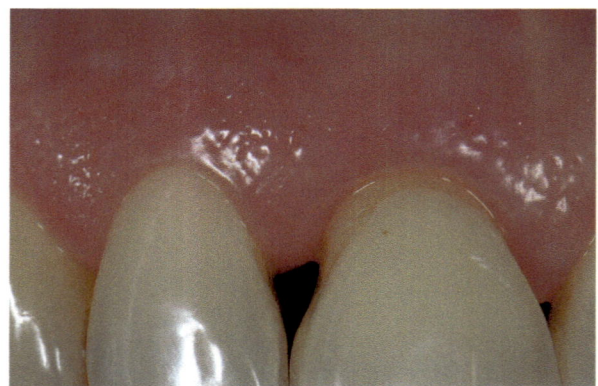

Fig. 6 Thick phenotype with no or minimal gingival recession and a well-preserved convex and wide interdental papilla

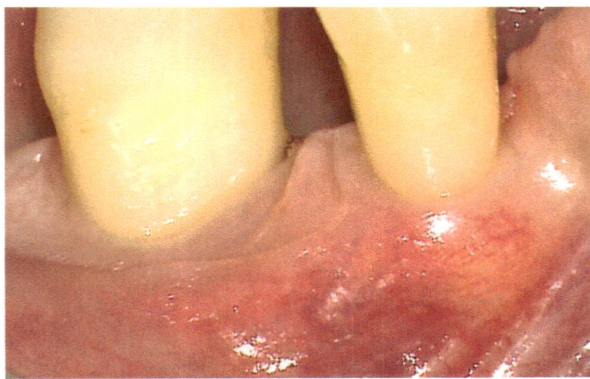

Fig. 7 Thin phenotype: risk for soft tissue contraction

Fig. 8 Buccal gingival recession: coronal limit for regeneration

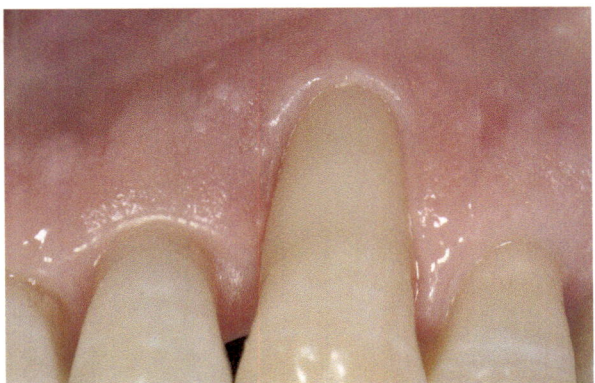

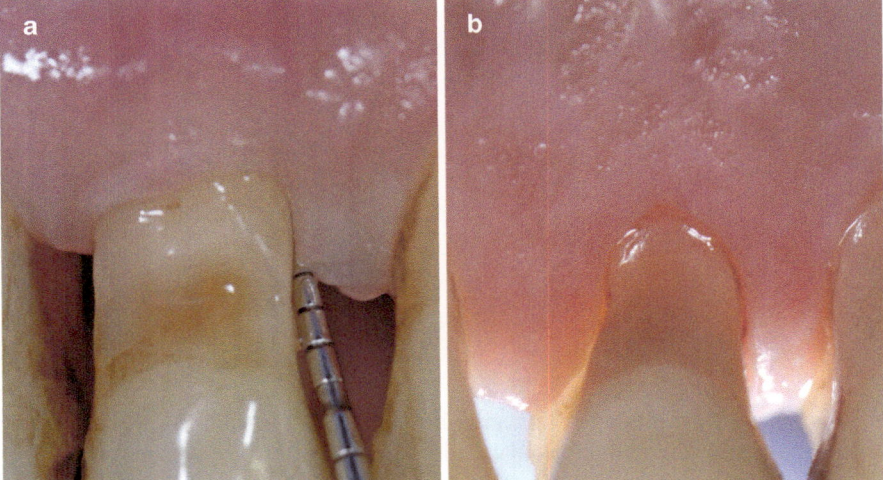

Fig. 9 (**a, b**) Buccal and lingual gingival recession: coronal limit for regeneration

- A concave papilla or the presence of a soft tissue crater is a condition that will render papilla preservation very demanding, sometimes impossible (Fig. 11). Not unfrequently, these conditions are the consequence of a very aggressive non-surgical approach that should be carefully avoided. Nonsurgical debridement and root planing in a site amenable to regeneration should be performed with the aim of the best decontamination and minimal soft tissue trauma. The use of an operative microscope and microsurgical instruments could greatly help this relevant step.

This accurate diagnosis is necessary to select the type of surgical approach and the regenerative materials to be applied to the given clinical condition. In fact, different surgical approaches have been developed through time that incorporate clear

Fig. 10 Thin papilla

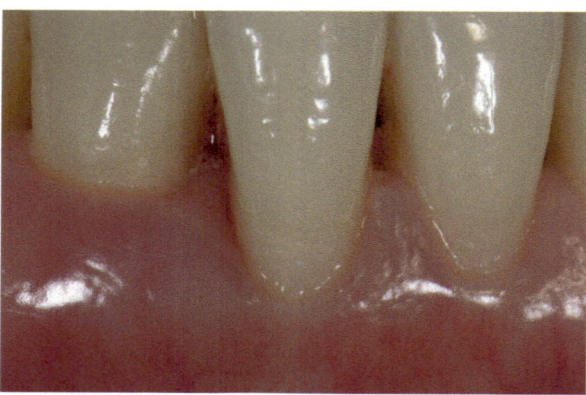

Fig. 11 Concave papilla

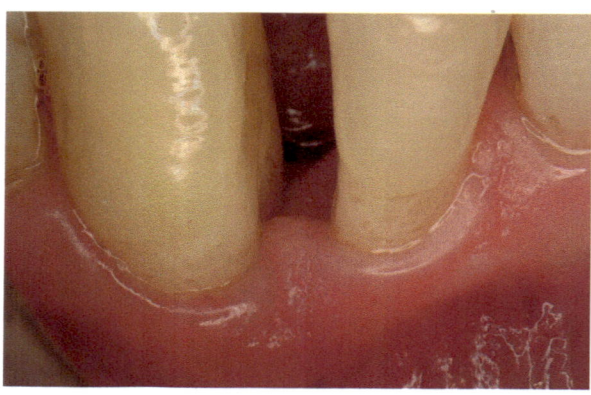

differences in terms of flap design and suturing technique. All the proposed surgical techniques have a common foundation in the attempt to fully preserve the defect-associated interdental papillae and the buccal and lingual keratinized gingiva performing intrasulcular incisions and rising full-thickness flaps.

3.2.4 Biologic Foundation of Periodontal Regeneration

The main objective of the surgical approach to periodontal regeneration is to design a flap and apply a suturing technique resulting in the stable primary closure of the wound margins. Flap design and extension should also allow for accurate defect and root surface debridement. The choice of the surgical approach and the selection of the regenerative material should be guided by soft and hard tissue morphology and by some factors that play a relevant role in the healing dynamics of periodontal regeneration:

a. *Space* for the formation of the blood clot at the interface between the flap and the root surface [34, 56–60]

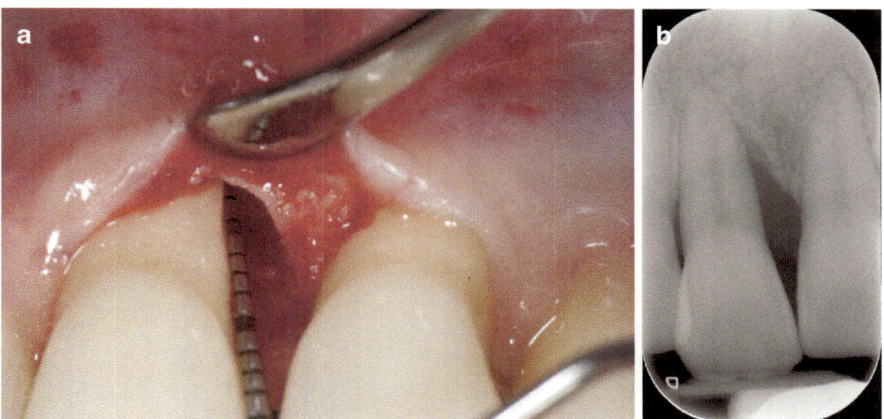

Fig. 12 (**a**, **b**) Containing, narrow two- to three-wall intrabony defect

b. *Stability of the blood* clot to maintain its adhesion with the root surface and prevent the apical migration of a long junctional epithelium [61–63]
c. *Soft tissue protection* of the treated area to prevent bacterial contamination [49, 64–67]

Space and blood clot stability are self-expressed by the defect morphology in the so-called containing defects, the narrow two and three walls in particular (Fig. 12a, b) [64, 68–71]. Space and blood clot stability can be further improved applying peculiar surgical flap designs based on the principles of minimally invasive surgery [38, 72]. The ideal design of a minimally extended envelope-like full-thickness flap will grant the greatest flap stability. Any increment in extension, or application of vertical releasing incisions, or periosteal fenestrations will increase flap mobility and its instability: this will have a negative impact on the stability of the blood clot. The "non-containing defects," like the large one wall, or the defects extending to the buccal/lingual aspects and associated with bone dehiscence do not afford adequate support to the soft tissues and adequate stability to the blood clot (Fig. 13a, b). Such a severe and complex morphology will also require the elevation of more ample and more flexible flaps to get access to the defect, introducing an additional component of instability. The challenge created by the complexity of the defect morphology and by the design of the flap has to be counteracted with the application of regenerative biomaterials, like barriers or fillers or combinations thereof, able to support the soft tissues and to stabilize the blood clot [49]. Blood clot stability, as reported above, is also influenced by tooth mobility: teeth with high mobility are to be stabilized before or immediately after the regenerative surgery [36, 73]. It has to be reminded that application of biomaterials like fillers and or membranes is associated with an increase of the postsurgical side effects, flap failure in particular [49, 66]. This is to be taken into account limiting the use of these materials only to the cases

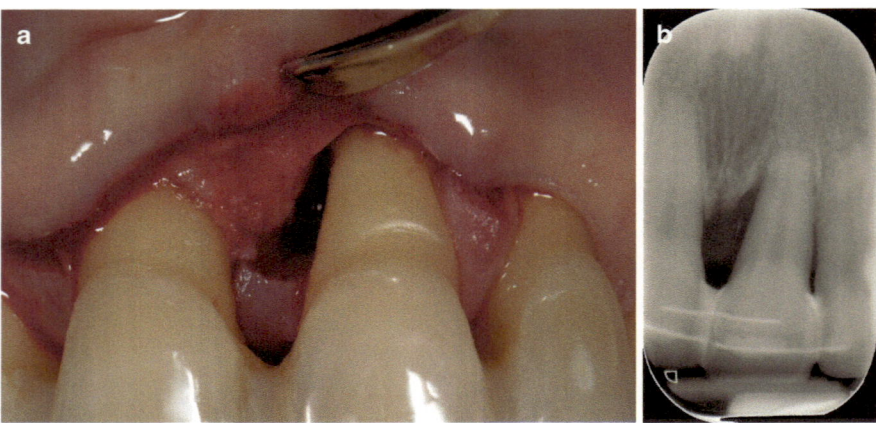

Fig. 13 (**a, b**) Non-containing, one-wall intrabony defect

that really require their application. Protection of the surgical site must be provided with an appropriate flap design and suturing approach selected among the surgical procedures that have so far been proposed including papilla preservation flaps [33–35, 74] and minimally invasive surgical approaches [29, 37, 39, 75].

4   Microsurgical Phase: Treatment of Intrabony and Furcation Defects

4.1   Workflow During PRT Utilizing the Operating Microscope

Clinical application of regenerative PRT utilizing the OM is an orchestrated effort involving all members of the microsurgical team. As previously described in more detail in chapter "Practical Considerations in Incorporating Microsurgery to Daily Workflow" of this book, workflow is optimized to maximize efficiency of movements and accuracy in execution of tasks. Positioning of the microscope, microsurgeon, assistant(s), patient, visual support media (co-observation binoculars/broadcasting monitors) must be choreographed to meet not only ergonomic comfort but to facilitate excellent delivery of care by everyone involved. The members of the microsurgical team must be completely engaged, focused on problem-solving and on seeking maximum productivity in goal achievement.

The following description of events is favored by the authors of this chapter in light of their own clinical experience. Modifications are always feasible, and ultimately, the microsurgeon and the support team will make decisions based on what mechanics of work will enhance delivery of care for everyone involved. A six-handed instrumentation system is favored as an ideal method to gain efficiency in operational flow during microscope-assisted PRT. A primary assistant will be seated in close proximity to the patient and microsurgeon, and a supporting secondary assistant will be seated on the side of the operator, opposite to the primary assistant, or contiguous to the primary assistant to avoid congestion, gain improved visual access, and be ready to support the microsurgeon and the primary assistant's logistic needs. For guiding principles on microsurgeon, assistant(s), and patient positioning, refer to chapter "Practical Considerations in Incorporating Microsurgery to Daily Workflow" of this book.

All microscope-assisted PRT procedures start by meticulous preplanning utilizing available diagnostic data such as patients' medical and dental history, clinical charting, and radiographic information available. Anatomical topography of the osseous defect will dictate the sequence of events to be adopted during the surgical intervention. As previously described in this chapter, if the intraosseous defect is of unilateral nature, meaning only the buccal or the palatal/lingual aspect of the target area is involved, operational maneuvers will be limited to single-sided flaps providing access without much positional disruption. Incisions are performed with instruments that allow precise cutting, such as mini-blades and ophthalmic knives mounted on light rounded handles conducive to facilitate finger-guided movements as opposed to wrist/arm-based displacements. The primary assistant will be ready to control hemorrhage associated with incision tracing by utilizing suctioning devices in combination with copious hydration delivered by the secondary assistant in order to help evacuate blood and clear the surgical field to facilitate visualization. The secondary assistant is ready to transfer instruments to the microsurgeon and support microscope positioning demands in an effort to minimize unnecessary, cumbersome, interrupting, and time-consuming handling of the operating microscope by the microsurgeon. The goal of the assisting team is to enhance execution of surgical operational movements by the microsurgeon in the oral cavity, which means maximizing both movement efficiency and time spent operating. Any adjustments of foot controls and operating microscope macro and micro motions are to be delegated to the supporting personnel.

4.2   The Biologically Driven Flap Design

Here a stepwise approach is illustrated to describe the use of the operating microscope and microsurgical instruments and materials in the treatment of intrabony and furcation defects. As for the intrabony defects, a "treatment model" will be described with the aim to provide the readers with solutions for the treatment of the many different morphologic presentations. As for the multirooted teeth with furcation involvement, two different presentations will be discussed: (1) the so-called key hole, characterized by a horizontal bone destruction at buccal and/or lingual furcation of lower molars and buccal of upper molars; (2) a combination of furcation involvement and vertical bone destruction at any furcation entrance.

Surgical access to intrabony and furcation defects and type of regenerative biomaterial should be selected according to the soft and hard tissue morphology.

In general, flap design should satisfy the following requirements:

1. Complete preservation of the interdental papilla and marginal soft tissues.
2. Elevation of full-thickness envelope-like flaps with enough mesio-distal extension to provide proper access to the defect and allow for thorough debridement and application of the selected regenerative material.
3. Application of periosteal incision and vertical releasing incisions to increase flap mobility, only when an ample coronal advancement is warranted.
4. Application of internal mattress sutures or sling sutures to obtain and maintain passive primary closure of the flap on top of the regenerative biomaterial during the early healing phase.

4.3   Technical Tips: Flap Design, Defect Debridement, Biomaterial Application, Suturing

When applying regeneration to any type of defect, it is suggested to have the patient rinsing with chlorhexidine 0.2% for 1 min and perform a full-mouth prophylaxis with slow-speed rubber cup and paste to reduce the bacterial oral burden. Anesthesia should be delivered far away from gingival margin and interdental papilla with low dose of vasoconstrictor (i.e., 1:100,000 epinephrine) to reduce unwanted postsurgical problems with revascularization of the flap edges.

4.3.1   Intrabony Defects

The following stepwise decisional process can guide clinicians to select the regenerative strategy of intrabony defects:

Step 1. Surgical access to intrabony defects is selected among three different modalities of incision (Flowchart 3). A horizontal incision as described in the MPPT [34] is chosen when the width of the interdental space is ≥2mm. A diagonal incision

Flowchart 3 Incision modalities for surgical access. Modified papilla preservation technique (MPPT); simplified papilla preservation flap (SPPF)

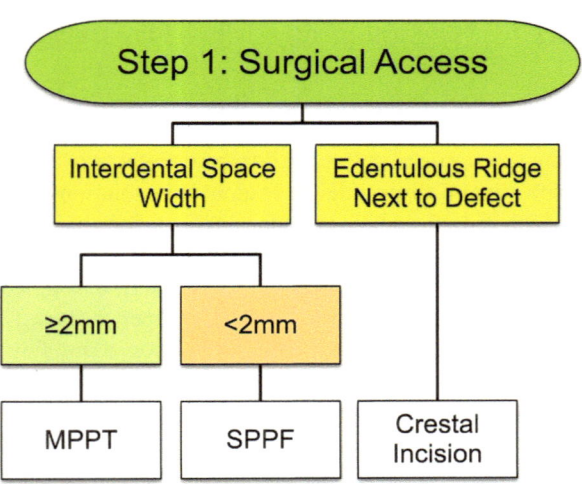

as described in the SPPF [35] is chosen whenever the width of the interdental space is <2 mm. A crestal incision is applied when the defect is allocated next to an edentulous area [49].

Step 2. Flap design (Flowchart 4). Extension and design of the flap is selected according to the defect morphology with two main objectives in mind: on one side, creating the conditions for defect debridement and for regenerative material allocation, and on the other side, the need for minimal invasiveness to favor wound stability and increase the healing potential. A balance among these different and sometimes conflicting requirements must be found. The accurate selection of the appropriate regenerative material will contribute to model the best regenerative strategy. Different scenarios can be depicted. (A) When the defect involves only one interproximal aspect, a minimally invasive approach with the elevation of a full thickness buccal flap is indicated without any need for papilla refection and lingual flap elevation [38]. Mesio-distal extension will be limited to the mid-buccal scalloping contour of the two teeth neighboring the defect. Corono-apical elevation of the full-thickness flap should be limited to the exposure of 1–2 mm of the residual buccal bone crest. A key point in deciding the application of the M-MIST is the possibility to debride the defect and the root surface through the tiny buccal window. If the defect is not cleansable from the buccal window, the interdental papilla should be elevated. (B) A buccal extension of the periodontal breakdown associated with a buccal bone dehiscence and the loss of the interproximal buccal bony wall (two-wall intrabony) will indicate a larger mesio-distal and corono-apical extension to increase flap reflection and reach the edge of the bone crest. The buccal extension of the flap might be preferably obtained involving the next interproximal space tracing a beveled buccal incision of the papilla. An alternative solution could be a vertical releasing incision. (C) The involvement of both the interproximal aspects with or

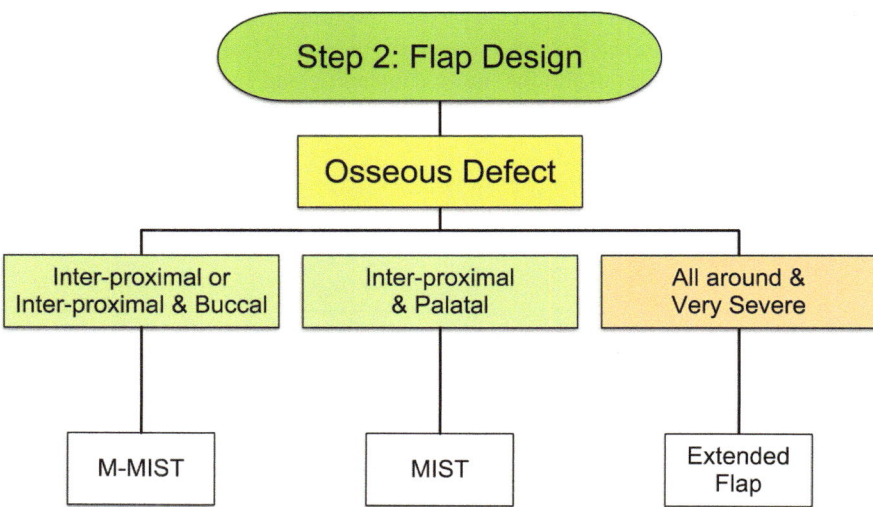

Flowchart 4 Flap design. Minimally invasive surgical technique (MIST); modified minimally invasive surgical technique (M-MIST)

without a buccal bone dehiscence indicates the application of an extended buccal flap without any need for papilla refection and lingual flap elevation (M-MIST). (D) The involvement of the palatal/lingual aspect indicates the elevation of the interdental papilla along with a palatal/lingual flap. The buccal and the lingual flap will be minimally extended according to the MIST principles when the buccal and the lingual/palatal extension of the defect is limited [37]. (E) A large flap, extended to the neighboring teeth and eventually including vertical releasing incision, will be chosen in the presence of a very severe and very deep defect, especially when associated with palatal/lingual dehiscence that require ample flap reflection for debridement. Frequently, these ample buccal flaps require a periosteal fenestration to increase flap mobility and coronal advancement to facilitate passive primary closure on top of membrane and/or biomaterial.

Step 3. Selection of the regenerative material (Flowchart 5). It is based on the defect morphology and on the type of flap design. Overall, amelogenins alone are preferred in containing defects with a prevalent three-wall morphology or in narrow two-wall defects, while the use of membranes and/or fillers is indicated in noncontaining defects, like the one wall or the large two walls, and in the presence of associated buccal and/or palatal/lingual dehiscence. As discussed above, the flap design is also guided by the defect morphology, so both the selection of the surgical approach and of the regenerative material have a common background. If a M-MIST approach is applied, amelogenins or no regenerative materials are the elective choices. The presence of a buccal dehiscence and/or the loss of part or all the interproximal bony wall especially in a wide defect might indicate the application of a filler. If a MIST approach is applied, amelogenins are indicated in narrow, containing defects or in combination with a filler in larger, non-containing defects. When a large flap is elevated, soft tissue support and stability of the blood clot should be improved by applying barriers or fillers, combinations of barriers and fillers, or combinations of amelogenins/growth factors and fillers. It has to be reminded that the application of biomaterials and especially the overfill of the defect will make passive primary closure of the flap more demanding and frequently will require a periosteal fenestration to coronally advance the buccal flap.

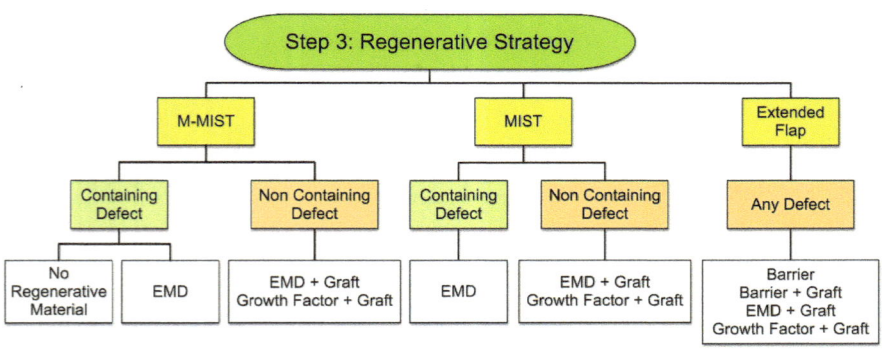

Flowchart 5 Regenerative material selection. Enamel matrix derivative (EMD); minimally invasive surgical technique (MIST); modified minimally invasive surgical technique (M-MIST)

Step 4. Suturing strategy (Flowchart 6). It is chosen according to the type of regenerative strategy applied. A single internal modified mattress suture is suggested when a full-thickness buccal flap without periosteal fenestration is chosen. A multiple-layer suturing approach, as described in the MPPT, is indicated when a large buccal flap with a periosteal incision is advanced to cover a barrier or a graft or a combination thereof [49]. Single interproximal additional interrupted sutures might be applied to improve papilla primary closure, as well as to seal vertical releasing incisions.

• When approaching the surgical area with the microscope, a stable position should be found that enables a clear vision of the buccal aspect following the ergonomic indications discussed in another chapter of this book. The best angle of vision to begin surgery and apply the buccal incision of the papilla is about 60–50° with respect to the buccal gingival surface.

The surgical approach starts with the incision of the papilla. The type of incision should be carefully planned, according to the following indications: when the papilla is ≥2 mm wide, a horizontal incision on the buccal aspect of the defect-associated papilla will be preferred (MPPT) [34]; when the interdental papilla is narrower than 2 mm, a diagonal incision will be chosen (SPPF) [35]. The incision is always buccal, irrespective to the prevalent position of the defect and is traced with a microblade. When applying a horizontal incision, the microblade is oriented perpendicular to the gingival surface. The "90 degrees" incision provides an ample, flat connective tissue surface supporting epithelium for the primary closure of the papilla. It is extremely important to avoid a "beveled" incision of the papillary tissue: the bevel will produce a thin edge of the papilla made of sole epithelium deprived of the vascularized connective tissue and will easily necrotize. This unwanted side effect will cause a failure of the primary intention seal of the wound. Position of the incision at the buccal side of the papilla is also critical and highly depending upon the papilla morphology. Two different scenarios can be depicted: (1) Papilla completely or almost completely preserved with a contact point (Fig. 14a). The incision should not be performed too coronal, i.e., close to the tip of the papilla, where most of the volume is occupied by epithelium; similarly, the

Flowchart 6 Selection of suturing technique. Minimally invasive surgical technique (MIST); modified minimally invasive surgical technique (M-MIST)

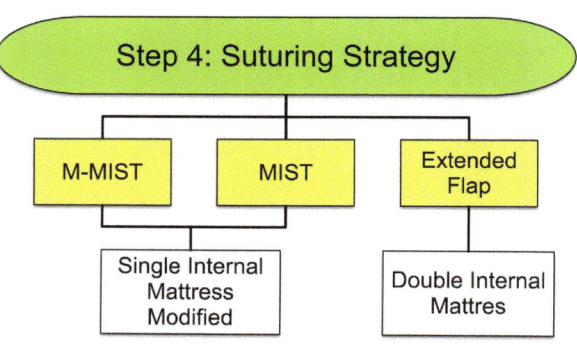

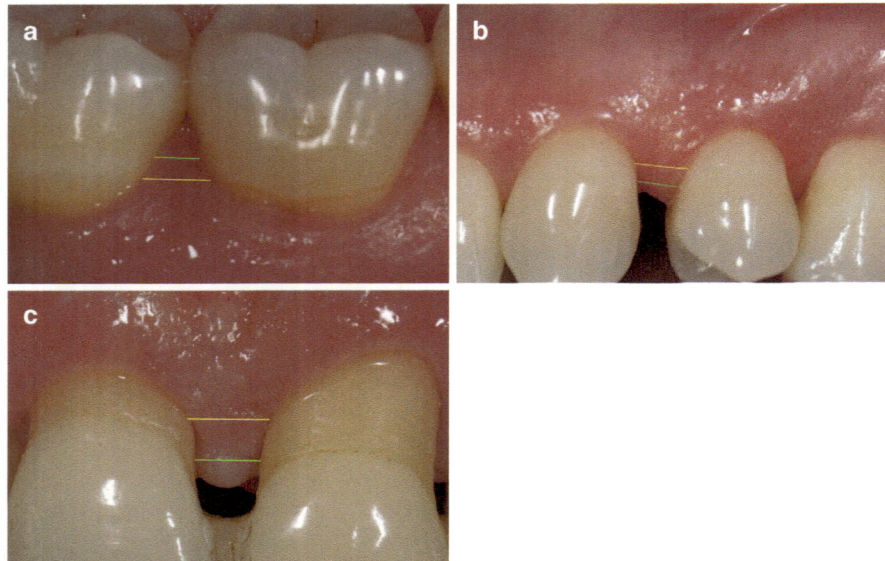

Fig. 14 (**a–c**) Wide interproximal spaces indicating a horizontal incision according to the MPPT. The yellow and the green lines indicate the apical and the coronal limit within which the incision should be traced. (**a**) Papilla completely or almost completely preserved with a contact point; (**b**) papilla completely or almost completely preserved with a diastema; (**c**) papilla retracted

incision should never be placed too apically, i.e., in the area where the scalloping buccal contour starts. The ideal incision line should be placed in the area contained within the described limits. (2) Papilla completely or almost completely preserved with a diastema (Fig. 14b) or papilla retracted (Fig. 14c). The apical limit is the same as in the previous example; the coronal limit however can be extended to the top of the papilla that will offer an ample surface of epithelium supported by connective tissue.

When the interdental site is narrower than 2mm, a diagonal incision will be performed. This condition is more frequently observed when the papilla is completely or almost completely preserved. The incision of the narrow papilla starts in the buccal sulcus of the defect-associated tooth and is continued in the sulcus of the interdental space until the blade can advance; when the crown of the two approximal teeth forbids further sulcular advancement in the interproximal space, the microblade is slightly rotated to diagonally cut the papilla through the interdental space. The blade has to reach the interdental root surface of the crest-associated tooth (Fig. 15).

- The primary horizontal or diagonal incision of the papilla in most of the instances will end into the body of the interproximal connective tissue and will not reach any bone plate (Fig. 16a–x). The primary incision of the papilla should be followed by short intrasulcular buccal incisions extended to the mid-buccal aspect of the two approximal teeth. When completed, a gentle buccal leaning traction of

Fig. 15 Narrow interproximal space indicating a diagonal incision according to the SPPF

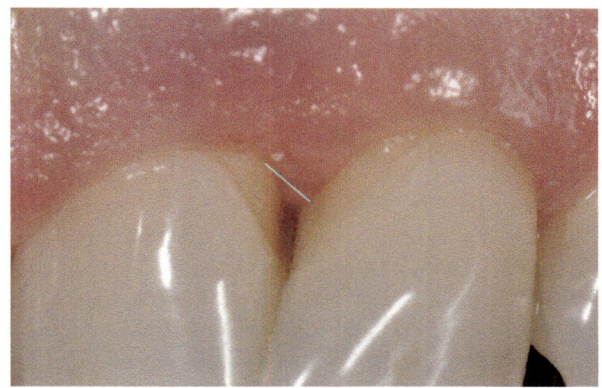

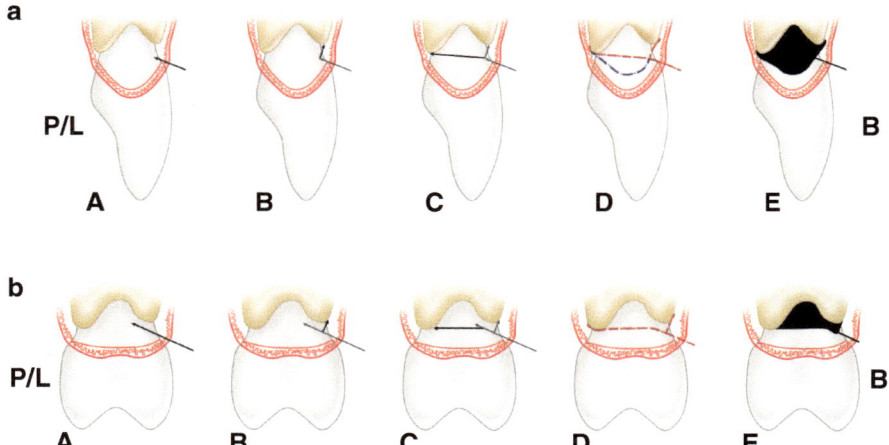

Fig. 16 (a, b) Graphic representation of the incision lines in the interproximal space. (A) Blade enters perpendicular to the gingival surface (B) Blade is repositioned so it aims at the buccal alveolar crest. (C) Blade is then redirected to the buccal aspect of the palatal alveolar crest. (D) Incision design. (Blue dotted line on anterior teeth: additional soft tissue excising allowed by papilla shape). (E) Space for regeneration. *B* buccal, *P/L* palatal-lingual

the gingiva with a periosteal elevator will enable the insertion of the microblade through the primary interproximal incision with a different angle aiming at the buccal bone crest. It is suggested to change the posture of the operative microscope taking a more "occlusal" position ("endodontic" position) that will enable a direct vision of the microblade dissecting the connective tissue. It is also suggested to preferably start the dissection at the buccal interproximal aspect of the crest-associated tooth where normally the bone crest is the most coronal and easy to reach. When positioned on the most coronal portion of the crest, the microblade will follow the edge of the crest gently cutting toward the defect-associated tooth. The buccal flap will be then elevated full thickness to expose just the coronal edge of the buccal bone crest. The mesio-distal extension of the buccal flap will be determined by the defect morphology and the type of regenerative material: a more extended defect and/or the decision to use a barrier will indicate a larger mesio-distal and corono-apical extension of the flap (Figs. 17a–i, 18a–k, and 19a–k). When a more ample flap is indicated, the neighboring papillae will be involved with a beveled buccal incision to separate the buccal flap from the body of the papilla. The latter will be left untouched to host the flap when sutured back at the end of surgery. When the neighboring interproximal spaces are involved with osseous defects, the associated papilla will be approached with a papilla preservation technique following the steps described above.

- Without modifying the microscope position, a sharp dissection between the papillary tissue and the granulation tissue should be performed (Fig. 16a–x). This incision should be carefully planned according to the following principles: (1) the dissection should preserve at least 2mm of the connective tissue coupled to the papilla; (2) the microblade should be directed toward the buccal surface of the palatal bony wall, preferably aiming at the most coronal portion of the palatal crest; (3) the crest of the palatal bony wall should thereby be carefully detected before running the blade through: a scenario in which the palatal bony wall is resorbed will require an inclination of the blade toward the palatal bottom of the defect, while when the bony wall is still present the microblade will be inclined more coronally; (4) the insertion of a periodontal probe through the granulation tissue to check for the position of the edge of the palatal crest is a possible solution; a second possibility could be planning a sequential series of incisions that will aim first at the palatal bottom of the defect and then more coronal in few steps until reaching the edge of the crest.

- It is also suggested to perform a sharp dissection of the granulation tissue from the bony walls: this will facilitate its removal with curettes. The use of microscissors might be of great help in trimming small portions of granulation tissue. Here the surgical approach could take two different paths: (1) elevation of the sole buccal flap (M-MIST) or (2) elevation of the preserved papilla with the palatal flap (MIST or large PPF). When M-MIST is indicated, the defect debridement and root planning will be performed through the buccal window (Fig. 20a–i). Here the contribution of the operative microscope becomes of outmost relevance to increase visual acuity and allow for a perfect decontamination and instrumentation of the defect and the root surface. Micro-curettes and tiny tips of mechanic instruments are necessary. The introduction of micro-mirrors will contribute to facilitate the vision of dark corners. One of the key issues when instrumenting under the papilla is to carefully avoid any trauma to the supracrestal fibers that connect the papilla to the root surface of the crestal tooth on top of the bone crest. Another issue is to carefully plan the amount of connective tissue to be removed from the apical side of the papillary body: the more tissue is taken away, the larger the room for regeneration, but the thinner the connective tissue supporting the papilla and granting its survival. Balancing these elements is critical to obtain as much space for regeneration as possible and to comply with the need for primary closure of the wound. When a *MIST* or a *Large PPF* is indicated, the defect

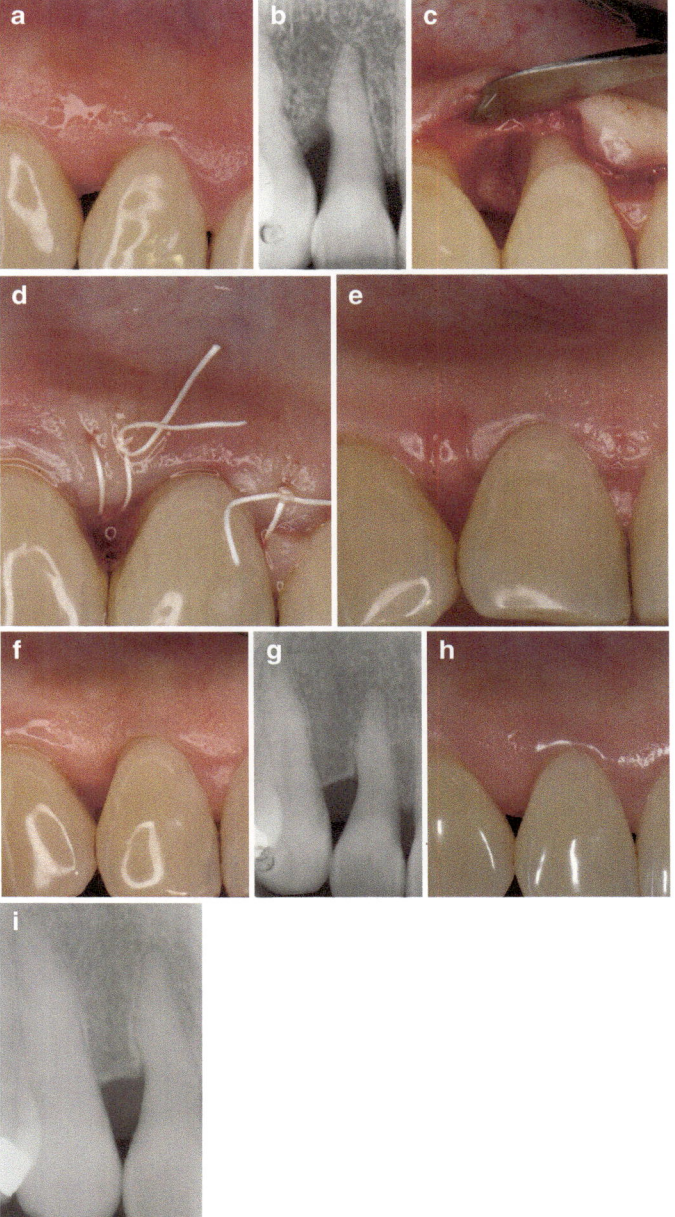

Fig. 17 (**a–i**) Upper right lateral incisor presenting with a distal two- to three-wall intrabony defect associated with a small buccal bone dehiscence (**a–c**). The defect morphology and extension indicated the flap design: horizontal incision of the wide distal papilla according to the MPPT principles, preservation of the distal papilla and extension of the buccal flap to the mesial papilla according to the MIST principles. After amelogenins delivery, primary closure was obtained with a horizontal modified internal mattress suture (**d**). Primary closure maintained at 1 week when sutures were removed (**e**). One-year resolution of the defect (**f, g**). Stability of the site after 10 years (**h, i**)

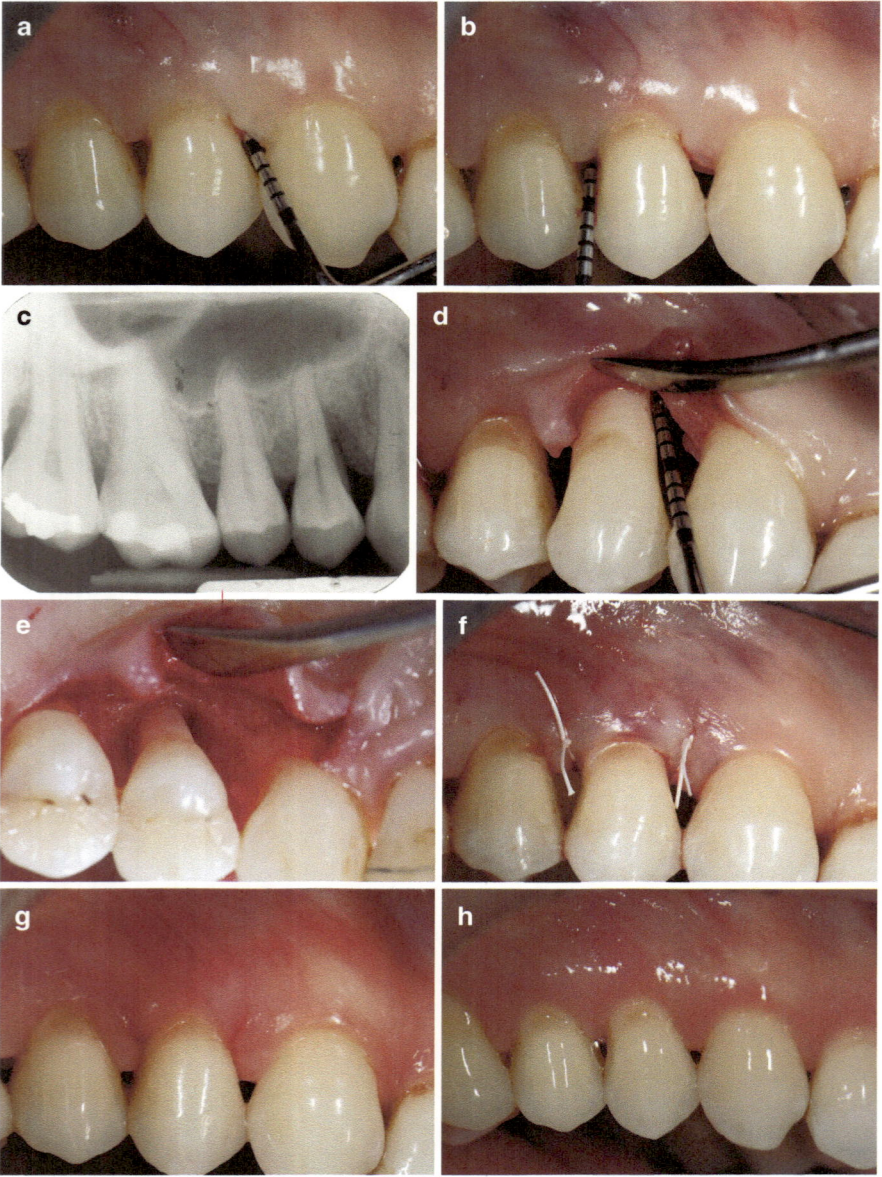

Fig. 18 (**a–k**) Upper right first premolar presenting with deep pockets and an intrabony defect involving the mesial, the distal, and the palatal aspect (**a–c**). The defect morphology and extension indicated the flap design: horizontal incision of both the wide mesial and distal papilla according to the MPPT principles, elevation of the mesial and distal papilla along with a palatal flap according to the MIST principles (**d, e**). After amelogenins delivery, primary closure was obtained with two vertical modified internal mattress sutures (**f**). Primary closure maintained at 1 week when sutures were removed (**g**). One-year complete resolution of the distal defect and partial resolution of the mesial one (**h, i**). Clinical and radiographic images at the 11-year follow-up (**j, k**)

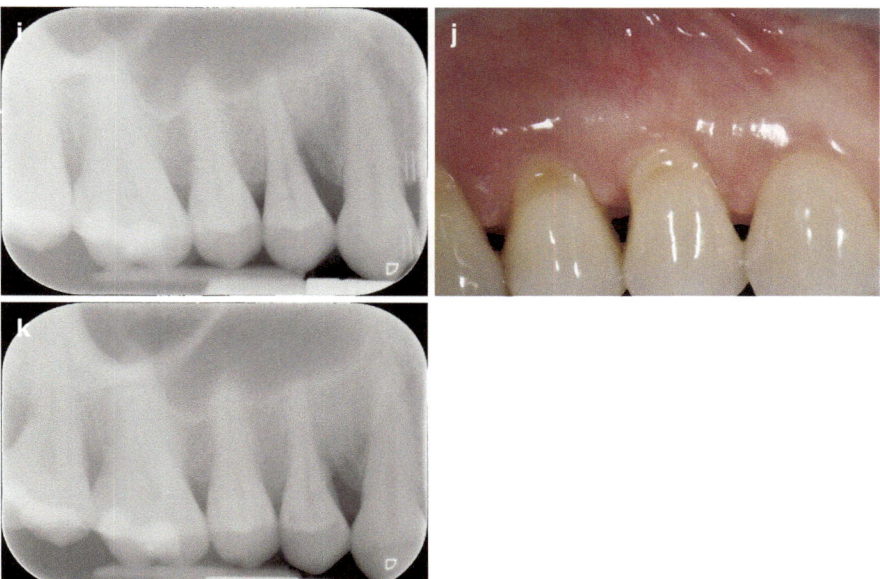

Fig. 18 (continued)

debridement and root planning will be completed after the elevation of the papilla. The partial removal of granulation tissue performed from the buccal side will expose the bone surfaces of the defect and facilitate the palatal/lingual elevation of the papilla.

- When the elevation of the papilla is indicated, the microblade will be positioned in the interproximal sulcus of the crest-associated tooth to cut the supracrestal fibers and separate the papilla from the root surface. The mobility of the papilla should be tested from buccal: if the previous steps have been carefully completed, the papilla should rotate almost completely toward the palatal/lingual side.
- The position of the microscope should now be modified to work on the lingual/palatal aspect and perform the intrasulcular incisions. The mesio-distal extension, as on the buccal aspect, will be determined by the defect morphology and the type of regenerative material: a complex and extended defect and/or the decision to use a barrier will indicate a larger mesio-distal and corono-apical extension of the flap. Special care should be devoted to the completion of the interproximal sulcular incision to completely separate the papilla from the crest-associated root surface. The rotation of the papilla will be tested by applying a small periosteal elevator from a side: should palatal rotation require force, consider the need to complete fibers dissection with the microblade. The papilla rotation can also be facilitated inserting the periosteal elevator between the base of the papilla and the palatal/lingual bone to create a tunnel. The full-thickness

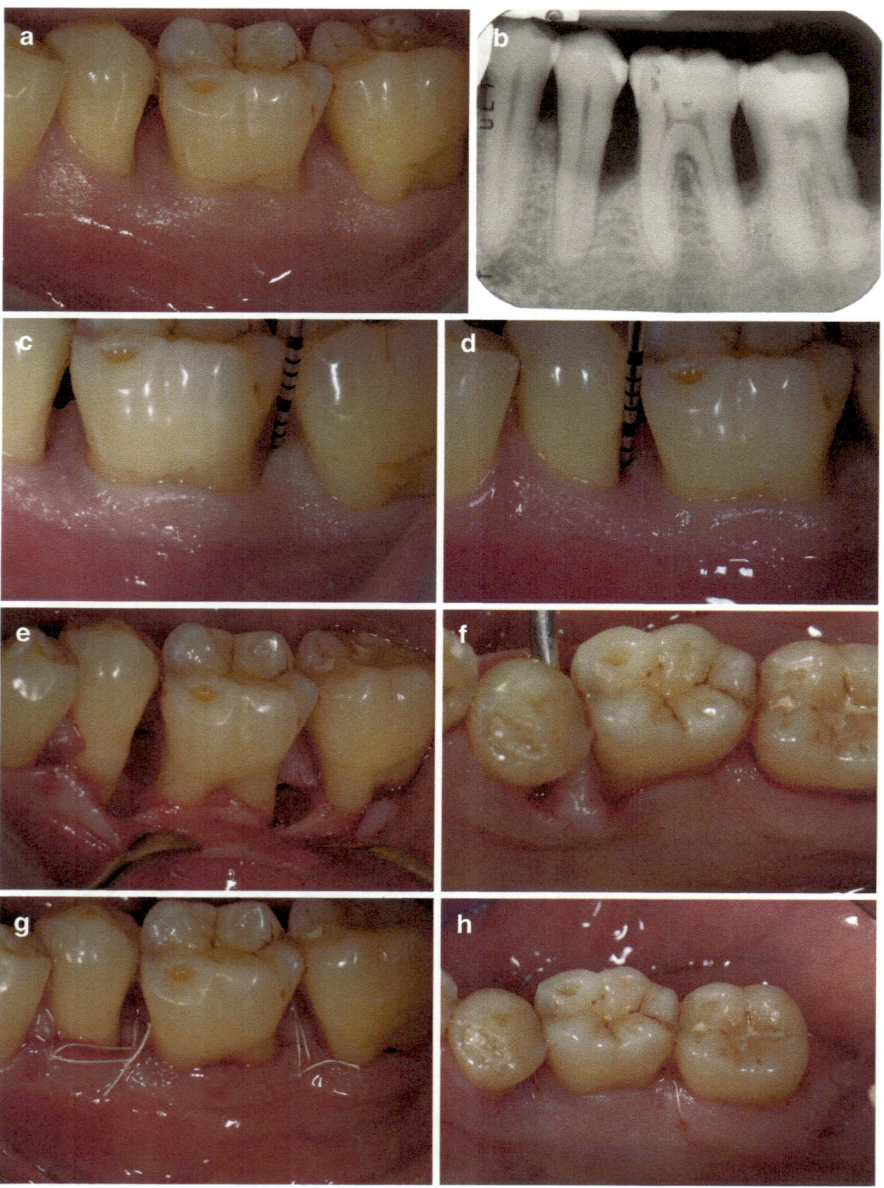

Fig. 19 (**a–k**) Lower left second premolar and first molar presenting with deep distal pockets associated with intrabony defects (**a–c**). The distal defect of the premolar extends to the palatal aspect. The buccal flap was extended from the mesial papilla of the premolar to the buccal sulcus of the second molar (**e**). The interproximal defect distal to the first molar was accessed without elevation of the papilla, according to the M-MIST principles, while the papilla between the premolar and the molar was elevated with a short lingual flap according to the MIST principles to get access to the lingual component of the defect (**f**). After amelogenins delivery, primary closure was obtained with vertical modified internal mattress sutures (**g**, **h**). Primary closure maintained at 1 week when sutures were removed (**i**). Clinical and radiographic images at the 9-year follow-up (**j**, **k**)

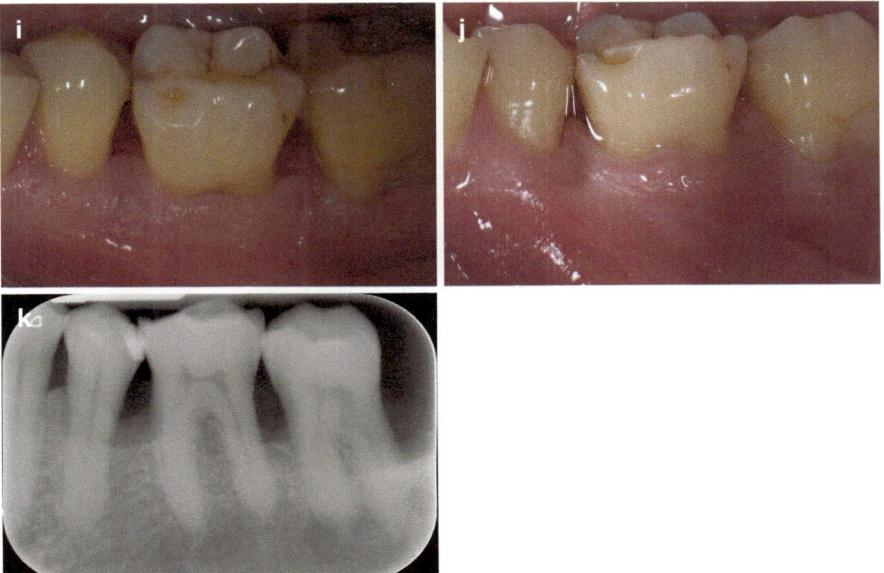

Fig. 19 (continued)

palatal/lingual flap will be risen to expose the coronal edge of the bone crest. Debridement will be completed on this aspect.

- At completion of palatal/lingual debridement, a buccal working position should be resumed to check the accuracy of the instrumentation with high magnification. It is reminded that debridement of the defect-associated root should involve all the exposed root surface from CEJ to periodontal ligament toward the bottom and the sides of the defect. By doing so, some supracrestal fibers will be removed along with root cementum. However, the main aim of defect instrumentation is to ensure a complete debridement of the exposed root surface: this absolute need overcomes the potential damage resulting by removal of some apical fibers. It has to be added that, when applying regeneration, we believe that regeneration will occur and the fibers removed from bottom and sides of the defect will be regenerated. A completely different approach should be used for the crest associated root surface. Here the bone crest is topped with supracrestal fibers that should not be removed: instrumentation to bone crest would cause attachment loss and a postsurgical crest resorption with a reduction of the regenerative space. These fibers do not have any possibility to be predictably regenerated, being out of the regenerative room. The ample variability of the width of the supracrestal connective tissue does not allow for an average determination of the supracrestal space forbidden to root planing. It is strongly suggested to carefully determine the attachment level before surgery and confirm this level during surgery inspecting the root surface with high magnification: it is often possible to detect the

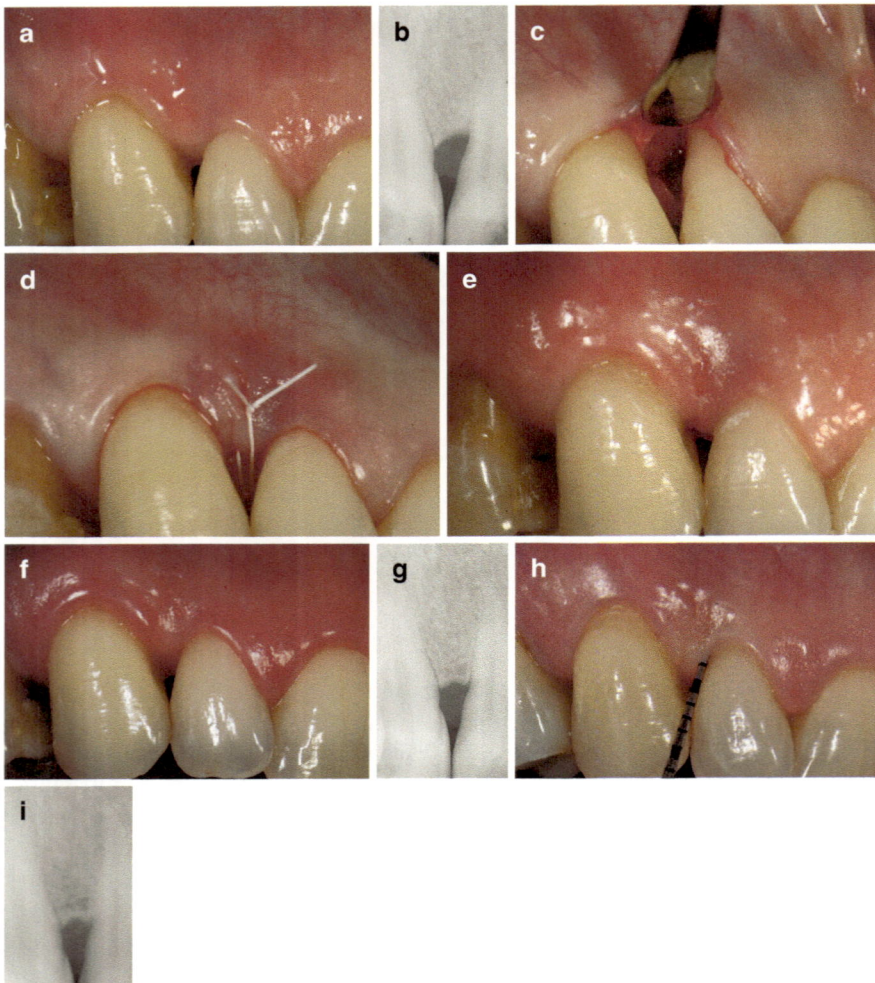

Fig. 20 (**a–i**) Upper right lateral incisor presenting with a distal two- to three-wall intrabony defect (**a–c**). The defect morphology and extension indicated the flap design: diagonal incision of the narrow papilla according to the SPPF principles, elevation of the buccal flap without papilla reflection according to the M-MIST principles. After amelogenins delivery, primary closure was obtained with a vertical modified internal mattress suture (**d**). Primary closure maintained at 1 week when sutures were removed (**e**). One-year resolution of the defect (**f, g**). Stability of the site after 12 years (**h, i**)

fibers adhering to the root cementum. Instrumentation should be performed coronally to the detected fibers (Fig. 21a–h).

- The choice of the regenerative biomaterial will influence the next steps of the surgical procedure. The application of biologicals (i.e., amelogenins or growth factors) or bone grafts within the intrabony component without over-filling the

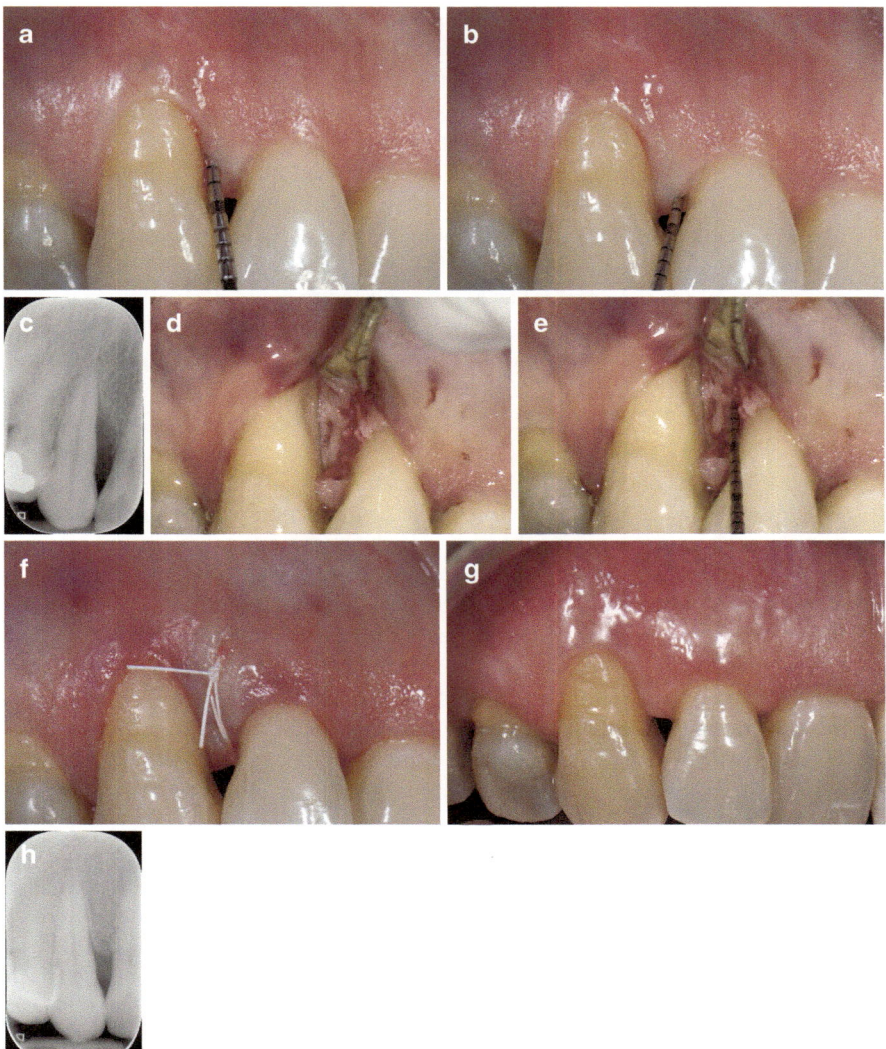

Fig. 21 (**a–h**) Upper right cuspid presenting with a 10 mm CAL associated with a deep mesial intrabony defect; a 4 mm CAL was measured at the crestal tooth (**a–c**). The defect was accessed with a buccal flap without papilla reflection according to the M-MIST principles (**d**). Debridement of the distal side of the lateral incisor (crestal tooth) was performed coronally to the supracrestal fibers: the tip of the probe on the crestal bone shows the presence of 3 mm supracrestal fibers, confirming the presurgical CAL measurement (**e**). After amelogenins delivery, primary closure was obtained with a vertical modified internal mattress suture (**f**). One-year complete resolution of the defect (**g, h**)

defect does not require further extension or mobilization of the flap. The use of barriers and/or fillers involving the supracrestal space generally requires a coronal advancement of the flap to allow for passive primary closure. Flap mobility is increased with a buccal periosteal incision. Sometimes, vertical releasing incisions can be added, but only when strictly necessary: the flap should preferably be envelope-like. Biologicals should be introduced on clean and dry root surfaces. The application of EDTA for 2' is strongly suggested before the application of amelogenins. This product should be carefully washed away. Bone grafts or other biomaterials should be introduced with the aim of filling the intrabony component of the defect; it is strongly suggested to avoid the compaction of the particles to leave enough space for the blood: the more particles filling the space, the less space for the blood and for the regenerative cells, causing sort of "bio-obstruction" that will delay the regenerative process. When combining biologicals and bone-like materials, the biologicals will be delivered first and grafts introduced afterward. Application of a barrier requires few steps. A custom-made shape should be obtained, the more frequent being a saddle-shape; the barrier should be extended 3–5 mm on top of the bone surrounding the defect; application should be made entering the barrier in the interproximal space and inserting the palatal/lingual portion under the flap; the buccal portion will be kept lifted to allow for the introduction of grafts when a combination approach is indicated; finally, the buccal portion of the barrier is introduced under the buccal flap.

- Flaps are repositioned or coronally positioned on top of the regenerative materials and sutured to provide a stable passive primary flap closure. This step is the most demanding in terms of operative posture, since it requires frequent change of position from buccal to lingual and back. It is suggested to take an "occlusal" position with the microscope that will allow for buccal and lingual vision through minimal movement. A key point is the proper position of the suture bites: the suture should bite at a distance of at least 2 mm from the edge of the wound or the gingival margin and two neighboring sutures should stay at a distance of at least 3 mm. Reducing this distance will increase the probability for the sutures to lose tension in the first week of healing with a high risk for flap failure. This happens for the early inflammation around the suture material due to bacterial colonization, that cause a reduction of the consistency of the connective tissue. A second key point is to reach a perfect "tension" when tightening the nod; this is obtained when the suture is no longer loose and is not causing overpressure on top of the gingival tissue. The material of choice to reach this balance is PTFE: this type of suture requires three single counter-throws to be locked and allows for a controlled refinement of tension after the application of the second throw. The closure is ideally provided with a multiple layer suturing approach when the buccal flap is coronally advanced. The first apical suture is a horizontal internal crossed mattress suture that will facilitate the coronal advancement of the buccal flap. This suture is preferably applied very close to the muco-gingival junction to leave enough space for the application of the second suture. The second more coronal one is a vertical internal mattress that will close the papilla in the absence of tension. In some instance, a third simple suture is positioned at the edge of the

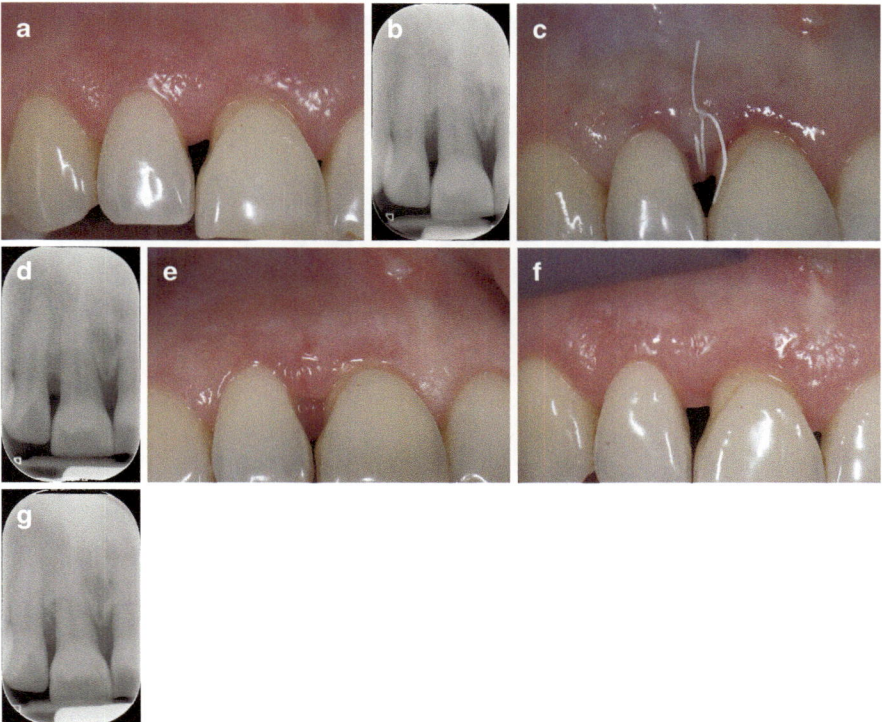

Fig. 22 (a–g) Upper right central incisor presenting with a distal one- to three-wall intrabony defect extending to the palatal aspect (**a, b**). The defect has been accessed with a MIST approach, debrided, and filled with a combination of amelogenins and deproteinized bovine bone mineral (Video 1). Primary closure with a vertical modified internal mattress suture (**c**). Postsurgical radiograph (**d**). Suture removal at 1 week (**e**). Clinical and radiographic images at 1 year (**f, g**)

papilla to optimize primary closure. When the procedure does not require a coronal advancement of the flap, an internal mattress modified suture is indicated. The neighboring papillae, when involved, are stabilized with interproximal interrupted sutures.

An example of the MIST surgical approach is shown in Video 1 (Fig. 22a–g). An example of the M-MIST surgical approach is shown in Video 2 (Fig. 23a–h).

- *Flaps with crestal incision*
  In some *instance*, the intrabony defect may involve a tooth with an adjacent edentulous ridge [49]. The crestal incision is traced in the mid-crestal area, perpendicular to the ridge surface, and its extension has to overcome by 2–3 mm the extension of the defect (Fig. 24a–i). The incision is then continued in the sulcus of the defect-associated tooth and eventually extended to the neighboring teeth as described above. Full-thickness buccal and lingual flaps are elevated as

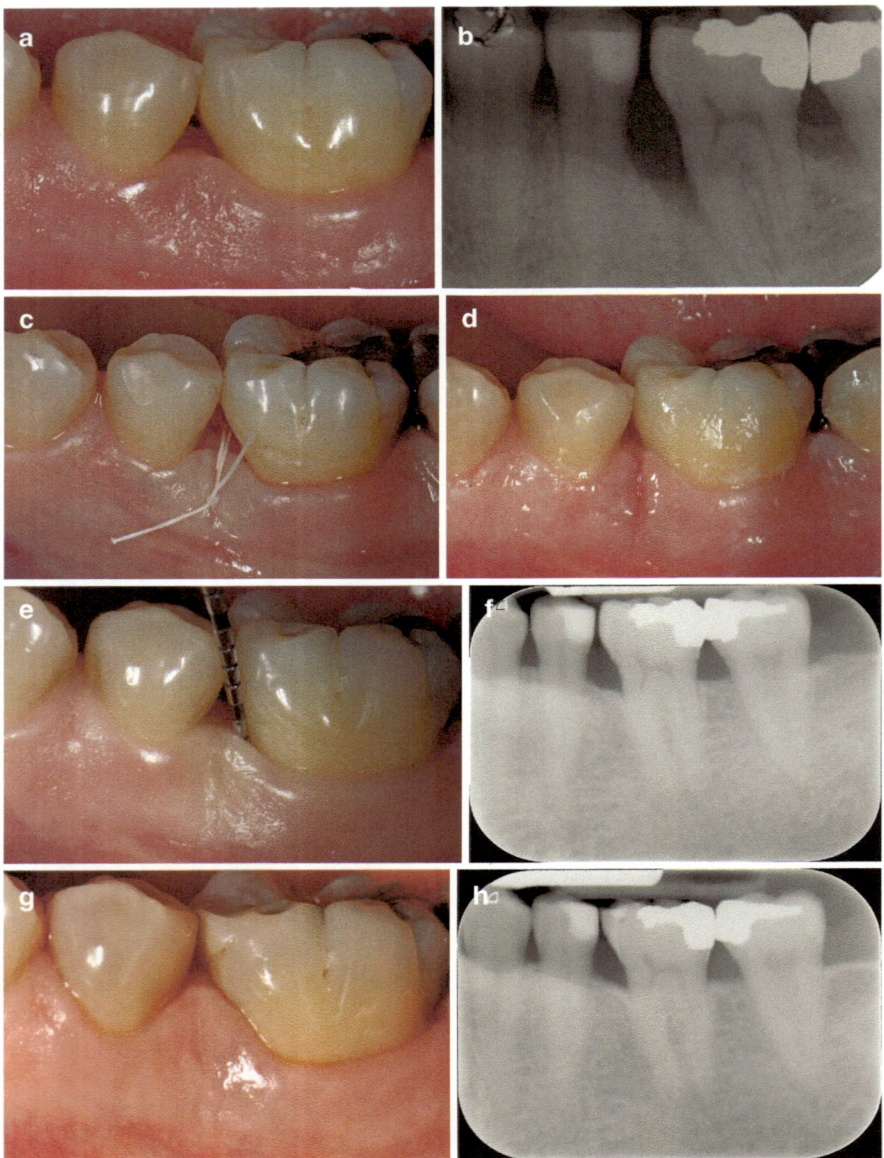

Fig. 23 (**a–h**) Lower left first molar presenting with a mesial three-wall intrabony defect (**a, b**). The defect has been accessed with a M-MIST approach, debrided and treated with amelogenins (Video 2). Primary closure with a vertical modified internal mattress suture (**c**). Suture removal at 1 week (**d**). Clinical and radiographic images showing the complete resolution of the defect at 1 year (**e, f**). Clinical and radiographic images at 10 years (**g, h**)

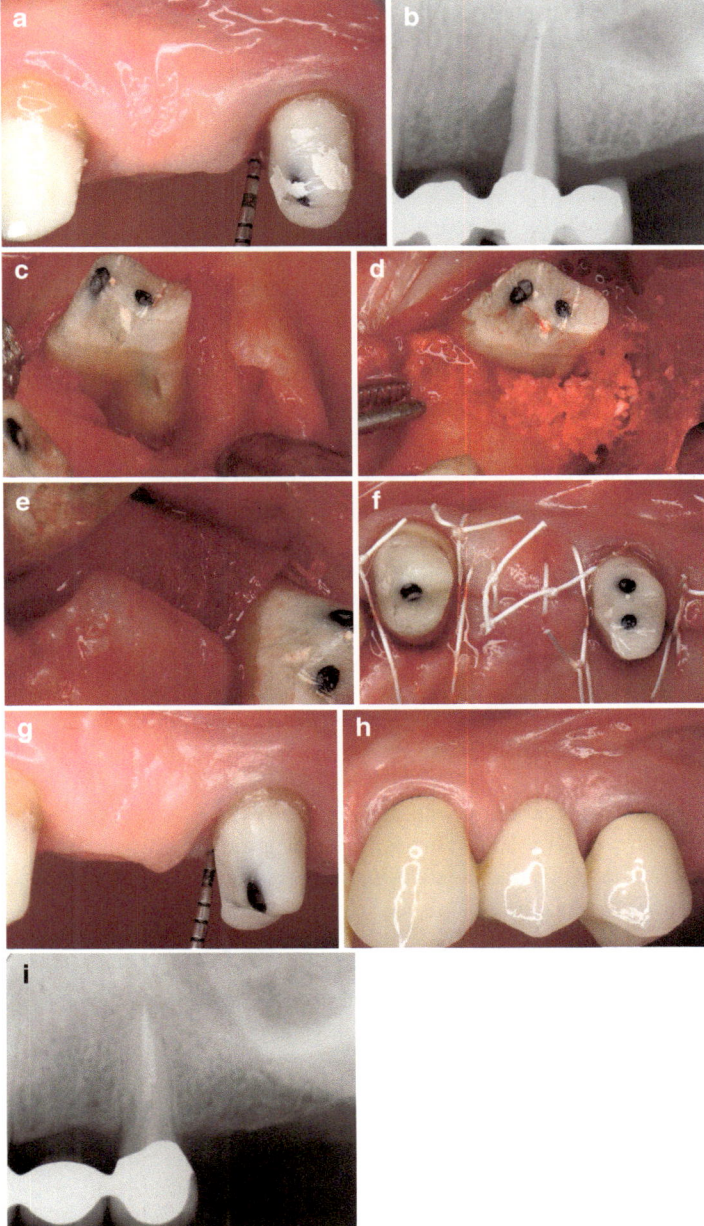

Fig. 24 (a–g) Upper right second premolar, bridge abutment, presenting with a 7 mm pocket associated with a deep intrabony defect involving the mesial, palatal, and distal aspects of the tooth (a, b). The site was accessed with a crestal incision and the elevation of buccal and lingual flaps (c). Deproteinized bovine bone mineral (d) and a bioresorbable barrier were positioned (e) and the flap closed with multiple sutures (f). Normal probing depth at 1 year (g). Clinical and radiographic images at the 8-year follow-up visit (h, i)

described for MPPT, followed by a periosteal incision and vertical releasing incisions, when necessary to increase flap mobility. Defect debridement, regenerative materials placement, and flap primary closure with sutures follow the same rules as described above.

- *The entire papilla preservation technique (EPP)*

    Recently, a novel technique, the Entire Papilla Preservation Technique (EPP) has been proposed for the treatment of isolated intrabony defects [76, 77]. The "EPP" is a tunnel-like approach of the defect-associated interdental papilla performed from the buccal aspect. Following a buccal intra-crevicular incision, a beveled vertical releasing incision is performed in the buccal gingiva of the neighboring interdental space and extended just beyond the mucogingival line to provide appropriate mechanical access to the intrabony defect. A microsurgical periosteal elevator is used to elevate a buccal full-thickness mucoperiosteal flap extending from the vertical incision to the defect-associated papilla. A specifically designed angled tunnel elevator facilitates the interdental tunnel preparation under the papillary tissue. The interdental papilla is gently elevated in full-thickness manner up to the intact palatal/lingual bone crest. Granulation tissue is removed from the inner aspect of the defect-associated interdental papilla with micro-scissors or microblade. Excessive thinning of the papilla must be avoided in order not to compromise the blood supply. The defect and root surface are debrided and planed. Regenerative materials like EMD and/or bone substitutes can be placed into the intrabony defect. A collagen barrier can be utilized to contain the biomaterial. Internal mattress and interrupted sutures are applied for optimal wound closure. The application of EPP is indicated in isolated interproximal intrabony defects. The ample involvement of the palatal side of a tooth makes this approach not applicable. It is a matter of fact that a two-wall intrabony with a missing buccal bony wall and a relatively well-preserved lingual wall is the best indication for EPP. This approach is greatly facilitated by the use of an operative microscope that is positioned to face the buccal aspect and kept stable for most of the procedure.

4.3.2 Key-Hole Furcation Defects

Key-hole class II furcations in the lower molars and at the buccal aspect of the upper molars can be predictably regenerated when some morphologic conditions are satisfied (Fig. 25a–j). Absence of gingival recession, thick gingival phenotype, preservation of the interproximal bone peaks coronal to the furcation roof, minimal vertical bone destruction around each root, and divergency angle of the roots allowing for furcation area debridement are main elements. Flap design for the "key hole" was described more than 30 years ago [41, 42]. The mucogingival condition indicates the design of the buccal or lingual flap. If the gingiva is not retracted and the furcation entrance is fully covered, a full-thickness envelope-like flap will be preferred; in the presence of a gingival recession that uncovers in part or completely the furcation entrance, a periosteal fenestration will be planned to coronally advance the flap; the preferred design will be envelope-like: a vertical releasing incision can be added only when necessary to increase flap mobility. Following intrasulcular incisions, the flap is

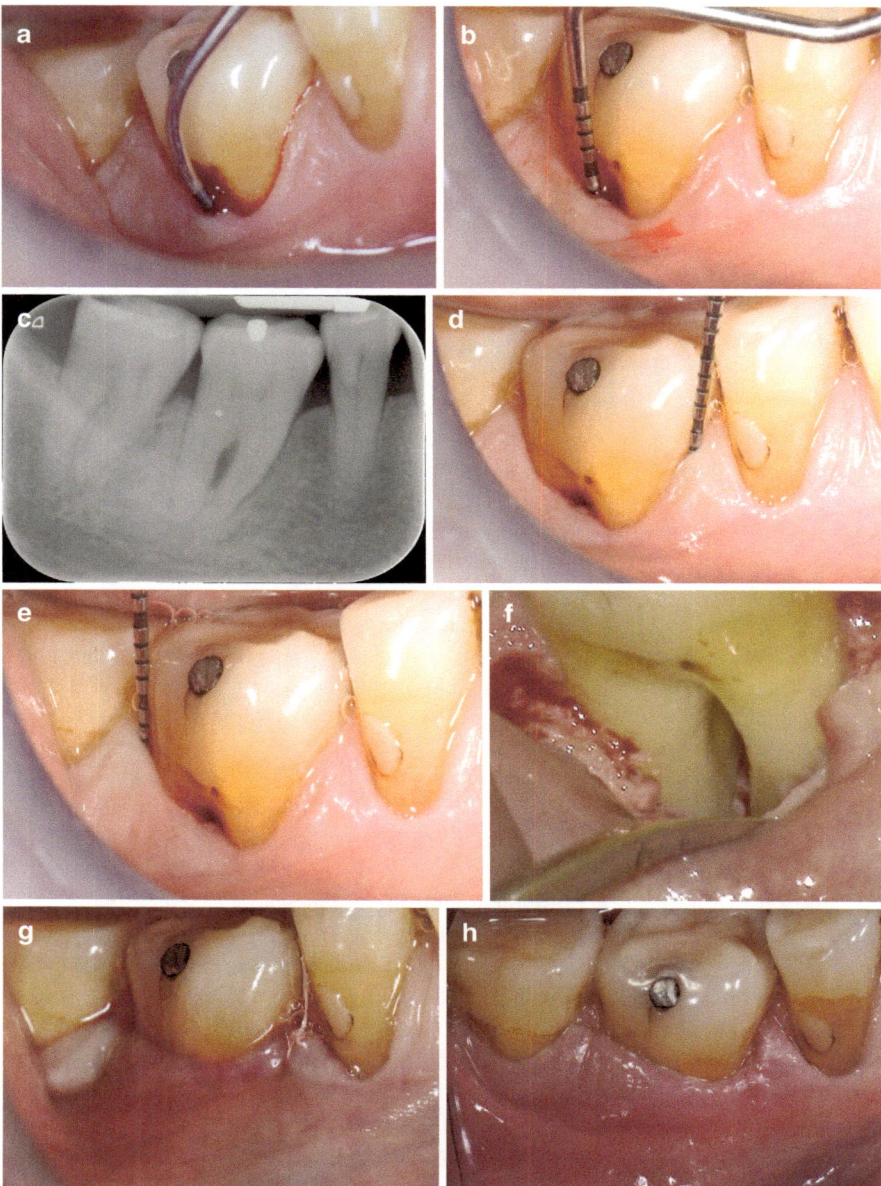

Fig. 25 (**a–j**) Lower right first molar presenting with a deep Class II buccal furcation involvement associated with a 10 mm vertical CAL (**a, b**). The interproximal bone peaks (**c**) and the interproximal attachment levels (**d, e**) are coronal to the furcation roof. The defect was accessed with a buccal envelope flap and carefully debrided (**f**). After application of amelogenins, the furcation area was filled with deproteinized bovine bone mineral. The flap was coronally advanced with a sling suture (**g**). Suture removal at 1 week (**h**). Clinical and radiographic images showing the resolution of the furcation involvement at 1 year (**i, j**)

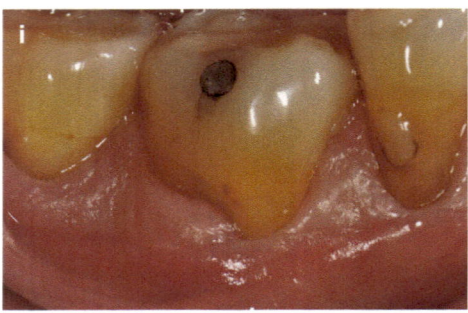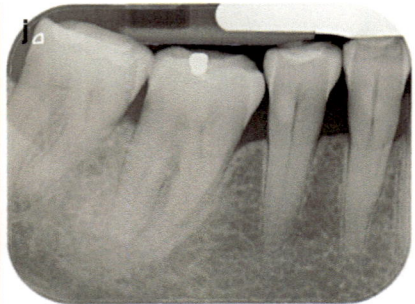

Fig. 25 (continued)

extended mesio-distally to involve the two neighboring interproximal spaces. A full-thickness flap is raised to expose the residual bone crest and give access to the furcation area for debridement. The granulation tissue is carefully removed to expose the root surfaces and the alveolar bone. The root surfaces are carefully scaled and planed using hand and power-driven instruments and rotating, flame-shaped diamond burs. It is also suggested to use diamond-coated tips on air-driven instruments. Special care should be devoted to clear the roof of the furcation, often characterized by the presence of furrows, cemento-enamel projections, enamel pearls, or other irregularities retaining biofilm and calculus. The application of diamond coated instruments aims at the elimination of these plaque-retaining irregularities creating a smooth, regular surface of the furcation roof. The use of micromirrors and high magnification is of great value to guide this meticulous approach and to check for its successful completion.

The regenerative material of choice (a bioresorbable barrier, a bone graft, a biologically active agent, or a combination approach) is positioned at the furcation area. A recent systematic review concluded that best outcomes in terms of horizontal clinical attachment level gain is expected using bone replacement grafts (BRG), followed by a combination of bioresorbable membrane and BRG and, finally, application of amelogenins [78]. Highest ranking of vertical attachment level gain is expected when using either BRG or a combination of bioresorbable membrane and BRG. When a barrier is used, it is adjusted to cover the entrance (buccal or lingual) of the furcation area, the adjacent root surfaces (from the disto-buccal/lingual line angle of the distal root to the mesio-buccal/lingual line angle of the mesial root), and a 3- to 5-mm-wide surface of the alveolar bone apical to the bone crest. The membrane can be retained in position by sutures placed around the crown of the molar using a sling technique. When a graft is preferred, it is positioned to completely fill the furcation area and slightly overfill the entrance. Biologically active agents are delivered into the furcation area. A combination approach requires the positioning of different biomaterials according to the properties of each material.

Following placement of the regenerative material, the mucoperiosteal flap is repositioned to completely cover the furcation and the biomaterials. When a periosteal incision is made, the flap is coronally advanced. The flap is preferably secured with sling sutures. Additional interdental sutures can be applied. An example of this surgical approach is shown in Video 3 (Fig. 26a–g).

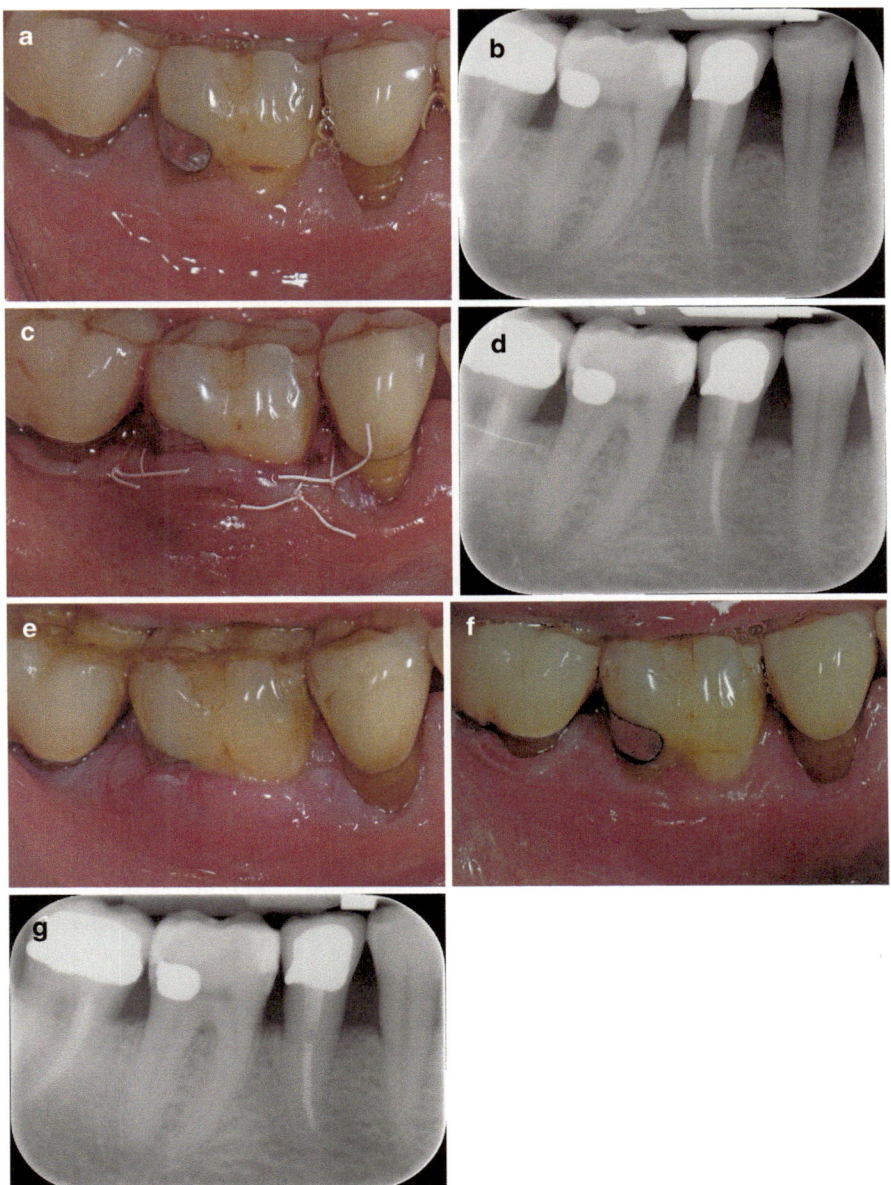

Fig. 26 (a–g) Lower right first molar presenting with a deep Class II buccal furcation involvement (a, b). The interproximal bone peaks are at the level of the furcation roof. The defect was accessed with a buccal envelope flap and carefully debrided; a bioresorbable barrier was positioned and stabilized with a sling ligature and the furcation area filled with deproteinized bovine bone mineral (Video 3). The flap was coronally advanced with a sling suture (c). Postsurgical radiograph (d). Suture removal at 1 week (e). Clinical and radiographic images showing the resolution of the furcation involvement at the 2-year re-evaluation (f, g)

4.3.3 Combined Intrabony and Furcation Defects

Compromised molars are frequently characterized by a pattern of periodontal break-down that involves both apical and interradicular spread of attachment and bone loss. The morphology of bone destruction can result in a combination of horizontal breakdown in the furcation area and vertical breakdown around the single roots. The peculiar anatomy of a combined furcation and intrabony defect requires a surgical approach different with respect to the traditional buccal or lingual flap for a key-hole defect. Cortellini et al. proposed the application of papilla preservation flaps (PPF) [79]. The design of PPF is selected upon the width of the interdental space. A horizontal incision according to the principles of the modified papilla preservation technique (MPPT [34]) is traced at the buccal aspect of the defect associated papilla when the width of the interdental space is ≥2mm, while a diagonal incision is applied when the interdental space is <2 mm (simplified papilla preservation flap, SPPF [39]). Flaps are designed to obtain adequate access to the defect limiting as much as possible flap extension and thus preserving optimal wound stability accord-ing to the concepts of minimally invasive surgery, as previously described for intrabony defects [5]. The choice of how far to extend the flap in a mesio-distal and bucco-lingual direction is dependent upon the morphology of the combined defect. Whenever possible, only the full-thickness buccal flap is elevated (M-MIST [38]) and the defect/furcation debrided through the buccal window (Fig. 27a–f). When the defect extends toward the oral aspect of the tooth, the preserved papilla is ele-vated along with the full-thickness lingual flap (MIST [37]). An example of this surgical approach is shown in Video 4 (Fig. 28a–g). The full-thickness flaps are elevated to expose the crest of bone surrounding the intrabony defect and to gain access to the involved inter-radicular space. Vertical releasing incisions are traced only when needed to gain access. Defects and furcation area are thoroughly debrided with a combination of micro-curettes and fine sonic tips. In the presence of furrows, the roof of the furcation is further instrumented with the aid of diamond tips mounted on a sonic device. Cleanliness of the furcation roof is carefully inspected at 30× magnification with the aid of micromirrors. The regenerative material and the suture strategy follow the same rules described above for regeneration of intrabony defects and furcations.

5   Errors Most Frequently Committed/Actions to Avoid

Do not apply regeneration when:

- Patient is burdened by high levels of residual plaque >25%
- Periodontal disease is not under control (i.e. FMBS >25%)
- Patient is heavy smoker (>20 cigarettes/day)
- In the presence of uncontrolled diabetes and/or high level of stress
- If the endodontic condition is not under control
- In the presence of high mobility impossible to control
- When periodontal tissues associated with the defect are inflamed
- When patient does not grant high levels of compliance with all the procedure

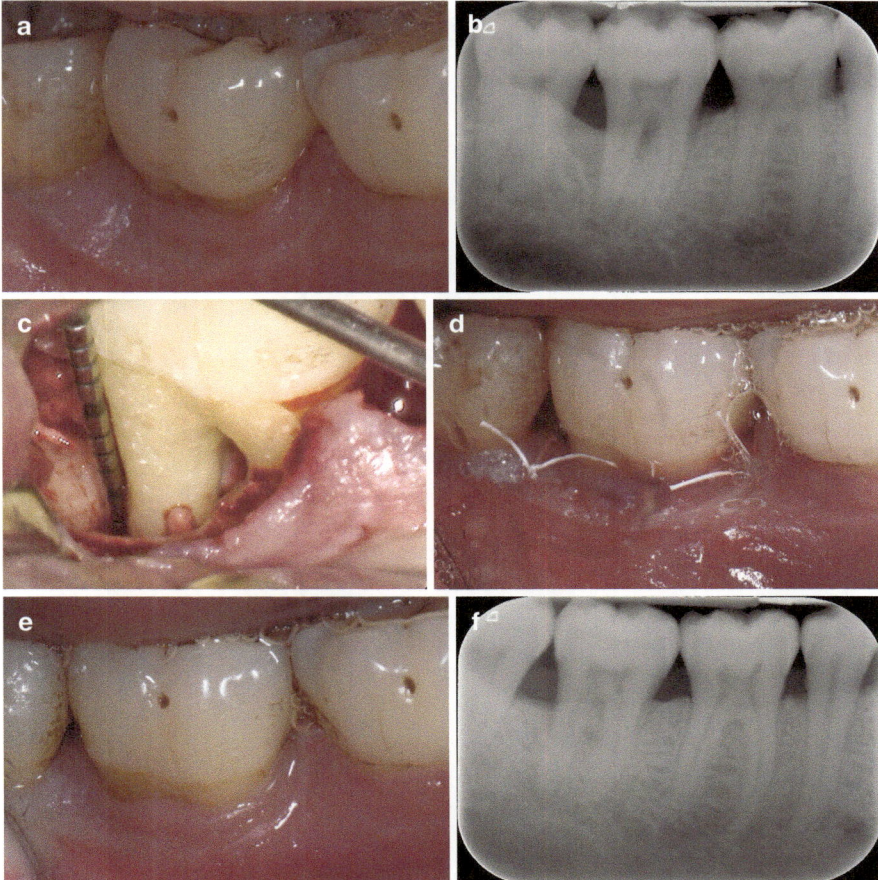

Fig. 27 (**a–f**) Lower right second molar presenting with a deep Class II buccal furcation involvement associated with a deep intrabony defect involving the distal root (**a, b**). The papilla between first and second molar was preserved according to the MIST approach and the buccal flap extended to the papilla between the first molar and the second premolar. The defect and the furcation were carefully debrided (**c**). After placement of amelogenins, the flap was closed with modified internal mattress sutures (**d**). Clinical and radiographic images showing the resolution of intrabony defect and of the furcation involvement at the 5-year re-evaluation (**e, f**)

When applying regeneration:

- Do not inject high dosages of anesthetic at the gingival margin and papilla
- Do not apply horizontal interproximal incision when the papilla is <2 mm
- Do not bevel the papillary incision
- Do not undermine the gingival margin and the KT with paramarginal incisions
- Use sharp instead of blunt dissection
- Do not instrument the supracrestal fibers coronal to the bone crest

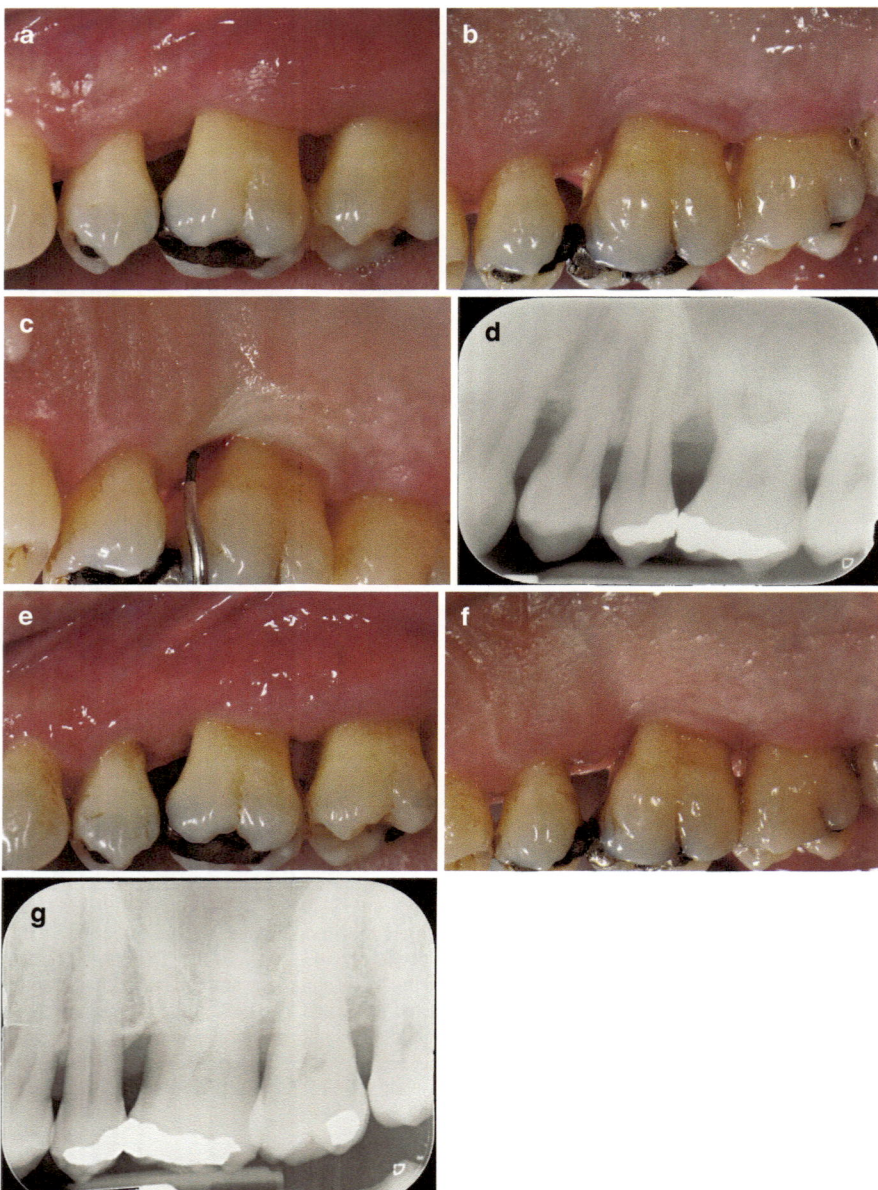

Fig. 28 (**a–f**) Upper left first molar presenting with a deep Class II mesial furcation involvement associated with an intrabony defect involving the mesial root (**a–d**). The interproximal bone peak distal to the second premolar is coronal to the furcation roof. The papilla between the molar and the premolar was approached with a buccal horizontal incision (MPPT), the defect accessed with a small palatal flap (MIST) and carefully debrided; a combination of amelogenins and deproteinized bovine bone mineral was positioned to fill the intrabony component and the furcation defect (Video 4). The flap was closed with a modified internal mattress suture. Clinical and radiographic images showing the resolution of intrabony defect and of the furcation involvement at 1 year (**e–g**)

- Avoid saliva contamination of the regenerative biomaterials
- Apply the regenerative biomaterials in a clean environment
- Do not overfill the defect when applying bone-like particles
- If you overfill, release the buccal flap
- Do not try to close the wound applying over-tension with the sutures
- Ensure that at the end of suturing, the wound is closed primary intension

---

6   Postsurgical Protocols and Complications

Postsurgical and early home care protocols are directly derived from the experiences developed in several controlled clinical trials [49].

After completion of surgery, patients are generally recalled after 1, 3, and 5 weeks for suture removal and control of the surgical site. This sequence can be modified according to needs. For example, when nonresorbable barriers are used, they must be removed after 5–6 weeks, and subsequently, the patients are further recalled for suture removal and control.

1. End of surgery. After primary closure of the wound patient is dismissed with prescriptions and indications:
   a. An empirical protocol for the control of bacterial contamination consisting of systemic antibiotics, when deemed necessary especially associated with the implantation of biomaterials, and 0.12% chlorhexidine mouth rinsing three times per day. Chlorhexidine is continued for some weeks, until the patient can resume full oral hygiene.
   b. An analgesic, preferably ibuprofen 600 mg at the end or immediately before surgery. A second compulsory dose is administered after 8 h. More tablets, according to patient needs. Acetaminophen or other analgesics can be prescribed to patients who cannot take non-steroidal anti-inflammatory drugs (NSAIDS).
   c. The following recommendations are given to the patients: refrain from mechanical brushing of the treated area; soft food intake avoiding the surgical site; steer clear of any action that involves pressure or trauma in the oral cavity (i.e., playing a trumpet); refrain from straining physical exercise for 1 week.
2. *Control at 1 week.* Sutures are removed after 1–2 weeks. Suture removal has to be done carefully to reduce the risk of damages to the delicate healing wound. The wound has to be carefully controlled to ascertain the primary closure or the presence of complications. Main possible complications include: redness or edema of the marginal soft tissues, wound failure and its severity, retraction of the gingival margin, regenerative material exposure, purulence. The regenerated area has to be carefully and gently debrided to remove soft deposits without any interference with the soft tissues. Curettes, dental floss, and slow-speed rubber cups are normally used. A full-mouth prophylaxis to decrease the overall bacterial load is also suggested. Patients are instructed to use a postsurgical soft toothbrush soaked in chlorhexidine to gently wipe the treated site. No interdental cleaning is allowed as well as any masticatory function in the treated area.

Complications. The presence of redness or edema is a minor issue if the primary closure is maintained. In the presence of a flap failure, especially when biomaterials are exposed, it is suggested to carefully clean the site with some tissue/cotton pellet and chlorhexidine. Exposed granules of biomaterial should be removed. Presence of pus indicates a relevant infection in the area possibly due to either an endodontic problem or a severe contamination of the implanted biomaterial. If the problem is endodontic, endo-treatment is indicated; if it is dependent upon severe contamination of biomaterials, their early removal might be necessary. The presence of complications indicates the need for an additional control after 1 week.

3. *Control after 3 weeks*. Some of the actions of week 1 are repeated: the regenerated area is carefully and gently debrided to remove soft deposits without any interference with the soft tissues. Curettes, dental floss, and slow-speed rubber cups are normally used. A full-mouth prophylaxis to decrease the overall bacterial load is also suggested. Patients are requested to continue chlorhexidine and avoid traumatisms to the regenerated area. The persistence of complications suggests a more careful behavior of the patient and more control visits.
4. *Control after 5 weeks*. The actions of week 1 are repeated, including debridement of the regenerated area and full-mouth prophylaxis. At this stage, the patient is instructed to resume full oral hygiene with a regular toothbrush, including interdental cleaning. Chlorhexidine is discontinued, and all masticatory restrictions are lifted.
5. Nonresorbable membranes are conventionally removed after 5–6 weeks. Patients can resume full oral hygiene and masticatory function in the treated area 2–4 weeks after membrane removal or when bioresorbable membranes are fully resorbed.
6. At the end of the "early healing phase," patients are enrolled in a 3-month supportive periodontal care regimen. General suggestion to avoid any invasive clinical action, like hard subgingival instrumentation, restorative dentistry, orthodontics, and additional surgery, for a period of about 9 months is also part of a strategy that is aimed at optimizing the clinical outcomes of periodontal regeneration.

It is evident that the most frequent postsurgical complication is the early flap failure. This has a negative impact on the clinical outcomes. It is therefore very important to select a regenerative strategy that is minimally burdened by such a negative event. In particular, the adoption of papilla preservation flaps or minimally invasive surgical procedures has by far reduced the probability for early flap failure (Table 3).

7 Surgical and Postsurgical Patient Morbidity

Few studies reported on intrasurgical and postsurgical patient outcomes.

As related to the *surgical phase*, few patients reported mild perception of intraoperative pain and described the intervention as "demanding" in two multicenter

Table 3 Primary closure of the wound during the first 6 weeks of healing

Type of flap	Surgical approach	Primary closure (6 weeks) (%)
Access flap [80, 81]	Macrosurgery	0
MPPT [34]	Macrosurgery	73
SPPF [35]	Macrosurgery	67
MPPT–SPPF [82]	Microsurgery	92.3
MIST [37]	Microsurgery	95
M-MIST [38]	Microsurgery	97.8

Data from different regenerative flap approaches
Access flap design without papilla preservation, *MPPT* modified papilla preservation technique, *SPPF* simplified papilla preservation flap, *MIST* minimally invasive surgical technique, *M-MIST* modified minimally invasive surgical technique

Table 4 Data from three clinical studies are reported

Type of flap	SPPF/MPPT + EMD	MIST + EMD	M-MIST + EMD
Surgical chair time (min)	80 ± 34	58 ± 11	54.2 ± 7.4
Postoperative discomfort (%)	47.5	17.5	13.3
Postoperative pain (%)	50	30	0
Pain intensity (VAS)	28 ± 20	19 ± 10	0
No. of pain killers intake	4.3 ± 4.5	1.1 ± 2	–
	Tonetti et al. [90]	Cortellini et al. [37]	Cortellini and Tonetti [86]

Patients have been treated with three different regenerative surgical approaches but with the same regenerative material (amelogenins). Pain intensity has been evaluated with a visual analogic scale (VAS) from 0 to 100
EMD amelogenins, *MPPT/SPPF* modified/simplified papilla preservation flap, *MIST* minimally invasive surgical technique, *M-MIST* modified minimally invasive surgical technique

RCTs. The surgical approaches were large papilla preservation flaps associated with bioresorbable barriers [82] and amelogenins [83]. The *intraoperative* discomfort and pain perception reportedly are extremely low in patients treated with minimally invasive surgery, in particular when treated with M-MIST [37, 38, 84]. The reduced morbidity can be explained, at least in part, with the reduced flap extension and chair time of minimally invasive approaches as compared with large papilla preservation flaps (Table 4). Obviously, the rigorous application of the operative field preparation, proper planning of the surgical intervention, proper anesthesia, and application of the surgical steps make it possible to reduce the intraoperative patient morbidity.

In the *postoperative phase*, discomfort and pain are the most relevant issues. The impact of different surgical approaches can be observed in Table 4 reporting patient outcomes collected in three studies in which defects were treated with amelogenins but with three different surgical approaches: large papilla preservation flaps [85], MIST [37], and M-MIST [86]. Postoperative discomfort is by far reduced in minimally invasive surgery as well as postoperative pain, in particular in patients treated with M-MIST. Reduced postoperative pain is associated with reduced need for pain killer intake.

8 Long-Term Outcomes of Regeneration

The outcomes obtained with periodontal regeneration (attachment and bone gain) can be maintained over an extended period of time, as demonstrated by several long-term studies [87–95]. Long-term stability is influenced by some key factors, such as: (1) participation into a supportive periodontal care program; (2) high quality of oral hygiene; (3) low level of bacterial recolonization of the treatment site; (4) no cigarette smoking.

The cited studies demonstrate that failing to follow the above-mentioned criteria increases the probability for disease recurrence, attachment loss, and finally tooth loss. The Cortellini and Tonetti study [90] evaluated the long-term tooth survival in a population of 175 patients treated with periodontal regeneration. In this study tooth survival was 96%. The six teeth that were lost were in the mouth of smokers not participating into a regular SPC. More recently, a 10-year RCT showed 88% survival of teeth treated with regeneration that at baseline were considered "hopeless," i.e., to be extracted and replaced [79] and a 20-year RTC demonstrated that patients under regular SPC, with good oral hygiene and nonsmokers can maintain the teeth treated with regeneration up to 20 years [89].

9 Summary

Microscope-assisted periodontal regenerative therapy is a true reality in the field of periodontal regeneration. Minimally invasive surgery is best applicable through the use of operating microscopes and microsurgical instruments and materials. Cohort studies and randomized controlled clinical trials have demonstrated the potential of minimally invasive surgery to greatly improve the periodontal conditions of sites associated with intrabony and furcation defects, proving its efficacy. The expected clinical improvements are associated with very limited patient morbidity during the surgical procedure, as well as in the postoperative period.

This advanced concept requires:

1. A well-organized setting of the private office in order to create a proper treatment flow for the patients
2. The adoption of stepwise decisional algorithms to select the proper clinical approach
3. The adoption of proper instruments and materials
4. The completion of an advanced training educational program

10 Key Points

1. Minimally invasive procedures have shown constant evolution since the introduction of this concept in medicine in the 1990. Microscope assisted periodontal regenerative therapy is a derivative of this paradigm shift.

2. Microscope assisted periodontal regenerative therapy has a track of well documented long term success when addressing intrabony and furcation defects or a combination of both.
3. Microscope assisted periodontal regenerative therapy is a biologically driven process that benefits from magnification and coaxial illumination to facilitate flap design and incision tracing, soft tissue manipulation, root surface preparation, biomaterial allocation, blood clot protection and approximation of wound margins.
4. Adherence to post-operative care protocols is a critical component for the success of microscope assisted periodontal regenerative therapy.
5. Pursuing advanced training, utilizing armamentarium designed for microsurgical therapy, following clinical decision algorithms to sort out the appropriate treatment execution and establishing operational workflows are the cornerstones of the concept behind microscope assisted periodontal regenerative therapy.

References

1. Glossary of Periodontal Terms. American Academy of Periodontology, Chicago, Ill. 2021. https://members.perio.org/libraries/glossary?ssopc=1. Accessed June 2022.
2. Mellonig JT. Periodontal regeneration: bone grafts. In: Nevins M, Mellonig JT, editors. Periodontal therapy clinical approaches and evidence of success. Chicago: Quintessence; 1998. p. 233–48.
3. Shanelec DA. Periodontal microsurgery. J Esthet Restor Dent. 2003;15:402–8.
4. Tibbetts LS, Shanelec D. Principles and practice of periodontal microsurgery. Int J Microdent. 2009;1:13–24.
5. Cortellini P. Minimally invasive surgical techniques in periodontal regeneration. J Evid Based Dent Pract. 2012;12:89–100.
6. Prichard J. Regeneration of bone following periodontal therapy; report of cases. Oral Surg Oral Med Oral Pathol. 1957;10:247–52.
7. Patur B, Glickman I. Clinical and roentgenographic evaluation of the post-treatment healing of infrabony pockets. J Periodontol. 1962;33:164–71.
8. Listgarten MA, Rosenberg MM. Histological study of repair following new attachment procedures in human periodontal lesions. J Periodontol. 1979;50:333–44.
9. Nabers CL, O'Leary TJ. Autogenous bone transplants in the treatment of osseous defects. J Periodontol. 1965;36:5–14.
10. Mann W. Autogenous transplant in the treatment of an Intrabony pocket. Periodontics. 1964;2:205–8.
11. Ellegaard B, Löe H. New attachment of periodontal tissues after treatment of Intrabony lesions. J Periodontol. 1971;42:648–52.
12. Schallhorn RG. Eradication of bifurcation defects utilizing frozen autogenous hip marrow implants. Periodontal Abstr. 1967;15:101–5.
13. Dragoo MR, Sullivan HC. A clinical and histological evaluation of autogenous iliac bone grafts in humans. II. External root resorption. J Periodontol. 1973;44:614–25.
14. Ellegaard B, Karring T, Listgarten M, Löe H. New attachment after treatment of interradicular lesions. J Periodontol. 1973;44:209–17.
15. Bowers GM, Chadroff B, Carnevale R, Mellonig J, Corio R, Emerson J, Stevens M, Romberg E. Histologic evaluation of new attachment apparatus formation in humans. Part III. J Periodontol. 1989;60:683–93.

16. Bowers GM, Chadroff B, Carnevale R, Mellonig J, Corio R, Emerson J, Stevens M, Romberg E. Histologic evaluation of new attachment apparatus formation in humans. Part I. J Periodontol. 1989;60:664–74.
17. Mellonig JT. Freeze-dried bone allografts in periodontal reconstructive surgery. Dent Clin N Am. 1991;35:505–20.
18. Emmings FG. Chemically modified osseous material for the restoration of bone defects. J Periodontol. 1974;45:385–90.
19. Nielsen IM, Ellegaard B, Karring T. Kielbone in new attachment attempts in Humans. J Periodontol. 1981;52:723–8.
20. Yukna RA. Syntehtic grafts and regeneration. In: Polson AM, editor. Periodontal regeneration: current status and directions. Chicago: Quintessence; 1994. p. 103–12.
21. Nyman S, Lindhe J, Karring T, Rylander H. New attachment following surgical treatment of human periodontal disease. J Clin Periodontol. 1982;9:290–6.
22. Heijl L. Periodontal regeneration with enamel matrix derivative in one human experimental defect. A case report. J Clin Periodontol. 1997;24(2):693–6.
23. Harrel SK, Wilson TG, Nunn ME. Prospective assessment of the use of enamel matrix proteins with minimally invasive surgery. J Periodontol. 2005;76:380–4.
24. Cortellini P, Tonetti MS. A minimally invasive surgical technique with an enamel matrix derivative in the regenerative treatment of intra-bony defects: a novel approach to limit morbidity. J Clin Periodontol. 2007;34:87–93.
25. Ribeiro FV, Casarin RC, Palma MA, Júnior FH, Sallum EA, Casati MZ. Clinical and patient-centered outcomes after minimally invasive non-surgical or surgical approaches for the treatment of intrabony defects: a randomized clinical trial. J Periodontol. 2011;82:1256–66.
26. Nevins M, Giannobile WV, McGuire MK, Kao RT, Mellonig JT, Hinrichs JE, et al. Platelet-derived growth factor stimulates bone fill and rate of attachment level gain: results of a large multicenter randomized controlled trial. J Periodontol. 2005;76:2205–15.
27. Kitamura M, Nakashima K, Kowashi Y, Fujii T, Shimauchi H, Sasano T, et al. Periodontal tissue regeneration using fibroblast growth factor-2: randomized controlled phase II clinical trial. PLoS One. 2008;2(3):e2611.
28. Fitzpatrick JM, Wickham JE. Minimally invasive surgery. Br J Surg. 1990;77:721–2.
29. Harrel SK, Rees TD. Granulation tissue removal in routine and minimally invasive procedures. Compend Contin Educ Dent. 1995;16:960.
30. Harrel SK. A minimally invasive approach for bone grafting. Int J Periodont Rest Dent. 1998;18:161–9.
31. Harrel SK. A minimally invasive surgical approach for periodontal regeneration: surgical technique and observations. J Periodontol. 1999;70:1547–57.
32. Harrel SK, Nunn M, Belling CM. Long-term results of a minimally invasive surgical approach for bone grafting. J Periodontol. 1999;70:1558–63.
33. Takei HH, Han TJ, Carranza FA Jr, Kenney EB, Lekovic V. Flap technique for periodontal bone implants. Papilla preservation technique. J Periodontol. 1985;56:204–10.
34. Cortellini P, Pini Prato G, Tonetti MS. The modified papilla preservation technique. A new surgical approach for interproximal regenerative procedures. J Periodontol. 1995;66:261–6.
35. Cortellini P, Pini Prato G, Tonetti MS. The simplified papilla preservation flap. A Novel surgical approach for the management of soft tissues in regenerative procedures. Int J Periodontics Restorative Dent. 1999;19:589–99.
36. Cortellini P, Tonetti MS. Microsurgical approach to periodontal regeneration. Initial evaluation in a case cohort. J Periodontol. 2001;72:559–69.
37. Cortellini P, Tonetti MS. A minimally invasive surgical technique (MIST) with enamel matrix derivate in the regenerative treatment of intrabony defects: a novel approach to limit morbidity. J Clin Periodontol. 2007;34:87–93.
38. Cortellini P, Tonetti MS. Improved wound stability with a modified minimally invasive surgically technique in the regenerative treatment of isolated interdental intrabony defects. J Clin Periodontol. 2009;36:157–63.

39. Harrel SK, Wilson TG Jr, Rivera-Hidalgo F. A videoscope for use in minimally invasive peri-odontal surgery. J Clin Periodontol. 2013;40:868–74.
40. Harrel SK, Nunn ME, Abraham CM, Rivera-Hidalgo F, Shulman JD, Tunnell JC. Videoscope assisted minimally invasive surgery (VMIS): 36-month results. J Periodontol. 2017;88:528–35.
41. Pontoriero R, Lindhe J, Nyman S, Karring T, Rosenberg E, Sanavi F. Guided tissue regenera-tion in degree II furcation-involved mandibular molars. A clinical study. J Clin Periodontol. 1988;15:247–54.
42. Martin M, Gantes B, Garrett S, Egelberg J. Treatment of periodontal furcation defects. (I). Review of the literature and description of a regenerative surgical technique. J Clin Periodontol. 1988;15:227–31.
43. Andersson B, Bratthall G, Kullendorff B, Gröndahl K, Rohlin M, Attström R. Treatment of furcation defects. Guided tissue regeneration versus coronally positioned flap in mandibular molars; a pilot study. J Clin Periodontol. 1994;21:211–6.
44. Jepsen S, Heinz B, Jepsen K, Arjomand M, Hoffmann T, Richter S, Reich E, Sculean A, Gonzales JR, Bödeker RH, Meyle J. A randomized clinical trial comparing enamel matrix derivative and membrane treatment of buccal Class II furcation involvement in mandibular molars. Part I: study design and results for primary outcomes. J Periodontol. 2004;75:1150–60.
45. Aslan S, Buduneli N, Cortellini P. Clinical outcomes of the entire papilla preservation tech-nique with and without biomaterials in the treatment of isolated intrabony defects: a random-ized controlled clinical trial. J Clin Periodontol. 2020;47:470–8.
46. Nibali L, Koidou VP, Nieri M, Barbato L, Pagliaro U, Cairo F. Regenerative surgery versus access flap for the treatment of intra-bony periodontal defects: a systematic review and meta-analysis. J Clin Periodontol. 2020;47(22):320–51.
47. Jepsen S, Gennai S, Hirschfeld J, Kalemaj Z, Buti J, Graziani F. Regenerative surgical treat-ment of furcation defects: a systematic review and Bayesian network meta-analysis of random-ized clinical trials. J Clin Periodontol. 2019;47(22):269–374.
48. Sanz M, Herrera D, Kebschull M, et al. Treatment of stage I–III periodontitis—the EFP S3 level clinical practice guideline. J Clin Periodontol. 2020;47:4–60.
49. Cortellini P, Tonetti M. Clinical concepts for regenerative therapy in intrabony defects. Periodontol. 2000;2015(68):282–307.
50. Cortellini P, Tonetti MS. Clinical performance of a regenerative strategy for intrabony defects: scientific evidence and clinical experience. J Periodontol. 2005;76:341–50.
51. Cortellini P, Bowers GM. Periodontal regeneration of intrabony defects: an evidence-cased treatment approach. Int J Periodont Rest Dent. 1995;15:128–45.
52. Cortellini P, Tonetti M. Evaluation of the effect of tooth vitality on regenerative outcomes in intrabony defects. J Clin Periodontol. 2001;28:672–9.
53. Cortellini P, Bissada NF. Mucogingival conditions in the natural dentition: narrative review, case definitions, and diagnostic considerations. J Periodontol. 2018;89(1):204–13.
54. Jepsen S, Caton JG, Albandar JM, Bissada NF, Bouchard P, Cortellini P, Demirel K, de Sanctis M, Ercoli C, Fan J, Geurs NC, Hughes FJ, Jin L, Kantarci A, Lalla E, Madianos PN, Matthews D, McGuire MK, Mills MP, Preshaw PM, Reynolds MA, Sculean A, Susin C, West NX, Yamazaki K. Periodontal manifestations of systemic diseases and developmental and acquired conditions: Consensus report of workgroup 3 of the 2017 World Workshop on the Classification of Periodontal and Peri-Implant Diseases and Conditions. J Periodontol. 2018;89(1):237–48.
55. Papapanou PN, Tonetti MS. Diagnosis and epidemiology of periodontal osseous lesions. Periodontol. 2000;2000(22):8–21.
56. Haney JM, Nilveus RE, McMillan PJ, Wikesjo UME. Periodontal repair in dogs: expanded polytetrafluoroethylene barrier mem- brane support wound stabilisation and enhance bone regeneration. J Periodontol. 1993;64:883–90.
57. Sigurdsson TJ, Hardwick R, Bogle GC, Wikesjo UME. Periodontal repair in dogs: space pro-vision by reinforced ePTFE membranes enhances bone and cementum regeneration in large supraalveolar defects. J Periodontol. 1994;65:350–6.
58. Cortellini P, Pini-Prato G, Tonetti M. Periodontal regeneration of human infrabony defects with titanium reinforced membranes. A controlled clinical trial. J Periodontol. 1995;66:797–803.

59. Wikesjo UME, Lim WH, Thomson RC, Cook AD, Hardwick WR. Periodontal repair in dogs: gingival tissue occlusion, a critical requirement for guided tissue regeneration. J Clin Periodontol. 2003;30:655–64.
60. Kim CS, Choi SH, Chai JK, Cho KS, Moon IS, Wikesjo UME, Kim CK. Periodontal repair in surgically created intrabony defects in dogs. Influence of the number on bone walls on healing response. J Periodontol. 2004;75:229–35.
61. Linghorne WJ, O'Connel DC. Studies in the regeneration and reattachment of supporting structures of teeth. I. Soft tissue reattachment. J Dent Res. 1950;29:419–28.
62. Hiatt WH, Stallard RE, Butler ED, Badget B. Repair following mucoperiosteal flap surgery with full gingival retention. J Periodontol. 1968;39:11–6.
63. Wikesjo UME, Nilveus R. Perio- dontal repair in dogs: effect of wound stabilisation on healing. J Periodontol. 1990;61:719–24.
64. Selvig K, Kersten B, Wikesjö UME. Surgical treatment of intrabony periodontal defects using expanded polytetrafluoroethylene barrier membranes: influence of defect configuration on healing response. J Periodontol. 1993;64:730–3.
65. DeSanctis M, Clauser C, Zucchelli G. Bacterial colonization of barrier material and periodontal regeneration. J Clin Periodontol. 1996;23:1039–46.
66. Sanz M, Tonetti MS, Zabalegui I, Sicilia A, Blanco J, Rebelo H, Rasperini G, Merli M, Cortellini P, Suvan JE. Treatment of intrabony defects with enamel matrix proteins or barrier membranes: results from a multicenter practice-based clinical trial. J Periodontol. 2004;75:726–33.
67. Polimeni G, Xiropaidis VX, Wikesjo UME. Biology and principles of periodontal wound healing/regeneration. Periodontology. 2000;41:30–47.
68. Goldman H, Cohen W. The infrabony pocket: classification and treatment. J Periodontol. 1958;29:272–91.
69. Cortellini P, Tonetti M. Radiographic defect angle influences the outcome of GTR therapy in intrabony defects. J Dent Res. 1999;78:381.
70. Tsitoura E, Tucker R, Suvan J, Laurell L, Cortellini P, Tonetti M. Baseline radiographic defect angle of the intrabony defect as a prognostic indicator in regenerative periodontal surgery with enamel matrix derivative. J Clin Periodontol. 2004;31:643–7.
71. Linares A, Cortellini P, Lang NP, Suvan J, Tonetti MS. and European Research Group on Periodontology (ErgoPerio). Guided tissue regeneration/deproteinized bovine bone mineral or papilla preservation flaps alone for treatment of intrabony defects. II: radiographic predictors and outcomes. J Clin Periodontol. 2006;33:351–8.
72. Cortellini P, Tonetti MS. Minimally invasive surgical technique (M.I.S.T.) and enamel matrix derivative (EMD) in intrabony defects. (I) clinical outcomes and intra-operative and postoperative morbidity. J Clin Periodontol. 2007;34:1082–8.
73. Trejo PM, Weltman RL. Favourable periodontal regenerative outcomes from teeth with presurgical mobility: a retrospective study. J Clin Periodontol. 2004;75:1532–8.
74. Murphy KG. Interproximal tissue maintenance in GTR procedures: description of a surgical technique and 1-year reentry results. Int J Periodont Rest Dent. 1996;16:463–77.
75. Trombeli L, Farina R, Franceschetti G, Calura G. Single-flap approach with buccal access in periodontal reconstructive procedures. J Periodontol. 2009;80:353–60.
76. Aslan S, Buduneli N, Cortellini P. Entire papilla preservation technique: a novel surgical approach for regenerative treatment of deep and wide intrabony defects. Int J Periodontics Restorative Dent. 2017;37:227–33.
77. Aslan S, Buduneli N, Cortellini P. Entire papilla preservation technique in the regenerative treatment of deep intrabony defects: 1-year results. J Clin Periodontol. 2017;44:926–32.
78. Jepsen S, Gennai S, Hirschfeld J, Kalemaj Z, Buti J, Graziani F. Regenerative surgical treatment of furcation defects: a systematic review and Bayesian network meta-analysis of randomized clinical trials. J Clin Periodontol. 2020;47(22):352–74.
79. Cortellini P, Cortellini S, Tonetti MS. Papilla preservation flaps for periodontal regeneration of molars severely compromised by combined furcation and intrabony defects: retrospective analysis of a registry-based cohort. J Periodontol. 2020;91:165–73.

80. Cortellini P, Pini-Prato G, Tonetti M. Periodontal regeneration of human infrabony defects. I. Clinical measures. J Periodontol. 1993;64:254–60.
81. Cortellini P, Pini-Prato G, Tonetti M. Periodontal regeneration of human intrabony defects with bioresorbable membranes. A controlled clinical trial. J Periodontol. 1996;67:217–23.
82. Cortellini P, Tonetti MS, Lang NP, Suvan JE, Zucchelli G, Vangsted T, Silvestri M, Rossi R, McClain P, Fonzar A, Dubravec D, Adriaens P. The simplified papilla preservation flap in the regenerative treatment of deep intrabony defects: clinical outcomes and postoperative morbidity. J Periodontol. 2001;72:1701–12.
83. Tonetti MS, Lang NP, Suvan JE, Adriaens P, Dubravec D, Fonzar A, Fourmousis I, Mayfield L, Rossi R, Silvestri M, Tiedemann C, Topoll H, Vangsted T, Wallkamm B. Enamel matrix proteins in the regenerative therapy of deep intrabony defects. A multicenter randomized controlled clinical trial. J Clin Periodontol. 2002;29:317–25.
84. Cortellini P, Nieri M, Pini Prato GP, Tonetti MS. Single minimally invasive surgical technique (MIST) with enamel matrix derivative (EMD) to treat multiple adjacent intrabony defects. Clinical outcomes and patient morbidity. J Clin Periodontol. 2008;35:605–13.
85. Tonetti MS, Cortellini P, Lang NP, Suvan JE, Adriaens P, Dubravec D, Fonzar A, Fourmousis I, Rasperini G, Rossi R, Silvestri M, Topoll H, Wallkamm B, Zybutz M. Clinical outcomes following treatment of human intrabony defects with GTR/bone replacement material or access flap alone. A multicenter randomized controlled clinical trial. J Clin Periodontol. 2004;31:770–6.
86. Cortellini P, Tonetti MS. Clinical and radiographic outcomes of the modified minimally invasive surgical technique with and without regenerative materials: a randomized- controlled trial in intra-bony defects. J Clin Peridontol. 2011;38:365–73.
87. Cortellini P, Pini-Prato G, Tonetti M. Periodontal regeneration of human infrabony defects. V. Effect of oral hygiene on long term stability. J Clin Periodontol. 1994;21:606–10.
88. Cortellini P, Pini-Prato G, Tonetti M. Long term stability of clinical attachment following guided tissue regeneration and conventional therapy. J Clin Periodontol. 1996;23:106–11.
89. Cortellini P, Buti J, Pini Prato G, Tonetti MS. Periodontal regeneration compared with access flap surgery in human intra-bony defects 20-year follow-up of a randomized clinical trial: tooth retention, periodontitis recurrence and costs. J Clin Periodontol. 2017;44:58–66.
90. Cortellini P, Tonetti MS. Long-term tooth survival following regenerative treatment of intrabony defects. J Periodontol. 2004;75:672–8.
91. Sculean A, Kiss A, Miliauskaite A, Schwarz F, Arweiler NB, Hannig M. Ten-year results following treatment of intra-bony defects with enamel matrix proteins and guided tissue regeneration. J Clin Periodontol. 2008;35:817–24.
92. Nickles K, Ratka-Kruger P, Neukranz E, Raetzke P, Eickholz P. Open flap debridement and guided tissue regeneration after 10 years in infrabony defects. J Clin Periodontol. 2009;36:976–83.
93. Pretzl B, Kim TS, Steinbrenner H, Dorfer C, Himmer K, Eickholz P. Guided tissue regeneration with bioabsorbable barriers III 10-year results in infrabony defects. J Clin Periodontol. 2009;36:349–56.
94. Nygaard-Østby P, Bakke V, Nesdal O, Susin C, Wikesjö UME. Periodontal healing following reconstructive surgery: effect of guided tissue regeneration using a bioresorbable barrier device when combined with autogenous bone grafting. A randomized controlled trial 10-year follow-up. J Clin Periodontol. 2010;37:366–73.
95. Pini Prato G, Cortellini P. Thirty-year stability after regeneration of a deep intrabony defect: a case report. J Clin Periodontol. 2016;43:857–62.

Microscope-Assisted Preprosthetic Surgery

Kotaro Nakata

Contents

Abstract

In recent years, esthetic dentistry has continued to evolve with our patients' demands. In addition to the harmony of facial features and smiles, it has become possible to achieve extremely advanced esthetic results including improving soft tissue quality and quantity. For that reason, we need to have the option of surgical management of soft tissues applying periodontal plastic surgery (PPS) when performing prosthetic restoration. As a pretreatment for prosthetic restoration, a soft tissue with the required amount and morphology around the implant and natural teeth is constructed in harmony with the surrounding tissue. Diagnosis and pre-operative examinations are very important before the treatments. Clinical parameters include the periodontal phenotype, the amount of keratinized gingiva, position of gingival margin, the height of interdental papilla, etc. Applying PPS options to gain esthetics and long-term function after prosthetic restoration are often needed. The application of microsurgery is an effective method because

K. Nakata (✉)
Kyoto Prefectural University of Medicine, Kyoto, Japan
e-mail: info@nakata-dental.com

351

these PPS procedures requires extremely delicate and precise surgical procedures. This chapter presents practical clinical examples and verifies the advantages of microsurgery.

Keywords

Microsurgery · Preprosthetic surgery · Periodontal plastic surgery · Prosthodontics

1 Introduction

In this chapter, we will primarily discuss the effectiveness of using operating microscope (OM) for preprosthetic surgery (PPS) in the esthetic area. PPS is applied not only to natural teeth but also to teeth that have already or will undergo prosthetic restoration. In the 1980s, Schallhorn introduced mucogingival surgery as a preprosthetic procedure [1]. Recently, various periodontal plastic surgeries, which are more frequent and diverse, have been applied as preprosthetic treatment. These procedures help to establish adequate amount of sound tooth structure, supracrestal attachment tissues (SAT), keratinized mucosa, symmetrical gingival margin level, regeneration of papillae, etc. for oral health, comfort, function, and esthetics [2]. A multifaceted approach and close collaboration between periodontists and prosthodontists are required [3]. In recent years, new dental technology and materials have continued to evolve. We have entered an era in which not only the esthetics of restorations but also the esthetics of the surrounding tissue is required. Microsurgery allows for accurate and delicate tissue handling in these transitional areas such as gingival margins and papilla tissue, potentially resulting in improved wound healing and clinical outcomes. This chapter will demonstrate how microscope can be used in four main preprosthetic periodontal plastic procedures, including free gingival graft (FGG)/connective tissue graft (CTG), open/closed periodontal plastic surgery techniques ± CTG, crown lengthening, and papilla regeneration (Table 1).

2 Donor Site Evaluation and Harvesting Techniques for Free Gingival Graft (FGG)/Connective Tissue Graft (CTG)

A positive clinical outcome of FGG/CTG harvesting requires a thorough understanding of the anatomy of the donor site, tissue integration, and vascular

Table 1 The four primary procedures and indications related to preprosthetic surgery

Procedures	Indications
Free gingival graft (FGG)/connective tissue graft (CTG)	To increase keratinized mucosa width; may be used for root coverage
Open/closed periodontal plastic surgery techniques ± CTG	Root coverage, increase tissue thickness
Crown lengthening	To increase tooth structure; to level gingival margin; to create SAT space
Papilla regeneration	To regenerate interdental papilla

regeneration processes. Basically, the donor site can be from the hard palate or from the maxillary tuberosity. The maxillary tuberosity, compared to the hard palate, may be away from the branches of the greater palatine vessels, thus may be safer. Additionally, patients in general experienced less postoperative discomfort and complications [4, 5]. The tuberosity tissues are thicker and may maintain the volume better. However, Zuhr et al. [6] suggested that the connective tissue from the maxillary tuberosity is denser, and richer in collagen than the palatal tissue. Therefore, it may negatively affect wound healing and is more likely to cause necrosis. Even though postoperative absorption is low, it is necessary to pay attention to the blood supply to prevent necrosis during transplantation. The collection method is the same as the distal wedge method, that is to thin the tissue at the maxillary tuberosity. The incision design could be in triangular shape (Fig. 1) or rectangular shape (Fig. 2). If the second molar is present, it may not be a suitable donor site due to the lack of the mesial-distal length of the maxillary tuberosity. The presence of a third molar poses a challenge for collection. If the patient has small mouth opening and limited access, soft tissue collection at this location can be difficult.

Harvest from the palatal mucosa is in general a preferred choice as a donor site because it is suitable to almost all patients. The palatal mucosa has a connective tissue layer covered by keratinized epithelium, immediately below which is a submucosal layer of fat and glandular tissue between the palatine bone. The thickness of the palatal mucosa varies from patient to patient, but it

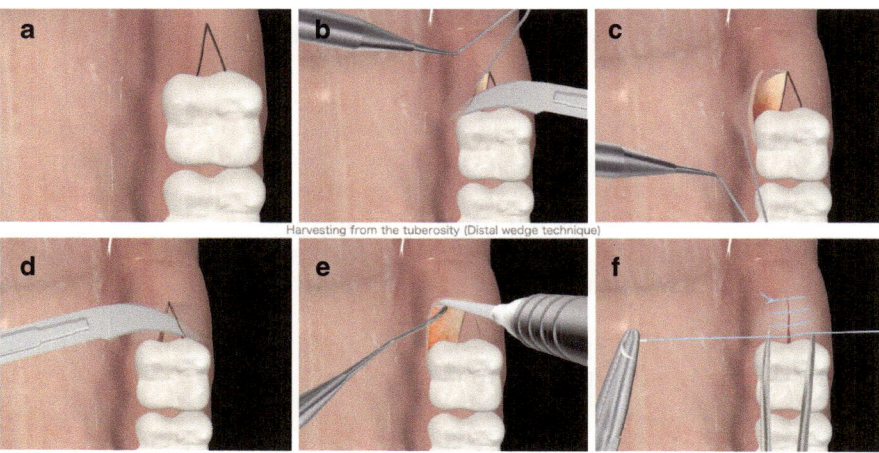

Fig. 1 Triangular-shaped incision for tissue harvest from the tuberosity. (**a**) Measure the gingival thickness in the tuberosity by bone sounding and mark the gingiva with the shape of a triangle. (**b**) Using a 12D scalpel from a triangle, remove the epithelium into a trapezoidal shape to expose connective tissue. (**c**) The state where the formation of the palatal mucosa is completed. (**d**) Subsequently, the buccal side is formed in the same manner. (**e**) Separate connective tissue from bone with an elevator. (**f**) After the graft has been collected, it is sutured, and the wound is closed. The epithelium remaining on the graft is removed by trimming

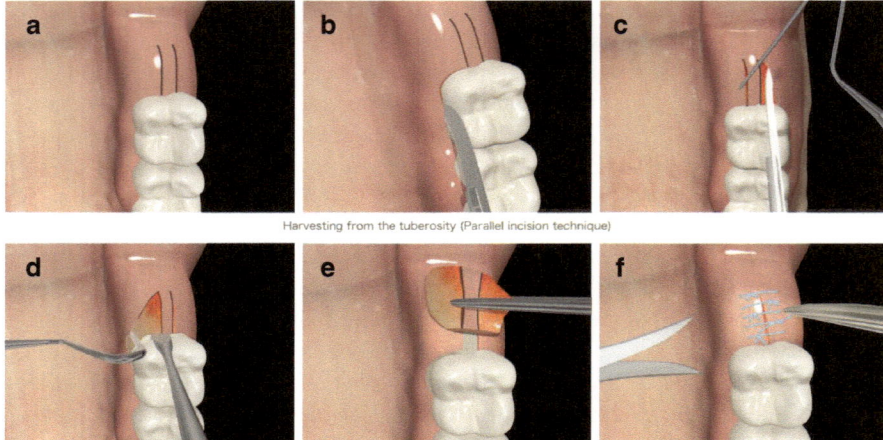

Fig. 2 Rectangular-shaped incision for tissue harvest from the tuberosity. (**a**) Mark the gingiva with two parallel incision lines (2–3 mm wide) that reach the alveolar mucosa. (**b**) Line the parallel incision line and widen the incision in the connecting 7th gingival sulcus. (**c**) Using a 12D scalpel, cut the subepithelial area into a trapezoidal shape from the parallel incision line to the palate and buccal side to form a connective tissue graft. (**d**) The graft is separated from the bone using a periosteal elevator. (**e**) The epithelial part of the collected graft is trimmed and transferred to the recipient site. (**f**) Close the wound using intermittent or simple continuous sutures

is desirable that the full thickness is 3 mm or more to be usable as a donor location. Location wise, the area from the 2nd premolar to 2nd molar might be suitable, in contrast to the 1st premolar site, where there is insufficient collagen tissue and thicker adipose and glandular tissues [7]. Various harvesting techniques have been developed over the past few decades. Edel [8] showed the trapdoor technique to collect CTG. This method is relatively easy to harvest CTG and is still used today, but it tends to cause partial necrosis on the epithelial side because the vertical incisions compromised the blood flow. Langer and Langer [9] presented a double-incision approach without a vertical incision. Hurzeler [10] proposed a single-incision technique that heals quickly and causes less discomfort and pain after surgery (Figs. 3 and 4). Another method is to first collect FGG, followed by de-epithelialization extra-orally. Table 2 summarized the advantages and disadvantages of the abovementioned techniques for harvesting soft tissues from the palate.

3 Root Coverage Procedures: Recipient Site Consideration and Preparation

Table 3 summarizes the two general surgical procedures, open and closed techniques for PPS in consideration for the recipient site preparation [11]. As a flap design for PPS, the method of performing tension reduction using a conventional envelope

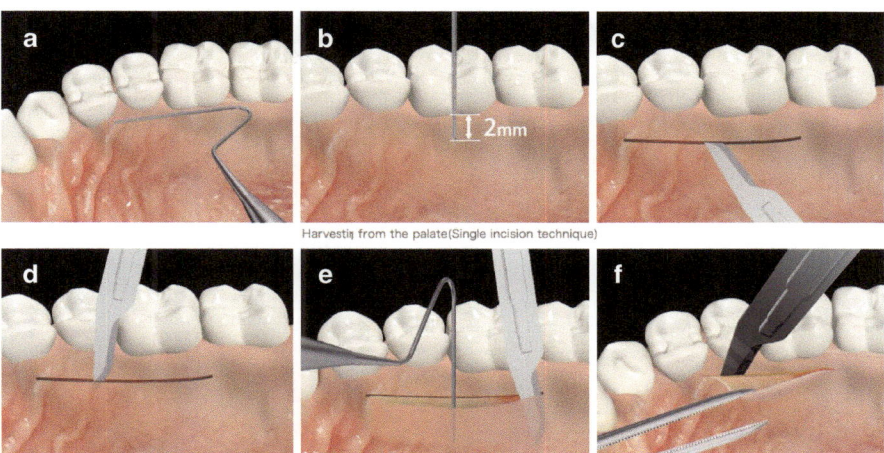

Fig. 3 Single incision technique for palatal tissue harvesting. The single incision technique is a typical technique for harvesting connective tissue from the palate. (**a**, **b**) Measurement with a probe, the initial incision is drawn approximately 2.0 mm apical to the gingival margin. (**c**) The incision line is drawn perpendicular to the palatal mucosa to the depth of 1–1.5 mm. (**d**) The incision might extend mesial to the first premolar and distal to the first molar in general, be cautious about the branches of the greater palatine artery. Then the scalpel is oriented parallel to the surface of the palatal tissue. (**e**) While visually recognizing the scalpel blade that is transparent from above the epithelium, a partial thickness incision is made to uniform depth at a depth of 0.5–1 mm from the epithelium. (**f**) The depth of the partial thickness incision should be calculated in respect to the length of the scalpel blade to reduce the risk injuring the artery

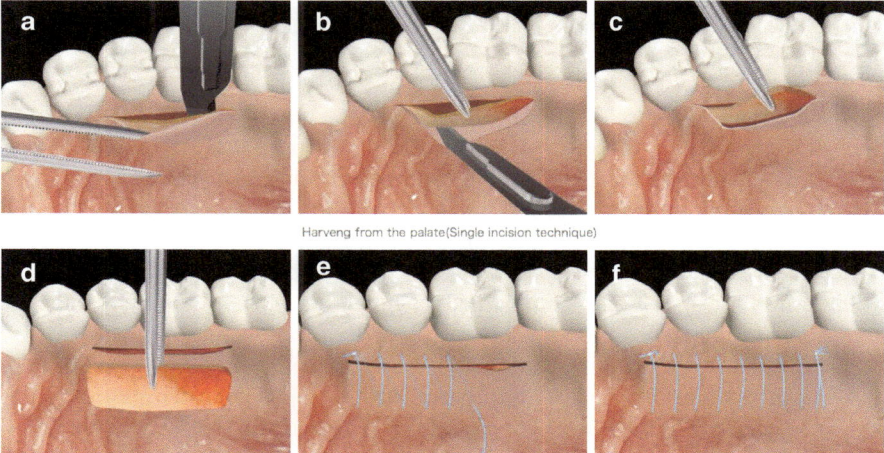

Fig. 4 Continuing from Fig. 3 for single incision to harvest palatal tissue. (**a**) Proceed with the periosteal incision at a deeper position parallel to the surface of the palatal mucosa while still leaving the periosteum on the bone. (**b**, **c**) Carefully separate the required amount of connective tissue to be harvested. (**d**, **e**, **f**) With compression hemostasis, a single incision is closed with a simple continuous suture using a 6-0 or 7-0 suture

Table 2 Advantages and disadvantages of the abovementioned techniques for harvesting soft tissues from the palate

Tissue harvesting methods	Advantages	Disadvantages
Trapdoor	Full access to the underlying CTG	Compromise healing due to vertical incisions Possible uneven graft thickness
Double incision	Include the epithelial layer	Limited access Possible uneven graft thickness
Single incision	Minimally invasive	Limited access Possible uneven graft thickness
De-epithelialization of FGG	Fast Better control of the graft thickness	2nd intension healing Extra step of de-epithelialization extra-orally Harder for bleeding control

Table 3 Two major techniques used based on recipient-site considerations

Open Technique (Trapezoidal flap, Triangular flap, etc.)	Closed Technique (Envelope Flap, tunneling flap,etc.)
Easier to perform	More difficult to prepare (blind technique)
Allows for direct visualization of dissection for uniform recipient site preparation	Immobilization of graft is more technique sensitive
Facilitates coronal advancement (>4mm)	Limits coronal advancement (≦4mm) Limited indication when the vestibular depth is minimal
Use of releasing incisions sacrifices circulation	Preserves circulation to area
May require secondary gingivoplasty	Allows for superior esthetics

incision with or without a vertical incision is called an open flap technique. The open flap technique is termed when the flap is advanced using intrasulcular/submarginal incisions to form a coronally advanced flap (CAF) (Fig. 5). This method is easier for access to the periosteum on the recipient bed, and for security of the tissue transplant. The modern treatment of root coverage procedure is based on the CAF named by Pini Prato [12] in 1999. Many modified techniques have been proposed with CAF alone or in combination with other procedures. There are methods in which CAF is used alone, in combination with some treatment (mainly transplantation), and in combination with biologics (Fig. 1). Examples of the open approach are the original Langer method [9], modified Langer method [13], and sling and tag method [14]. This technique is indicated when the flap needs to be extended greatly toward coronally, such as in cases where the exposed root surface or the implant abutment needs to be covered. When combining a CTG, it is beneficial that the flap covers the graft for ensuring adequate blood supply, and minimal compression to the underlying graft. However, the vertical incision is surgically invasive, blocks blood flow, and

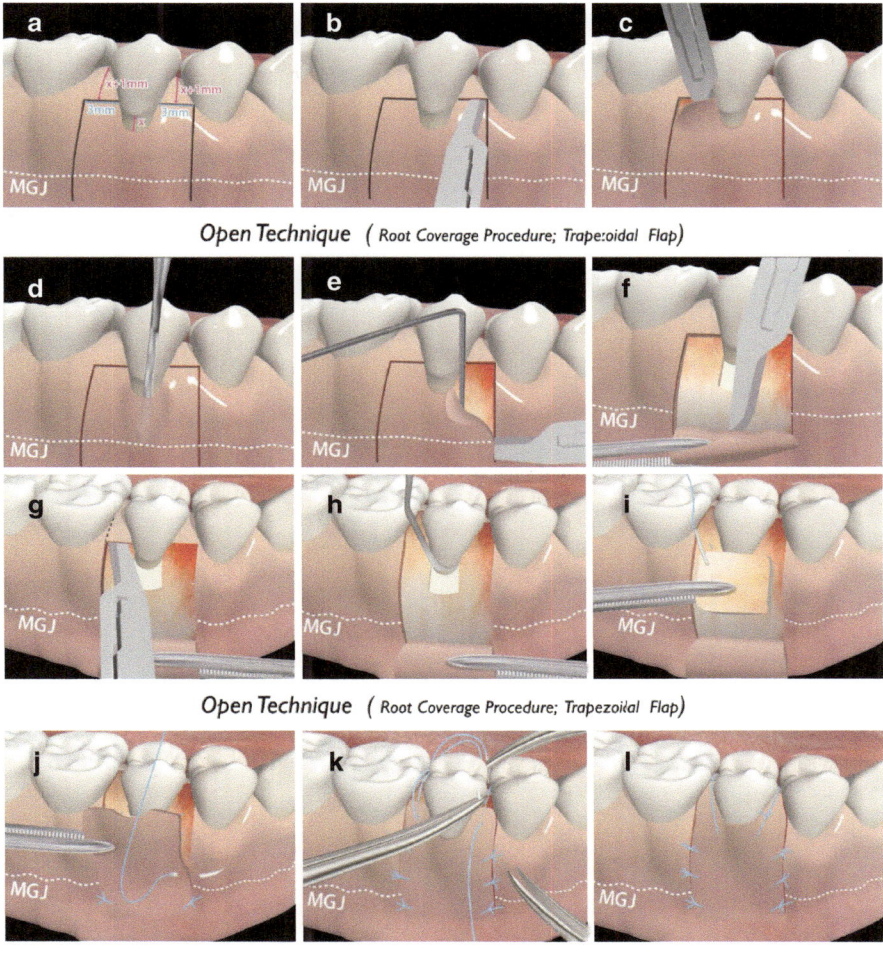

Fig. 5 Open technique for soft tissue augmentation. (**a**) The horizontal incision is located at $(x + 1)$ mm to the papilla tip; whereas x = the midfacial recession amount). (**b, c**) Full-thickness incision is made at the horizontal and vertical incisions. (**d**) Intrasulcular incision is made. (**e, f**) Full-thickness flap reflection and flap releasing beyond MGJ. (**g**) De-epithelialization of the papillae. (**h**) Mechanical root surface treatment when indicated. (**i**) Security of the CTG to the recipient bed. (**j–l**) Suturing of the flap with interrupted and slight sutures

takes longer time to heal. Furthermore, there is a risk of scarring after surgery, and there are drawbacks such as the need for secondary gingival surgery.

Alternatively, the closed technique without vertical releasing incisions can be applied (Fig. 6). Azzi et al. introduced a technique that has the advantage of covering the graft, referred to the so-called movable cover flap without incision lines as a "pouch & tunnel technique." It can be applied in root coverage, with stable graft underneath the flap [15–18]. Examples of the closed approach include the envelop

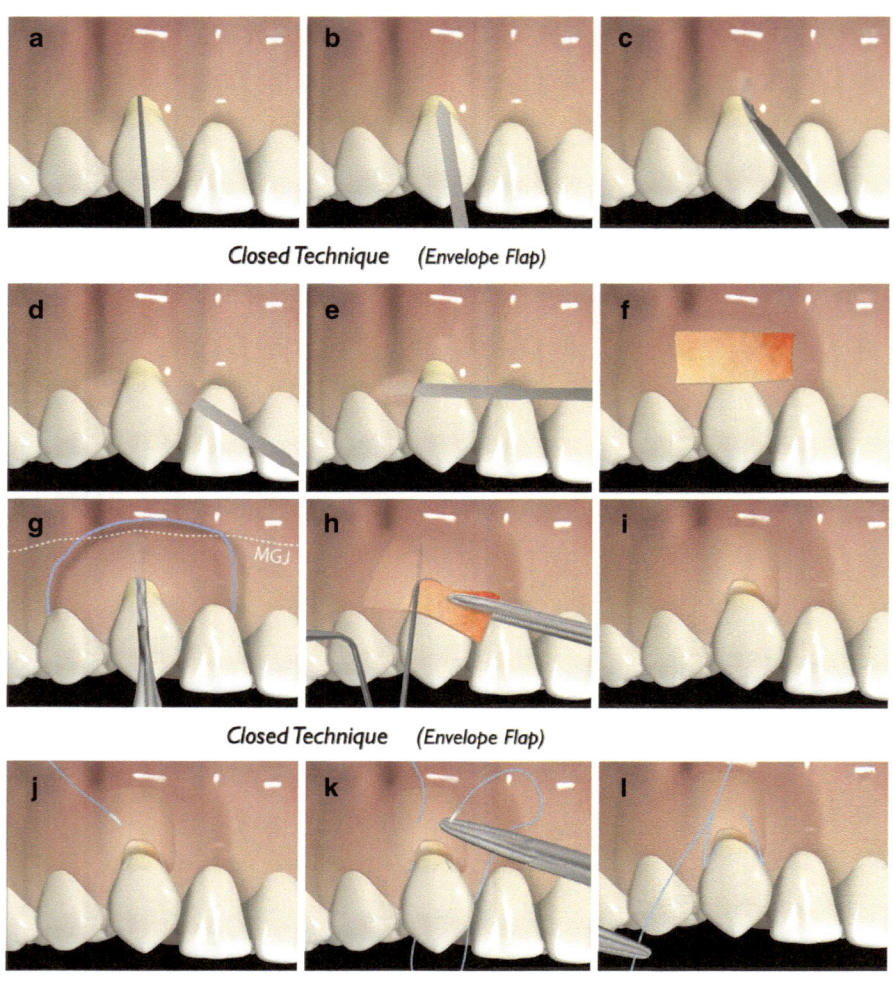

Fig. 6 Closed/envelope technique for soft tissue augmentation. (**a**) Measurement of the defect with a probe. (**b**) Intrasulcular incision with a microblade. (**c**) Flap releasing in a closed approach. (**d**, **e**) Papilla releasing. (**f**) CTG/tissue substitute harvest and placement. (**g**) The flap releasing extends to adjacent tooth and apical to MGJ. (**h**, **i**) Placement of the graft. (**j**–**l**) A sling suture is placed for securing the graft and flap

technique and tunneling technique. The closed technique that avoids a vertical incision facilitates blood flow to the surgical site and is likely to have more esthetic results [11]. Also called a "blind technique," it is generally considered more difficult to perform, but is less invasive with a shorter healing time. However, contrary to the open technique, it is difficult to reliably dissect the muscular tissue, and the amount of coronal advancement can be less.

Since the closed approach is technique sensitive and requires delicate handling, microsurgery has a distinct advantage. When approaching the gingival margin or

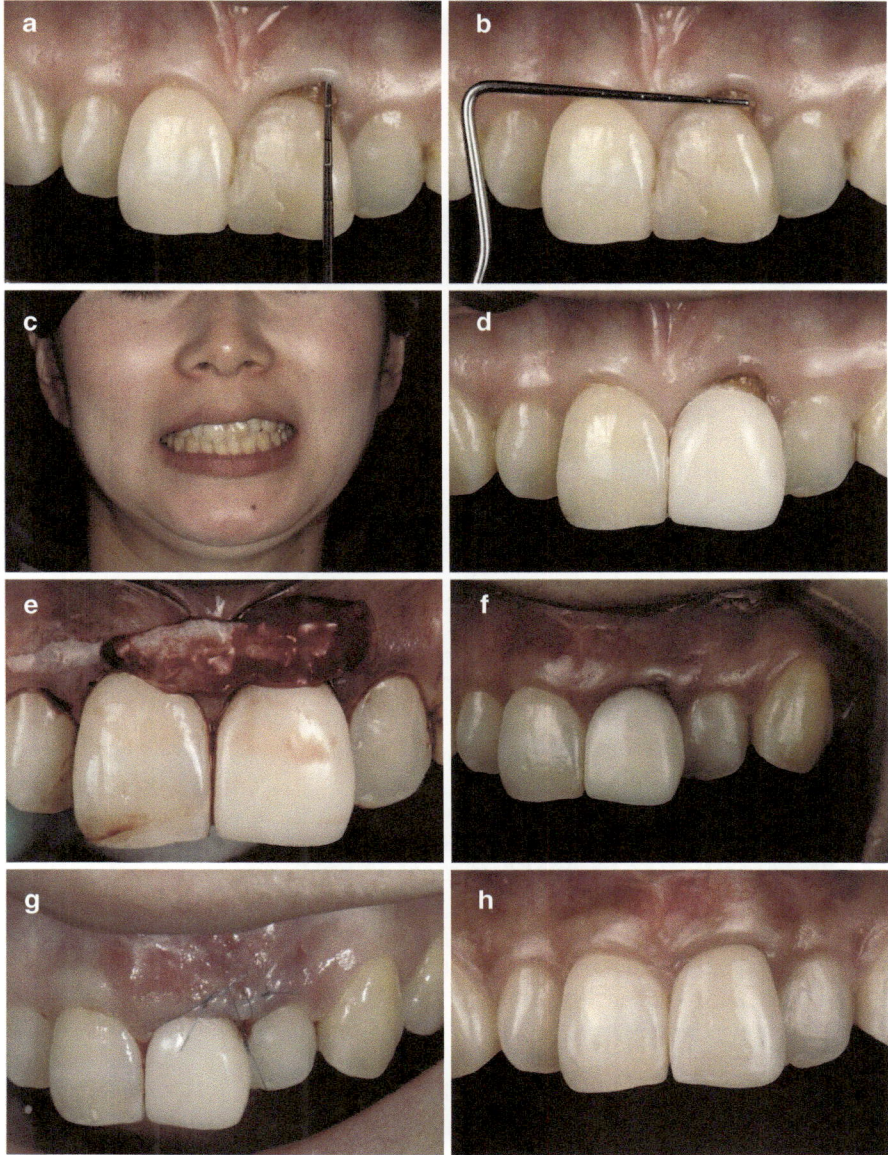

Fig. 7 (**a–j**) A case (case 1) treated with a closed technique and CTG for improving prosthetic outcomes. Please see the text for details

interdental papilla, great care can be taken to avoid damaging the tissue by higher magnification and illumination provided by the OM.

Case 1 presented an example of soft tissue augmentation before prosthetic reconstruction (Fig. 7a–k). The patient is a 40-year-old woman. She came to the clinic

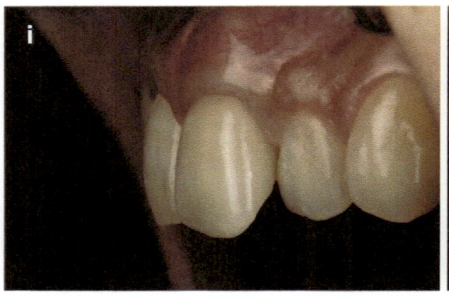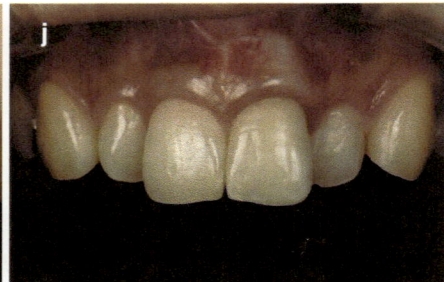

Fig. 7 (continued)

with an esthetic problem of the maxillary left central incisor (Tooth #9) (Fig. 7a–c). She had a trauma at that region and the incisal edge was fractured and restored with composite resin. At that time, pulpectomy was also performed. Gingival recession of 2 mm was also observed on #9 (Fig. 7a). The exposed root surface was rough and recession width was wide. (Fig. 7b). The patient was not interested in orthodontic treatment. Therefore, a root coverage procedure was proposed. A provisional crown was placed (Fig. 7d). A tunneling technique with connective tissue harvested from the palate was performed to correct the recession on teeth #8 and #9 (Fig. 7e). Two months after the surgery, some improvement was seen, but not sufficient (Fig. 7f). A revision surgery was performed (Fig. 7g).

The provisional restoration was replaced with a final prosthesis on tooth #9 (Fig. 7h, i). Two years after installing the final prosthesis, tissue health and harmony were achieved (Fig. 7j).

4   Preprosthetic Gingival Augmentation

Gingival recession causes esthetic and functional problems not only in natural teeth and prosthetic restoration procedures but also in implant restoration. Restoring this is one of the most difficult procedures in PPS. Valderhaug [19] in a long-term clinical trial showed gingival recession was 40% 1 year after restoration and 70% 10 years after restoration of 300 crown restorations with subgingival margins. Furthermore, Tao et al. [20] compared gingival phenotypes, and because of 5 years of follow-up with 100 metal ceramic single crowns showed gingival recession was more pronounced in thin biotypes, with 1.09 ± 0.22 mm and 0.31 ± 0.16 mm for thin and thick biotype, respectively. Seven crowns with thin biotype were evaluated as unsuccessful due to esthetic problems. These results indicate that the frequency of gingival recession after prosthetic restoration is unfortunately common, especially in thin gingival phenotypes. Zuhr et al. [18] found that gingival overgrowth is an effective procedure for soft tissue stability and prevention of recession when the prosthesis margin needs to be set below the margin in patients with thin biotypes. Therefore, it is indicated to prophylactically thicken the gingiva for successful treatment outcomes in selected cases, especially when there is a risk of postoperative gingival recession. The timing of transition to provisional restoration is based on the time when epithelial attachment and connective tissue attachment, which are the concepts of biological width, are reconstructed and matured, as in the case of the next surgical crown lengthening. Therefore, it is necessary to observe the stability of the gingiva by long-term provisional restoration for this gingival overgrowth.

Case 2 (Fig. 8): This patient is a 21-year-old, college student. She visited the clinic with the chief complaint of esthetic problem of the maxillary right central

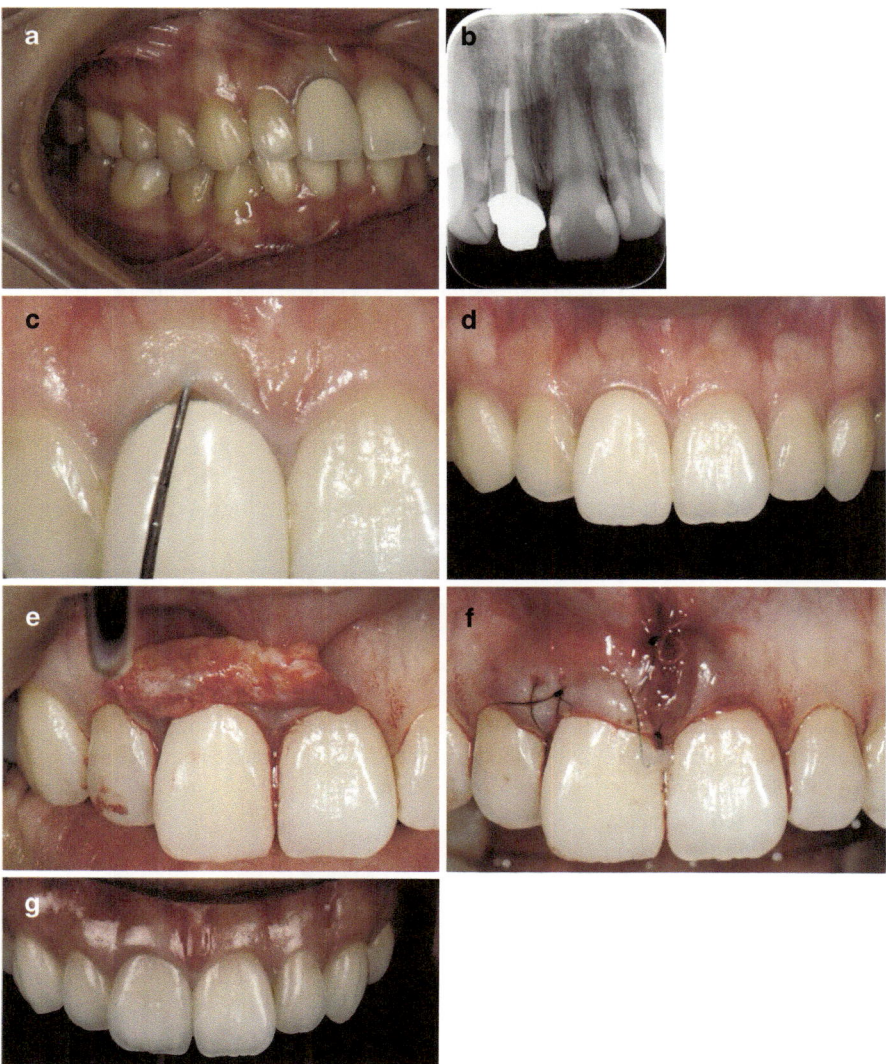

Fig. 8 A case (case 2) presenting CTG to improve gingival thickness and esthetics before restoration

incisor restored with a crown, with gingival discoloration (Fig. 8a). The X-ray showed satisfactory root canal treatment (Fig. 8b). In the close-up view, coloring of the crown margin was observed, and the attachment of the upper lip frenum was high (Fig. 8c). When tooth #8 was replaced with a provisional crown, the discoloration improved, but the crown was slightly longer than tooth #9 due to slight recession (Fig. 8d).

Connective tissue was harvested from the palate by the single incision technique. Then, after trying it on the recipient site, trimming and adjustment were performed under magnification. The graft was then fixed to the recipient bed performed by tunneling flap (Fig. 8e). The frenum was removed at the same time, and two interrupted sling sutures were performed (Fig. 8f). Eight months after the final prosthesis was placed, a satisfactory esthetic outcome was achieved (Fig. 8g).

Case 3 (Fig. 9): This patient visited the clinic complaining of esthetic problems of the mandibular anterior teeth after the completion of surgical orthodontic treatment (Fig. 9a). There is evidence of severe clinical attachment loss in this problematic region, confirmed by horizontal bone defect extending to 1/2 of the roots (Fig. 9b). The plan was to improve the thickness of the gingiva, after which single crowns were placed. Partial thickness flap was performed with scalloped incisions in the papillae and a connective tissue graft was placed in the right side (Fig. 9c). Healing at 3 months after the surgery showed thickening of the gingiva (Fig. 9d). Three months after the surgery on the right side, the same procedure was performed on the left side (Fig. 9e, f). Two years after the surgery, provisional restorations were placed (Fig. 9g, h). The gingiva was in harmony with the restorations. When the final prostheses were placed, long interproximal contacts were able to close the open space between the teeth with esthetically appealing gingiva (Fig. 9i).

5 Surgical Crown Lengthening

Crown lengthening is a surgical procedure used to build a prosthetic and esthetically pleasing gingival morphology. Subsequent prosthetic restorations are as important as the surgery itself, such as setting margins, adjusting provisional restoration subgingival contours, and timing of final restoration. Cases in which extension of crown length is required can be broadly divided into prosthetic/functional requirements and esthetic requirements.

Prosthetic requirements are indicated when (1) there is not enough tooth structure for restoration, e.g., subgingival caries or fracture, and (2) realigning the occlusal plane disturbed by tooth extrusion is needed. On the other hand, as an esthetic requirement, the teeth appear short, and the gingiva is overexposed while smiling, so-called gummy smile. The etiology of "gummy smile" is multifactorial (Table 4); therefore, prudent examination and correct diagnosis are important. "Altered passive eruption" is common and can be addressed with crown lengthening. It is estimated to occur in approximately 10% of the population. During normal passive eruption, the gingiva-alveolar complex moves apically to establish supracrestal attachment tissue (SAT). When this normal process does not occur, it is called

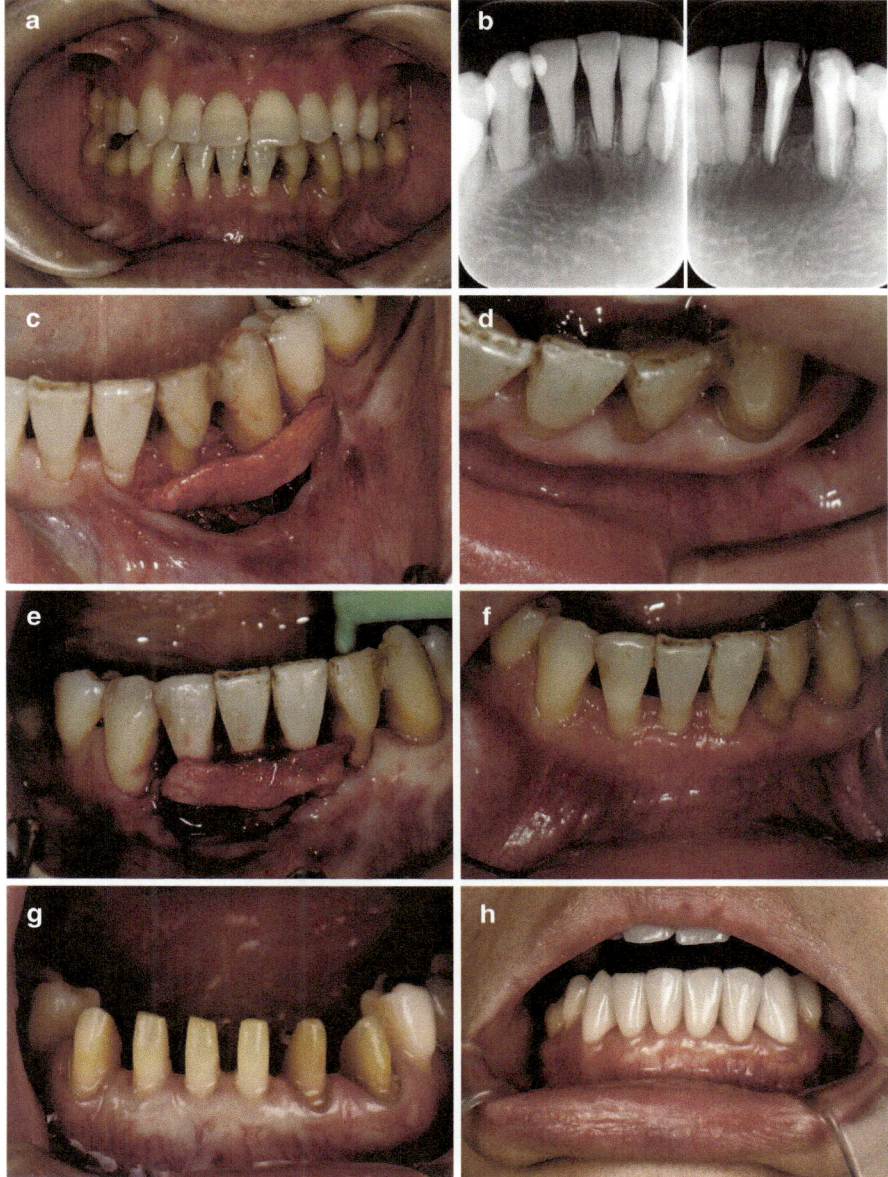

Fig. 9 Example of preprosthetic soft tissue augmentation in the mandibular anterior region

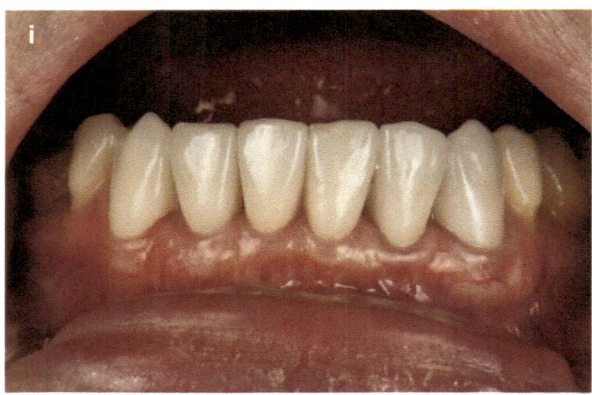

Fig. 9 (continued)

Table 4 The main etiologic factors of excessive gingiva display and possible solutions

Etiology	Solutions
Skeletal (long lower face)	Orthognathic surgery
Muscular (hypermobile lip)	Lip repositioning surgery; Botox application
Dental (tooth attrition)	Crown lengthening followed by restorations
Altered passive eruption	Crown lengthening with/without restoration

altered passive eruption [21, 22]. Altered passive eruption is classified into four types according to the width of the keratinized gingiva and the positional relationship between the alveolar crest and CEJ [23].

Case 4 (Fig. 10): A healthy 34-year-old female patient and a non-smoker presented at our clinic with complaints of pain in tooth #7 and gingival swelling. The labial gingiva receded with pus discharge from the periodontal pocket, and a vertical root fracture was suspected (Fig. 10a). Uneven gingival margins were observed, due to altered passive eruption in the maxillary anterior region. A decision was made to replace tooth #7 with a dental implant and crown lengthening of the area (Fig. 10b, c). Three months after #7 extraction and socket augmentation and the crown lengthening, an implant was placed under OM. Four months after implant placement, the second surgery was simply applied with a minor roll technique. Temporary restoration (Fig. 10d, e), final restoration (Fig. 10f), and the radiograph showed satisfactory outcomes (Fig. 10g).

Case 5 (Fig. 11): A healthy 40-year-old female came to the clinic with a complaint of unesthetic appearance in her maxillary anterior teeth. Resin facing cast crowns were placed on teeth #8 and #9 (Fig. 11a). The gingival line of anterior teeth

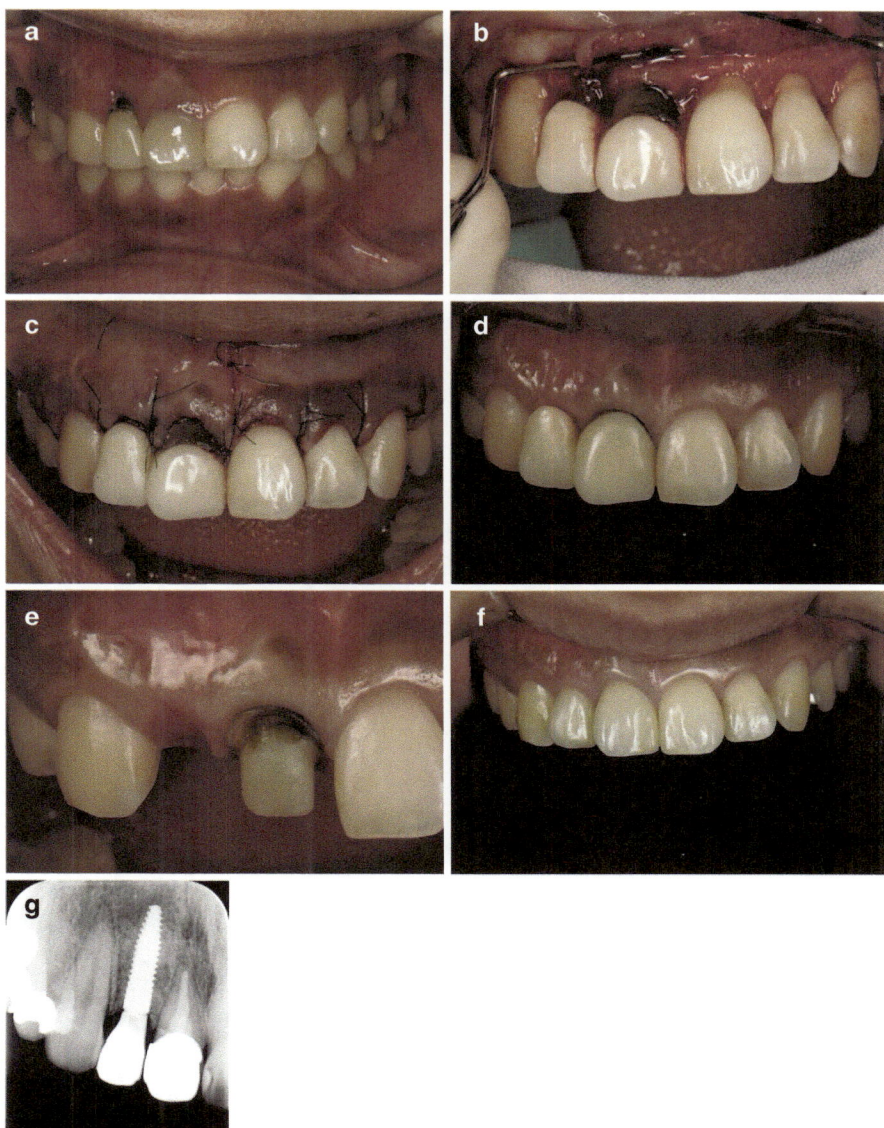

Fig. 10 A combination of crown lengthening and implant therapy for restoring anterior esthetics. See Case 4 for details

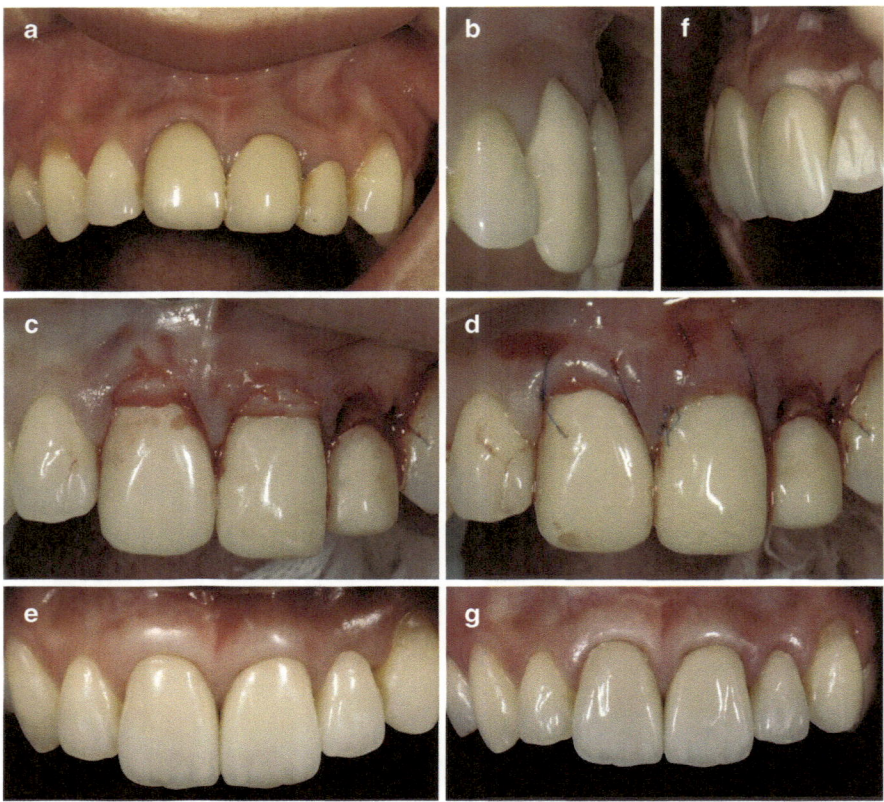

Fig. 11 Soft tissue augmentation to improve the thickness and contour around maxillary anterior teeth. Please see Case 5 for details

was uneven with slight crowding. The patient was not interested in orthodontic treatment. It was then decided to improve the esthetics as much as possible by pros-thetic restorations. As a preprosthetic treatment, CTG was planned to be placed on #8 and #9, along with #10 crown lengthening. All planned prostheses were replaced with provisional restorations before the scheduled surgery (Fig. 11b). An intrasulcu-lar incision was placed with a microblade and tunneling in the closed technique. Only distal papilla of #10 was elevated to ensure access to the alveolar crest for crown lengthening. Ostectomy of the bone was performed using round diamond burs. At this time as well, care must be taken not to damage the roots as much as possible under microscope. This is a procedure that can only be performed precisely under enlargement. Periodontal fibers remaining on the root surface must be removed carefully with ultrasonic devices. Collection of CTG was performed using the single incision technique. The CTG was placed on the labial side and the grafts are fixed with 6-0 sling sutures (Fig. 11c, d). The contour and the gingival margin improved compared to before surgery. Eight months after the surgery, the final prosthetic restorations were placed. At 1 year, the patient was very pleased with the results (Fig. 11e–g).

6 Papilla Reconstruction

A short papilla that does not fill the interdental space can be an esthetic concern. Factors to be considered include the space size and morphology, tooth positioning, periodontal phenotype, and the level of the alveolar crest. It might be improved by prosthetic treatment and/or orthodontic treatment. When it comes to surgical reconstruction, many different surgical procedures have been reported using autologous tissue, and various results have been shown [15, 24–29]. However, most of these studies are case series with a short-term outcome, and the reconstruction of the lost interdental papilla cannot be predictable. The primary challenges are due to limited blood supply and inability of the tissue transplant to keep the volume in this constrained space. Zuhr et al. [18] suggest that the grafts used for papilla reconstruction should be harvested from the maxillary tuberosity, which is rich in collagen fibers.

Case 6 (Fig. 12): The patient is a 50-year-old woman with a complaint of an esthetic issue in the maxillary anterior teeth. In particular, she was dissatisfied with the coloring of teeth #7 and #8 and the black triangle between the teeth (Fig. 12a). On X-ray, the crestal bone between #7 and #8 was higher, and the interdental distance was considered wide (Fig. 12b). Both the teeth were restored with composite resin. Gingival recession was also observed in both the teeth (Fig. 12c). Under local anesthesia, the root surface was flattened to promote reattachment before the scheduled root coverage and papilla reconstruction surgery (Fig. 12d). The tunneling procedure was performed, followed by placement of the two CTGs harvested from the palate on the labial side and under the papilla (Fig. 12e). Enamel Matrix Derivative (EMD) was also applied on the root surface after 24% of EDTA for 2 min to enhance the effect of reattachment to the root surface. The flap was repositioned coronally with interrupted sling sutures (Fig. 12f). Two months after the surgery, the restorative phase was initiated (Fig. 12g). At this point, the margin of the provisional restoration was determined. Four years after the surgery, the esthetic result was maintained, even though there was slight gingival redness on tooth #7 (Fig. 12h). The radiograph showed stable bone crestal level and re-established interdental contacts between teeth #7 and #8.

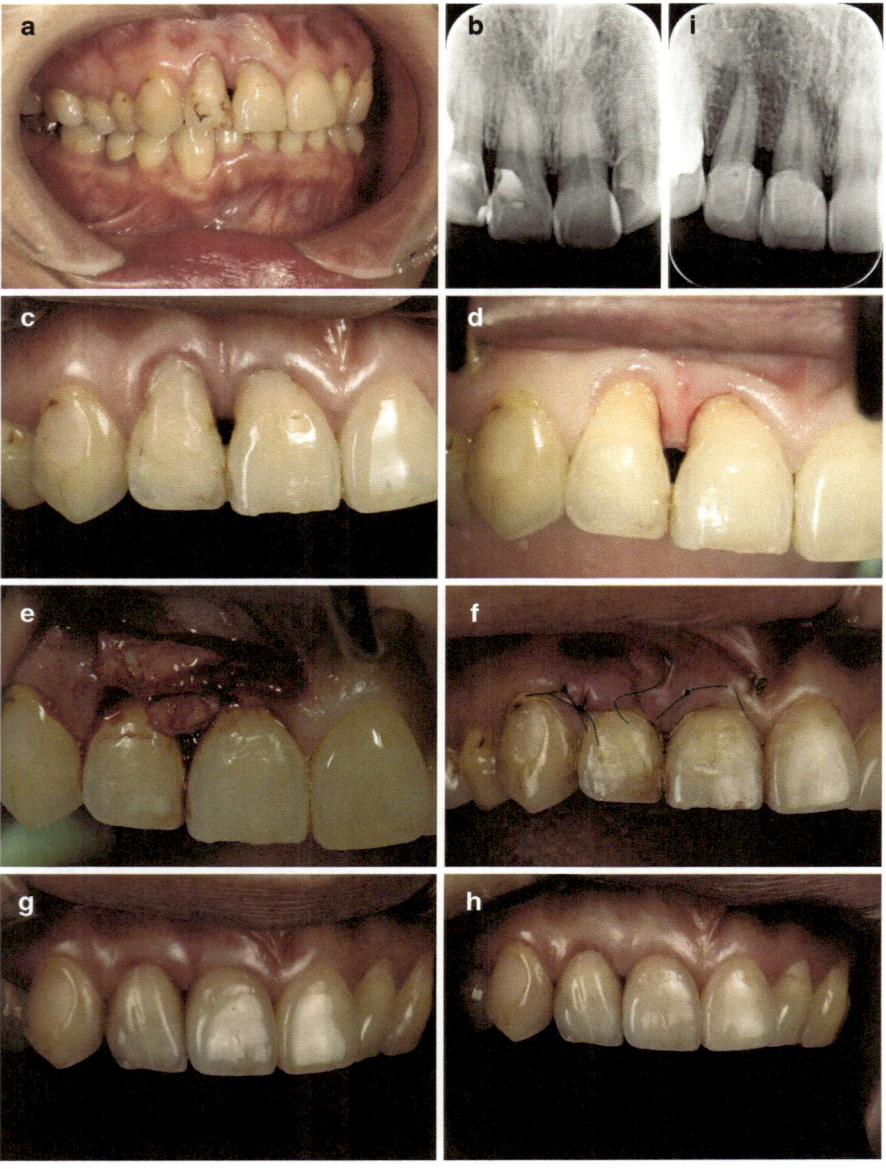

Fig. 12 Pre-prosthetic surgical papilla reconstruction for improve esthetics. Please see Case 6 for details

7 Conclusion

The appearance of restorations has become so vivid and natural tooth-like thanks to the evolution of materials and technology sciences. It is also the result of the great laboratory work from dental technicians. To further improve the esthetic outcome, healthy and esthetically pleasing periodontal tissues should be established. The field of periodontal plastic surgery is evolving in this aspect. In recent years, microscope-assisted periodontal plastic surgery has achieved improved clinical outcomes by allowing minimally invasive, precise, and delicate touch to periodontal hard and soft tissues. This chapter serves as a testimony to this and to encourage fellow dentists to join us for this exciting journey.

8 Key Points

1. Preprosthetic surgical procedures can improve the esthetic and functional outcomes. These procedures deal with the transition zone, requiring precise and gentle handling of soft and hard tissues. Therefore, applying operating microscope would be beneficial for these delicate procedures.
2. Commonly applied preprosthetic surgical procedures include (1) free gingival graft/connective tissue graft for increasing zone of keratinized mucosa, (2) root coverage with closed or open technique, (3) functional or esthetic crown lengthening, and (4) papilla reconstructive procedures.
3. A free gingival graft/connective tissue graft can be collected from the maxillary tuberosity or the palate. Harvesting from the palate is the most common because of the availability. Tuberosity tissue may contain higher collagen, providing volume stability but at the same time harder to become vascularized.
4. The closed technique for root coverage can be effective performed under microscope, which is considered less traumatic, compared to the open technique, and can promote better wound stability.
5. Etiologies of excessive gingival display may include skeletal discrepancy, hypermobile lip, altered passive eruption, and tooth attrition. Altered passive eruption can be effectively treated with a crown lengthening procedure.
6. Papilla reconstruction is still challenging and unpredictable; however, with a combination of restorations and surgical papilla reconstruction the esthetic outcome may be improved.

References

1. Schallhorn RG. Specialty perspective: periodontal therapy overview. Int J Prosthodont. 1988;1(1):107–15.
2. Padbury A Jr, Eber R, Wang HL. Interactions between the gingiva and the margin of restorations. J Clin Periodontol. 2003;30(5):379–85.
3. Burkhardt R, Lang NP. Coverage of localized gingival recessions: comparison of micro- and macrosurgical techniques. J Clin Periodontol. 2005;32(3):287–93.

4. Studer SP, Allen EP, Rees TC, et al. The thickness of masticatory mucosa in the human hard palate and tuberosity as potential donor sites for ridge augmentation procedures. J Periodontol. 1997;68:145–51.
5. Tavelli L, Barootchi S, Greenwell H, Wang HL. Is a soft tissue graft harvested from the maxillary tuberosity the approach of choice in an isolated site? J Periodontol. 2019;90(8):821–5.
6. Zuhr O, Bäumer D, Hürzeler MB. The addition of soft tissue replacement grafts in plastic periodontal and implant surgery: critical elements in design and execution. J Clin Periodontol. 2014;41(Suppl 15):S123–42.
7. Zucchelli G, 沼部幸博, 中田光太郎, 他:イラストで見る天 然歯のための審美形成外科. 第1版. 東京:クインテッセンス出版, 425–35, 2014.
8. Edel A. Clinical evaluation of free connective tissue grafts used to increase the width of keratinised gingiva. J Clin Periodontol. 1974;1(4):185–96.
9. Langer B, Langer L. Subepithelial connective tissue graft technique for root coverage. J Periodontol. 1985;56(12):715–20.
10. Hürzeler MB, Weng D. A single-incision technique to harvest subepithelial connective tissue grafts from the palate. Int J Periodontics Restorative Dent. 1999;19:279–87.
11. Sclar AG. Soft tissue and esthetic considerations in implant therapy. Batavia, IL: Quintessence Publishing Co, Inc; 2003. p. 114–5.
12. Pini-Prato G, Baldi C, Pagliaro U, Nieri M, Saletta D, Rotundo R, Cortellini P. Coronally advanced flap procedure for root coverage. Treatment of root surface: root planning versus polishing. J Periodontol. 1999;70(9):1064–76.
13. Langer L, Langer B. The subepithelial connective tissue graft for treatment of gingival recession. Dent Clin North Am. 1993;37(2):243–64. Review.
14. Huang LH, Wang HL. Sling and tag suturing technique for coronally advanced flap. Int J Periodontics Restorative Dent. 2007;27(4):379–85.
15. Azzi R, Takei HH, Etienne D, Carranza FA. Root coverage and papilla reconstruction using autogenous osseous and connective tissue grafts. Int J Periodontics Restorative Dent. 2001;21(2):141–7.
16. Azzi R, Etienne D, Takei H, Fenech P. Surgical thickening of the existing gingiva and reconstruction of interdental papillae around implant-supported restorations. Int J Periodontics Restorative Dent. 2002;22(1):71–7.
17. Azzi R, Etienne D, Takei H, Carranza F. Bone regeneration using the pouch-and-tunnel technique. Int J Periodontics Restorative Dent. 2009;29(5):515–21.
18. Zuhr O, Hurzeler M. ペリオとインプラントのための審美形成外科. クインテッセンス出版.
19. Valderhaug J. Periodontal conditions and carious lesions following the insertion of fixed prostheses: a 10-year follow-up study. Int Dent J. 1980;30(4):296–304.
20. Tao J, Wu Y, Chen J, Su J. A follow-up study of up to 5 years of metal-ceramic crowns in maxillary central incisors for different gingival biotypes. Int J Periodontics Restorative Dent. 2014;34(5):e85–92. https://doi.org/10.11607/prd.2024.
21. Dolt AH, Robbins J. Altered passive eruption: an etiology of short clinical crowns. Quintessence Int. 1997;28:363–72.
22. Garber DA, Salama MA. The aesthetic smile: diagnosis and treatment. Periodontol 2000. 1996;11:18–28.
23. Coslet J, Vanarsdall R, Weisgold A. Diagnosis and classification of delayed passive eruption of the dentogingival junction in the adult. Alpha Omegan. 1977;70:24–8.
24. Beagle JR. Surgical reconstruction of the interdental papilla: case report. Int J Periodontics Restorative Dent. 1992;12(2):145–51.
25. Azzi R, Etienne D, Sauvan JL, Miller PD. Root coverage and papilla reconstruction in Class IV recession: a case report. Int J Periodontics Restorative Dent. 1999;19(5):449–55.
26. Evian CI, Corn H, Rosenberg ES. Retained interdental papilla procedure for maintaining anterior esthetics. Compend Contin Educ Dent. 1985;6(1):58–64.

27. Han TJ, Takei HH. Progress in gingival papilla reconstruction. Periodontol 2000. 1996;11:65–8.
28. Nemcovsky CE. Interproximal papilla augmentation procedure: a novel surgical approach and clinical evaluation of 10 consecutive procedures. Int J Periodontics Restorative Dent. 2001;21(6):553–9.
29. Azzi R, Etienne D, Carranza F. Surgical reconstruction of the interdental papilla. Int J Periodontics Restorative Dent. 1998;18(5):466–73.

Microsurgery in Guided Bone Regeneration

Lizette Llamosa-Cáñez

Contents

Supplementary Information The online version contains supplementary material available at [https://doi.org/10.1007/978-3-030-96874-8_11].

L. Llamosa-Cáñez (✉)
Private practice in Periodontal Medicine and Microscopic Implantology, Institute of Surgery, Hospital Zambrano Hellion, Nuevo León, Mexico

Clinical Professor, Tecnologico de Monterrey, School of Medicine and Health Science, Periodontology Department, Monterrey, Nuevo León, Mexico
e-mail: lizette.llamosa@tecsalud.mx

Abstract

Guided bone regeneration (GBR) is the process of replacing lost tissues with elements to restore normal function and structure for ideal three-dimensional placement of dental implants. GBR is based on guided tissue regeneration and has common mechanical and biological principles; their similarities are obvious throughout the evolution of bone regeneration concepts. There are four fundamental biological principles for successful GBR: primary wound closure, adequate blood supply, clot stability, and space maintenance.

Microsurgery was introduced in Periodontology in 1992 for the improvement of surgical techniques. It was made possible by the advancements in visual acuity obtained through the microscope. Microsurgery helps develop motor skills by improving surgical capacity, reduces tissue trauma, and contributes to the primary closure of the wound.

The proposed use of the microscope in GBR can aid precision in surgical execution. It has been shown that microsurgery contributes to improved healing and treatment outcomes in other areas of Periodontology.

This chapter provides a detailed description of GBR techniques using a surgical microscope (MO) along with information on the elements essential for the application of this technology. The principles of magnification and coaxial light and fundamentals of microsurgery are used for the execution of incisions, release of flaps, preparation of the surgical bed, handling of biomaterials, and membrane fixation, complementing the techniques for flap closure and soft tissue management in regenerative therapy.

Keywords

Bone regeneration · Microsurgery · Microscopic periodontal surgery
Microsurgery in bone regeneration therapy · Microsurgery in process augmentation · Microsurgical flap · Microsurgical regenerative therapies

1   Introduction

Regenerative therapy replaces tissues lost by injury or disease with new elements of
high organizational disposition to restore normal function and structure.
Augmentation procedures for the maxillaries have evolved to offer predictable
results. Under optimal conditions, the reconstruction of the original structure and
function of the bone tissue can occur.

Predictable success of guided bone regeneration (GBR) depends mainly on four
important biologic principles: primary wound closure, adequate blood supply, clot
stability, and space maintenance. [1] This chapter discusses the microsurgical
approach in regenerative therapy, with an emphasis on the precision and additional
clinical benefits it offers.

1.1   History of Guided Bone Regeneration

GBR is based on guided tissue regeneration, and they have common mechanical and
biological principles; [2] their similarities can be observed throughout the evolution
of the concepts of osseous regeneration [3, 4].

Several authors have reported difficulties in the placement of prostheses at edentulous sites due to post-extraction alveolar ridge resorption. This resorption is more
accentuated on the buccal bone plate of both maxillaries. The buccal bone is thinner
in most cases and undergoes post-extraction resorption, complicating prosthetic
rehabilitation [5–7]. On many occasions, the use of dental materials was shown to
resolve the esthetic concerns associated with these deficiencies. Further, implementing surgical soft tissue techniques can improve both esthetic and functional
outcomes; [8] however, the lost structures cannot be completely restored. With the
development of implantology, bone regeneration has become a priority.

Several studies have described morphological changes in the post-extraction
healing of alveolar tissue [6, 7, 9]. Araujo and Lindhe demonstrated the occurrence
of significant three-dimensional alteration of the alveolar ridge within 4–8 months
after extraction, with a reduced buccal and lingual ridge height; the vestibular region
was most affected [10]. The researchers also described horizontal bone loss accompanying the destruction of the alveolar height. Prospective clinical studies and systematic reviews have demonstrated significant variation in the post-extraction
changes within the first 12 months, although the first 3 months are the most critical
[11, 12]. The situation is further compromised when the alveolus loses height

because of trauma, periodontal disease, periapical pathologies, or damage caused during the extraction [11, 13].

An understanding of osseous deficiencies, tissue management, and regenerative materials is necessary to determine the clinical prognosis of GBR [14]. The developed techniques comply with biological and functional demands and have improved the treatment outcomes to satisfactory levels [15]. Microsurgery can further improve the outcomes of these techniques and allow better predictability.

1.2   Development of Microscopic Surgery and its Application in Regenerative Bone Therapy

Microsurgery improves the execution of each surgical step in GBR and allows more predictable results than conventional bone regeneration surgery. These improvements result from the precision, accuracy, and gentle treatment of tissues made possible under magnification, in addition to improved techniques for autogenous tissue procurement, membrane fixation, and wound closure.

1.2.1   History

Microsurgery was introduced in periodontics in 1992, [16] and its application has since evolved with introduction in different aspects of periodontal treatment [17–24]. In 1962, osseous reconstructive microscopic surgery was introduced in traumatology for vascularized bone flap transfers for the reconstruction of traumatic tibial defects [25]. Therefore, GBR has been performed under the microscope for benefits already demonstrated in other areas of medicine, such as traumatology, since the 1970s, and in several areas of periodontics, since the 1990s [26].

Microscope is a modern surgical accessory and a critical factor for the success of the most complex medical surgeries performed today. The emergence of this tool reflects the advances in the principles of optics [27].

Currently, there is no scientific evidence to support the benefits of microsurgery in GBR. Research results are based primarily on patients' subjective opinions and the observations of the microsurgeon performing the procedure. Microscopic surgery is still in its early stages of development in periodontics and implantology and is considered an area of great potential for prospective analyses comparing macro and microsurgical techniques to demonstrate the benefits of the latter.

1.3   Importance of the Surgical Microscope in GBR

The microsurgical approach enhances the efficiency of the operator with consistent treatment outcomes [28].

The application of microsurgical principles starts by evaluating the surgical site indicated for augmentation. Further, preparation of tissues with nonsurgical therapy under magnification can give better results than treatment without magnification.

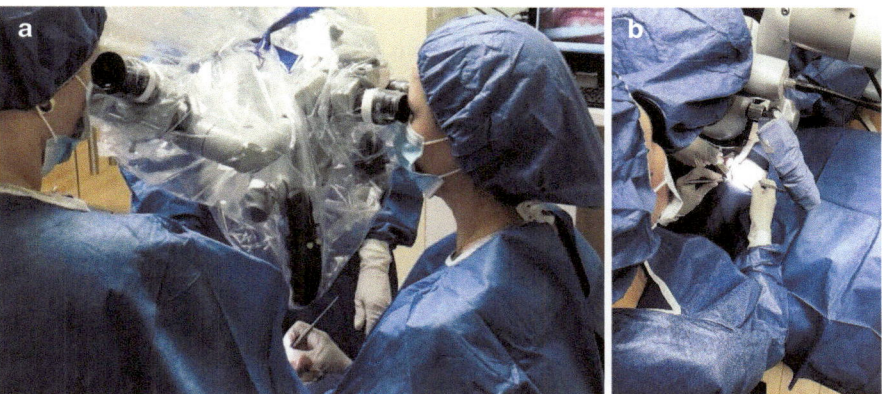

Fig. 1 (**a**, **b**) Microscope-assisted guided bone regeneration

Microscope-assisted GBR can enhance the surgeon's performance by enabling precise placement of surgical incisions and elevation of the flap using microsurgical instruments designed to induce minimal tissue trauma. Magnification and illumination allow suitable handling of materials, and microsurgical suturing techniques produce less tissue damage and promote primary wound closure [17, 28, 29] Video 1 and Fig. 1a, b.

2 Biological Basis and Anatomical Consideration During Microscope-Assisted GBR

The restoration of lost or absent tissue requires comprehension of the biological structures to be regenerated. A predictable procedure should consider the biological mechanisms of bone regeneration. A range of techniques have been proposed to induce bone formation and restore alveolar defects, for example, osteoinduction by bone grafts or growth factors, osteoconduction by bone grafts substitutes that serve as scaffolds for new bone formation, osteodistraction, forced extrusion orthodontics, and GBR using membranes as barriers. However, regardless of the selected technique, the biological foundation and microsurgical principles must be respected and adhered to.

2.1 Ridge Deformity Classifications

Residual deformities have been described and classified using different systems with further subdivisions based on the aspects of deformity and tissue absence.

Horizontal (Class I) defects include those with a loss of the bucco-palatal/lingual contour with an adequate apico-coronal ridge dimensions. Vertical (Class II) defects represent the loss of the apico-coronal tissue contour with adequate bucco-palatal/

lingual ridge dimensions, and Class III defects include deficiency of both apico-coronal and bucco-palatal/lingual dimensions [8].

Another proposed classification relates the severity of the defect to the dimensions of the adjacent ridge. The defects are classified as low (less than 3 mm), moderate (3–6 mm), and advanced (more than 6 mm) [30]. These classifications aid the analysis of intra-arch defects. The surgeon must also consider the inter-arch alveolar ridge relationship during treatment planning to achieve adequate surgical results for prosthetic treatment [31].

The classification systems help the microsurgeon to define the clinical problem and assist further decision-making and treatment planning. The evolution of dental implant therapy has further contributed to the modification of the available classification systems [32] Figs. 2a, b, 3a, b, 4a, b, 5a, b, 6a, b and 7a, b.

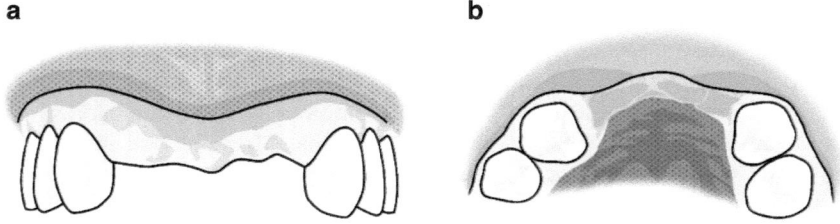

Fig. 2 (**a**) Buccal view of the horizontal defect. (**b**) Occlusal view of the horizontal defect

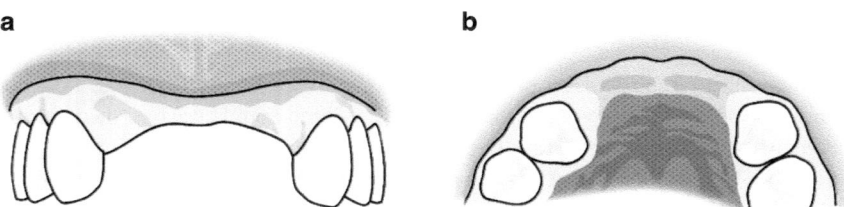

Fig. 3 (**a**) Buccal view of the vertical defect. (**b**) Occlusal view of the vertical defect

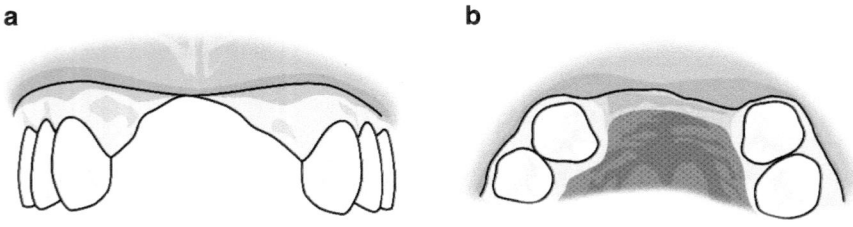

Fig. 4 (**a**) Buccal view of the horizontal and vertical deficiency. (**b**) Occlusal view of the horizontal and vertical deficiency

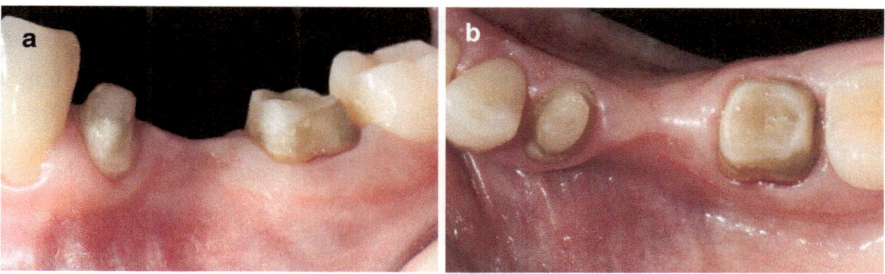

Fig. 5 (**a, b**) Buccal and occlusal view of the defect involving loss of buccolingual contour with an adequate apico-coronal ridge dimension

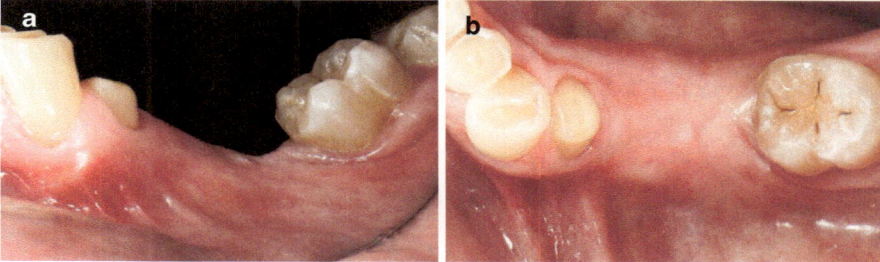

Fig. 6 (**a, b**) Buccal and occlusal view of the defect involving loss of apico-coronal tissue contour with an adequate buccolingual ridge dimension

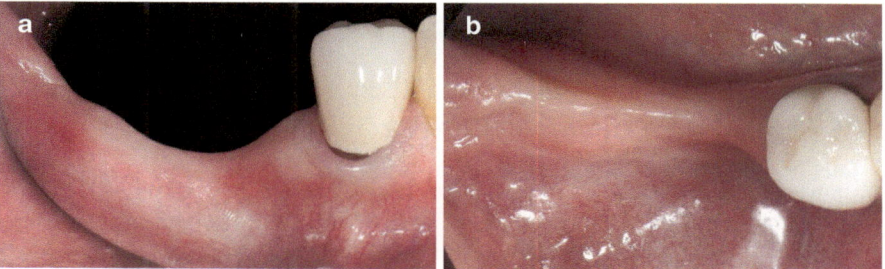

Fig. 7 (**a, b**) Defects involving deficiency of both apico-coronal and buccolingual dimensions

2.2 Physiology of Bone Regeneration, Histology, and Participating Cells

Bone regeneration aims to achieve the original structure with a reparative process similar to physiological regeneration but with certain limitations. The minimum conditions required for success include ample blood supply and mechanical stability.

Osseous tissue has an internal layer of endosteum covering the medullar area. It contains osteoprogenitor cells and periosteum, an external fibrous layer of dense connective tissue that has vascular and lymphatic vessels and nerves, in addition to an osteogenic layer formed by several types of cells, elastic fibers, and blood vessels. Cellular richness is capable of promoting growth and bone remodeling. The bone tissue has an intercellular matrix rich in collagen and is also composed of dispersed cells, 25% water, and 25% protein and mineral salts. In osseous tissue, there are five different types of cells which regulate bone formation, maintenance, and repair: osteoblasts, bone-lining cells, osteomorphs, osteoclasts that cover bone surfaces, and osteocytes found within the bone matrix [33–37].

Bone regeneration involves restoration of the lost tissue with cells of the same lineage through osteogenesis, osteoconduction, and osteoinduction through a series of angiogenesis processes and migration and proliferation of undifferentiated cells that transform into osteoblasts. Osteoid production, mineralization, and remodeling occur [33].

There is an intimate relationship between blood vessel formation (angiogenesis) and new bone formation [38]. Bone regeneration significantly depends on these events. Angiogenesis is the physiological process of formation of new blood vessels from the existing vessels, and therefore, the residual bone and periosteum must be treated with special care during surgery; this is possible with enhanced magnification provided by the operating microscope.

2.3   Intra-Operative Visualization of Anatomical Structures

Microsurgery improves soft and hard tissue management, offering better visualization and recognition of anatomical structures during incision placement and flap elevation, where soft tissue integrity is essential. The illumination and magnification can be adjusted according to the needs of the microsurgeon. They aid preservation of the anatomical structures during separation and detachment of tissues, helping to obtain an intact flap of the desired thickness, maintain periosteal integrity, and avoid tissue perforation [22].

2.4   Anatomical Considerations for GBR

Knowledge of the maxillary and mandibular anatomy allows the microsurgeon to locate muscular insertions, neurovascular pathways, spaces occupied by glandular structures, and the oral mucosa. Thus, a thorough understanding of the surgical anatomy provides a solid foundation for the performance of regenerative surgery [39, 40, 41, 43].

2.4.1   Anatomical Considerations: Musculature

Maxilla
Muscles are attached to the external surface of the maxillae. During GBR, vestibular flap release involves the release of the underlying muscular structures. Using microsurgical techniques, the microsurgeon can perform this action without perforating the mucosa. (Graph 1).

Mandible
The mandible, especially its posterior part, is considered high risk. The clinical experience of the microsurgeon is therefore essential. Microsurgery requires

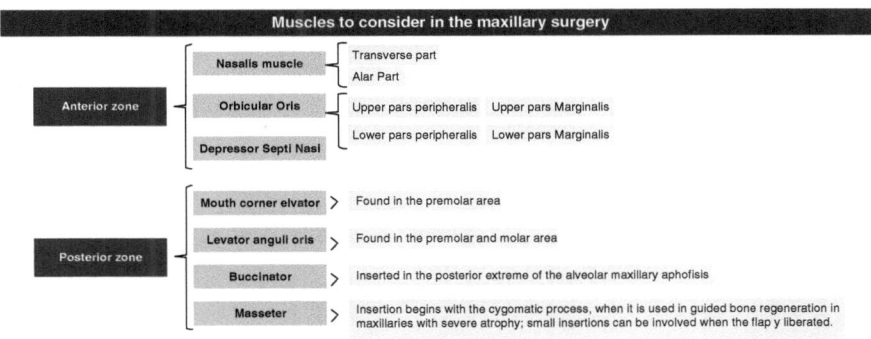

Graph 1 Muscle anatomical considerations in the maxilla

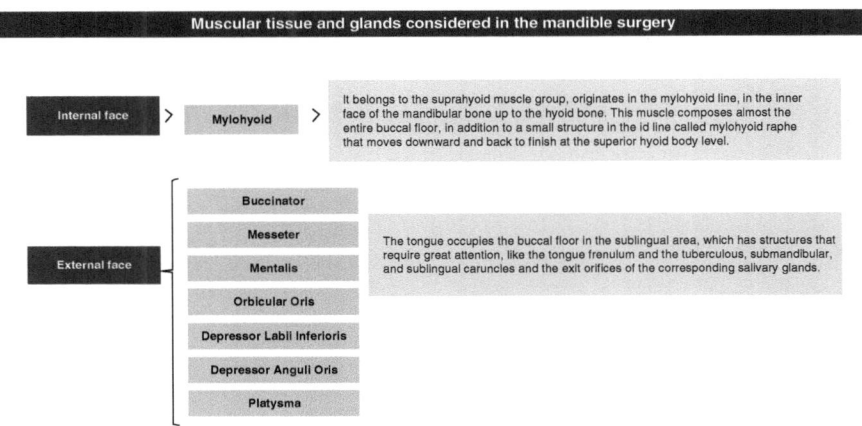

Graph 2 Muscle anatomical considerations in the mandible

knowledge and training with a steep learning curve; it allows gradual refinement of the surgical procedures.

The floor of the oral cavity, formed by the mylohyoid muscle, requires special consideration as it is a critical area for the release of the lingual flap. Further, a small tendinous structure, called the mylohyoid raphe, is present in the midline.

The tongue occupies the buccal floor in the sublingual area. The structures including the frenulum and its insertions, mandibular tubercles, and openings of the ducts of the corresponding salivary glands require attention during surgery. The muscles inserted on the external surface of the mandible must be considered when releasing the vestibular microsurgical flap. (Graph 2).

2.4.2 Anatomical Considerations: Vasculature

The maxillaries obtain their vascular supply through branches from the external carotid artery. Three of these branches most relevant to maxillary and mandibular GBR microsurgery are: maxillary, lingual, and facial arteries. During regenerative surgery, the microscope, providing illumination and magnification, is useful while

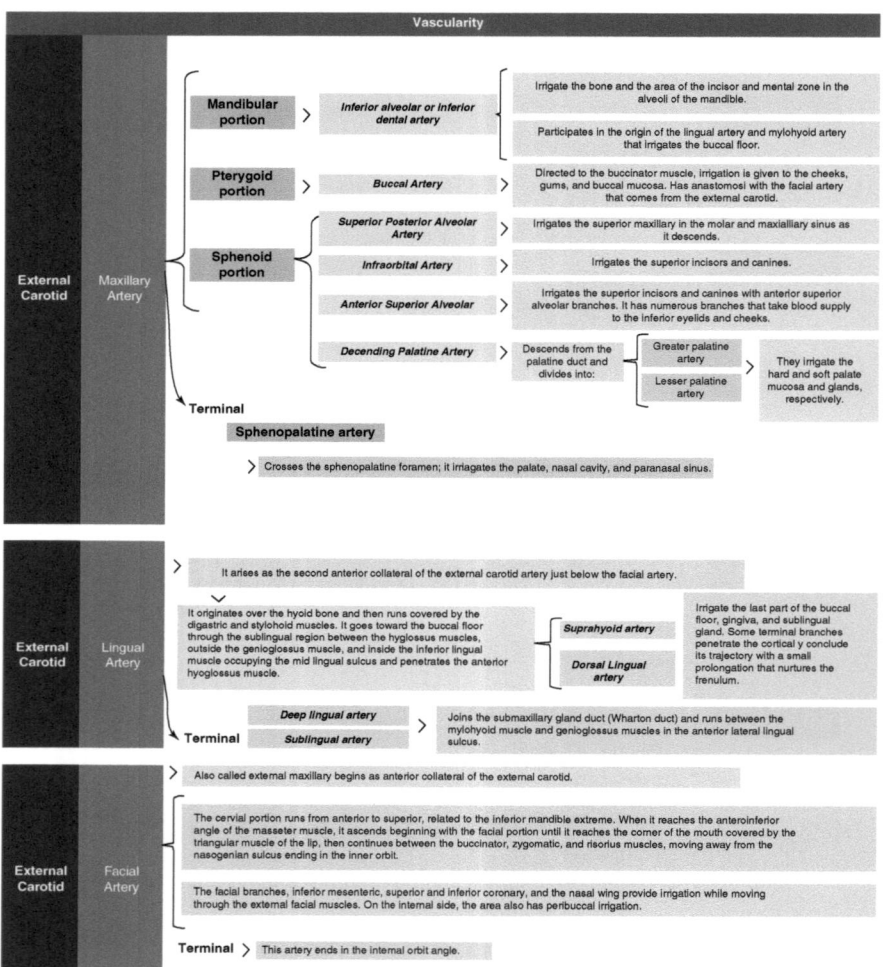

Graph 3 Vascular anatomical considerations in guided bone regeneration

operating close to these vasculature structures and handling flaps and periosteum incisions, preventing surgical complications. (Graph 3).

2.4.3 Anatomical Considerations: Innervation

Prior knowledge of the innervation of the surgical area is necessary, as the preservation of its integrity is essential to preventing complications. The microscope can help visualize areas with severe defects, aiding in the identification of nerve bundles and prevention of intraoperative damage to them.

The trigeminal nerve or V cranial nerve (a mixed nerve) innervates the maxilla and mandible. The use of microscope can enable careful handling of the anatomical structures (Graph 4a–c).

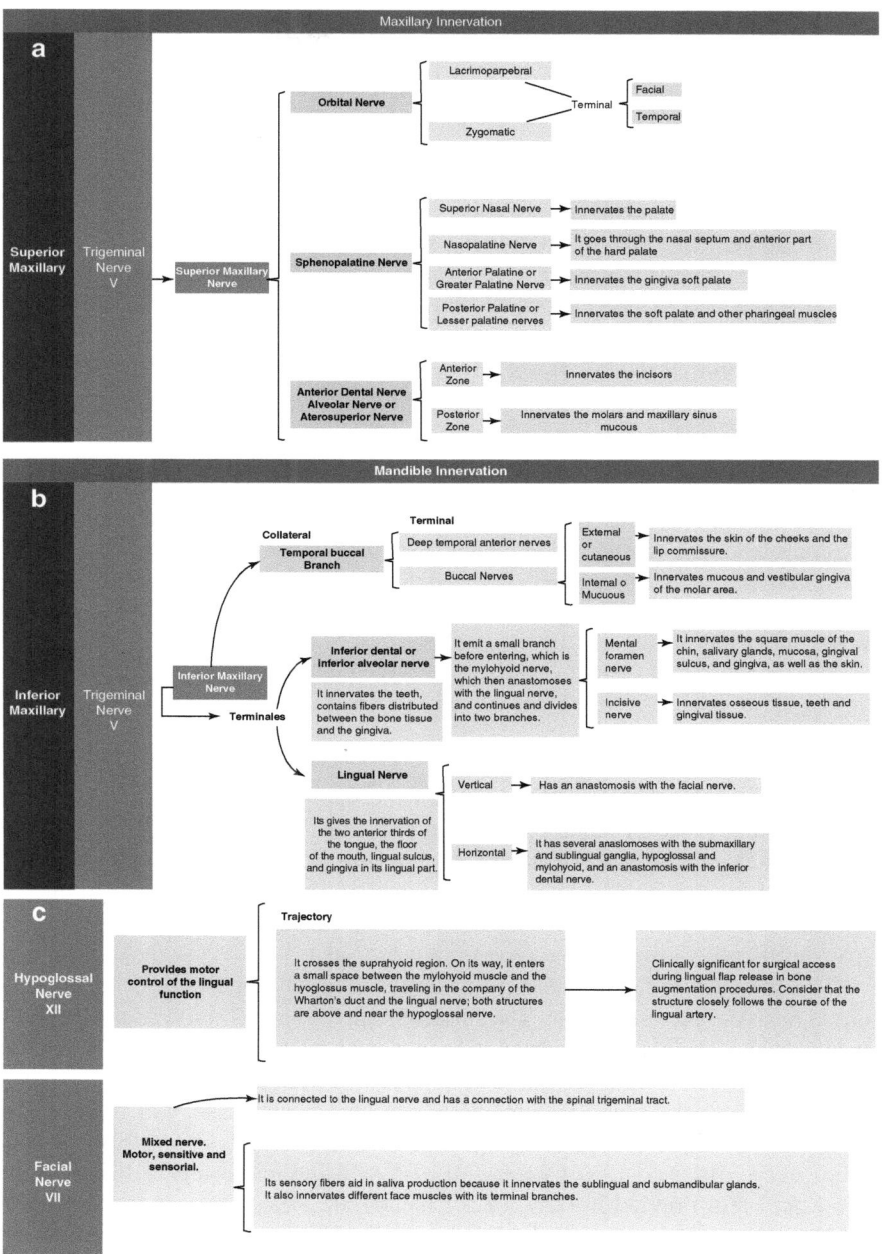

Graph 4 (**a**) Innervation in the maxilla related to guided bone regeneration. (**b**) Innervation in the mandible related to guided bone regeneration. (**c**) Hypoglossal and facial nerve ramifications

3   Microsurgical Soft Tissue Management

Soft tissue management offers numerous advantages in GBR. The knowledge of existing surgical techniques is necessary for refinement of the procedures. Training of the surgeon improves the execution of the techniques and gradually decreases the time taken to perform them. The improvements in the technical results obtained with microsurgical and macrosurgical approaches have been compared, demonstrating advantages in terms of vascularity, healing, and the clinical parameters. The microscopic approach decreases tissue trauma due to the protocols and refined precision because of magnification, which enables improvements in the division and release of the flaps [22].

The selection of the flap design, incisions, materials, and microsurgical instruments differs with each area in the oral cavity. Different degrees of magnification are applied depending on the indication of the surgery. A presurgical appointment for microscopic examination is part of the evaluation and treatment planning process; it is scheduled after non-surgical periodontal therapy with adequate inflammation control criteria that require dental corrections and optimal hygiene. Using different field and augmentation depths, the surgeon observes the tissue quality at the defect site and evaluate the height and thickness of the keratinized tissue, frenulum insertions, vestibular depth, and muscular tone; this data, with the other diagnostic tools, aid in defining the incision area.

3.1   Incision Design

It is necessary to determine the design of the flap before placing the incision to ensure maintenance of flap closure during healing. The planning for flap closure starts even before the placement of dental implants [42]. Thus, determining the type of osseous deficiency, selection of the bone augmentation technique, anatomic references, bone peaks adjacent to the defect, estimated bone gain, and degree of anticipated difficulty of the surgical procedure is crucial.

The primary incision (crestal incision) is placed crestally, in a mesio-distal direction at the edentulous site. The surgical scalpel is held firmly, perpendicular to the tissue and a single lightly penetrating incision is placed, touching the bone along the incision line. A secondary incision is repeated over the first, ensuring penetration of the scalpel through the complete thickness of the tissue, which protects its integrity with the inner face. The surgeon makes the main incision with a 15C blade (Hu-Friedy Mfg. Co., LLC Chicago, IL, USA) using microsurgery blades MB64 and MB67 (Hu-Friedy Mfg. Co., LLC Chicago, IL, USA) in the areas close to the teeth, extending as intracrevicular incision on the buccal and palatal/lingual aspects of the adjacent teeth. The surgeon begins the incisions on the distal aspect of the most distal tooth included in the flap design, moving mesially. Using angled microsurgery blades ensures a complete cut while placing intracrevicular incisions. This area has complicated access, and indirect vision is necessary to ensure incision integrity.

The surgeon places the principal or crestal incision in keratinized tissue. This incision will depend on the position of the center of the mandibular ridge, but exceptions may occur. In the maxilla, it is recommended to place the incision slightly buccally. This is because the palatal mucosa is firmly adherent, while the lingual mucosa of the mandibular ridge is associated with movable mucosa and muscular tissue that favors passive advance [42, 43].

Secondary incisions (releasing) allow visibility and accessibility to instruments and increase flap mobility, contributing to tension-free closure [43]. The extension of the horizontal releasing incision improves access and, if using non-resorbable membranes, helps avoid vascular compromise [44]. In the edentulous areas, releasing incisions must be placed 8–10 mm distal to the membrane borders, up to 2 mm distal to the retromolar pad. It is preferable to place the vertical incisions one or two teeth away from the defect site on the buccal aspect and two to three teeth away from the lingual/palatal site; therefore, the length of the flap varies based on the case and region of interest. An example of the horizontal length of the flap being greater occurs when surgeons do not place vertical releasing incisions.

The same criteria apply to the vertical releasing incisions at mesial, distal, or both sides of the area requiring augmentation. The incision should be placed at least one or two teeth away from the surgical site to protect the underlying bone and the vascularity of the flap. In adjacent buccal areas with teeth, the bone augmentation area must be distant in at least one or two teeth, and the complete incision is performed with a new 15C blade or with a microsurgical scalpel held perpendicular to the underlying bone. The trajectory begins at the gingival margin at the tooth angle, avoiding the interdental area or midsections with radicular prominences; [45] this incision is placed to achieve exact repositioning and may require greater magnification because the visual field should be more localized to improve precision. The vertical incision may have a hockey stick form initially, involving papillae, continuing straight with a total thickness [46]. Another variation includes a vertical incision placed to produce a surgical papilla positioned coronally, followed by a partial incision perpendicular to the tissue, without reaching the bone. The microsurgeon places the blade perpendicular to the gingival margin, forming the papilla diagonally with a slight angle to continue with the releasing incision of total thickness beyond the mucogingival line (video). In the posterior areas of the mandible, the distal releasing incision is made, moving obliquely toward the mandibular branch and ending lateral to the flap so as to preserve the lingual nerve.

On the lingual/palatal aspects, we place mesial and distal vertical releasing incisions in areas distant from the augmented site. The criteria are determined according to the requirement of the surgical site and the discretion of the microsurgeon since it involves increased difficulty [41, 45]. Videos 2, 3, 4 and Fig. 8a–e.

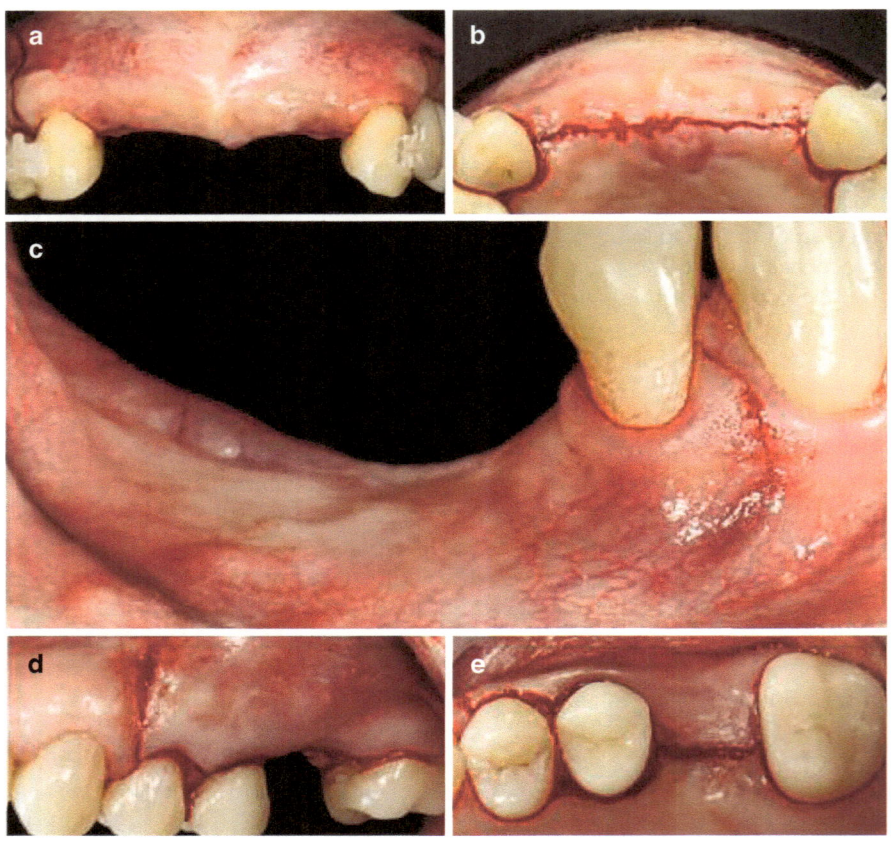

Fig. 8 (a–e) Primary (crestal) and secondary (releasing) incisions

3.2 Decision to Place Vertical Incisions

Vertical releasing incisions aid the coronal positioning of the flap and provide the visibility and accessibility necessary for the appropriate placement of the graft and membranes, also allowing the procurement of autologous bone.

Vascularity is an essential aspect of flap nutrition; a vertical incision could interrupt the vascular supply gingiva, the mucous vessels' microcirculation trajectory, and the periosteum. However, the microsurgical adaptation will aid revascularization, allowing for the incised tissue to heal rapidly (Video 5).

3.3 Steps in Flap Releasing: Layered Releasing Incision, Linear Incision, and Selectively Releasing Incision

3.3.1 Microsurgical reflection

It is described as *initial separation*, or the detachment of the adhered zone on the buccal and lingual/palatal sides. It is secondary to the periosteal incision in the buccal and lingual areas and releasing of muscular attachments in the upper and lower buccal areas and lower lingual areas. It is necessary to have magnification for the visualization of the instrument trajectory. In certain situations, the surgeon may take a closer look to perform adjustments. Additionally, adequate irrigation is essential to keep the tissues in the surgical area clean and hydrated, in addition to a microsurgical ejector with effective suction.

The surgeon makes the *initial separation* in the flap reflection, carefully elevating the periosteum with a microsurgical periosteal elevator throughout the length of the incision and firmly separating the adhered tissue. This separation is extended beyond the vertical and horizontal dimensions of the defect, on both the facial and lingual/palatal aspects.

For the secondary periosteum incision and the release of muscle fibers on the buccal aspect in the maxilla, the microsurgeon must take into account the anatomical areas at risk and move the blade in a coronal-buccal direction Fig. 9a–c The procedure is performed with a 15C scalpel starting from the distal areas, moving mesially along the length of the flap. The muscle fibers should be separated until significant flap mobility is achieved. The released extension is verified by advancing coronally until it reaches the occlusal aspect.

The posterior areas allow limited visibility. The microscope therefore offers excellent safety while performing the periosteal incision for flap liberation, allowing detachment of the flap with a single cut to prevent tissue damage in such areas Video 6 and Fig. 9d–f. The anterior area receives equal treatment, with the periosteal incision extending from side to side, connecting both vertical incisions. When the flap does not advance in both situations, additional subperiosteal cuts are necessary to separate the elastic fibers using microsurgery tissue scissors, and a periosteal instrument is used in a coronal pulling motion to separate the elastic fibers.

There is a compromised zone on the mandibular buccal aspect near the premolars by the mental foramen. The location of the foramen must be identified, and the periosteal incision should be placed cautiously using the inverse side of the scalpel blade, drawing a curve surrounding and continuing at the linear incision to protect the site during reflection and minimize the risk of paresthesia Fig. 10a–c.

The surgeon separates the muscle fibers in the lateral and bucco-coronal directions on the buccal aspect. In this particular area, magnification enables good execution Video 7.

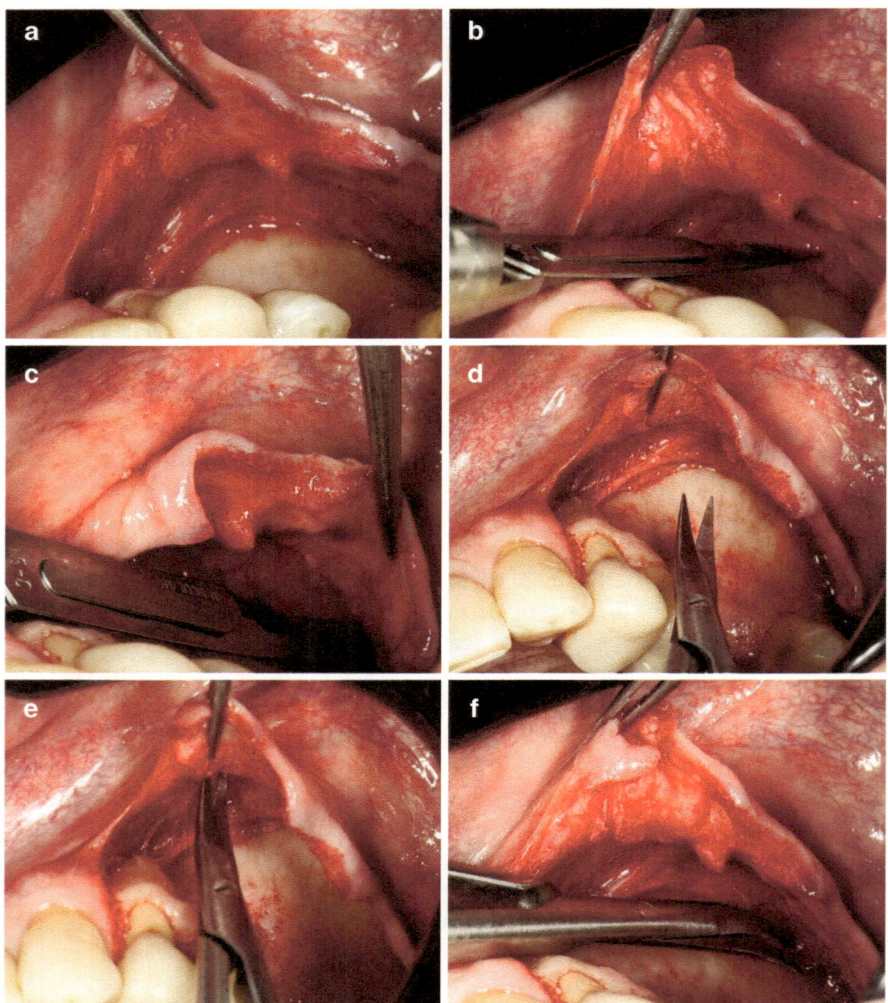

Fig. 9 (a–f) Secondary periosteal incisions and release of muscle fibers

The lingual area is considered high risk because of the anatomical structures and possible complications [47]. A microscope allows the observation of different tissues with a clear definition. Magnification aided by the coaxial light offers a clear image of the insertion of the mylohyoid for correct dissection and allowing careful manipulation around the neuro-lingual sublingual artery branching from the lingual artery in this area.

The molar area is located at the highest position of the buccal floor, closer to the neurovascular bundle. Thus, the mylohyoid muscle fibers are released using a blunt instrument with a soft movement in the coronal direction extending mesially. There

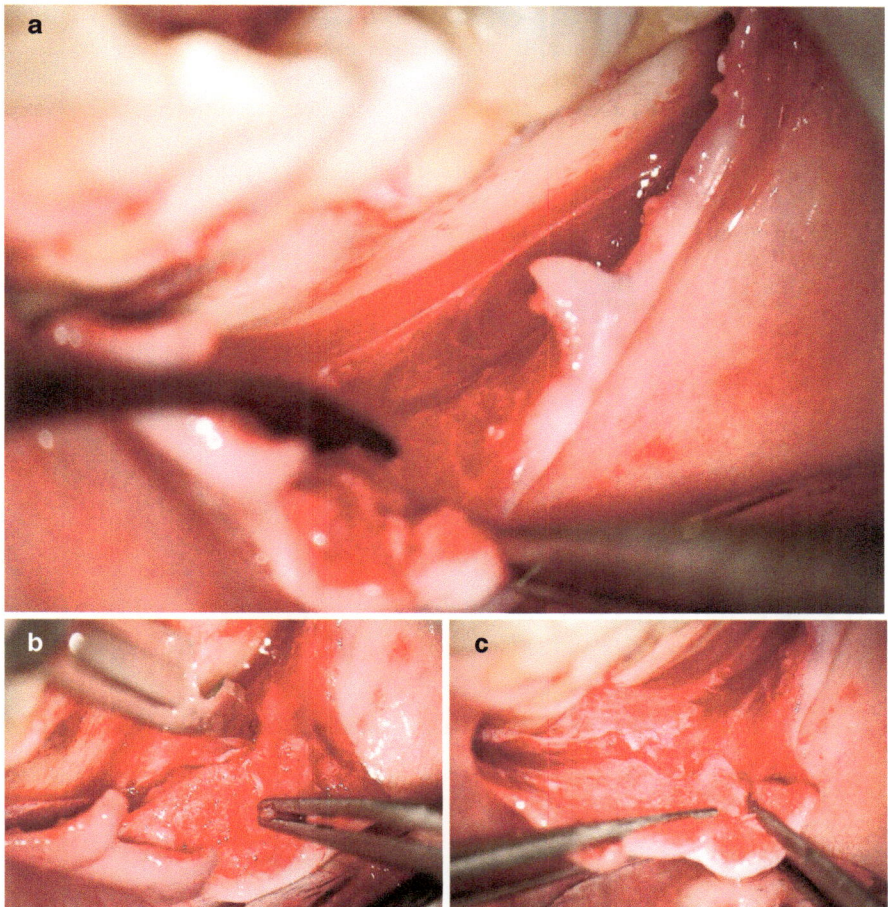

Fig. 10 (**a–c**) Secondary periosteal incisions and release of muscle fibers in the mandibular premolar region

is a deep muscular insertion at the premolar level, and the surgeon may be able to release it with a soft sweeping motion in the coronal direction [41, 44].

Therefore, the effective release of the lingual muscle fibers will compensate for the limited release of the buccal flap in the mental nerve area, allowing flap closure [44, 47].

Another option for lingual flap release in the posterior mandibular region is to reflect the flap using a wet gauze positioned between the osseous and the soft tissue, with moderate pressure over the gauze [48] (Video 8). Then, the mylohyoid muscle fibers can be gently separated, using posterior sweeping movements with a blunt instrument [48]. The adequate release of muscle fibers using any technique allows to obtain hemostatic control on reflection of the flap, which is another benefit of microsurgery and having support when inexperienced at high-risk procedures. The use of microscope significantly improves the surgeon's performance.

The palatal tissue does not have elastic properties. Therefore, its integrity must be preserved during the separation. Inappropriate manipulation can damage the tissue, complicating closure. The anatomical situation contributes to the increased difficulty. Thus, the surgeon must treat the anterior and posterior zones differently. The buccal tissues move palatally during closure because the density and insertion of the palatal mucosa prevents its displacement. A double internal incision can be made on the palatal area to allow the rotation of the underlying connective tissue in a coronal direction to aid flap closure [43, 48] (Figs. 11, 12, 13, 14, 15, 16, 17, 18, 19, 20, 21, 22).

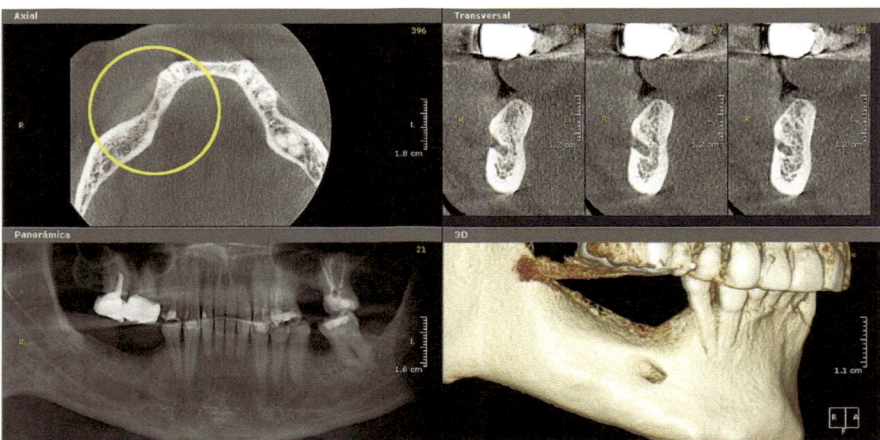

Fig. 11 Axial, transverse, panoramic, and 3D cone beam images showing apico-coronal and buccolingual deficiencies in the right posterior region of the mandibular alveolar process

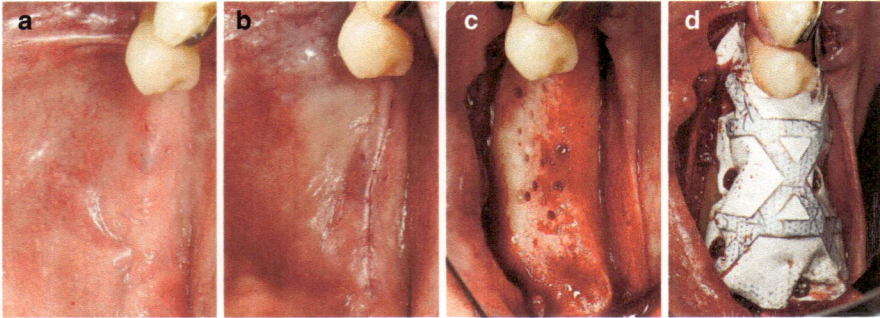

Fig. 12 Occlusal microsurgical guided bone regeneration in the right posterior mandible. (**a**) Preoperative image. (**b**) Primary incision (supracrestal). (**c**) Buccal and lingual microsurgical release and bone screening. (**d**) Graft placement (autologous and deproteinized bovine bone and placement of a nonabsorbable PTFE ™ dense, titanium-reinforced Cytoplast ™ membrane, with Pro-fix ™ fixation system screws)

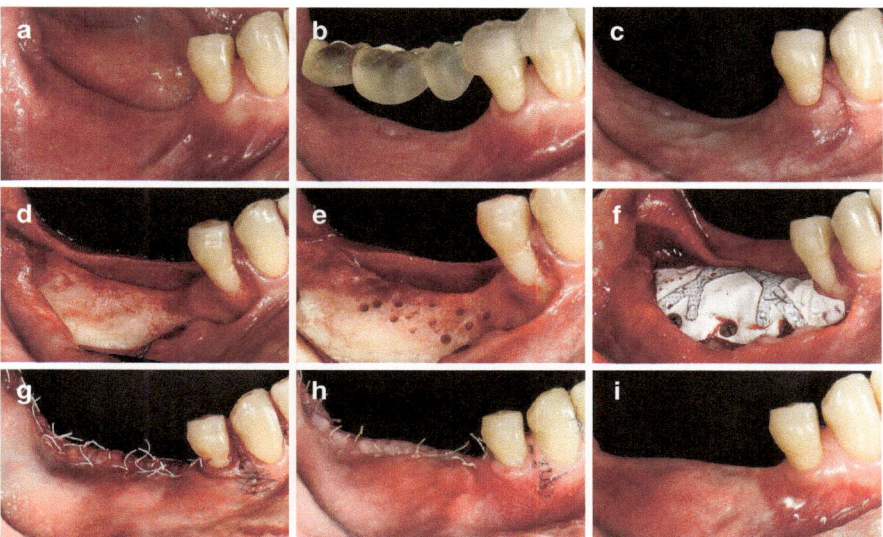

Fig. 13 Intraoral microsurgical guided bone regeneration of the right posterior mandible. (**a**) Initial image of the defect in the posterior right mandible. (**b**) Surgical guide. (**c**) Buccal view: primary (supracrestal) and secondary (vertical) incisions. (**d**) Buccal and lingual microsurgical release. (**e**) Bone screening. (**f**) Buccal view: graft placement (autologous and deproteinized bovine bone and placement of cytoplast™ dense non-absorbable PTFE™ membrane reinforced with titanium, with Pro-fix™ fixation system screws). (**g**) Flap closure at the primary incision with horizontal mattress sutures and individual interrupted knots, complemented with individual microsurgical knots for closure along the vertical incisions. (**h**) After 2 weeks of healing. (**i**) After 6 weeks of healing

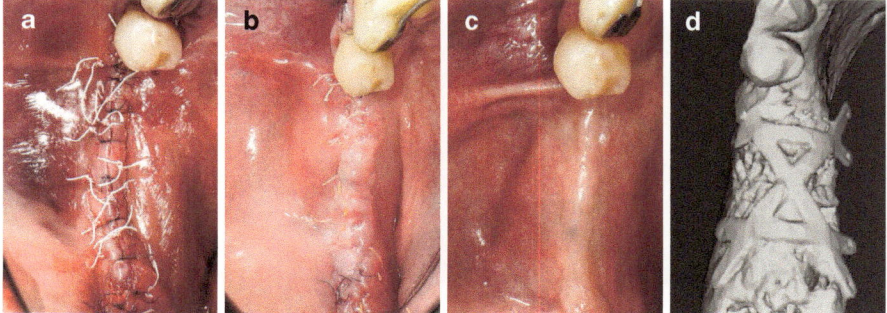

Fig. 14 Occlusal microsurgical guided bone regeneration of the right posterior mandible. (**a**) Flap closure at the primary incision with horizontal mattress sutures and individual interrupted knots, complemented with individual microsurgical knots. (**b**) Occlusal view after 2 weeks of healing. (**c**) Occlusal view 6 weeks into healing. (**d**) Digital imaging for guided surgical treatment planning

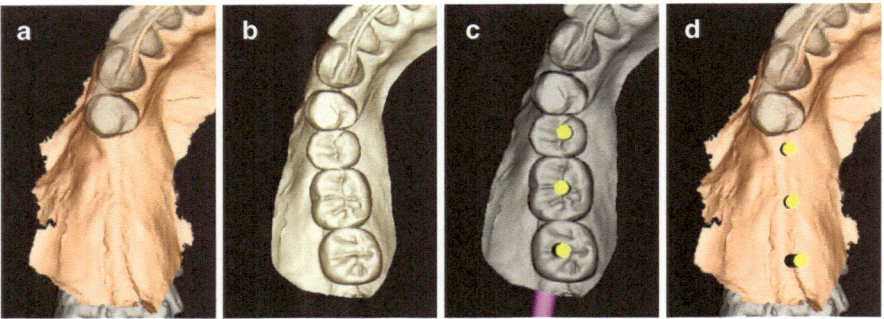

Fig. 15 (**a–d**) Digital imaging for guided surgical treatment planning using coDiagnostiX™

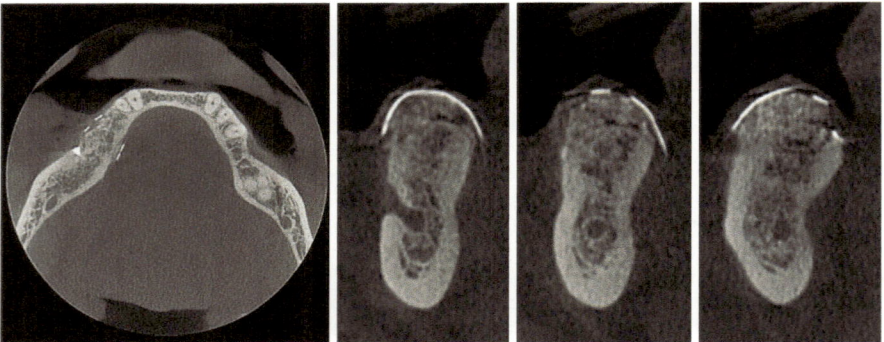

Fig. 16 Axial, sagittal, and 3D cone beam images showing an apico-coronal

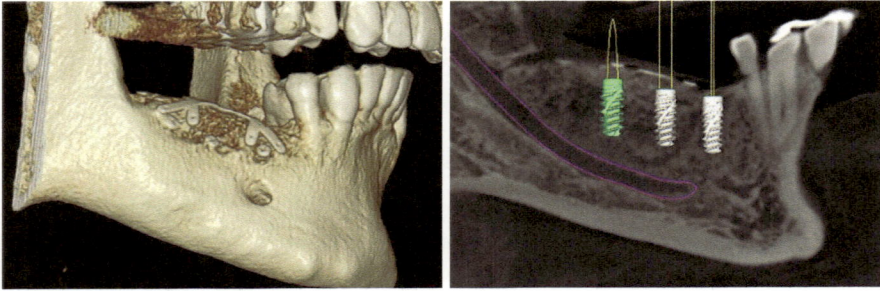

Fig. 17 Buccolingual gain in edentulous alveolar processes of the right posterior mandible and treatment planning using coDiagnostiX™

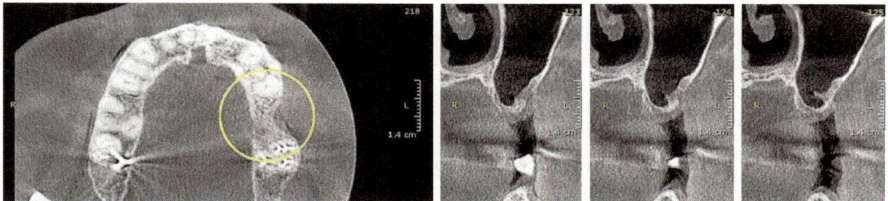

Fig. 18 Axial cone beam images showing bone loss in the bucco-palatal direction in the posterior maxilla, sagittal images with advanced vertical loss, and collapse of the maxillary sinus

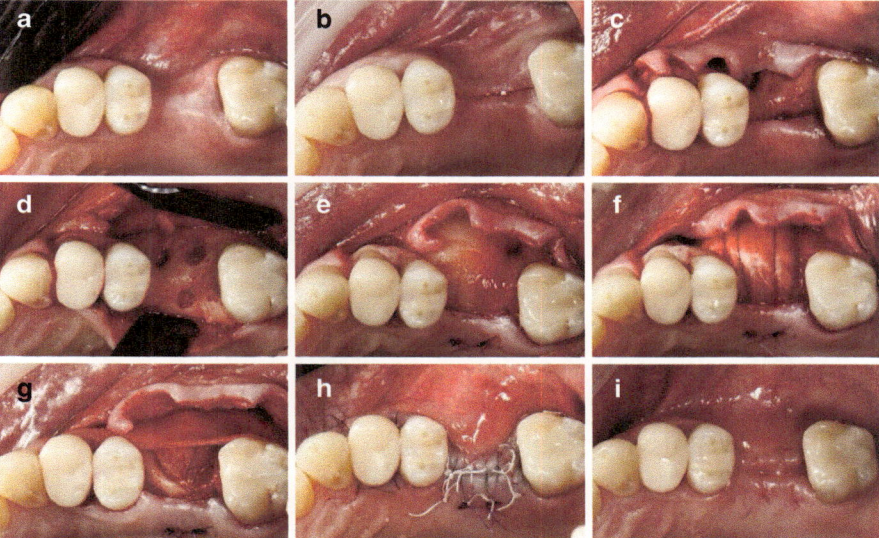

Fig. 19 Microsurgical guided bone regeneration. Occlusal views of the left posterior maxillary dentition. (**a**) Preoperative image. (**b**) Primary incision (supracrestal). (**c**) Buccal and palatal microsurgical release. (**d**) Occlusal view of receptor bed showing bone defects. (**e**) Placement of the autologous membrane of leucocyte and platelet-rich fibrin (L-PRF) on a mixture of xenograft (inorganic bovine Bio.Oss® cancellous bone substitute) and allograft Puros® cancellous particulate allograft bone. (**f**) Occlusal view of the long-lasting absorbable membrane (botiss Jasonz®), with horizontal suspensory sutures using absorbable Polyglycolic acid and caprolactone 5-0 (RESORBA®, Glycolon™ Manufacturing) sutures. (**g**) Management of soft tissue on regeneration using an allograft (acellular dermal matrix) placed before flap closure. (**h**) Flap closure at the primary incisions with horizontal mattress sutures and individual interrupted knots, complemented with individual microsurgical knots. (**i**) Occlusal view 2 weeks into healing

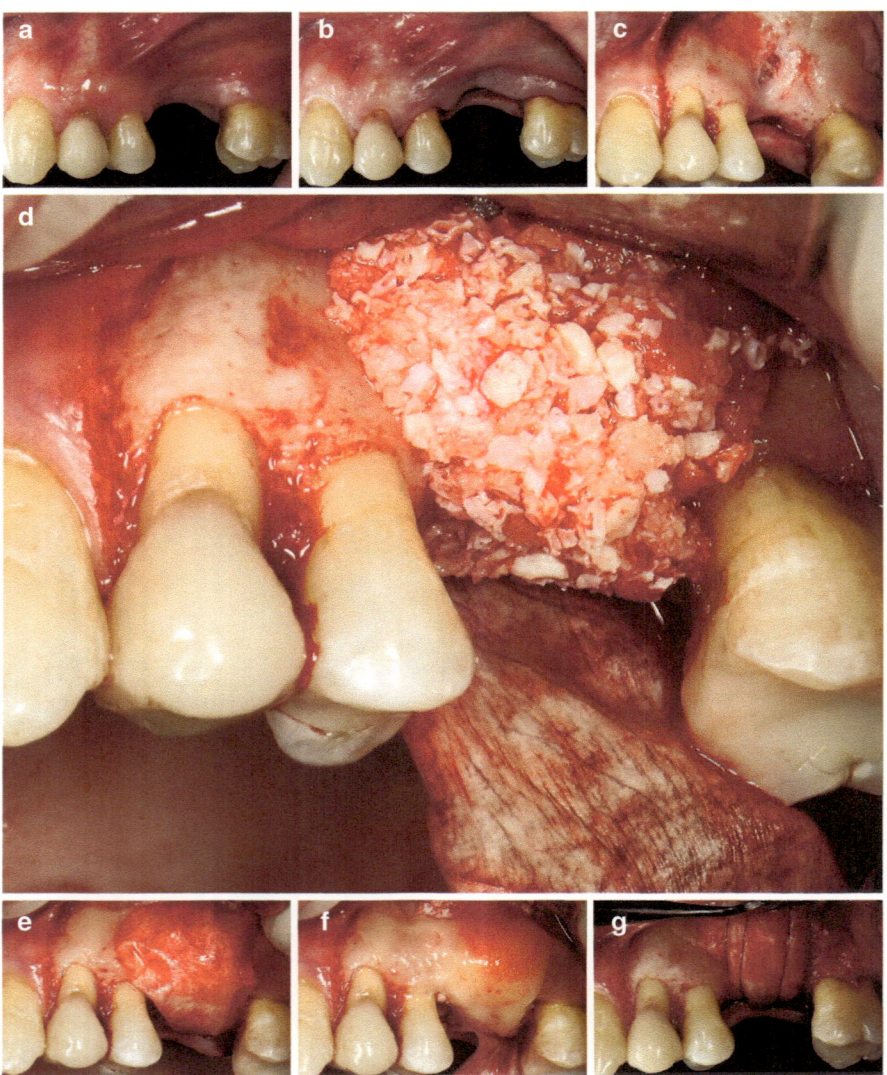

Fig. 20 Intraoral microsurgical guided bone regeneration. Buccal views of the left posterior maxillary dentition. (**a**) Initial image of the horizontal and vertical defect in the upper right first molar area. (**b**) Buccal view: crestal and vertical releasing incisions. (**c**) Elevation of a full-thickness mucoperiosteal flap reveals the receptor bed with bone fenestration communicating with the maxillary sinus. (**d**) Placement of xenograft (Bio.Oss® bovine inorganic spongious bone substitute), cancellous bone allograft (Puros®), and autologous membrane fibrin rich in crushed platelets (L-PRF) in a uniform mixture with adaptation to the bone defect before placement of the membrane. (**e**) Placement of an autologous membrane of L-PRF. (**f**) Placement of a long-lasting absorbable membrane (botiss Jasonz®). (**g**) Membrane fixation with horizontal suspensory sutures using resorbable suture of polyglycolic acid and caprolactone 5-0 (RESORBA®, Glycolon™ Manufacturing)

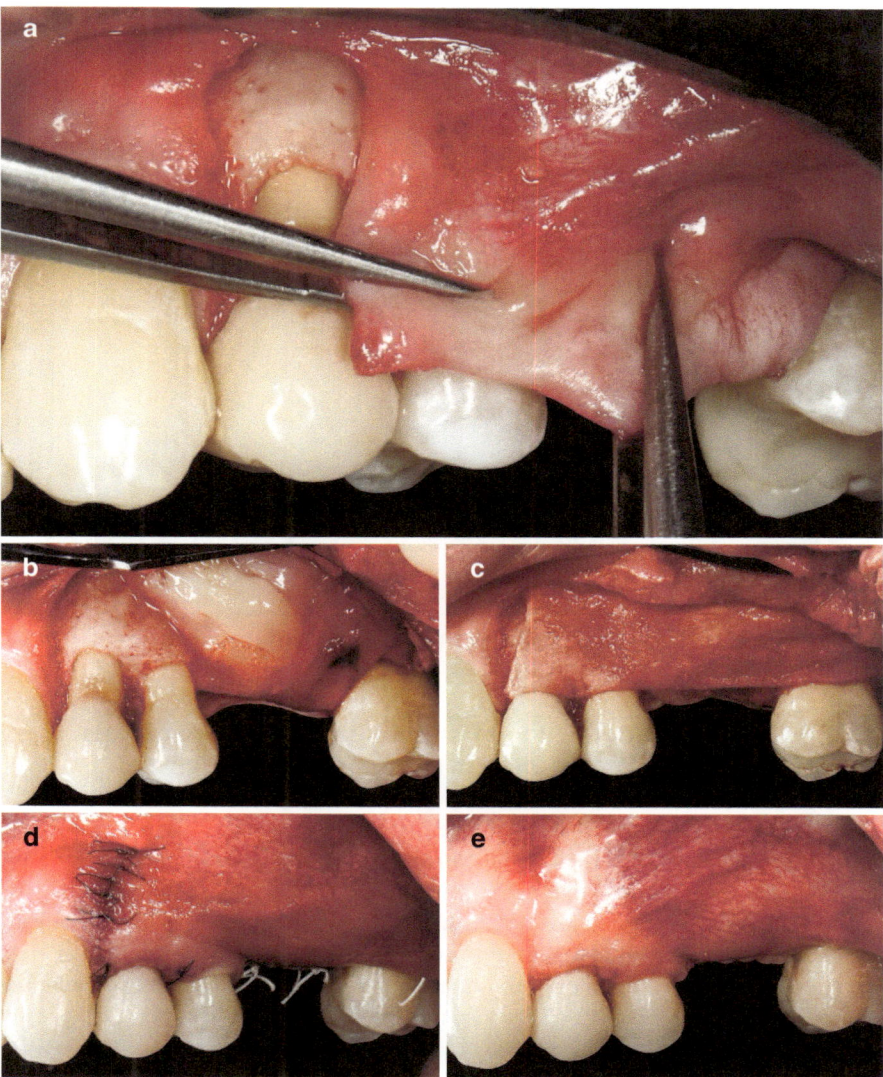

Fig. 21 (**a–e**) (**a**) The extension and release of the flap are verified by advancing it coronally. (**b**) Placement of an autologous membrane of leucocyte and platelet-rich fibrin (L-PRF) on the regenerative materials. (**c**) Soft tissue management by placement of an allograft (acellular dermal matrix) before closure and fixation with microsurgical (8-0) polyglycolic acid sutures. (**d**) Flap closure at the primary incisions with horizontal mattress sutures and individual interrupted knots, complemented with individual microsurgical knots for closure along the vertical incisions. (**e**) Buccal view 2 weeks postoperatively

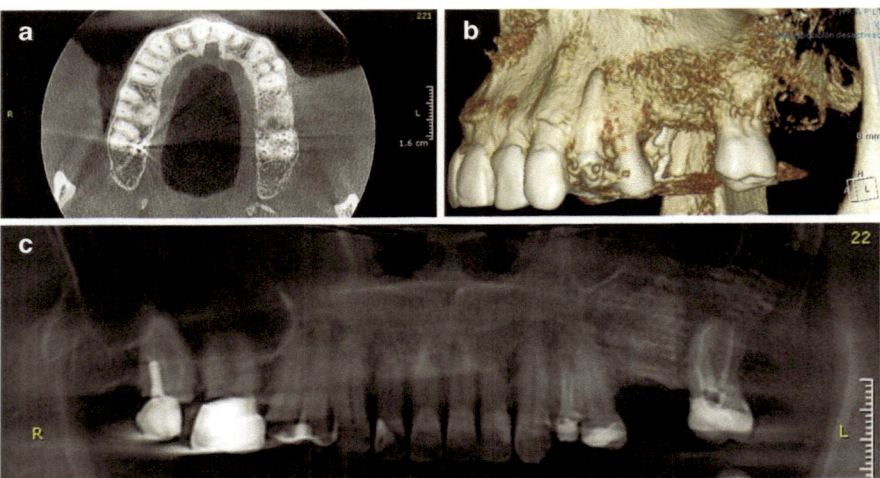

Fig. 22 (**a–c**) Cone beam images show the results of guided bone regeneration, with ridge gain in both directions and bone gain following sinus elevation

4 Special Considerations in Material Selection and Placement

4.1 Selection and Management of Regenerative Materials and Their Combination in Microsurgery

Impeccable management of regenerative materials is essential when working with microscopic techniques. The magnification and resulting optimum accuracy allow compliance with the strict biological principles for manipulation, autologous bone collection, mixture preparation, and membrane fixation. Material selection depends on the operator's approach to scientific evidence. The purpose of regenerative materials is to induce formation of high-quality bone tissue that allows osseointegration of the dental implants intended for masticatory use [49].

4.2 Autologous Bone Graft, Allografts, Xenografts, and Membranes

Intraoral autologous bone is considered the best grafting material, and its properties comply with the primordial biological requirements of regeneration, such as osteogenesis, osteoconduction, and osteoinduction [50] Fig. 23a. A donor site is required, and the graft is procured in the particulate form or as a block, depending on the selected technique. The posterior mandible is an ideal location to obtain the graft. However, there are also tuberosities, symphysis, mandibular tori, and peripheral supporting bone. Some instruments and attachments are ideal to effectively

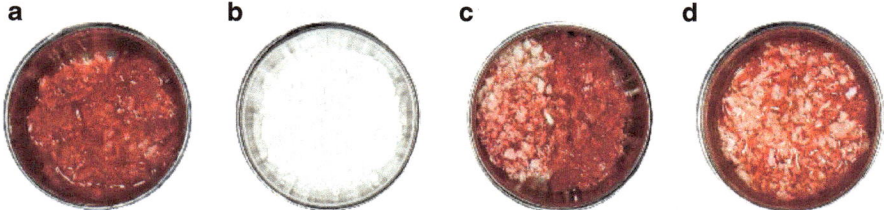

Fig. 23 (**a–d**) (**a**) Intraoral autologous bone graft. (**b**) Xenograft: inorganic bovine-mineral tissue, deproteinized and cancellous (Bio.Oss®) substitute for natural bone. (**c**) Mixed graft: mixture of autologous bone graft and xenograft inorganic bovine Bio.Oss®. (**d**) Sticky bone: mixture of autologous bone graft and xenograft inorganic bovine (Bio.Oss®) with crushed platelet-rich autologous membrane fibrin (L-PRF)

obtain particulate bone. Microscopic surgery aids in this approach by protecting the adjacent tissue and providing visibility, which helps to control the quantity of the bone material obtained. The experience of the technician is an essential factor to consider.

Autologous bone is the gold standard in bone regeneration. Nevertheless, literature also describes other bone-filling material options that prevent donor-site morbidity and are used in different clinical situations.

4.2.1 Xenografts

There is scientific evidence that supports the use of inorganic bovine bone as a substitute for natural bone. It has osteoinductive properties and provides a scaffold that aids bone formation with its orientation and structure. It is used for horizontal and vertical bone augmentation, preserving bone volume in the long term. Technological advancements have helped to develop this graft to facilitate biological interactions and subsequent bone regeneration [51]. The inorganic bovine-mineral tissue is deproteinized and cancellous, with a form and surface that favors contact with the blood clot and has internal interconnected channels that facilitate vascular and cellular growth Fig. 23b.

4.2.2 Allografts

Allografts obtained from a human cadaver are mineralized and demineralized, depending on the processing of the graft. They are used for GBR due to the osteoconductive property of the mineralized cancellous graft. Allografts have a high regenerative capacity. However, long-term bone gain requires further investigation, especially in relation to the stability of vertical augmentation.

4.2.3 Mixed Grafts

Hard evidence demonstrates that combining graft materials in different proportions, especially autologous and deproteinized bovine bone, offer satisfactory results, with predictable bone regeneration and high success rates for both horizontal and vertical bone augmentation [52–54]. Videos 9, 10, 11 and Figs. 23a–d and 24a, b.

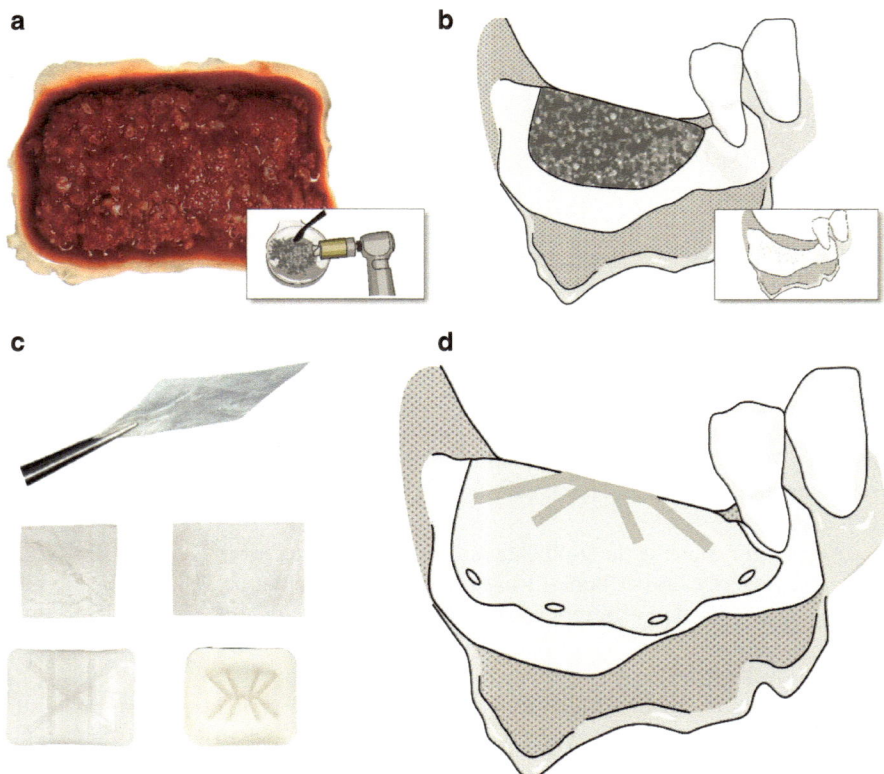

Fig. 24 (**a**.1) Sticky bone: mixture of autologous bone graft and xenograft inorganic bovine (Bio. Oss®) with crushed platelet-rich autologous membrane fibrin (L-PRF). (**a**.2) Trephine used to obtain autologous bone and its careful handling. (**b**.1) Placement of the graft (sticky bone) in the recipient bed. (**b**.2) Bone screening before graft placement. (**c**.1) Membranes can be resorbable and non-resorbable. Their selection is based on the defect morphology. (**d**) Example of fixation of a nonabsorbable membrane (nonabsorbable dense PTFE™ membrane reinforced with titanium with Pro-fix™ fixation system screws)

4.3   Use of Resorbable and Non-resorbable Membranes

Successful bone augmentation depends on four essential biological principles: wound closure, angiogenesis, maintenance, and wound stability [1].

The use of membranes in GBR depends on the principle of the exclusion of unwanted cells at the grafted site, creating a protected space for the blood clot-organized area, preventing collapse, and allowing migration of cellular osteoprogenitors and vessels, facilitating osteopromotion [4, 55, 56]. Membranes can be resorbable or non-resorbable and designed for simple management; they integrate with the surrounding tissue and allow nutrient permeation. The selection of the membrane depends on the size, morphology, and the severity of bone deficiency Fig. 24c, d.

Resorbable membranes with high biocompatibility integrate with tissues, improving vascularity for bone formation. They are easy to manage and are used in combination with particulate grafts in horizontal defects. There are different types of resorbable membranes: synthetic membranes, crosslinked collagen membranes with higher resorption times, and native collagen membrane with rapid biodegradation. Although indicated for horizontal defects, resorbable membranes can be used in unusual vertical defects, minimizing exposure risks [41, 53, 54].

Surgeons also use **non-resorbable membranes** for vertical augmentation treatments, where greater stability is required to support the graft. They maintain their structural integrity, require re-entry for removal, are biocompatible, and must be adequately adapted because they are susceptible to exposure complications. The standard membrane is composed of polytetrafluoroethylene (PTFE), high density or expanded. Titanium reinforcements are adequate for moderate to severe vertical augmentation [52, 55, 57].

4.4   Use of Dermis Allograft as Membrane

The use of acellular dermal matrix has been accepted for augmentation of soft tissues and is used in GRB to complement membranes for improvement of the soft tissues or as an occlusive membrane Videos 12, 13 and Fig. 25a–c. They offer rapid revascularization and cell growth and have a traditional method of fixation with tacks or suspensory sutures with additional microsurgical sutures to the

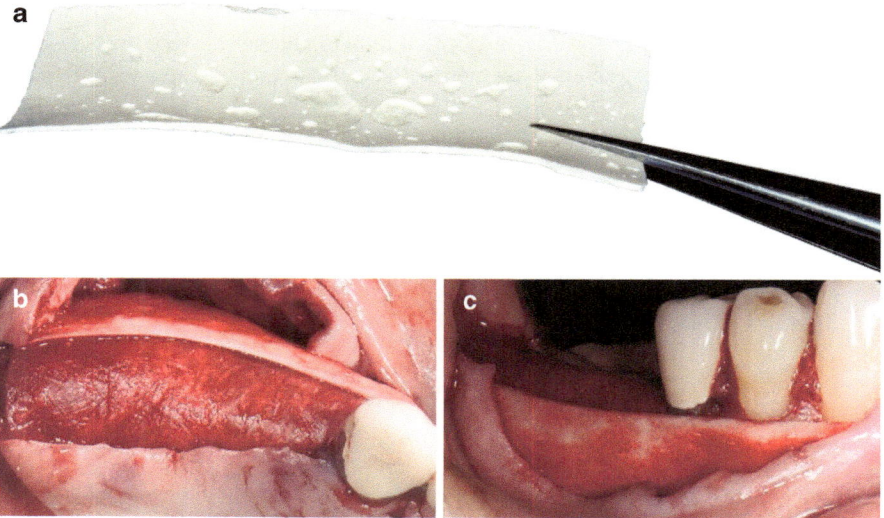

Fig. 25 (**a**) Acellular dermal matrix (AlloDerm™) for soft tissue application (**b, c**). Occlusal and buccal view: placement of the membrane for soft-tissue management in regenerative therapy

periosteum. Its use as a membrane has satisfactory results, with improved cicatrization patterns. However, further research is needed to support these observations [58, 59].

4.5 Use of Biologics

Biological mediators have received great acceptance in regenerative therapy. Different autologous blood concentrates increase the healing response for favorable results. Leucocyte and platelet-rich fibrin (L-PRF) is a commonly used mediator. It is a second-generation platelet concentrate used as a bone augmentation therapy adjunct. It offers continuous growth factors and other bioactive substances that protect and stimulate the surgical site; it can be used as a membrane, plug, or exudate, promoting tissue healing and imparting antibacterial effects [60–62]. The L-PRF has an application in periodontal therapy, in microsurgical bone augmentation, because of its biological properties. For example, the membranes can be sutured to cover grafts or regenerative materials, enabling close contact with the flap periosteum. It also protects the graft from complications, such as exposed membrane, and aids in soft tissue healing. The microsurgical suture preserves the integrity of the L-PRF membrane when fixed in the outermost area of the wound or bone clot during the first days of healing, and is used with composite bone grafts and *sticky bone*, among others, to offer stability and biological properties Videos 14, 15, 16 and Figs. 24a, 26e, 27c, 28, 29, 30, 31, 32, 33, 34, 35, 36, 37(e, g), 38, 39.

Other growth factors have gained attention in recent years. Development of tissue engineering has contributed to the use of biological factors that stimulate tissue formation in bone regeneration therapy. The safety and efficiency of the highly purified bioactive protein rhPDGF-BB (purified human platelet-derived growth factor) combined with an osteoinductive matrix (beta-tricalcium phosphate) GEM21S®

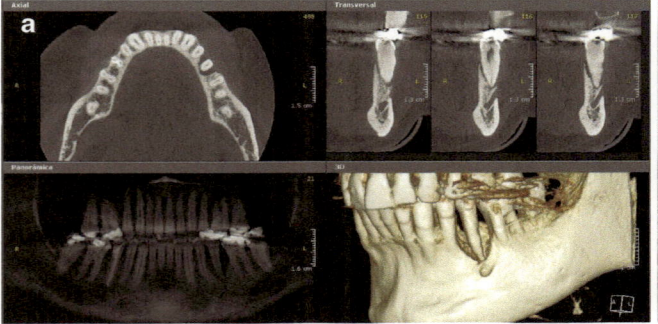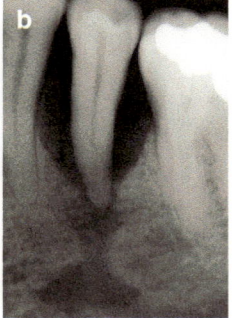

Fig. 26 (**a**) Axial, transverse, panoramic, and cone beam 3D images showing a severe vertical and horizontal defect in the lower left second premolar. Progressive bone loss is present close to the mental foramen. (**b**) Periapical radiograph shows the apical extent of the bone defect shaped like an hourglass

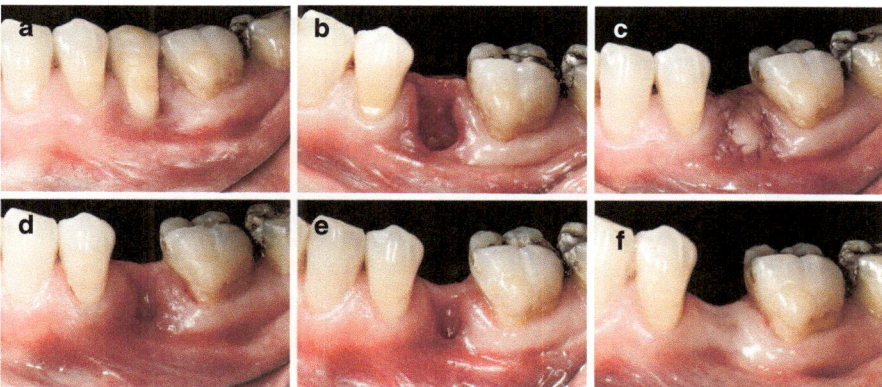

Fig. 27 Extraction of the lower left second premolar extraction and use of biological mediators with microsurgical techniques. (**a**) Preoperative image. (**b**) Result of the atraumatic extraction. (**c**) Fibrin plugs and membranes rich in leukocytes and platelets (L-PRF) are introduced into the alveolus and stabilized with a microsurgical suture. This helps preserve the integrity of the L-PRF membrane, maintaining its biological properties and promoting healing. (**d–f**) Buccal view two, four, and eight weeks into healing

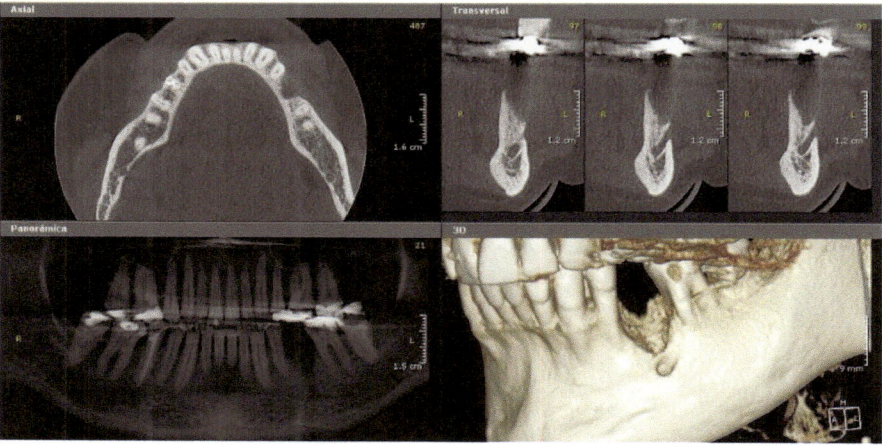

Fig. 28 The axial, transversal, panoramic, and cone beam 3D images show the residual post-extraction defect

Lynch Biologics, Franklin, TN 37064, has been demonstrated to cause a significant increase in regeneration, proliferation, and migration of osteoblasts and other periodontal cells.

The autogenous bone mixed with inorganic bovine bone-derived mineral (ABBM) and rhPDGF-BB has demonstrated significant potential for bone regeneration [63–65].

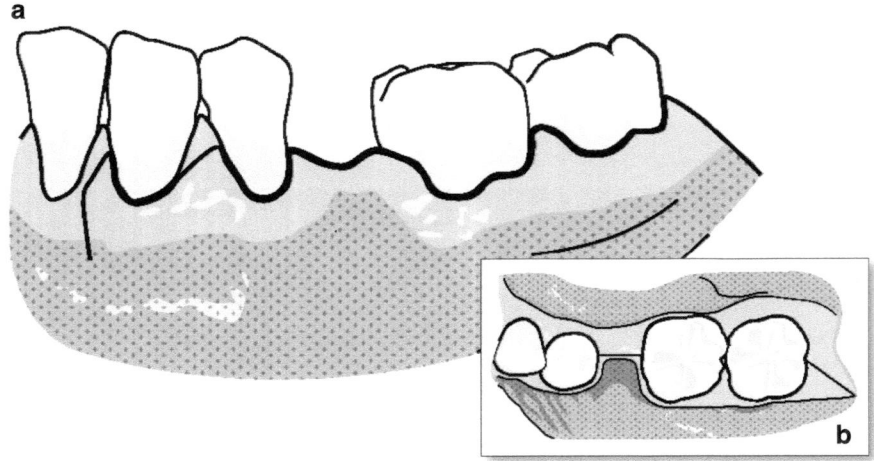

Fig. 29 (**a**, **b**) Design of the flap: primary incision and horizontal and vertical releasing incisions

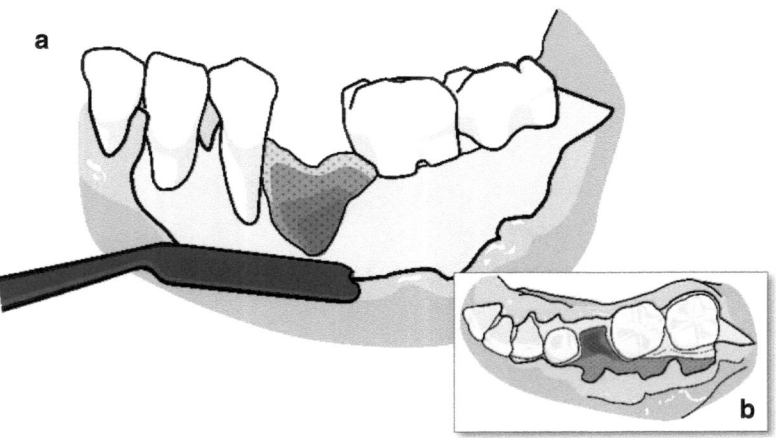

Fig. 30 (**a**, **b**) Full-thickness buccal and lingual flaps elevated to expose the deficient ridge

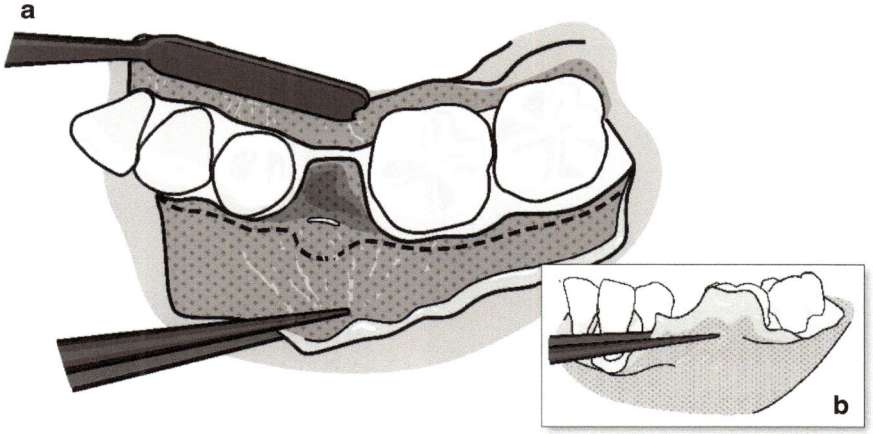

Fig. 31 (**a, b**) The drawings represent the line of the periosteal incision protecting the mental foramen area and the flexibility of the buccal flap after flap release

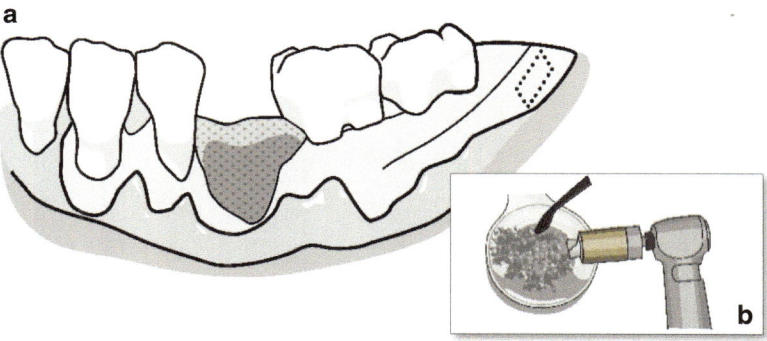

Fig. 32 (**a, b**) Representation of bone extraction from the mandibular ramus, which is an ideal donor site for autologous graft

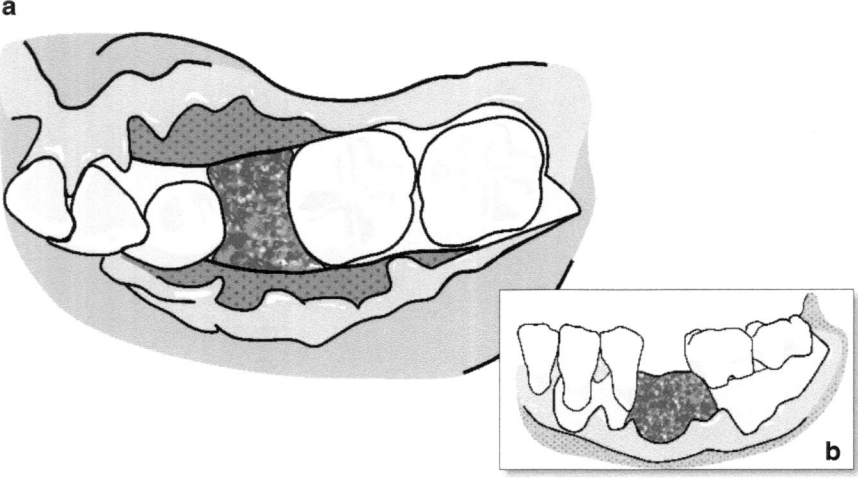

Fig. 33 (**a**, **b**) Placement of the graft (sticky bone) at the recipient bed

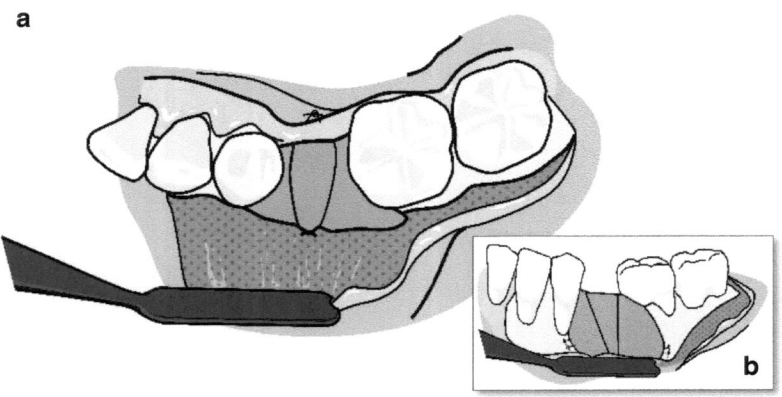

Fig. 34 (**a**, **b**) Membrane fixation with horizontal suspensory sutures, complementing the apical fixation with small-caliber microsurgical sutures (8-0, 9-0)

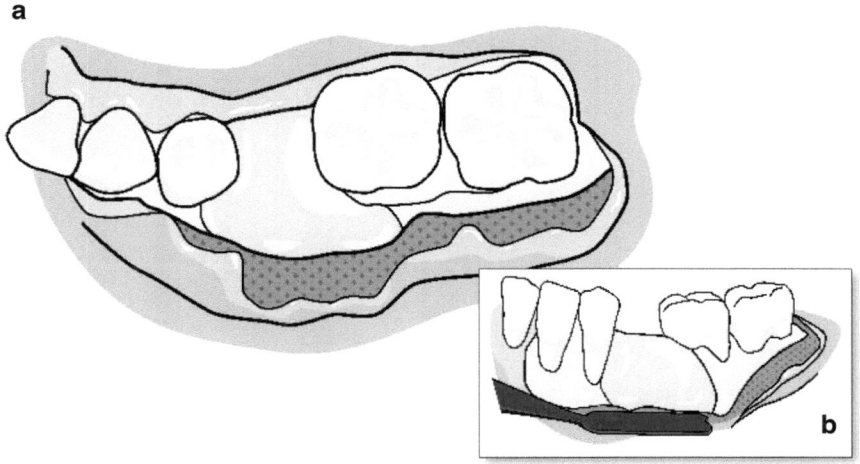

Fig. 35 (**a, b**) Placement of the L-PRF membrane over the regenerative materials before suturing of the microsurgical flap

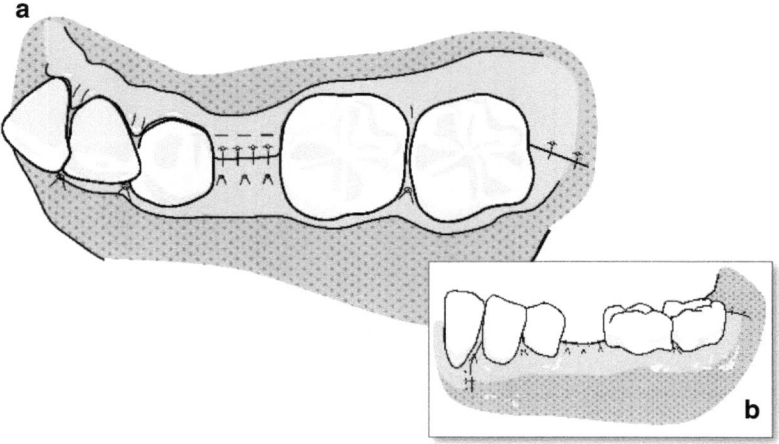

Fig. 36 (**a, b**) The main incision is closed with horizontal suspension mattress sutures, and interrupted sutures achieve optimal soft tissue closure. Interrupted microsurgical knots are placed along the vertical incisions

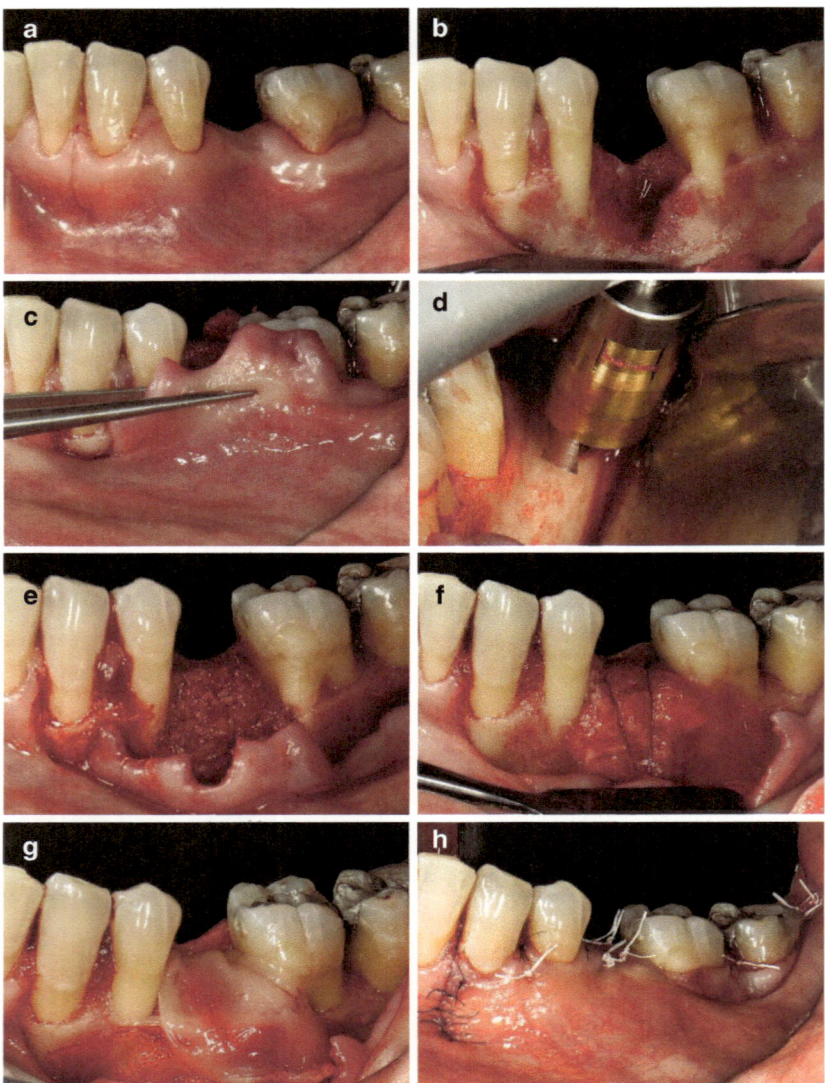

Fig. 37 Microsurgical guided bone regeneration images in a severe vertical-horizontal defect in the lower left second premolar region. (**a**) Primary incision and horizontal and vertical release incisions. (**b**) Microsurgical reflection. (**c**) The extension and release of the flap is verified by advancing it coronally. (**d**) Extraction of autologous bone from the mandibular branch. (**e**) Placement of the mixture of autologous bone and xenograft (Bio.Oss® bovine inorganic cancellous bone substitute) with autologous membrane L-PRF (sticky bone). (**f**) Placement of a long-lasting absorbable membrane (botiss Jasonz®). Membrane fixation with horizontal suspensory sutures using resorbable polyglycolic acid and caprolactone 5-0 sutures (RESORBA®, Glycolon™) complementing the apical fixation with small-caliber polyglycolic acid microsurgical sutures (8-0, 9-0). (**g**) Placement of an autologous membrane (L-PRF) on regenerative materials. (**h**) The main incision is closed with horizontal suspension mattress sutures, and interrupted sutures achieve optimal soft tissue closure. Interrupted microsurgical knots are placed along the vertical incisions

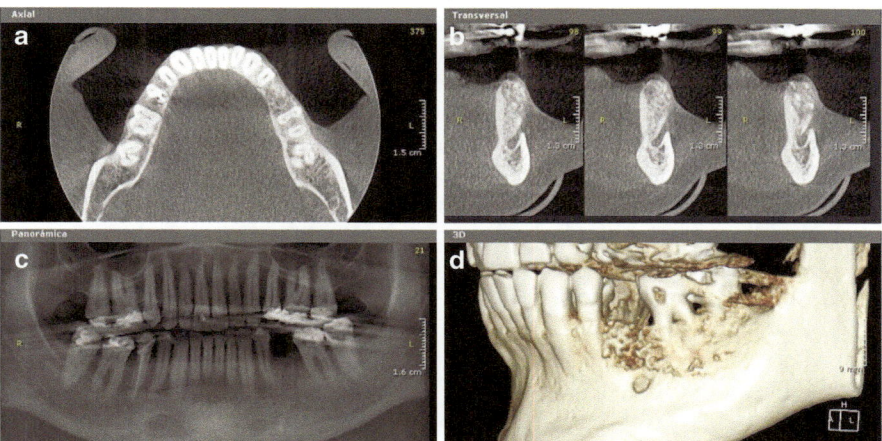

Fig. 38 (**a–d**) Axial, cross-sectional, panoramic, and cone beam 3D images showed healing 6 months after guided bone regeneration

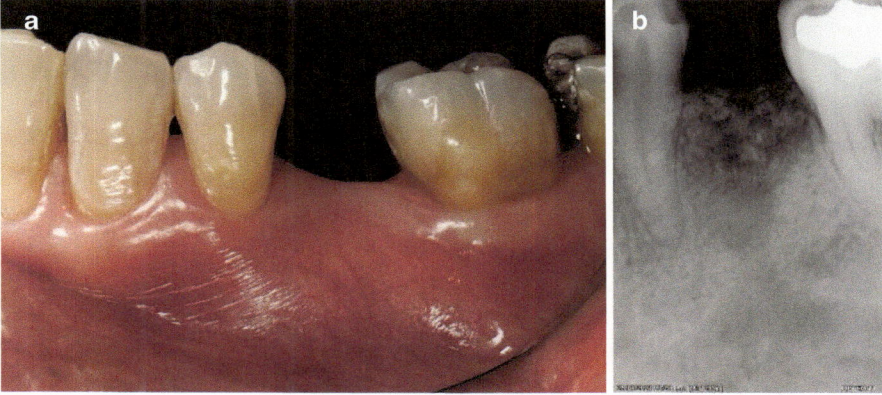

Fig. 39 (**a**) Six months following microsurgical regenerative therapy. (**b**) Progress of graft maturation seen on periapical radiograph

4.6 Membrane-Fixation Microsurgical Techniques

Performing the removal of granulation tissue and decortication under the microscope helps prepare the recipient site [66]. Visualization with a microscope also facilitates membrane adaptation, when it completely covers the defect, perhaps even 1–2 mm more and prevents contact with adjacent teeth, improving membrane fixation.

Non-resorbable membranes have complex handling characteristics, especially for fixation on the lingual or palatal site. The microsurgical access offered for condensed graft placement, with adaptation to the defect, is followed by efficient apical fixation of the membrane. The clarity provided by the microscope enhances the concentration and performance of the microsurgeon during this surgical step. There are different fixation kits for membranes, including tacks or mini-screws placed manually or with a low-speed power unit Fig. 40.

Resorbable membranes can be fixated with tacks, [53] but with resorbable suspensory horizontal sutures is usually adequate with Polyglycolic acid and caprolactone 5-0 (Glycolon™ Manufacturing: RESORBA® Nürnberg, Germany). Polyglycolic acid microsurgical sutures of a small caliber (8-0, 9-0) (Manufacturing USIOL®, Kentucky, USA) can contribute to the apical fixation of the membrane, with individual knots to the periosteum. The microsurgical technique enables suturing of an autologous membrane, L-PRF, to the periosteum on the apical and the lateral aspects of the surgical site with resorbable extra-fine sutures Videos 17, 18, 19 and Figs. 41a, b, 42, 43a, b, 44a, b.

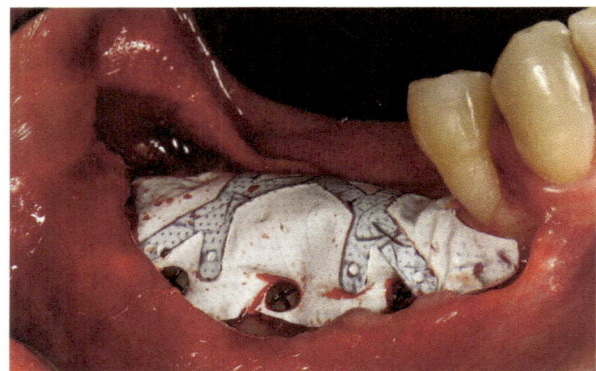

Fig. 40 Fixation of a non-resorbable PTFE™ membrane reinforced with titanium with screws from the Pro-fix™ fixation system

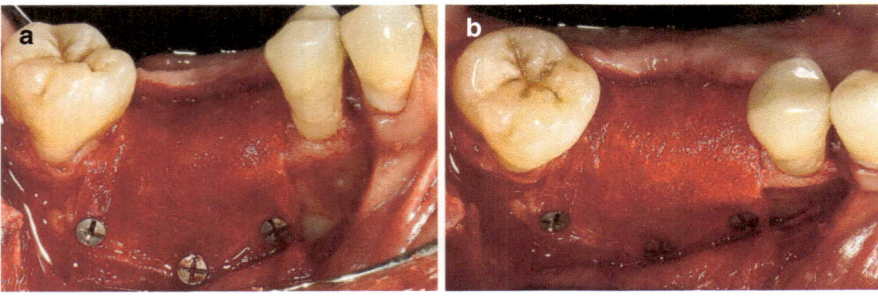

Fig. 41 (**a**, **b**) The buccal and occlusal images showed *Fixation* of absorbable membranes (BioMend Extend) with screws from the Pro-fix™ fixation system

Fig. 42 Resorbable membrane *fixation* (botiss Jasonz®) with suspensory sutures at the periosteum knotted on the palatal aspect of the flap

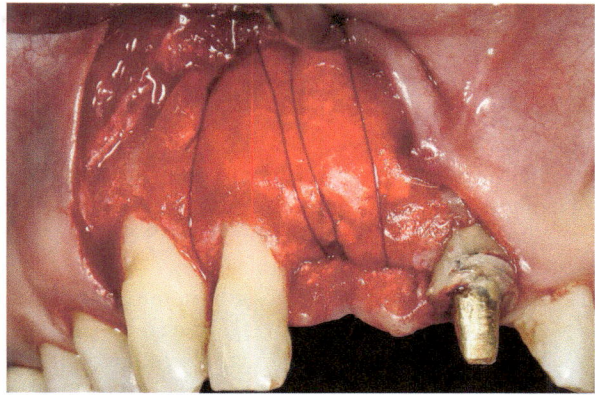

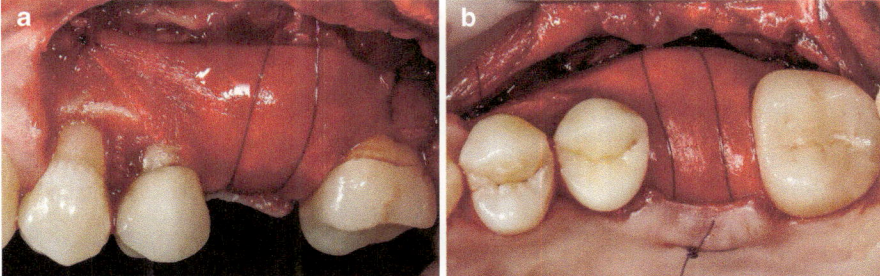

Fig. 43 (**a, b**). Buccal and occlusal views: resorbable membrane fixation (Geistlich Bio-Gide®) with suspensory suture to the periosteum complementing apical fixation with individual microsurgical knots

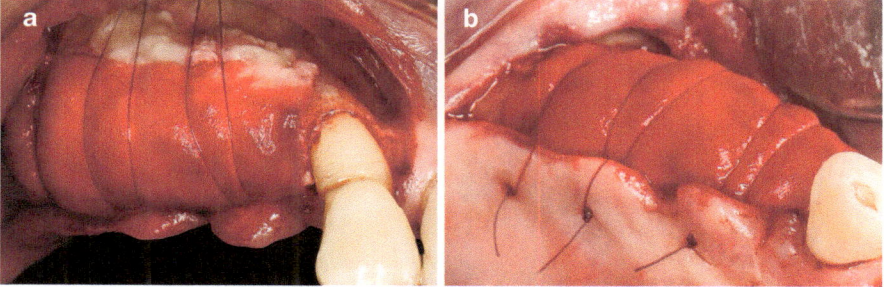

Fig. 44 (**a, b**) Buccal and palatal views: fixation of a resorbable membrane (Geistlich Bio-Gide®) with several vertical mattress sutures to the periosteum in a regenerative flap for vertical and horizontal augmentation in the posterior maxillary region

5   Microsurgical Sutures Specific to Bone Regeneration

A significant aspect of microsurgical GBR therapy is the primary closure of the wound; it is fundamental to preserving bone-graft integrity, thereby contributing to the success of the GBR procedure.

Suturing techniques in microsurgery require special instruments with unique handling characteristics. Active parts of these instruments help to place the microsurgical sutures and are approximately 18 cm long, with a design that provides support and comfort with controlled weight stability. The weight of any instrument should not exceed 20 g [17] to prevent muscle fatigue and allow balanced blocking forces while using the Castroviejo instruments.

These specifications assist the microsurgeon to effectively perform during flap closure. Also, the sutures of very small diameters are selected to reduce tissue trauma. The placement of sutures must be tension-free; when the tension exceeds during flap closure, the suture breaks [67]. Thus, the surgeon should use moderate force when tightening the knots to preserve the vascularity Figs. 45 and 46.

Fig. 45 The microsurgical instruments used in guided bone regeneration (Swiss Perio Kit for Hu-Friedy Selection Periodontal Microsurgery)

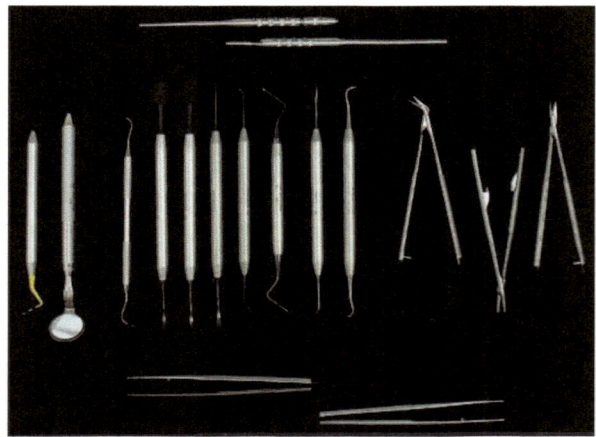

Fig. 46 The image shows a microsurgical needle holder with a correct grip, ensuring greater precision when suturing

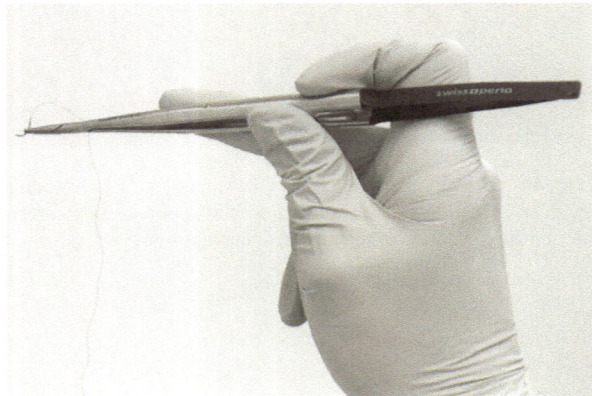

5.1   Microsurgical Knots [68]

The microsurgical approach to placing knots includes some crucial factors: ergonomic position of the microsurgeon, use of instruments with sufficient handgrip, adequate forearm support to reduce physiological tremor [69], suture material selection, and adequate tension handling. These are fundamental requirements of microsurgery.

The technique involves handling of the instruments with bimanual skill, using the dominant hand to support the microsurgical Castroviejo needle holder, and handling the microsurgical forceps with the other one. The needle, preferably of a fine diameter, is handled through the suture. A variety of knots exist; the knot with the *nomenclature 2 = 2,* used with microsurgical techniques, consists of one double loop to the right and one double loop to the left, completed by tying the part with a space created between the sutures in the central part of the knot [70].

This microsurgical knot (2 = 2) is placed across the vertical and horizontal incisions and with individual knots that complement suspensory sutures. These knots offer stability during wound healing, remaining intact during this period and providing resilience during the inflammatory processes related to healing. This microsurgical knot complies with the principles of periodontal microsurgery, and its advantages improve the effectiveness of GBR.

5.2   Suspensory Suture Technique

There is abundant scientific evidence to support the closure of the principal incision with suspensory horizontal mattress sutures in regenerative therapy. This suture is positioned on both the sides of the flap coronally, increasing the connective tissue contact on both sides and increasing the distance between the incision line and the membrane [44, 48, 50]. It is achieved by appropriately releasing the muscle fiber attachment to achieve passive displacement of the flap. Figure 47 presents the described technique. In addition to the required horizontal mattress, the regenerative flap receives a set of interrupted secondary sutures, microsurgical knots between

Fig. 47 Closure of the regenerative flap is performed with horizontal mattresses separated 3–4 mm from the incision, preferably within the keratinized tissue. Individual interrupted knots allow optimal soft tissue closure

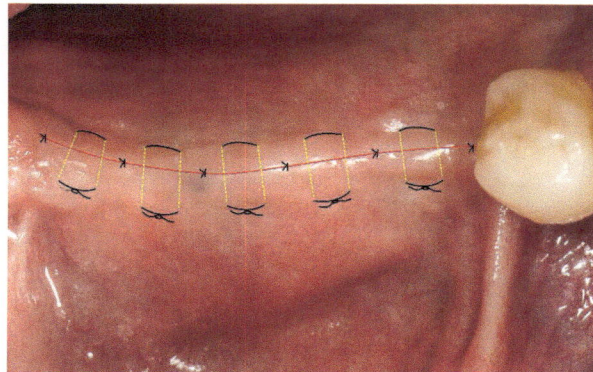

every individual knot to complement closure over the incision line Videos 20, 21 and Figs. 48 and 49.

The crossed horizontal mattress sutures are very effective in alveolar preservation regenerative therapy, complementing the individual microsurgical knots for closure. Video 22 and Figs. 50, 51, 52 and 53.

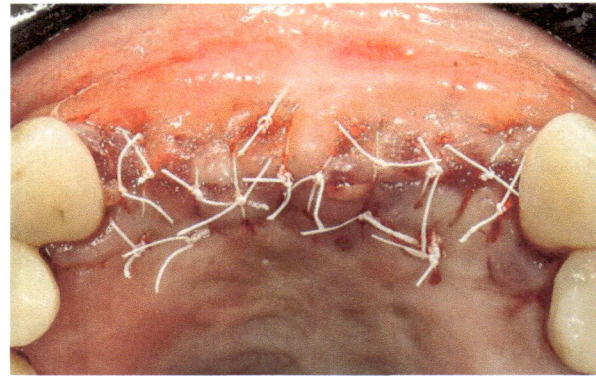

Fig. 48 The occlusal view shows the closure of the regenerative microsurgical flap with horizontal mattresses and interrupted individual knots

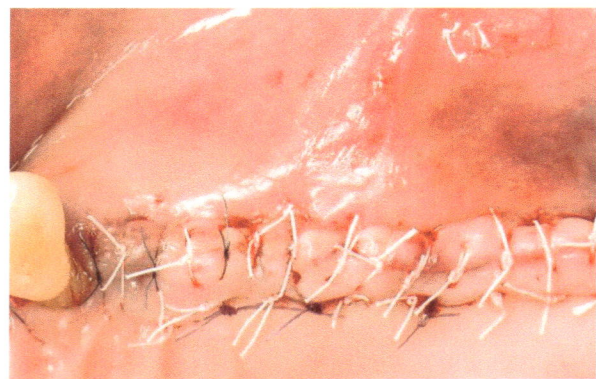

Fig. 49 Occlusal view of the tension-free flap closure using the double-layer suture technique, complemented with microsurgical sutures

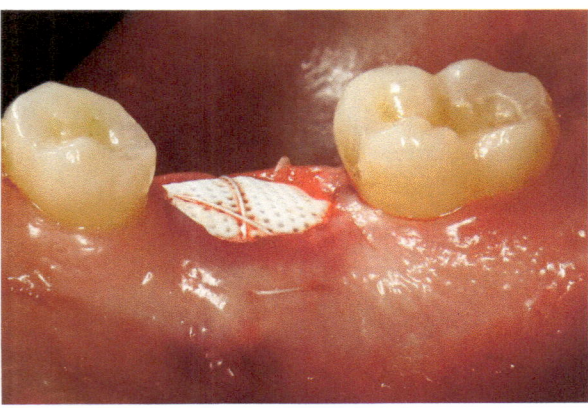

Fig. 50 Crossed horizontal mattress sutures for membrane *fixation* in microsurgical alveolar preservation therapy

Fig. 51 Occlusal images of bone preservation using microsurgical principles

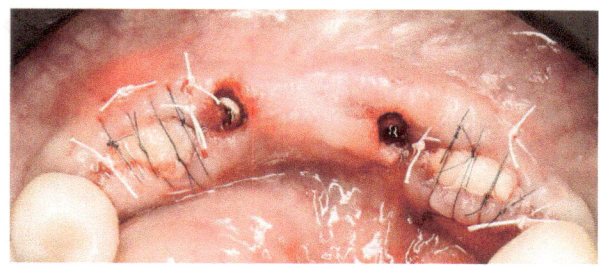

Fig. 52 Occlusal images of bone preservation using microsurgical principles

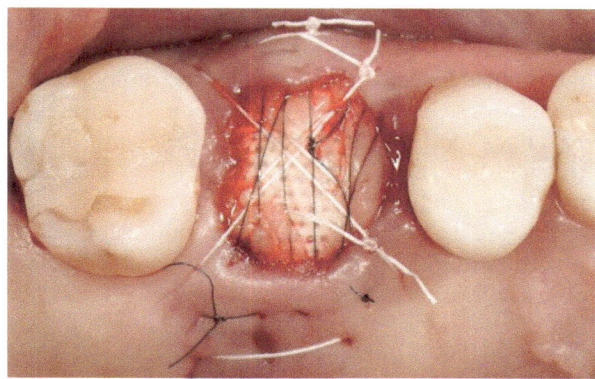

Fig. 53 Occlusal images of bone preservation using microsurgical principles

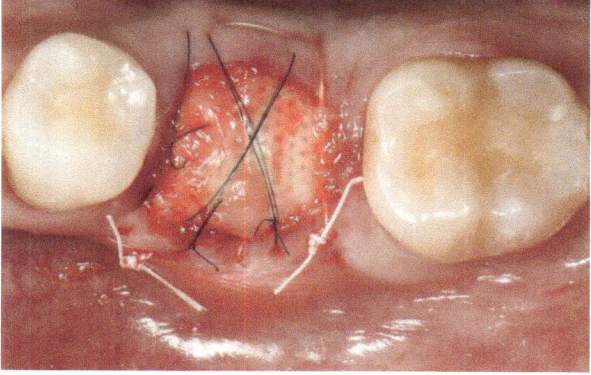

5.3   Different Suturing Materials

Knowledge of the biological aspects of different suturing materials, including their behavior and application, is part of preparation for microsurgery. The selected suturing material must be biocompatible, causing minimal tissue irritation and bacterial plaque accumulation. Suturing materials should have good quality and resistance, maintaining its strength until the wound has healed sufficiently to manage the tension with the help of the vascular changes in the healing tissue [22, 29, 67, 68].

The recommended suspensory suture for the primary incision (supra-ridge) is composed of PTFE (Cytoplast, manufactured by Osteogenics Biomedical, Inc., Texas, USA), which has all the required properties suitable for regenerative procedures, including strength and biocompatibility [44, 48, 50].

Surgeons can also use 6-0 nylon monofilament microsurgical sutures (Atramat®, manufactured by Obelis, Brussels, Belgium). For fragile tissues, 7-0 polyamide (Resolon™, manufactured by RESORBA® Nürnberg, Germany) and 3/8 reverse needles are both recommended.

According to the case, a second suture composed of interrupted knots can be placed with PTFE (Cytoplast) or monofilament 6-0 nylon (Atramat®). The microsurgical intermediate knots are placed using non-resorbable 7-0 polyamide (Resolon™). In the fragile tissues or critical areas, sutures are placed with even smaller needles than those described earlier, with 10-0 nylon threads (Atramat®).

A flap raised at an implant site for procedures aimed at gaining keratinized tissue and vestibular repositioning should be sutured with 7-0 polyamide (Resolon™), 8-0, 9-0 polyglycolic acid (USIOL®), or 5-0 glycolic acid copolymer and caprolactone (Glycolon™) sutures.

6   Post Microsurgical Management

Patient selection is essential and requires medical evaluation to determine health and adequate control of systemic diseases and oral hygiene. Smokers are required to quit smoking 1–2 weeks before the surgery and during the healing process (for a minimum of 3 weeks, and ideally for 6 weeks). Patients with a compromised medical status or a history of extensive surgeries under sedation are required to undergo hematic biometry, biochemical profile, and coagulation tests before surgery.

6.1   Postoperative Indications

Patients require a liquid diet for the first 72 h postoperatively, and sometimes for longer for patients who have undergone prolonged or complex surgery procedures.

A diet of soft foods should be administered for the following 10 days. The diet evolves according to the healing process.

During the first hours, patients are instructed to take bed rest and avoid facial muscle movement. Pausing activities that stimulate blood flow is essential, as is applying a cold dressing to the affected area 48–72 h after the surgery. Suspension of dental hygiene in the surgical and adjacent areas and the use of antiseptics are essential. Patients should use an antiseptic mouthwash with a neutral pH and an active substance including chlorine and oxygen (0.0015%) to contain the microbial spectrum. Also, rinsing with chlorhexidine gel or solution is prescribed for at least the first 15–21 days [71–73]. The surgeon usually prescribes amoxicillin with clavulanic acid (875/125 mg) once every 12 h for 7–10 days. In case of allergy to penicillin drugs, clindamycin is the next choice. Anti-inflammatory medication, such as potassium diclofenac, 50 ml every 12 h, starting the night before the microsurgery, is also prescribed. For prolonged surgeries, intravenous sedation with intake of steroid anti-inflammatories is recommended, and in cases of intra-operative pain, sublingual administration of 30 mg ketorolac is done.

6.2   Microsurgical Suture Removal

A microsurgical suture eliminates vertical incisions. Microsurgical knots across the main incision are evaluated using microscope magnification and removed on the fifth day under higher magnification, carefully cleaning the sutures before being cut to avoid introducing bacteria in the tissue. The suspensory sutures are removed between postoperative days 10 and 21 Video 23.

7   Microsurgical Management of Postoperative Complications

The risk of complications after microsurgery can be reduced by carefully following each step of the technique being performed. The use of microscopes helps achieve this, along with gentle handling of tissues, precision, realizing incisions, and protection of the periosteum. The suture must be placed tension-free, and materials that induce minimal tissue reaction are selected.

Membrane exposure is one of the most frequent complications affecting the outcomes of GBR procedures. In such a situation, the proliferation of pathogens can occur at the site of the failed regeneration [74]. Therefore, the surgeon should treat the incident immediately, following established protocols depending on the degree of exposure. Non-resorbable membrane exposures are more common and are classified according to the healing complications: Class I (<3 mm) and Class II (>3 mm), both without the presence of purulent exudate, can be treated locally with the application of chlorhexidine gel (0.12%) over the area 2–3 times a day [75]. Classes III and IV are advanced cases with infection; they require membrane elimination with antibiotic therapy. For the management of this complication, the author proposes the placement of an autologous L-PRF membrane over the exposed area and stabilizing it at the tissue surrounding the perforation by placing 8-0, 9-0 polyglycolic acid sutures (USIOL®). The results are usually observable within hours. For extensive exposures or development of infection, the surgeon must eliminate the contaminated membrane and place a native collagen resorbable membrane, placed over an autologous L-PRF membrane sutured as described above, with prescription of antibiotics and chlorhexidine gel for infection control Video 24.

8   Soft Tissue Management and Vestibular Repositioning After Bone Regeneration

Under ideal conditions, GBR provides the amount of bone necessary to comply with the clinical parameters of success. Peri-implant tissue health maintenance with low inflammation levels and stable marginal bone levels determine long-term graft integrity [76, 77]. Recent evidence describes total periodontium reconstruction, including that of soft tissue, in which combined augmentation of bone and soft tissue results in a positive inter-implant gingival contour [78]. Most analyses associate an increase in dental bacterial plaque accumulation with soft tissue inflammation, gingival recession, and marginal bone loss around implants when less than 2 mm of keratinized tissue is present [79–82]. However, controversy still exists regarding the role of soft tissue behavior, thickness, and height; keratinized tissue width; and their relation to these treatments. The treatment-related decisions are dependent on the surgeon's discretion. There is a specific clinical situation in which soft tissue augmentation with periodontal plastic surgery may be justified [83, 84]. The use of a surgical microscope has been described in periodontal plastic treatment before [17, 28]. This discipline is related to microsurgery as it requires technical finesse. We observe the benefits of this technology in soft tissue management using magnification. Evidence demonstrates that magnification increases the coordination between the surgeon's hand and arm motor muscles and improves cognitive abilities with training. These benefits increase on using microsurgical instruments and suturing materials designed to decrease trauma during tissue handling. In periodontal microsurgery, minimally invasive incisions reduce trauma, and using appropriate wound closure techniques prevents cellular necrosis, resulting in faster wound-healing as compared with macrosurgical procedures [22, 28].

8.1 Vestibular Deepening

The large displacement of the flap to achieve closure may result in vestibular loss and mucogingival alterations. Vestibular repositioning has a high degree of success when performed with simultaneous free gingival graft placement, which would result in a gain in keratinized tissue. The last step of GBR treatment precedes placement of the definite prosthesis, performed in the secondary stage or simultaneously with implantation if the technique allows it. Figures 54, 55, 56, 57, 58, 59, 60, 61, 62, 63, 64, 65a, b, 66a–c, 67a–j.

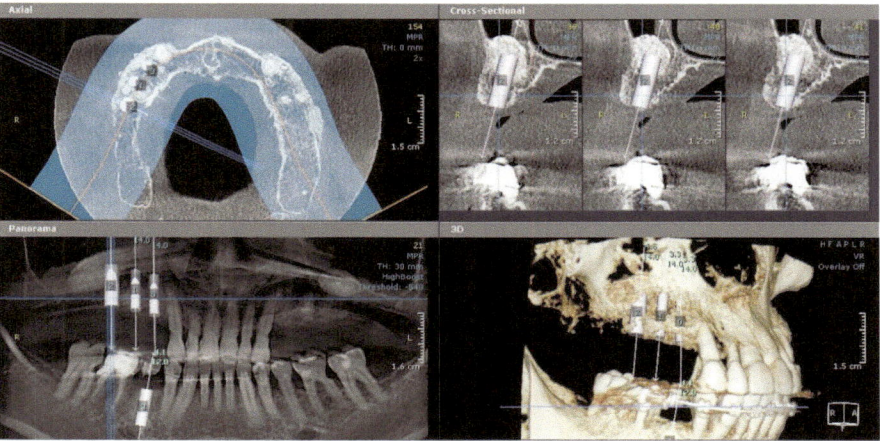

Fig. 54 Axial, cross-sectional, panoramic and cone beam 3D images demonstrating the results of guided bone regeneration, with maxillary sinus lift and planning for implant placement

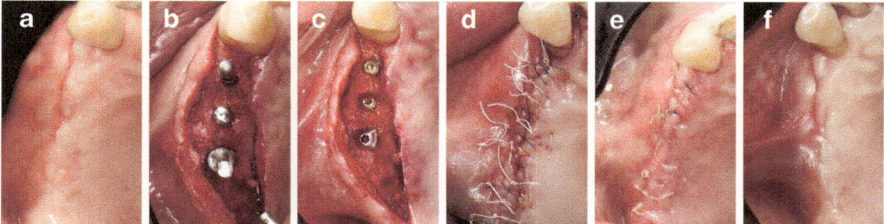

Fig. 55 (**a–f**) Occlusal images of implant placement surgery 9 months after microsurgical guided bone regeneration in the right posterior maxilla, showing a loss of vestibule with significant mucogingival distortion created by the surgical procedure

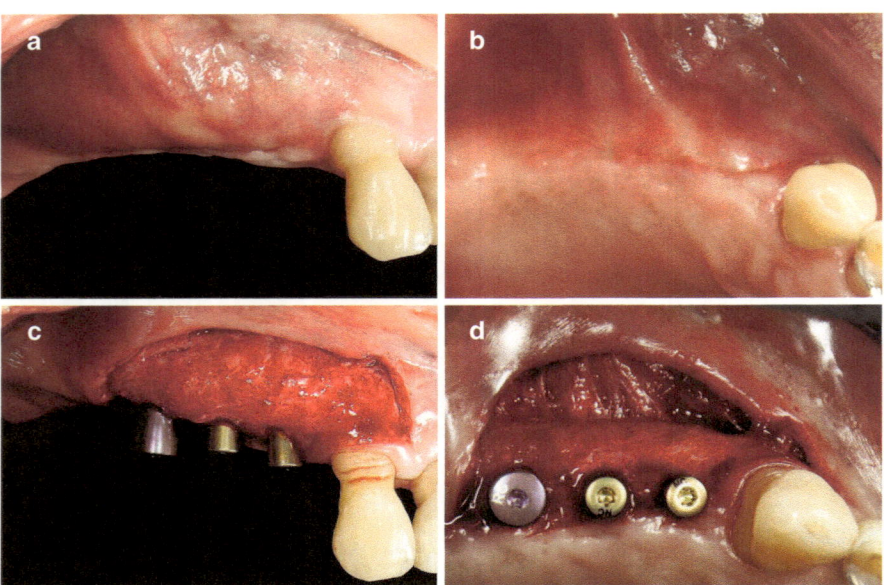

Fig. 56 (**a–d**) Soft tissue management and vestibular repositioning after bone regeneration. (**a, b**) Buccal and occlusal views show distortion of the mucogingival line after regenerative procedures and implant placement. (**c, d**) Buccal and occlusal views of microsurgical preparation of the surgical bed with a partial-thickness flap displacing the vestibule apically, with initiation of the incision on the occlusal aspect. Healing abutments were placed during second stage surgery

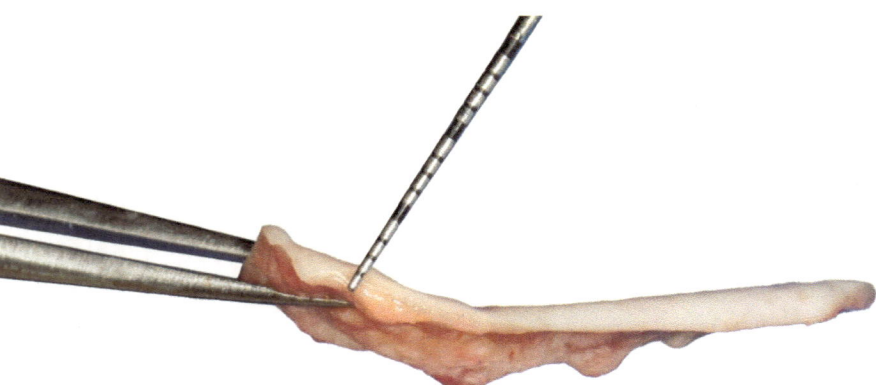

Fig. 57 Free gingival graft of an adequate thickness (less than 2 mm) obtained under magnification and trimmed for adaptation to the healing abutments

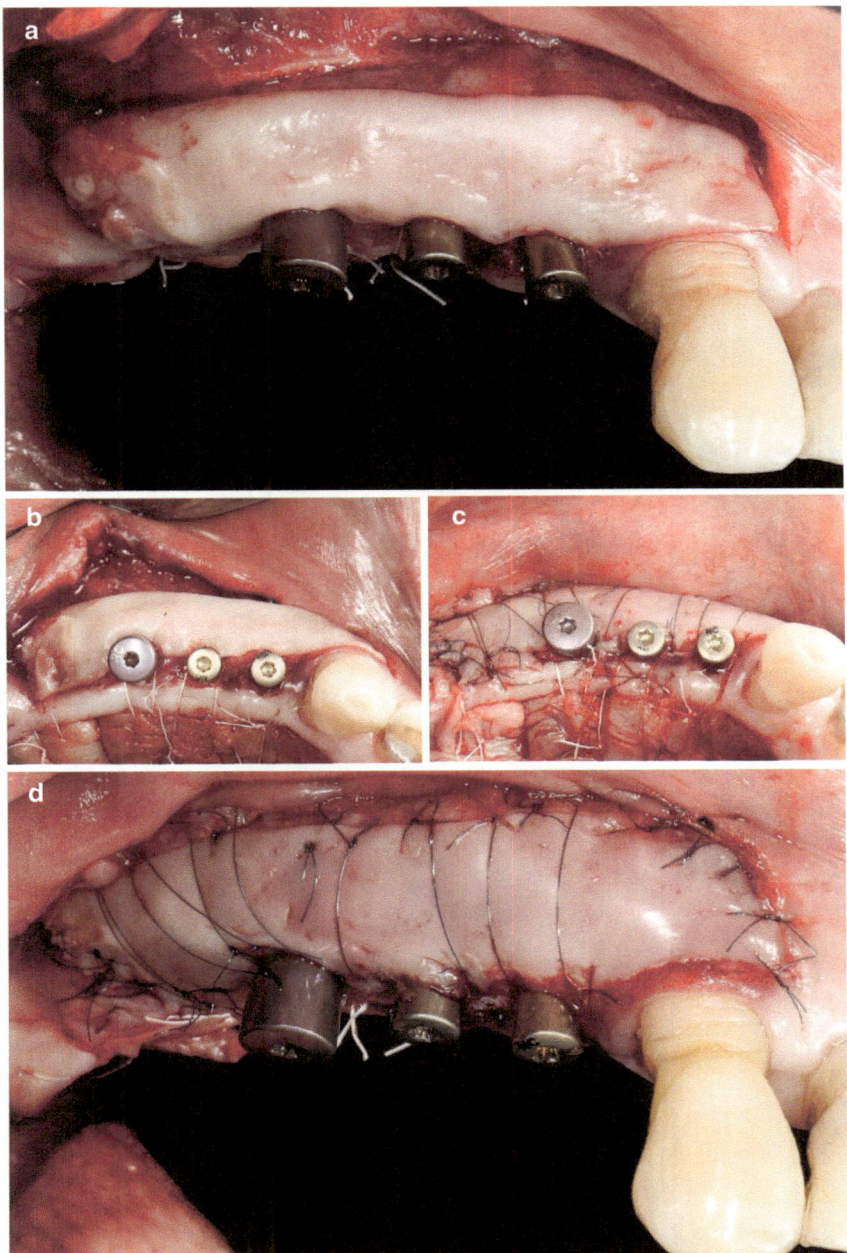

Fig. 58 (**a, b**). Buccal and occlusal images of free gingival graft placement, corroborating the extension and adaptation in the recipient site. (**c, d**). Buccal and occlusal view of graft stabilization with microsurgical suturing techniques using small-caliber polyamide 7-0 (Resolon™) and glycolic acid copolymer 5-0 and caprolactone (Glycolon™) sutures to the periosteum with apical displacement the vestibule

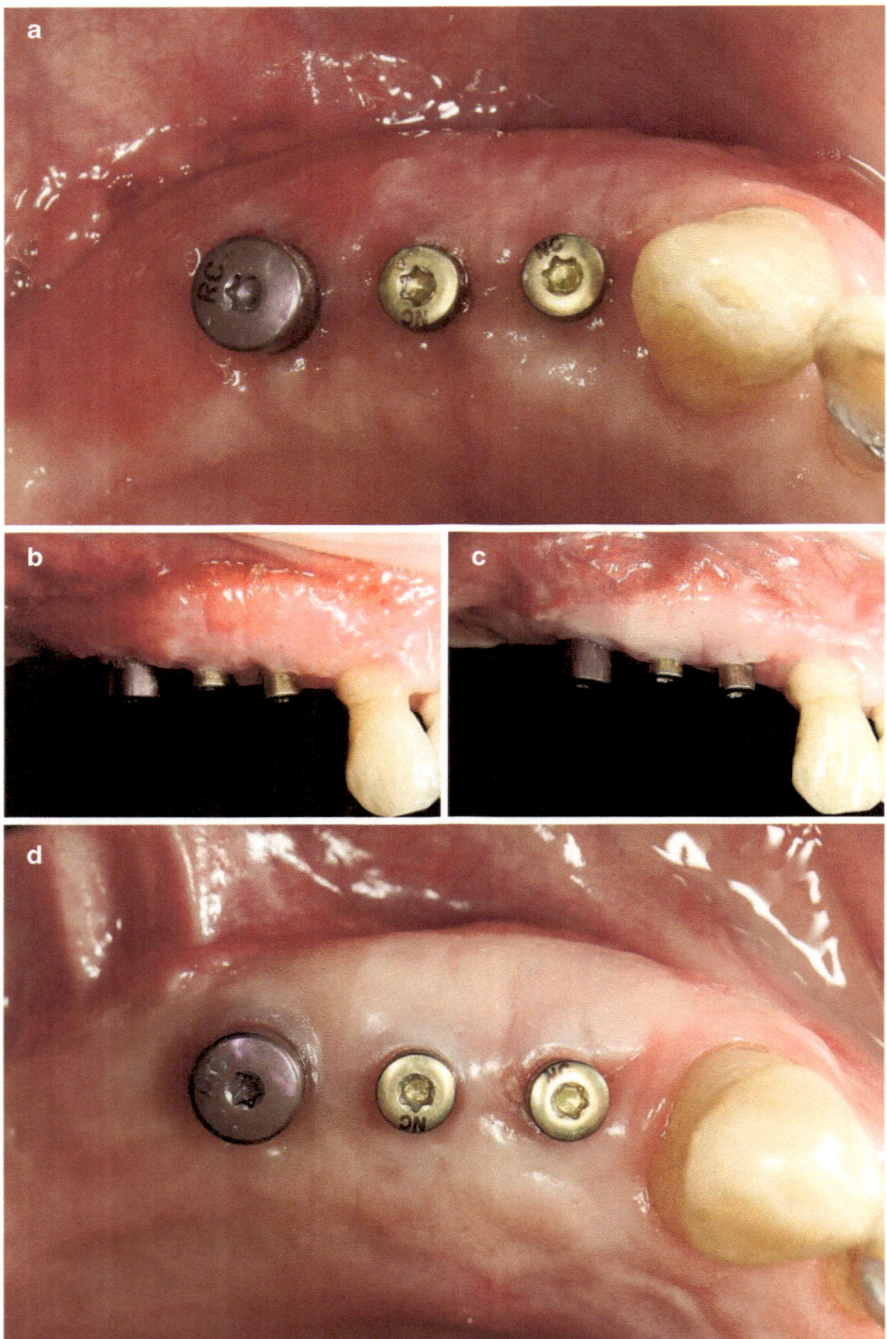

Fig. 59 (**a**, **b**). Buccal and occlusal images of the grafted site 3 weeks after graft placement. (**c**, **d**). Buccal and occlusal images show uniform integration of the graft 6 weeks postoperatively

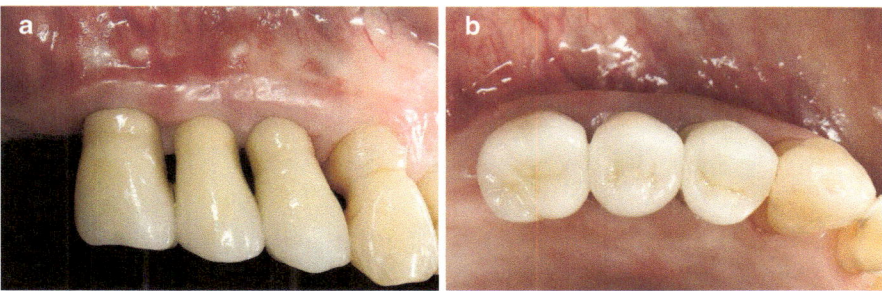

Fig. 60 (**a, b**) Buccal and occlusal views of the final restoration, vestibular repositioning, and soft tissue modification with increased keratinized tissue

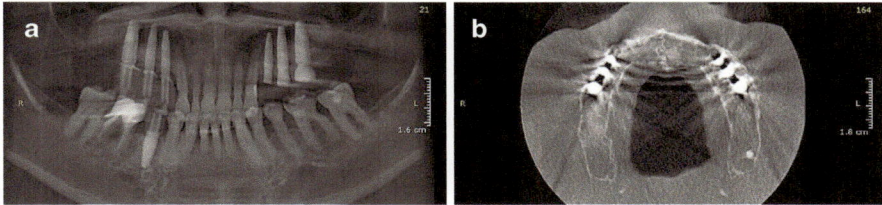

Fig. 61 (**a, b**) Panoramic and axial cone beam images showing the results of guided bone regeneration in posterior maxillary areas and planning for implant placement

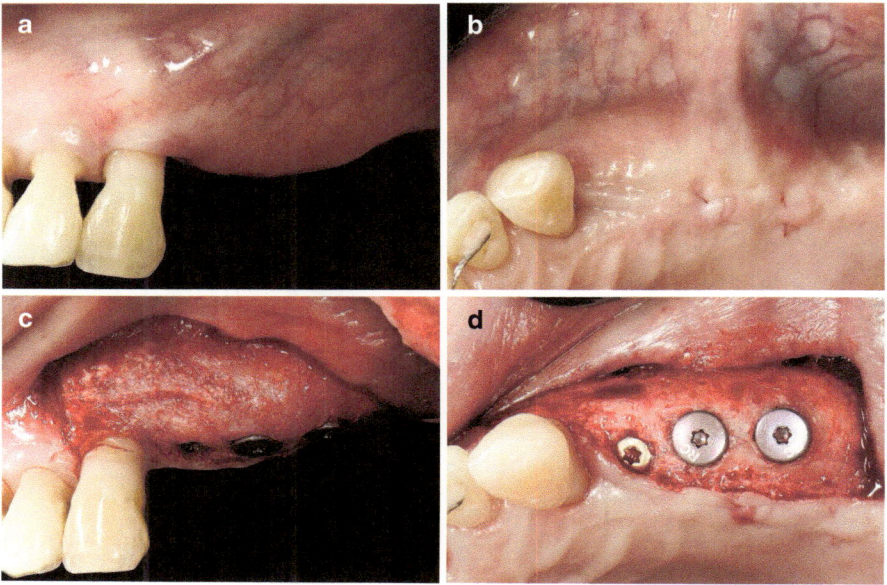

Fig. 62 (**a, b**). Buccal and occlusal views show distortion of the mucogingival line after regenerative procedures and implant placement in the left posterior maxilla. (**c, d**) Buccal and occlusal views of the microsurgical preparation of the surgical bed with a partial-thickness flap displacing the vestibule apically after initiating the incision in the occlusal aspect, performing the second stage by placing the healing abutments

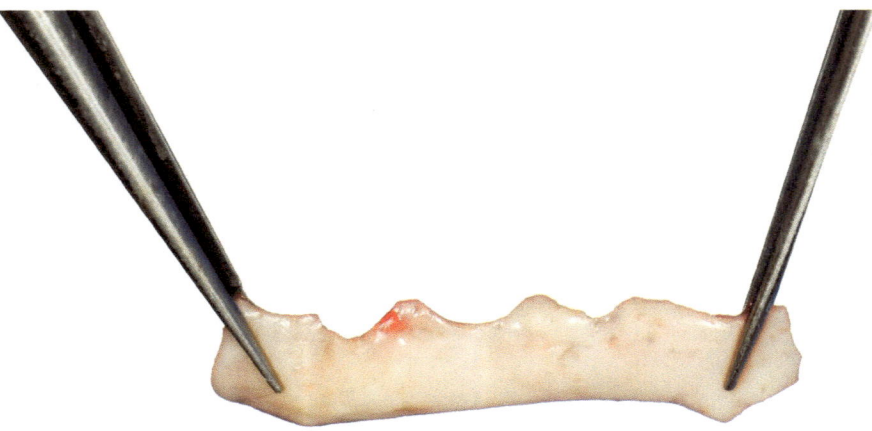

Fig. 63 The free gingival graft is taken under high magnification. The size of the graft depends on the horizontal and vertical extension of the recipient bed

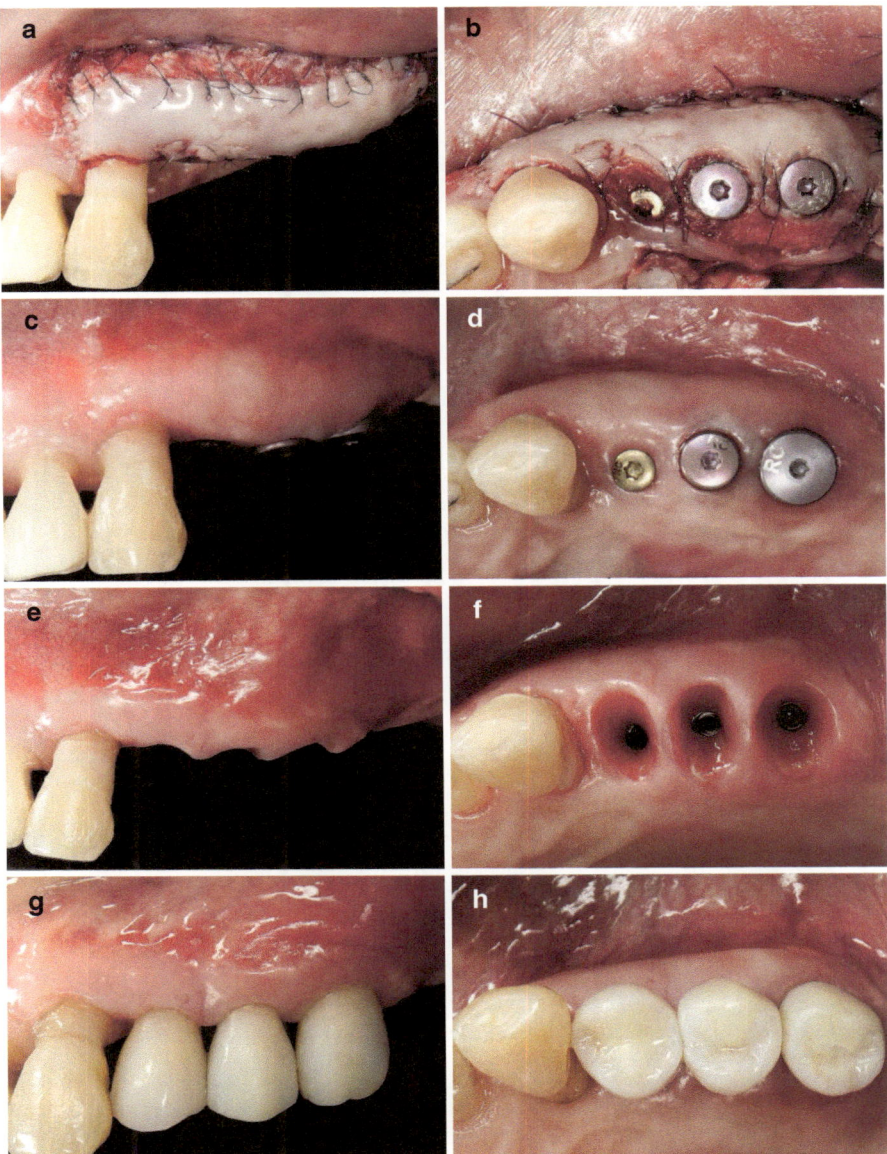

Fig. 64 (**a**, **b**) Buccal and occlusal images of the free gingival graft fixed with microsurgical suture techniques. Using 7-0 polyamide (Resolon™) at the occlusal, apical, and distal ends, 8-0 polyglycolic acid, 9-0 mesially (USIOL®), and glycolic acid and caprolactone copolymer (Glycolon®) apical to the periosteum 5-0™. (**c**, **d**). Buccal and occlusal view of the graft at six weeks of healing. (**e–h**) Buccal and occlusal view of the healed free gingival graft with a significant gain in keratinized tissue. Observe the formation of the emergence profiles 4 months after of using provisional restorations

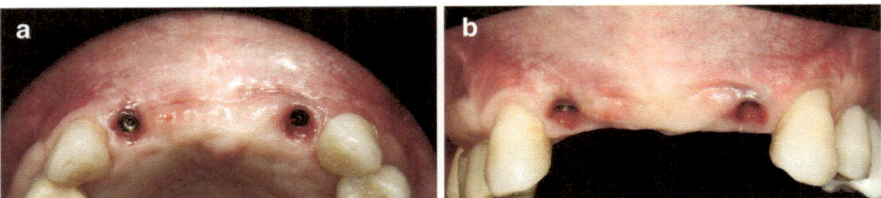

Fig. 65 (**a, b**) Buccal and occlusal views of a significant mucogingival distortion following guided bone regeneration in the anterior maxilla

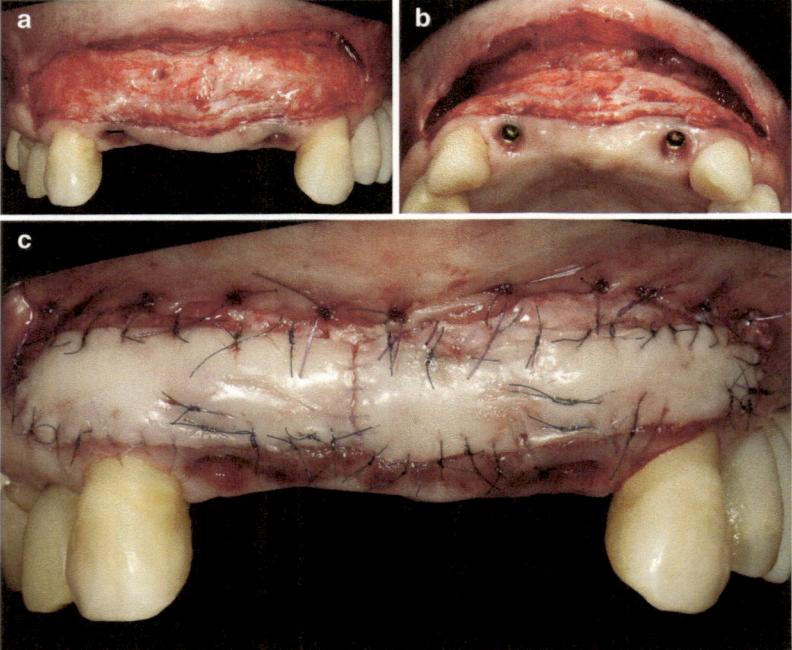

Fig. 66 (**a, b**) Buccal and occlusal views of the microsurgical partial-thickness flap bed preparation using an operating microscope. The releasing muscle attachments carefully result in a non-moving receptor bed. (**c**) The image shows a free gingival graft taken from the palate in two sections and sutured to each other with microsurgical sutures (8-0). The graft is then sutured to the recipient bed with individual microsurgical knots using 7-0 polyamide monofilament sutures (Resolon™) at the ends, 8-0, 9-0 polyglycolic acid sutures (USIOL®) and glycolic acid copolymer 5-0 and caprolactone (Glycolon™) sutures to the periosteum with apical displacement the vestibule

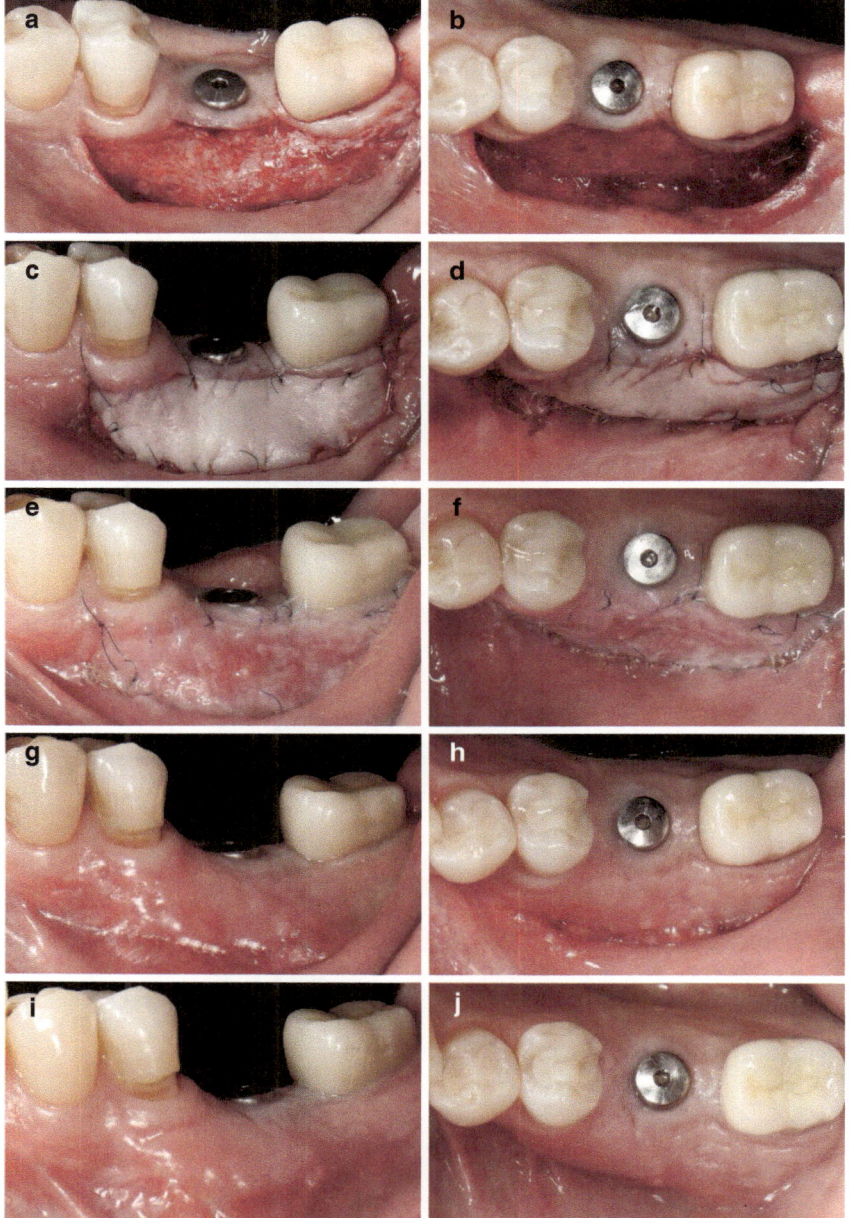

Fig. 67 (**a–j**) Soft tissue management and vestibular repositioning after bone regeneration in the lower left first molar (3.6). (**a, b**) Preparation of the bed respecting the margin of keratinized tissue. (**c, d**) Free gingiva graft fixation and adaptation with individual microsurgical knots using 7-0 polyamide monofilament suture (Resolon™) at the ends with 9-0 polyglycolic acid sutures (USIOL®). (**e, f**) Healing 12 days postoperatively. (**g, h**) Healing 26 days postoperatively. (**i, j**) Healing 40 days postoperatively. Note the significant gain in keratinized tissue and soft tissue integration

The integration of periodontal plastic surgery principles increases or modifies soft tissue, contributing to the functional and esthetic improvement in regenerative therapy. Trained surgeons utilize different techniques to perform this task, and there are many graft materials, such as free gingival grafts, connective tissue grafts, allografts, and xenografts that may be used. The selection of the technique and graft would depend on the chief objective and the available corresponding scientific evidence [85–87] (Figs. 68, 69, 70, 71, 72, 73, 74, 75, 76, 77, 78).

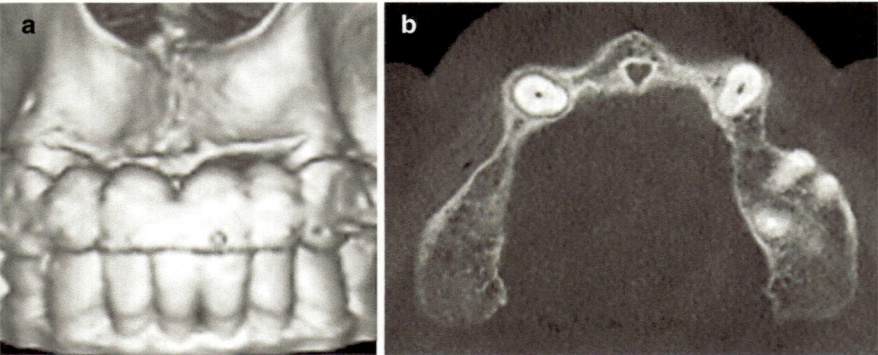

Fig. 68 (**a, b**) 3D and axial cone beam images of severe deficiency in the bucco-palatine direction in the anterior maxillary region

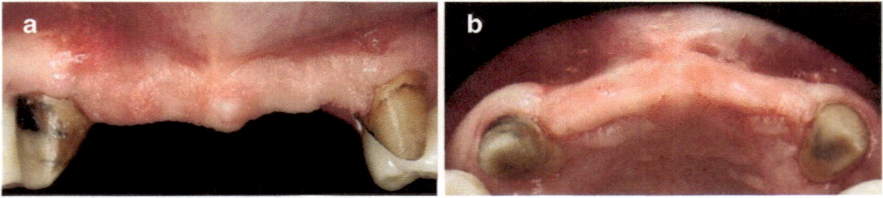

Fig. 69 (**a, b**) Buccal and occlusal images of horizontal ridge deficiency with integrity of the apico-coronal dimensions

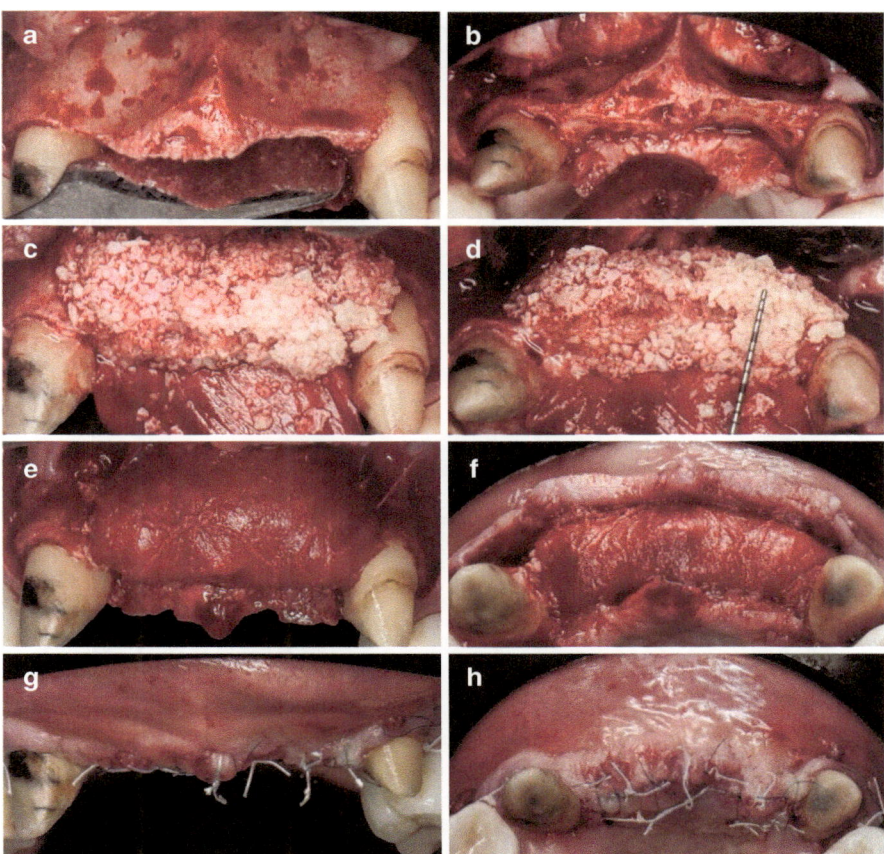

Fig. 70 (**a–h**). Representative case of horizontal augmentation in the anterior maxilla utilizing a microsurgical approach. (**a, b**) Buccal and occlusal view of a thin anterior superior ridge. (**c, d**) Buccal and occlusal view of the bone graft. (xenograft particulate anorganic bovine bone Bio.Oss® combined with cancellous bone allograft Puros®). (**e, f**) Placement and fixation of the membrane on the graft. (**g, h**) The flap is sutured with horizontal double mattresses complementing individual microsurgical knots

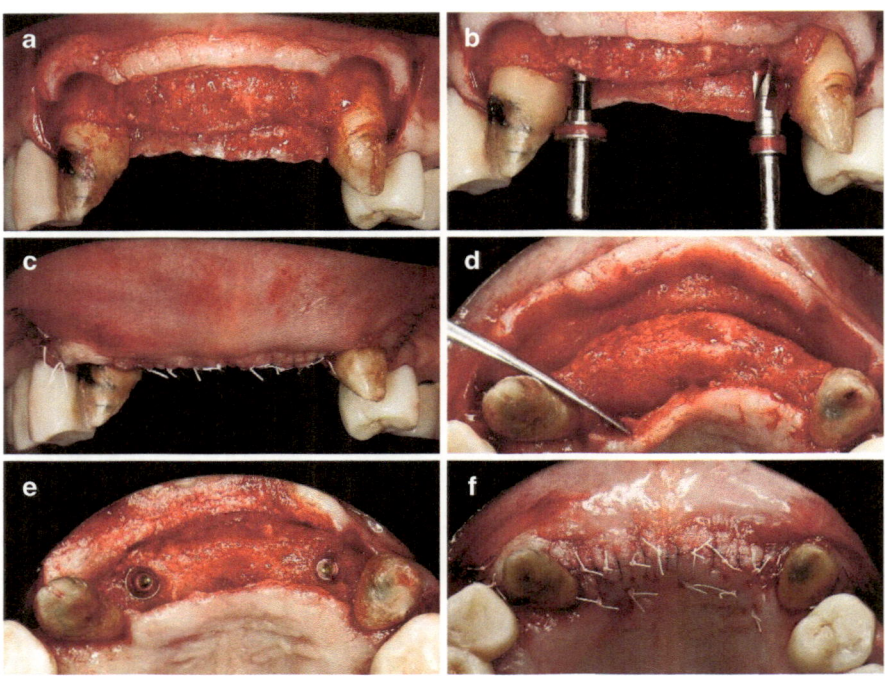

Fig. 71 (**a, d**) Buccal and occlusal views of the microsurgical flap showing the regenerated bone after 9 months of healing. (**b, e**) Buccal and occlusal views of implants placed in the regenerated bone. (**c, f**) Images of double-layered closure with individual microsurgical knots

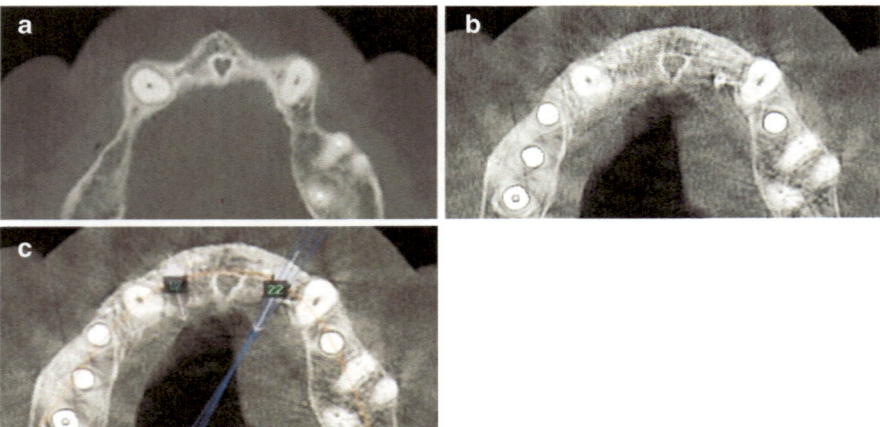

Fig. 72 (**a**) Axial image showing severe maxillary atrophy. (**b, c**) Images showing the results of guided bone regeneration and planning for implant placement

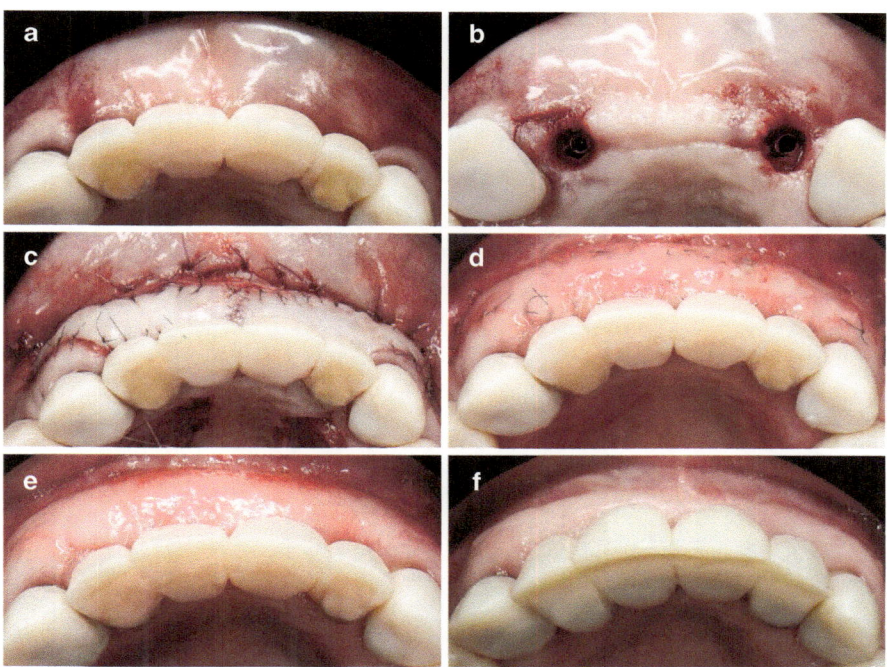

Fig. 73 (**a, b**) Occlusal image of significant mucogingival distortion created by guided bone regeneration in the anterior maxilla. (**c**) Vestibular deepening with simultaneous placement of a free gingival graft with a microsurgical approach. (**d, e, f**) Postoperative healing of the free gingival graft at 3 weeks, 2 months, and 1 year, respectively

Fig. 74 Buccal view 1 year after free gingival grafting and vestibular deepening

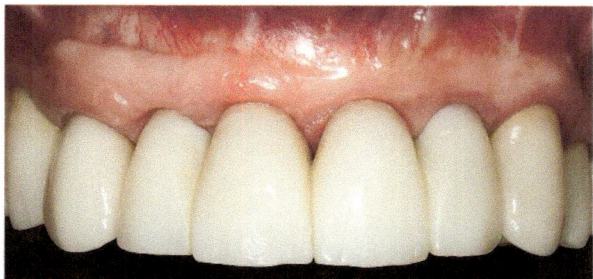

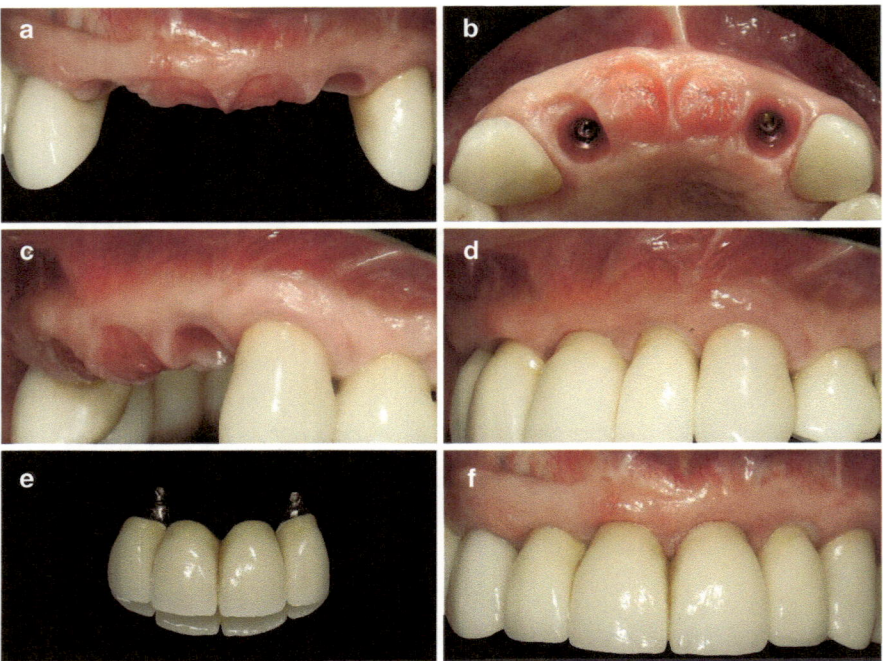

Fig. 75 (**a**, **b**, **c**) Buccal, occlusal, and lateral views showing the quality and maturation of the keratinized tissue after 1 year and 4 months of using provisional restorations and healing of the free gingival graft. (**d**, **f**) Lateral and vestibular view of the definitive restoration 2 years after microsurgical bone regeneration. (**e**) Implant-supported restoration

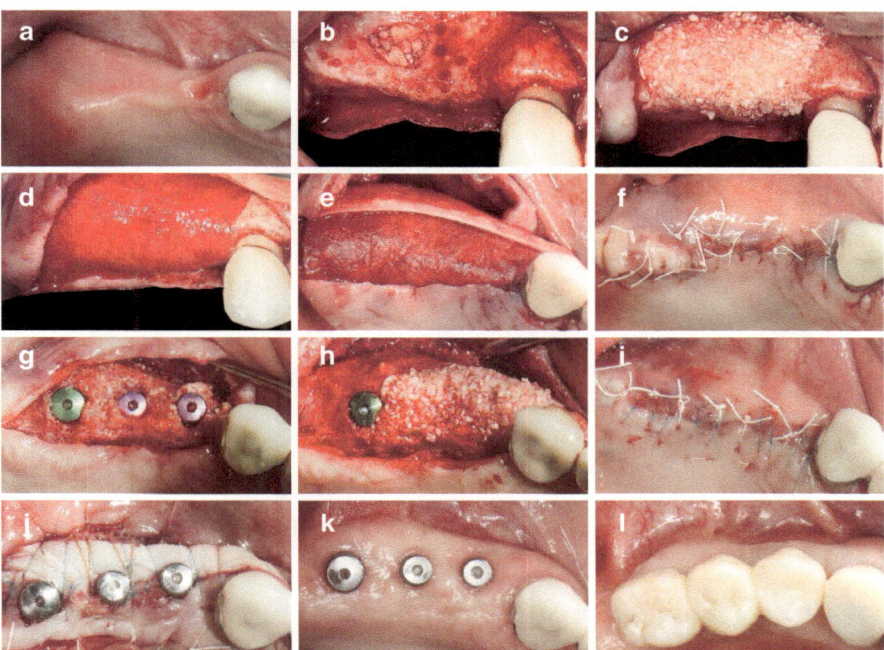

Fig. 76 Alveolar ridge augmentation with maxillary sinus elevation using a microsurgical approach. (**a**) The initial occlusal view shows a significant horizontal defect. (**b**) Buccal view of the defect area with elevated maxillary sinus shows the preparation of the recipient bone bed with multiple decorticalization holes. (**c**) Surgical image showing the placement of mixed xenograft (Bio.Oss® bovine inorganic cancellous bone substitute) and cancellous bone allograft (Puros®) and its adaption to the bone defect before membrane placement. (**d**) Buccal view of the membrane in place. (**e**) Occlusal images show a resorbable membrane (Geistlich Bio-Gide®) complemented with an acellular dermal matrix (AlloDerm™). (**f**) Closure of the flap at the primary incisions with horizontal mattress suture and individual interrupted knots. (**g, h**). Occlusal view of the implants in place and placement of bone substitute. (**i**) Occlusal view of tension-free flap closure. (**j**) Occlusal view of a free gingival graft placed around the implants. (**k**) Two months postoperatively. Note the significant gain in keratinized tissue and soft tissue integration. (**l**) Occlusal view of the temporary restorations placed and healing 1 year after free gingival grafting

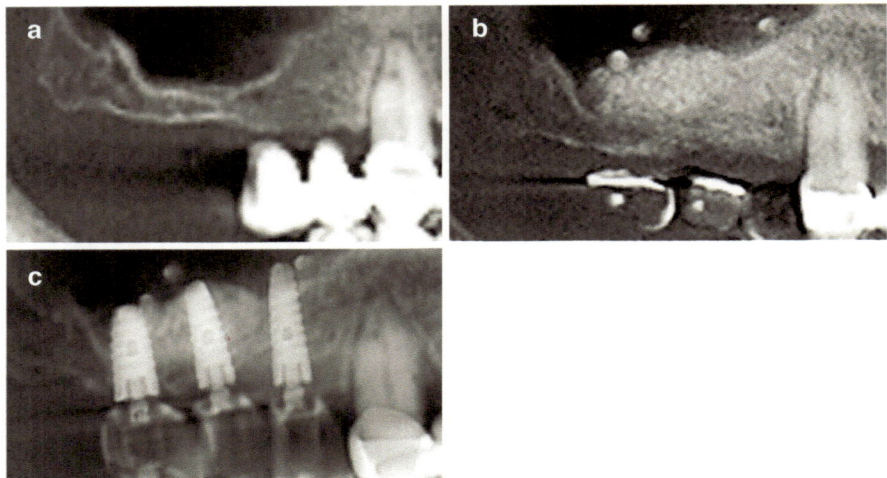

Fig. 77 (**a**) Preoperative radiograph. (**b**) Radiograph taken following guided bone regeneration and sinus lift. (**c**) Radiograph taken 1 year after implant loading

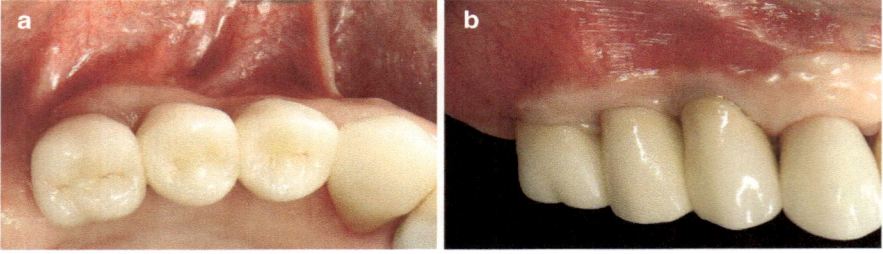

Fig. 78 (**a, b**). Occlusal and buccal views of the definitive restoration 2 years after microsurgical bone regeneration

8.2   Connective Tissue Grafts for Increased Thickness

Procedures using autogenous connective tissue grafts increase thickness and induce keratinization at sites indicated for or those that have undergone augmentation procedures. These procedures can precede regenerative surgery in areas with an extremely thin periodontal biotype to improve its management during regenerative microsurgery. It is also possible to perform it simultaneously or compensation treatment parallel to the prosthetic therapy with subgingival prothesis profiles, creating ideal gingival anatomy. References [88–90] show the application of microsurgical principles in connective tissue graft techniques Video 25 and Figs. 79, 80, 81, 82, 83, 84, 85, 86, 87a–g.

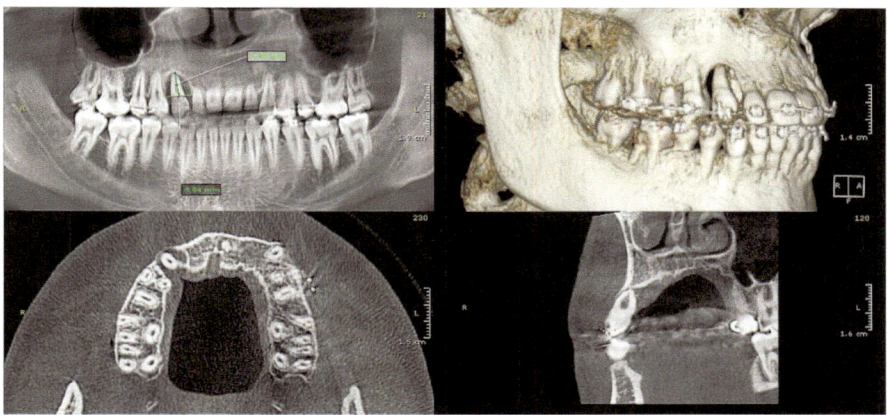

Fig. 79 Panoramic, axial, transverse, and cone beam 3D images, showing a severe vertical and horizontal defect in the area of the right upper canine

Fig. 80 Periapical radiograph showing apical extension of the severe circumferential bone defect at the right upper canine

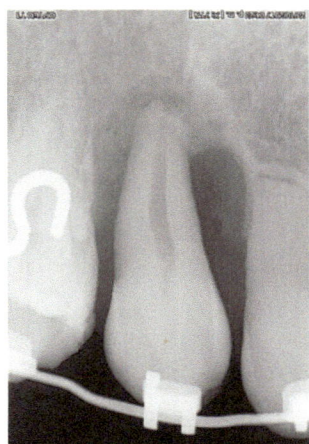

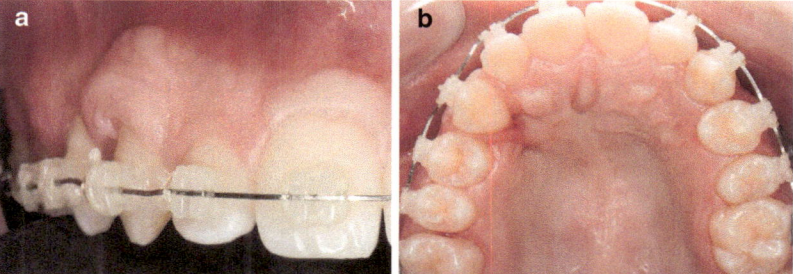

Fig. 81 (**a, b**). Buccal and occlusal clinical images taken preoperatively

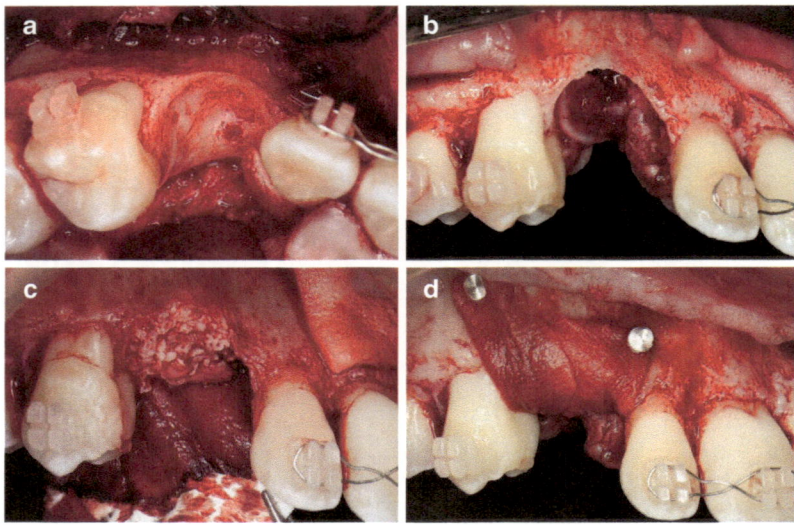

Fig. 82 (**a, b**). Occlusal and buccal images of the full thickness microsurgical flap after canine extraction showing loss of palatal alveolar bone as well as a pronounced vertical deficiency. (**c**) Placement of the mixture of autologous bone and xenograft (Bio.Oss® bovine inorganic cancellous bone substitute). (**d**) Buccal images show a resorbable membrane (Geistlich Bio-Gide®) immobilized with titanium pins

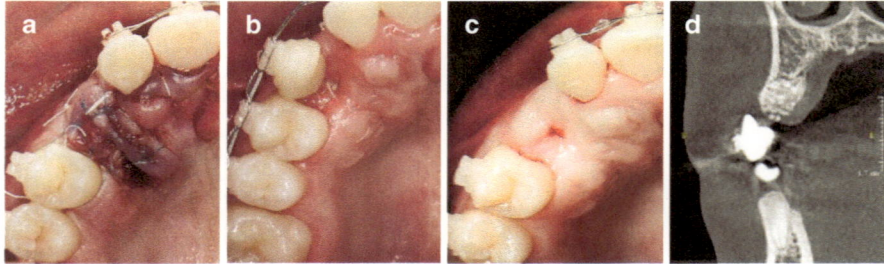

Fig. 83 (**a**) The flap is sutured with horizontal double mattresses complemented with individual microsurgical knots. (**b, c**) Healing at 3 and 6 weeks after guided bone regeneration. (**d**) The cross-sectional image showed progress in healing 7 months after guided bone regeneration and bone preservation

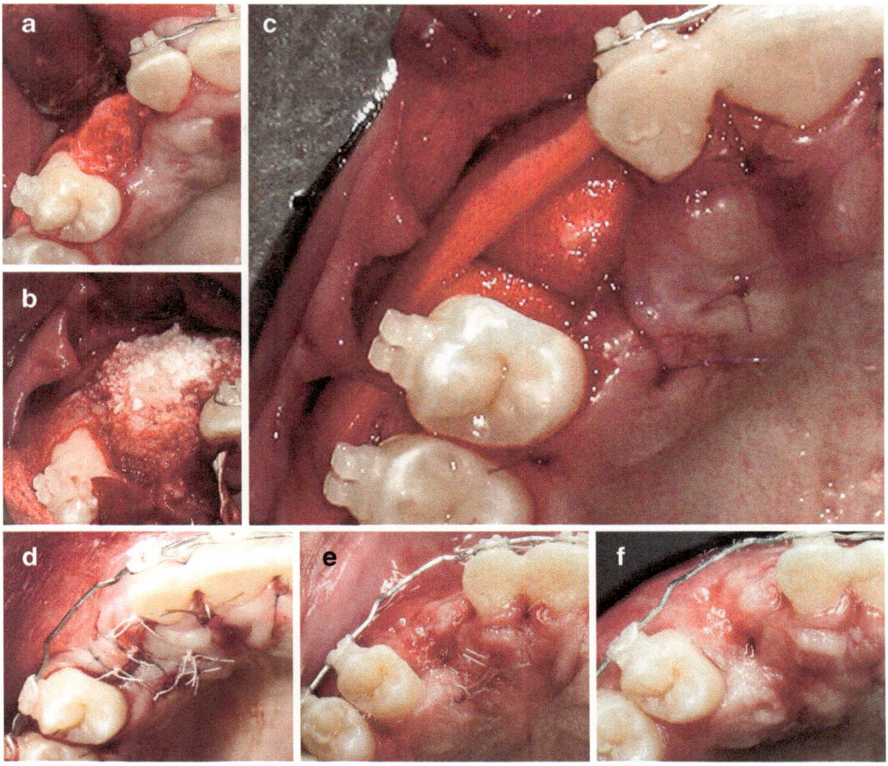

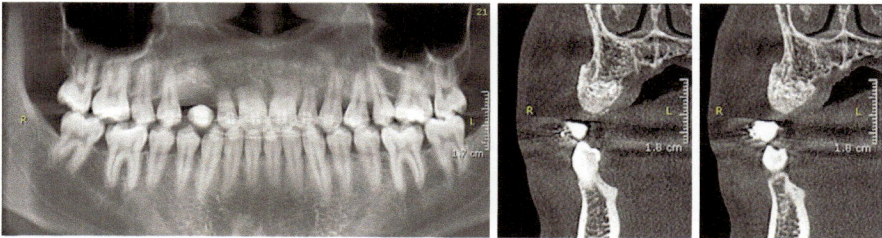

Fig. 84 (**a**) Occlusal image of the full-thickness flap showing the results of the first guided bone regeneration microsurgical procedure. (**b**) Bone graft placement with a mixture of xenograft (Bio. Oss® Bovine Inorganic Cancellous Bone Substitute) and cancellous bone allograft (Puros®). (**c**) Occlusal view shows resorbable membrane fixation (Geistlich Bio-Gide®) performed with suspension sutures for the periosteum and dermal matrix (AlloDerm®) for soft tissue augmentation. (**d**) The flap is sutured with horizontal double mattresses complementing the individual microsurgical knots. (**e**) Clinical view after one week of healing. (**f**) After 3 weeks of uneventful healing

Fig. 85 Cross-sectional and cone-beam panoramic images show healing 9 months after guided bone regeneration

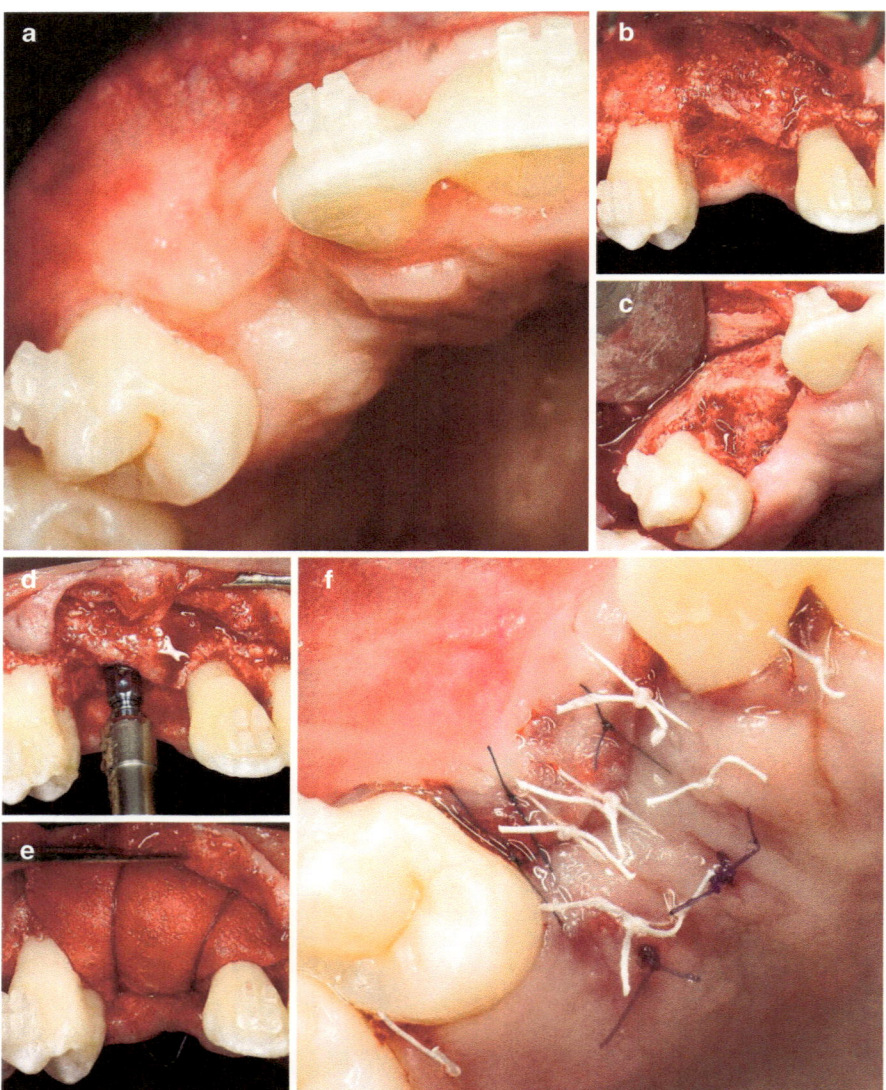

Fig. 86 (a) The occlusal image shows healing 9 months after microsurgical guided bone regeneration. (b, c) Buccal and occlusal views of regenerated bone. (d) Buccal view of implant placement. (e) Buccal images show that membrane placement after grafting increases buccal thickness. (f) The flap is sutured with horizontal double mattresses complemented with individual microsurgical knots

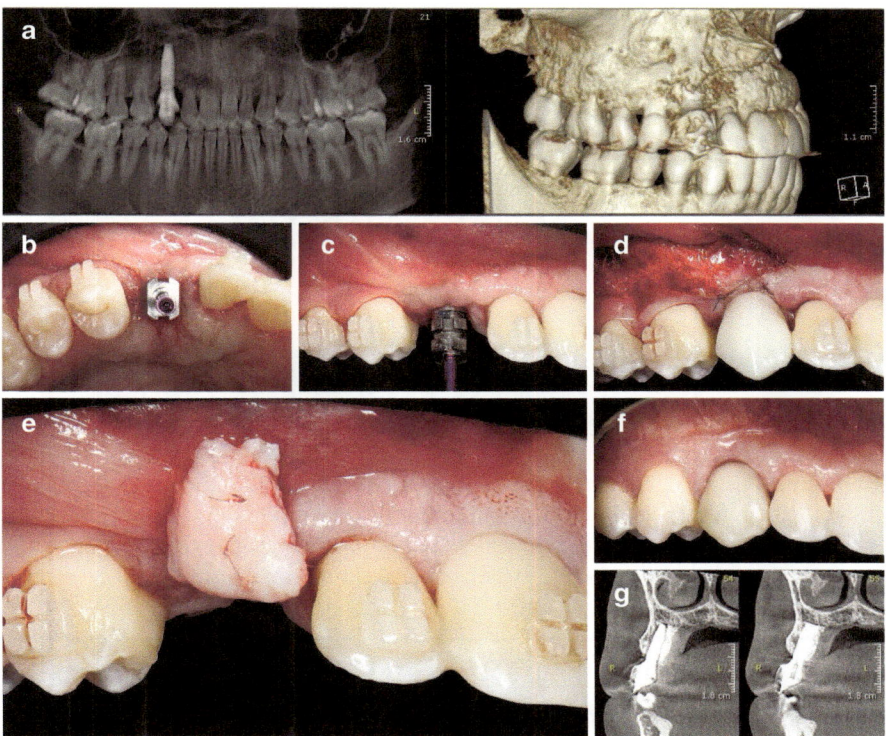

Fig. 87 (**a**) Panoramic and 3D cone beam images show healing four months after implant placement. (**b, c**) Occlusal and buccal images show significant mucogingival distortion following guided bone regeneration. (**d, e**) Vestibular repositioning and connective tissue graft placement are performed to improve soft tissue architecture, following which temporary restorations are placed. (**f**) Buccal image shows healing 6 months after connective tissue graft placement. (**g**) Three-dimensional cross-sectional images showing the results of microscope-assisted guided bone regeneration

8.3 Soft Tissue Grafts to Increase Keratinized Tissue

Free gingival grafts have a high success rate when discussing keratinized tissue in regenerated sites. Placement of a free gingival graft with an apically positioned flap has good predictability. A partial-thickness flap is raised at the previously augmented site. The extension of the horizontal and vertical incision reaches the regeneration site limits, where the surgeon should reposition the vestibule to recover its depth as the mucogingival loss. The bed is prepared by carefully releasing the tissue and muscular insertion with a microsurgical scalpel and microsurgical tissue scissors, resulting in a receptor bed without movement Videos 26, 27, 28. The technique of procuring the palatal graft depends on the bed's horizontal and vertical extension [86–91]. The recommended thickness of the graft is less than 2 mm. After procuring the graft from the donor site, an L-PRF autologous membrane is sutured over the wound to protect the area and aid the healing process Video 29. Adapting and suturing the graft to the receptor site begins with properly tied microsurgical 2 = 2 knots using monofilament suture 7-0 polyamide (Resolon™) at the extremes and polyglycolic acid 8-0, 9-0 (USIOL®) for completion. For apical fixation in the deepening of the vestibule where the muscle tone is strong, we recommend using the glycolic acid copolymer and caprolactone 5-0 (Glycolon™). Videos 30, 31, and 32.

8.4   Allografts, Xenografts, and Their Use

Substitute soft tissue allografts and xenografts can be used to gain soft tissue in regenerative therapy. Videos 12 and 13 However, vestibule repositioning and gain in keratinized tissue demonstrate the superiority of the autologous free gingival graft [85]. Although this material is useful, other evidence-based techniques have also shown to increase keratinized tissue by combining xenografts with autogenous tissue to reduce donor-site morbidity and achieve satisfactory results [87].

9   Ultra-Minimally Invasive GBR Techniques

At present, science and technology are evolving toward increasing the predictability of surgical treatments with minimally invasive procedures. Traditional bone regeneration techniques do not always comply with the requisites of minimally invasive flap surgery because they require flaps of greater dimensions. Bone regeneration microsurgery is minimally invasive because it allows the handling of tissues with greater precision and minimal damage. Periodontal microsurgery shares these attributes with medical microsurgery.

Microsurgery is an example of minimally invasive surgery applied to bone preservation and is performed conservatively without the need to raise flaps. When performed simultaneously with tooth extraction, it helps to preserve the keratinized tissue and achieve closure and fixation with different membranes and contributes to the application of microsurgical techniques to improve the handling of different materials (Video 22).

Other examples of minimally invasive procedures are those in which implant placement is performed simultaneous to regeneration techniques, with placement of bone grafts and membranes using different protocols, [92, 93] and conservative approaches with high precision under the microscope. (Video 33) Another minimally invasive technique proposed in recent years is the Subperiosteal Minimally Invasive esthetic Ridge Augmentation Technique, which consists of small incisions near the defect, creating a tunnel access for the regeneration of bone defects. These tunnels allow the placement of the graft without the need for flap reflection [94].

10   Conclusion

Microscope is an alternative modality that can be useful for clinicians in performing regenerative therapy, and it fulfills the essential requirements of GBR. Microsurgical principles offer tremendous support, facilitating and improving this complex therapy, and microsurgery promises ideal and predictable results.

11   Key Points

1. Guided bone regeneration (GBR) replaces lost tissues with elements to restore normal function and structure for the ideal three-dimensional placement of dental implants.
2. The microscope is a modern surgical accessory and a critical factor for the success of the most complex medical surgeries.
3. The microscope in GBR can aid precision in surgical execution. It has been shown that microsurgery contributes to improved healing and treatment outcomes in other areas of Periodontology.
4. Microsurgery helps develop motor skills by improving surgical capacity, reducing tissue trauma, and contributing to the wound's primary closure.
5. The microscope in GBR improves soft and hard tissue management, offering better visualization during incision placement, flap elevation, preparation of the surgical bed, and flap closure.
6. The microsurgical approach in GBR includes some crucial factors: ergonomic position of the microsurgeon, use of instruments with sufficient handgrip, adequate forearm support to reduce physiological tremor, suture material selection, and adequate tension handling. These are fundamental requirements of microsurgery.

Acknowledgments   The authors declare no conflicts of interest.

References

1. Wang HL, Boyapati L. "PASS" principles for predictable bone regeneration. Implant Dent. 2006;15(1):8–17. https://doi.org/10.1097/01.id.0000204762.39826.0f.
2. Nyman S, Karring T, Lindhe J, Plantén S. Healing following implantation of periodontitis-affected roots into gingival connective tissue. J Clin Periodontol. 1980;7(5):394–401. https://doi.org/10.1111/j.1600-051x.1980.tb02012.x.
3. Gottlow J, Nyman S, Lindhe J, Karring T, Wennstrom J. New attachment formation in the human periodontium by guided tissue regeneration. Case reports. J Clin Periodontol. 1986;13(6):604–16. https://doi.org/10.1111/j.1600-051X.1986.tb00854.X.
4. Schenk RK, Buser D, Hardwick WR, Dahlin C. Healing pattern of bone regeneration in membrane-protected defects: a histologic study in the canine mandible. Int J Oral Maxillofac Implants. 1994;9(1):13–29. PMID: 8150509
5. Pietrokovski J, Massler M. Ridge remodeling after tooth extraction in rats. J Dent Res. 1967;46(1):222–31.

6. Amler MH, Johnson PL, Salman I. Histological and histochemical investigation of human alveolar socket healing in undisturbed extraction wounds. J Am Dent Assoc. 1960;61:46–8. https://doi.org/10.14219/jada.archive.1960.0152.

7. Boyne PJ. Osseous repair of the postextraction alveolus in man. Oral Surg Oral Med Oral Pathol. 1966;21(6):805–13. https://doi.org/10.1016/0030-4220(66)90104-6.

8. Seibert JS. Reconstruction of deformed, partially edentulous ridges, using full thickness onlay grafts. Part I. technique and wound healing. Compend Contin Educ Dent. 1983;4(5):437–53. PMID: 6578906

9. Huebsch RF, Hansen LS. A histopathologic study of extraction wounds in dogs. Oral Surg Oral Med Oral Pathol. 1969;28:187–96. https://doi.org/10.1016/0030-4220(69)90286-2.

10. Araújo M, Lindhe J. Dimensional ridge alterations following tooth extraction. An experimental study in dog. J Clin Periodontol. 2005;32(2):212–8. https://doi.org/10.1111/j.1600-051x.2005.00642.x.

11. Schropp L, Wenzel A, Kostopoulos L, Karring T. Bone healing and soft tissue contour changes following single-tooth extraction: a clinical and radiographic 12-month prospective study. Int J Periodontics Restorative Dent. 2003;23(4):313–23. PMID: 12956475

12. Van der Weijden F, Dell'Acqua F, Slot DE. Alveolar bone dimensional changes of post-extraction sockets in humans: a systematic review. J Clin Periodontol. 2009;36(12):1048–58. https://doi.org/10.1111/j.1600-051X.2009.01482.x.

13. Iasella JM, Greenwell H, Miller RL, Hill M, Drisko C, Bohra AA, et al. Ridge preservation with freeze-dried bone allograft and a collagen membrane compared to extraction alone for implant site development: a clinical and histologic study in humans. J Periodontol. 2003;74(7):990–9. https://doi.org/10.1902/jop.2003.74.7.990.

14. Nevins M, Mellonig JT, Clem DS 3rd, Reiser GM, Buser DA. Implants in regenerated bone: long-term survival. Int J Periodontics Restorative Dent. 1998;18(1):34–45. PMID: 9558555

15. Simion M, Jovanovic SA, Tinti C, Benfenati SP. Long-term evaluation of osseointegrated implants inserted at the time or after vertical ridge augmentation. A retrospective study on 123 implants with 1-5 year follow-up. Clin Oral Implants Res. 2001;12(1):35–45. https://doi.org/10.1034/j.1600-0501.2001.012001035.x. PMID: 11168269

16. Shanelec DA, Tibbetts LS. Orlando, FL: 78th American Academy of Periodontology Annual Meeting; 1992. Nov 19, Periodontal microsurgery, continuing education course.

17. Burkhardt R, Hürzeler MB. Utilization of the surgical microscope for advanced plastic periodontal surgery. Pract Periodontics Aesthet Dent. 2000;12(2):171–80; quiz 182. PMID: 11404959

18. Cortellini P, Tonetti MS. Microsurgical approach to periodontal regeneration. Initial evaluation in a case cohort. J Periodontol. 2001;72(4):559–69. https://doi.org/10.1902/jop.2001.72.4.559.

19. Cortellini P, Tonetti MS. A minimally invasive surgical technique with an enamel matrix derivative in the regenerative treatment of intra-bony defects: a novel approach to limit morbidity. J Clin Periodontol. 2007;34(1):87–93. https://doi.org/10.1111/j.1600-051X.2006.01020.x.

20. Cortellini P. Minimally invasive surgical techniques in periodontal regeneration. J Evid Based Dent Pract. 2012;12(3):89–100. https://doi.org/10.1016/S1532-3382(12)70021-0.

21. Nordland WP, Sandhu HS. Microsurgical technique for augmentation of the interdental papilla: three case reports. Int J Periodontics Restorative Dent. 2008;28(6):543–9. PMID: 19146049

22. Burkhardt R, Lang NP. Coverage of localized gingival recessions: comparison of micro- and macrosurgical techniques. J Clin Periodontol. 2005;32(3):287–93. https://doi.org/10.1111/j.1600-051X.2005.00660.x.

23. Tavelli L, Borgonovo AE, Saleh MH, Ravidà A, Chan HL, Wang HL. Classification of sinus membrane perforations occurring during Transcrestal sinus floor elevation and related treatment. Int J Periodontics Restorative Dent. 2020;40(1):111–8. https://doi.org/10.11607/prd.3602.

24. Di Gianfilippo R, Wang IC, Steigmann L, Velasquez D, Wang HL, Chan HL. Efficacy of microsurgery and comparison to macrosurgery for gingival recession treatment: a systematic review with meta-analysis. Clin Oral Investig. 2021;25(7):4269–80. https://doi.org/10.1007/s00784-021-03954-0. Epub ahead of print

25. Spark DS, Wagels M, Taylor GI. Bone reconstruction: a history of vascularized bone transfer. Microsurgery. 2018;38(1):7–13. https://doi.org/10.1002/micr.30260.
26. Jacobson JH, Suarez EL. Microvascular surgery. Dis Chest. 1962;41:220–4. https://doi.org/10.1378/chest.41.2.220.
27. Uluç K, Kujoth GC, Başkaya MK. Operating microscopes: past, present, and future. Neurosurg Focus. 2009;27(3):E4. https://doi.org/10.3171/2009.6.FOCUS09120.
28. Tibbetts LS, Shanelec DA. Principles and practice of periodontal microsurgery. Int J Microdent. 2009;1:13–24.
29. de Campos GV, Bittencourt S, Sallum AW, Nociti Júnior FH, Sallum EA, Casati MZ. Achieving primary closure and enhancing aesthetics with periodontal microsurgery. Pract Proced Aesthet Dent. 2006;18(7):449–54.
30. Allen EP, Gainza CS, Farthing GG, Newbold DA. Improved technique for localized ridge augmentation. A report of 21 cases. J Periodontol. 1985;56(4):195–9. https://doi.org/10.1902/jop.1985.56.4.195.
31. Kao D, Fiorellini JP. Clasificación de la relación de la cresta alveolar interarcada. Rev Int Odontol Restaur Period. 2010;14(5):522–9.
32. Wang HL, Al-Shammari K. HVC ridge deficiency classification: a therapeutically oriented classification. Int J Periodontics Restorative Dent. 2002;22(4):335–43.
33. Bosshardt D, Schenk RK. Bone regeneration: biologic basis. In: 20 Years of Guided Bone regeneration in Implant Dentistry. 2nd ed. Batavia, Illinois: Quintessence; 2009. p. 15–45.
34. Davies J, Hosseini M. Histodynamics of endosseous wound healing. In: Davies JE, editor. Bone engineering. Atlanta, GA: Em Squared Inc.; 2000. p. 1–14.
35. Fernández-Tresguerres-Hernández-Gil I, MA AG, del Canto PM, Blanco JL. Physiological bases of bone regeneration I. Histology and physiology of bone tissue. Med Oral Patol Oral Cir Bucal. 2006;11:E47–51. © Medicina Oral S. L. C.I.F. B 96689336-ISSN 1698–6946
36. McDonal MM, Khoo WH, Ng PY, Xiao Y, Zamerli J, Thatcher P, Kyaw W, Pathmanandavel K, Grootveld AK, Moran I, Butt D, Nguyen A, Corr A, Warren S, Biro M, Butterfield N, Guilfoyle SE, Komla-Ebri D, Dack MRG, Dewhurst HF, Logan JG, Li Y, Mohanty ST, Byrne N, Terry RL, Simic MK, Chai R, Quinn JMW, Youlten S, Petttitt JA, Abi-Hanna D, Jain R, Weninger W, Lundberg M, Sun S, Ebetino FH, Timpson P, Lee WM, Baldock PA, Rogers MJ, Brink R, Williams GR, Bassett JHD, Kemp JP, Pavlos NJ, Croucher PI, Phan TG, Less S. Footnotes S. Osteoclasts recycle via osteomorphs during RANKL-stimulated bone resorption. Cell. 2021;184:1330–1347.E13. https://doi.org/10.1016/j.cell.2021.02.002.
37. Geneser F, Brüel A, et al. Geneser Histología. Edición: 4ª Ed. Singapore: Panamericana; 2015.
38. Schmid J, Wallkamm B, Hämmerle CH, Gogolewski S, Lang NP. The significance of angiogenesis in guided bone regeneration. A case report of a rabbit experiment. Clin Oral Implants Res. 1997;8(3):244–8. https://doi.org/10.1034/j.1600-0501.1997.080311.x.
39. Urban IA, Monje A, Wang HL, Lozada J, Gerber G, Baksa G. Mandibular regional anatomical landmarks and clinical implications for ridge augmentation. Int J Periodontics Restorative Dent. 2017;37(3):347–53. https://doi.org/10.11607/prd.3199.
40. Moore KL, Dalley AF II, Agur AMR, Gutiérrez A, Vasallo L, Fontán Fontán F, et al. Cabeza, Wolters Kluwer Anatomía con orientación clínica. 8a edición; 2018. p. 932–52.
41. Urban I. Principles of vertical and horizontal ridge augmentation in the posterior mandible. In: Vertical and horizontal ridge augmentation new perspectives. Batavia, IL: Quintessence Publishing; 2017. p. 39–60.
42. Elian N, Ehrlich B, Jalbout ZN, Classi AJ, Cho S-C, Kamer AR, et al. Advanced Concepts in Implant Dentistry: Creating the "Aesthetic Site Foundation." Dental Clinics of North America. Dent Clin N Am. 2007;51(2):547–63, xi-xii. https://doi.org/10.1016/j.cden.2007.03.001.
43. Joly JC, Carvalho PFM, Silva RC. Perio-Implantodontia Estética. Quintessence Editora: São Paulo; 2015.
44. Ronda M, Stacchi C. Management of a coronally advanced lingual flap in regenerative osseous surgery: a case series introducing a novel technique. Int J Periodontics Restorative Dent. 2011;31(5):505–13.

45. Zuhr O, Hurzeler M. Cirugia Plastica y Estética, Periodontal e Implantológica . Un enfoque microquiruúgico. Quintessence, São Paulo; 2011.
46. Tinti C, Parma-Benfenati S. Vertical ridge augmentation: surgical protocol and retrospective evaluation of 48 consecutively inserted implants. Int J Periodontics Restorative Dent. 1998;18(5):434–43. https://doi.org/10.11607/prd.00.0287.
47. Urban I, Traxler H, Romero-Bustillos M, Farkasdi S, Bartee B, Baksa G, et al. Effectiveness of two different lingual flap advancing techniques for vertical bone augmentation in the posterior mandible: a comparative, Split-mouth cadaver study. Int J Periodontics Restorative Dent. 2018;38(1):35–40. https://doi.org/10.11607/prd.3227.
48. Greenstein G, Greenstein B, Cavallaro J, Elian N, Tarnow D. Flap advancement: practical techniques to attain tension-free primary closure. J Periodontol. 2009;80(1):4–15. https://doi.org/10.1902/jop.2009.080344.
49. Sculean A, Nikolodakis D, Schwarz F. Regeneration of periodontal tissues: combinations of barrier membranes and grafting materials - biological foundation and preclinical evidence: a systematic review. J Clin Periodontol. 2008;35(8 Suppl):106–16. https://doi.org/10.1111/j.160051X.2008.01263.x.
50. Urban IA, Monje A, Lozada J, Wang HL. Principles for vertical ridge augmentation in the atrophic posterior mandible: a technical review. Int J Periodontics Restorative Dent. 2017;37(5):639–45. https://doi.org/10.11607/prd.3200.
51. Galindo-Moreno P, Hernndez-Corts P, Aneiros-Fernndez J, Camara M, Mesa F, Wallace S, et al. Morphological evidences of bio-Oss colonization by CD44-positive cells. Clin Oral Implants Res. 2014;25(3):366–71. https://doi.org/10.1111/clr.12112. Epub 2013 Jan 28
52. Simion M, Fontana F, Rasperini G, Maiorana C. Vertical ridge augmentation by expanded-polyetetrafluoroethylene membrane and a combination of intraoral autogenous bone graft and deproteinized anorganic bovine bone (bio Oss). Clin Oral Implants Res. 2007;18(5):620–9. https://doi.org/10.1111/j.1600-0501.2007.01389.x.
53. Urban IA, Nagursky H, Lozada JL, Nagy K. Horizontal ridge augmentation with a collagen membrane and a combination of particulated autogenous bone and anorganic bovine bone-derived mineral: a prospective case series in 25 patients. Int J Periodontics Restorative Dent. 2013;33(3):299–307. https://doi.org/10.11607/prd.1407.
54. Urban IA, Nagursky H, Lozada JL. Horizontal ridge augmentation with a Resorbable membrane and Particulated autogenous bone with or without Anorganic bovine bone-derived mineral: a prospective case series in 22 patients. Int J Oral Maxillofac Implants. 2011;26(2):404–14.
55. Jovanovic SA, Nevins M. Bone formation utilizing titanium-reinforced barrier membranes. Int J Periodontics Restorative Dent. 1995;15(1):56–69.
56. Hämmerle CH, Jung RE. Bone augmentation by means of barrier membranes. Periodontol. 2000;2003(33):36–53. https://doi.org/10.1046/j.0906-6713.2003.03304.x.
57. Urban IA, Lozada JL, Jovanovic SA, Nagursky H, Nagy K. Vertical ridge augmentation with titanium-reinforced, dense-PTFE membranes and a combination of particulated autogenous bone and anorganic bovine bone-derived mineral: a prospective case series in 19 patients. Int J Oral Maxillofac Implants. 2014;29(1):185–93. https://doi.org/10.11607/jomi.3346.
58. Novaes AB Jr, Souza SL. Acellular dermal matrix graft as a membrane for guided bone regeneration: a case report. Implant Dent. 2001;10(3):192–6. https://doi.org/10.1097/00008505-200107000-00009.
59. Borges GJ, Novaes AB Jr, Grisi MF, Palioto DB, Taba M Jr, de Souza SL. Acellular dermal matrix as a barrier in guided bone regeneration: a clinical, radiographic and histomorphometric study in dogs. Clin Oral Implants Res. 2009;20(10):1105–15. https://doi.org/10.1111/j.1600-0501.2009.01731.x. Epub 2009 Jun 10
60. Castro AB, Meschi N, Temmerman A, Pinto N, Lambrechts P, Teughels W, et al. Regenerative potential of leucocyte- and platelet-rich fibrin. Part B: sinus floor elevation, alveolar ridge preservation and implant therapy. A systematic review. J Clin Periodontol. 2017;44(2):225–34. https://doi.org/10.1111/jcpe.12658. Epub 2017 Jan 10
61. Castro AB, Meschi N, Temmerman A, Pinto N, Lambrechts P, Teughels W, et al. Regenerative potential of leucocyte- and platelet-rich fibrin. Part a: intra-bony defects, furcation defects

and periodontal plastic surgery. A systematic review and meta-analysis. J Clin Periodontol. 2017;44(1):67–82. https://doi.org/10.1111/jcpe.12643.

62. Castro AB, Herrero ER, Slomka V, Pinto N, Teughels W, Quirynen M. Antimicrobial capacity of leucocyte-and platelet rich fibrin against periodontal pathogens. Sci Rep. 2019;9(1):8188. https://doi.org/10.1038/s41598-019-44755-6.

63. Urban I, Caplanis N, Lozada JL. Simultaneous vertical guided bone regeneration and guided tissue regeneration in the posterior maxilla using recombinant human platelet-derived growth factor: a case report. J Oral Implantol. 2009;35(5):251–6. https://doi.org/10.1563/AAID-JOI-D-09-00004.1.

64. Nevins M, Giannobile WV, McGuire MK, Kao RT, Mellonig JT, Hinrichs JE, et al. Platelet-derived growth factor stimulates bone fill and rate of attachment level gain: results of a large multicenter randomized controlled trial. J Periodontol. 2005;76(12):2205–15. https://doi.org/10.1902/jop.2005.76.12.2205.

65. Simion M, Nevins M, Rocchietta I, Fontana F, Maschera E, Schupbach P, et al. Vertical ridge augmentation using an equine block infused with recombinant human platelet-derived growth factor-BB: a histologic study in a canine model. Int J Periodontics Restorative Dent. 2009;29(3):245–55.

66. Sebaoun JD, Kantarci A, Turner JW, Carvalho RS, Van Dyke TE, Ferguson DJ. Modeling of trabecular bone and lamina dura following selective alveolar decortication in rats. J Periodontol. 2008;79(9):1679–88. https://doi.org/10.1902/jop.2008.080024.

67. Burkhardt R, Preiss A, Joss A, Lang NP. Influence of suture tension to the tearing characteristics of the soft tissues: an in vitro experiment. Clin Oral Implants Res. 2008;19(3):314–9. https://doi.org/10.1111/j.1600-0501.2007.01352.x.

68. Burkhardt R, Lang NP. Influence of suturing on wound healing. Periodontol 2000. 2015;68(1):270–81. https://doi.org/10.1111/prd.12078.

69. Harwell RC, Ferguson RL. Physiologic tremor and microsurgery. Microsurgery. 1983;4(3):187–92. https://doi.org/10.1002/micr.1920040310.

70. Terra H, Aberg C. Tensile strengths of twelve types of knot employed in surgery, using different suture materials. Acta Chir Scand. 1976;142:1–7.

71. Gjermo P, Bonesvoll P, Rölla G. Relationship between plaque-inhibiting effect and retention of chlorhexidine in the human oral cavity. Arch Oral Biol. 1974;19(11):1031–4. https://doi.org/10.1016/0003-9969(74)90090-9.

72. Hamp SE, Rosling B, Lindhe J. Effect of chlorhexidine on gingival wound healing in the dog. A histometric study. J Clin Periodontol. 1975;2(3):143–52. https://doi.org/10.1111/j.1600-051x.1975.tb01736.x.

73. Heitz F, Heitz-Mayfield LJ, Lang NP. Effects of post-surgical cleansing protocols on early plaque control in periodontal and/or periimplant wound healing. J Clin Periodontol. 2004;31(11):1012–8. https://doi.org/10.1111/j.1600-051X.2004.00606.x.

74. Ling LJ, Hung SL, Lee CF, Chen YT, Wu KM. The influence of membrane exposure on the outcomes of guided tissue regeneration: clinical and microbiological aspects. J Periodontal Res. 2003;38(1):57–63. https://doi.org/10.1034/j.1600-0765.2003.01641.x.

75. Fontana F, Maschera E, Rocchietta I, Simion M. Clinical classification of complications in guided bone regeneration procedures by means of a nonresorbable membrane. Int J Periodontics Restorative Dent. 2011;31(3):265–73.

76. Thoma DS, Naenni N, Figuero E, Hammerle CHF, Schwarz F, Jung RE, et al. Effects of soft tissue augmentation procedures on peri-implant health or disease: a systematic review and meta-analysis. Clin Oral Implants Res. 2018;29(Suppl 15):32–49. https://doi.org/10.1111/clr.13114.

77. Linkevicius T, Apse P, Grybauskas S, Puisys A. The influence of soft tissue thickness on crestal bone changes around implants: a 1-year prospective controlled clinical trial. Int J Oral Maxillofac Implants. 2009;24(4):712–9.

78. Urban IA, Monje A, Wang HL. Vertical ridge augmentation and soft tissue reconstruction of the anterior atrophic maxillae: a case series. Int J Periodontics Restorative Dent. 2015;35(5):613–23. https://doi.org/10.11607/prd.2481.

79. Ladwein C, Schmelzeisen R, Nelson K, Fluegge TV, Fretwurst T. Is the presence of keratinized mucosa associated with periimplant tissue health? A clinical cross-sectional analysis. Int J Implant Dent. 2015;1(1):11. https://doi.org/10.1186/s40729-015-0009-z.

80. Roccuzzo M, Grasso G, Dalmasso P. Keratinized mucosa around implants in partially edentulous posterior mandible: 10-year results of a prospective comparative study. Clin Oral Implants Res. 2016;27(4):491–6. https://doi.org/10.1111/clr.12563.

81. Ueno D, Nagano T, Watanabe T, Shirakawa S, Yashima A, Gomi K. Effect of the keratinized mucosa width on the health status of Periimplant and contralateral periodontal tissues: a cross-sectional study. Implant Dent. 2016;25(6):796–801. https://doi.org/10.1097/ID.0000000000000483.

82. Monje A, Blasi G. Significance of keratinized mucosa/gingiva on peri-implant and adjacent periodontal conditions in erratic maintenance compliers. J Periodontol. 2019;90(5):445–53. https://doi.org/10.1002/JPER.18-0471. Epub 2018 Dec 7

83. Cairo F, Pagliaro U, Nieri M. Soft tissue management at implant sites. J Clin Periodontol. 2008;35(8 Suppl):163–7. https://doi.org/10.1111/j.1600-051X.2008.01266.x.

84. Chiu YW, Lee SY, Lin YC, Lai YL. Significance of the width of keratinized mucosa on peri-implant health. J Chin Med Assoc. 2015;78(7):389–94. https://doi.org/10.1016/j.jcma.2015.05.001.

85. Thoma DS, Benić GI, Zwahlen M, Hämmerle CH, Jung RE. A systematic review assessing soft tissue augmentation techniques. Clin Oral Implants Res. 2009;20(Suppl 4):146–65. https://doi.org/10.1111/j.1600-0501.2009.01784.x.

86. Zuhr O, Bäumer D, Hürzeler M. The addition of soft tissue replacement grafts in plastic periodontal and implant surgery: critical elements in design and execution. J Clin Periodontol. 2014;41(Suppl 15):S123–42. https://doi.org/10.1111/jcpe.12185.

87. Urban IA, Lozada JL, Nagy K, Sanz M. Treatment of severe mucogingival defects with a combination of strip gingival grafts and a xenogeneic collagen matrix: a prospective case series study. Int J Periodontics Restorative Dent. 2015;35(3):345–53. https://doi.org/10.11607/prd.2287.

88. Edel A. Clinical evaluation of free connective tissue grafts used to increase the width of keratinised gingiva. J Clin Periodontol. 1974;1(4):185–96. https://doi.org/10.1111/j.1600-051x.1974.tb01257.x.

89. Orsini M, Orsini G, Benlloch D, Aranda JJ, Lázaro P, Sanz M. Esthetic and dimensional evaluation of free connective tissue grafts in prosthetically treated patients: a 1-year clinical study. J Periodontol. 2004;75(3):470–7. https://doi.org/10.1902/jop.2004.75.3.470.

90. Silverstein LH, Kurtzman D, Garnick JJ, Trager PS, Waters PK. Connective tissue grafting for improved implant esthetics: clinical technique. Implant Dent. 1994;3(4):231–4. https://doi.org/10.1097/00008505-199412000-00003.

91. Bouri A Jr, Bissada N, Al-Zahrani MS, Faddoul F, Nouneh I. Width of keratinized gingiva and the health status of the supporting tissues around dental implants. Int J Oral Maxillofac Implants. 2008;23(2):323–6.

92. Chen ST, Wilson TG Jr, Hämmerle CHF. Immediate or early placement of implants following tooth extraction: review of biologic basis, clinical procedures, and outcomes. Int J Oral Maxillofac Implants. 2004;19(Suppl):12–25.

93. Wessing B, Urban I, Montero E, Zechner W, Hof M, Alández CHJ, Alández MN, Polizzi G, Meloni S, Sanz M. A multicenter randomized controlled clinical trial using a new reabsorbable non-cross-linked collagen membrane for guided bone regeneration at dehisced single implants sites: interim results of a bone augmentation procedure. Clin Oral Implants Res. 2016;28(11):e218–26. https://doi.org/10.1111/clr.12995.

94. Lee EA. Subperiosteal minimally invasive aesthetic ridge augmentation technique (SMART): a new standard for bone reconstruction of the jaws. Int J Periodontics Restorative Dent. 2017;37(2):165–73. https://doi.org/10.11607/prd.3171.

Microscope-Assisted Sinus Augmentation

Benyapha Sirinirund, Riccardo Scaini, Tiziano Testori,
Diego Velasquez-Plata, and Hsun-Liang (Albert) Chan

Contents

B. Sirinirund
Department of Periodontics and Oral Medicine, School of Dentistry, University of Michigan, Ann Arbor, MI, USA

Division of Periodontology, Department of Restorative Dentistry and Periodontology, Faculty of Dentistry, Chiang Mai University, Chiang Mai, Thailand

R. Scaini
IRCCS Istituto Ortopedico Galeazzi, Milan, Italy

Department of Biomedical, Surgical and Dental Sciences, Università degli Studi di Milano, Milan, Italy

T. Testori
Department of Periodontics and Oral Medicine, School of Dentistry, University of Michigan, Ann Arbor, MI, USA

IRCCS Istituto Ortopedico Galeazzi, Milan, Italy

Department of Biomedical, Surgical and Dental Sciences, Università degli Studi di Milano, Milan, Italy

D. Velasquez-Plata
Private Practice, Fenton, MI, USA

Department of Periodontics and Oral Medicine, School of Dentistry, University of Michigan, Ann Arbor, MI, USA

H.-L. (A.) Chan (✉)
Periodontics Graduate Program, School of Dentistry, University of Michigan, Ann Arbor, MI, USA
e-mail: hlchan@umich.edu

© The Author(s), under exclusive license to Springer Nature Switzerland AG 2022
H.-L. (A.) Chan, D. Velasquez-Plata (eds.), *Microsurgery in Periodontal and Implant Dentistry*, https://doi.org/10.1007/978-3-030-96874-8_12

Abstract

Sinus augmentation via vertical or lateral approach is commonly applied to increase the alveolar ridge height for standard-sized implant placement in the posterior maxilla. While enjoying satisfactory success rate, traditional methods without assistance of the operating microscope may create great surgical trauma and leave the Schneiderian membrane perforation unnoticed, which may be associated with a higher complication rate. Microscope-assisted sinus augmentation could enhance clinical outcomes with early detection of intraoperative complications, potentially accelerate wound healing, and minimize postoperative pain through minimally invasive surgical approaches made possible by the provided high-magnification and co-axial illumination. This chapter describes the fundamental knowledge related to sinus augmentation and details the rationales of how the operating microscope may improve the performance of sinus augmentation and possible enhanced clinical outcomes.

Keywords

Minimally invasive · Sinus augmentation · Sinus lift · Operating microscope

1 Introduction

Minimally invasive surgery with the adjunctive use of the operating microscope is growing in both periodontal and implant surgeries. The advancement of instruments, techniques, and materials helps surgeons to better manipulate, preserve the integrity of the Schneiderian membrane, and reduce complications of sinus augmentation surgeries. However, literature showing the benefits of the microscope and how it can be used to maximize clinical outcomes of sinus augmentation surgeries are scarce. This chapter explains the evolution of sinus augmentation procedures and highlights the importance of the operating microscope and how it can be used in minimally invasive surgical approaches for sinus lift surgeries.

2 Keys to Success in Sinus Augmentation Procedures

2.1 Historical Background and the Current Trend of Sinus Augmentation Surgery

Maxillary sinus augmentation was originally developed in the 1980s [1, 2], and surgical techniques along with bone replacements grafts and dental implants have evolved to increase the predictability and reduce intrasurgical and postoperative complications [3]. Lateral sinus augmentation consists in gain access to the maxillary sinus through an opening in the lateral osseous wall below the zygoma to elevate the Schneiderian membrane at the floor and lateral and medial wall of the sinus for gaining vertical height (more than 3–4 mm). Alternatively, when vertical ridge deficiency is less (less than 3–4 mm), vertical ridge augmentation could be used to lift the sinus membrane at the floor of the maxillary sinus [4]. The latter technique is a blind approach using osteotome or specially designed surgical drills to gain access to the inferior border of the maxillary sinus from the alveolar crest of the edentulous ridge.

Despite lateral and crestal approaches provide high implant survival rates, sinus membrane perforation was the most common intraoperative complication range from 0% to 58.2% and 0% to 21.4% for lateral and crestal approaches, respectively [5, 6]. The presence of sinus septa and severe vertical ridge deficiency has been reported to be the main risk factors for increasing sinus membrane perforation rates, and a higher prevalence of postoperative sinusitis associated with membrane perforation was observed [7]. Undetected sinus perforation could potentially result in postoperative sinusitis by contaminated particulate graft material escaping into the maxillary sinus and cause infection or blockage of the ostium. Therefore, key factors for the success of sinus augmentation and to reduce complications to a minimum are (1) adequate evaluation of sinus health and identification of sinus pathology if any, and (2) understanding sinus anatomy with optimal treatment planning.

2.2 The Rationale for Microscope-Assisted Sinus Augmentation

Careful Schneiderian membrane manipulation during sinus augmentation procedures is very crucial. Technological advancement in surgical instruments allows gentler management of the sinus membrane. Piezoelectric osteotomy was first introduced in 2001 for bony window preparation for lateral sinus augmentation [8]. The incidence of sinus membrane perforation has been shown to reduce significantly after the use of piezosurgery instruments for osteotomy preparation compared to conventional air-driven rotating burs [9].

The ability to visualize the sinus membrane during surgery is of paramount importance to reduce the incidence of sinus membrane perforation. The maxillary sinus is a closed, dark space with anatomical irregularities (e.g., sinus septa at the floor and/or continuing adjacent walls, oblique sinus floor, narrow-angle of palatonasal recess on the medial wall, narrow buccal and palatal alveolar wall) [7, 10–12]. After osteotomy window preparation in lateral sinus augmentation, an adjunctive use of an operating microscope could help surgeons to clinically visualize inside the sinus bony cavity and detect any pathology or irregularities of anatomical structures (Fig. 1). Furthermore, the elevation of the Schneiderian membrane with hand instruments, especially close to septa could be a very difficult task. For vertical sinus augmentation, evaluation of the Schneiderian membrane integrity through a small crestal osteotomy site is feasible with the operating microscope. Using traditional direct visualization and Valsalva maneuver to detect perforation of the Schneiderian membrane may be less predictable for the evaluation of the sinus membrane integrity. In addition, cone-beam computerized tomography (CBCT) and periapical radiographs are not also reliable methods to detect soft tissue perforations [13]. The use of the operative microscope has been demonstrated to have very high intraoperative detection accuracy (87.5%) that coincided with postoperative and radiographic and clinical assessment in a cadaveric study [14]. Again, the detection and accurate diagnosis of the size of the perforation in the middle of surgery with sufficient magnification and illumination of the operating microscope could guide clinicians to establish an optimal solution and avoid unforeseen postoperative severe complications [15].

Another advantage of microscope-assisted sinus augmentation is faster healing and less early implant failure. The operating microscope facilitates a minimally invasive surgical approach characterized by a conservative incision design, minimal flap elevation, smaller osteotomy site preparation approximately 5–6 mm in diameter, minimal elevation of the Schneiderian membrane, and less amount of particulate grafts in the sinus cavity. This minimally surgical approach resulted in low early failure and complication rates in lateral sinus augmentation, only 7 out of 124 patients (6%) had a perforation of the sinus membrane [16] and none of 6 cases

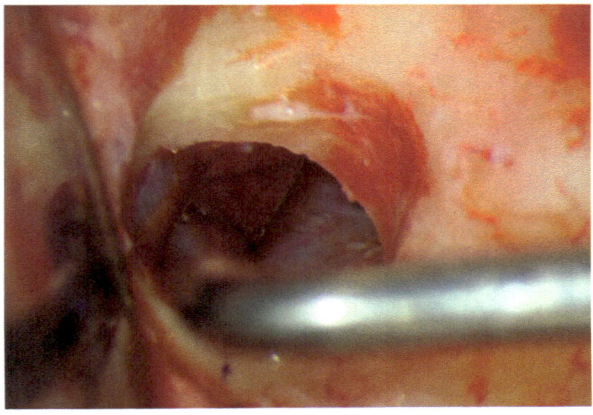

Fig. 1 Operating microscope help to clinically visualize inside the sinus bony cavity and detect any pathology or irregularities of anatomical structures if present

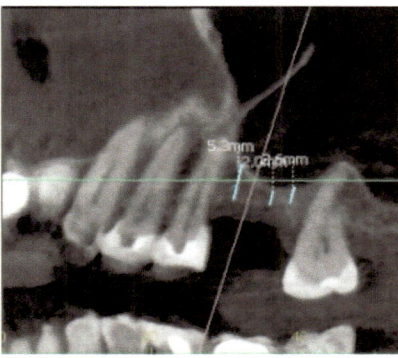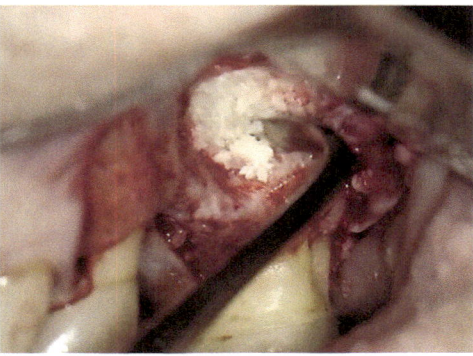

Fig. 2 Lateral sinus augmentation is possible in a limited space with the adjunctive use of the operating microscope

(0%) in a more recent case report [17]. Low failure rates could be explained by accelerated bone maturation, less residual bone graft particulates, a higher percentage of vital bone with the preservation of vascularized bony walls of the smaller osteotomy window [18]. Moreover, in a severely resorbed ridge with a vertical deficiency in a limited space (e.g., a single-tooth gap), the lateral sinus augmentation approach is feasible with the adjunctive use of the operating microscope (Fig. 2).

Lastly, microscope-assisted sinus augmentation could facilitate a minimally invasive, precise hard and soft tissue manipulation and result in minimal postoperative pain with high patient satisfaction due to smaller window size and minimal flap elevation [17, 19, 20].

3   Anatomical Considerations and Clinical Implications

The maxillary sinus is the largest of the paranasal cavities which include ethmoidal, frontal, and sphenoid sinuses and occupy most of the maxilla [21]. It is a pneumatic, quadrangular pyramid-shaped cavity with many walls:

- a medial wall facing the nasal cavity,
- a posterior wall facing the maxillary tuberosity,
- a vestibular (or lateral) wall that joins the mesial (or anterior) wall that appears concave due to the canine fossa.

The angle between the vestibular and mesial walls varies widely from individual to individual; in dolichocephalic patients, the transition is usually gradual (the internal angle between the two walls is wider with a clinical range of 140° to 170°), whereas in brachycephalic patients, it is less pronounced ranging from 100° to 140°.

- an upper wall serving as the orbital floor
- an inferior wall corresponding to the alveolar process functioning as the sinus floor

The maxillary sinus is the first of the paranasal sinuses to develop (65th to 70th day of gestation). Between 12 and 14 years of age with the eruption of permanent teeth, pneumatization of the sinus increases following the development of the mid-face. The process is completed with the eruption of the third permanent molar between the ages of 16 and 18 years and, when development is complete, in young adults, the average sinus volume is 12 mL but may range up to 25 mL. The sinus communicates with the homolateral nasal cavity via a natural ostium anterosuperior to the medial wall. Mucus is discharged by ciliary activity through the natural ostium, ethmoidal infundibulum, and semilunar hiatus (which encompass the osteo-meatal complex [OMC]) toward the middle meatus of the nasal cavity. The patency of the nasal cavity is a determining factor in the maintenance of normal sinus physiology.

The natural sinus ostium is usually oval shaped (7–11 mm by 2–6 mm). It is con-nected to the nasal cavity indirectly via a narrow, subtle vestibule termed the *eth-moidal infundibulum*. This slim antechamber situated at the level of the lateral nasal wall joins the middle meatus through a fissure called the *semilunar hiatus* (confined by the posterior, anteroinferior side of the ethmoidal bulla and posterior free margin of the uncinate process on the anterior side). This allows the sinus mucus to reach the medial surface of the middle concha and be transported toward the rhino pharyn-geal cavity and the underlying digestive tract. The narrowness of the ethmoidal antechamber brings mucus membranes close to each other so that under normal circumstances the transport of mucus is more efficient thanks to the synergic action of opposing cilia. The same structural peculiarity can cause the blockage of drain-age following even a slight swelling of the mucous membranes, arresting mucus transport and ventilation, and creating the conditions for the insurgence of sinus disease. All paranasal sinuses communicate with nasal cavities and therefore indi-rectly with each other. Their main function is to humidify and warm inhaled air. They also reduce the weight of facial bones, protect the base of the skull from pos-sible trauma, insulate the brain, and influence phonation (indirectly functioning like a voice box). Finally, the paranasal sinuses produce a large quantity of nitric oxide (NO), an important factor in regulating ciliary activity, with antibacterial properties.

3.1 Schneiderian Membrane

The maxillary sinus is lined by pseudostratified ciliated columnar epithelial cells on the internal side and periosteum on the sinus walls. The mucous membrane consist-ing of three layers with a thickness of 80–100 μm in a healthy patient:

- The first layer is a superficial layer corresponding to the respiratory epithelium (cylindrical, ciliated, pseudostratified), composed of basal cell units, columnar ciliates, and calciform cells (the so-called goblet cells attached to the basal membrane).
- The second layer is a middle layer corresponding to the lax connective tissue that can become edematous (lamina propria) in reaction to inflammation. It is

separated from the overlying basal membrane epithelium and entirely permeated by a dense network of blood vessels that ensure abundant nourishment of the mucosa. The lamina propria houses the serous mucous glands, which are very abundant at the level of the sinus ostium in particular.

– The third deep layer, corresponding to the periosteum, separates the connective tissue from the bony walls of the sinus.

The epithelium that lines the sinus continues into nasal mucosa that tends to be thicker, around 1 mm. The apical ciliated cells consist of 50–200 cilia, whereas nonciliated cells possess microvilli that increase the surface area. The mucus film lining the sinus mucosa consists of two overlapping layers: a deeper serous layer (*sol phase*) inside which the ciliary movement takes place, and a more superficial, denser layer (*gel phase*). Various contaminants (e.g., dust, environmental pollutants, germs) that may enter the sinus are trapped in the gel phase, transported by ciliary action to the natural ostium, and expelled from the nasal cavity. In the absence of sinus disease, this mechanism keeps the nasal cavity sterile. Under normal conditions, the mucociliary transport mechanism allows the renewal of the antral mucous film in 20–30 min with a flow rate of around 1 cm per minute. The mucus is the most important protection mechanism of the nasal sinus complex, 96% of which is water containing 3–4% glycoproteins: IgA-S, IgG, IgM, IgE, lysosome, lactoferrin, prostaglandins, leukotrienes, and histamine. It is produced by the glands associated with the mucosa and regulated mostly by the parasympathetic system and orthosympathetic system. In the parasympathetic system, fibers travel from the upper salivary nucleus and are conveyed through the greater petrosal nerve and sphenopalatine ganglion, whereas the orthosympathetic system involves mostly vascular action. Some neuropeptides, such as substance P, act on the nasal sinus mucosa causing hypersecretion, vasodilation, and plasma exudation. The quality and quantity of the mucus depend on hydration, environmental humidity, and consumption of drugs (e.g., atropine and similar substances). The ciliary apparatus under normal conditions has a beat rate of between 8 and 20 cycles per second; the inhaled air temperature directly influences such action (ideally 33 °C; reduced activity is observed under 18 °C and over 40 °C; no activity is detected under 12 °C and over 43 °C) as well as the pH (optimal between 7 and 8), oxygenation, osmotic pressure, metabolism, humidity, and hydration. Maxillary endoscopy shows that ciliary movement stops during sinus elevation, the duration and extent of which are currently unknown.

At the sinus level, the mucociliary transport has a genetically determined characteristic; it starts star-shaped at the sinus floor and progresses along the anterior, medial, posterior, and lateral walls and the sinus roof until the ostium opening. The maxillary sinus septa do not obstruct the flow of mucus, nor do the occasional narrow recesses created by the sinus walls. These are easily crossed by the gel layer thanks to a bridging phenomenon (e.g., direct flow from one peak to the other by the propulsive push created by the movement of epithelial cilia that line these recesses). Even perforations of around 1 mm in diameter do not impede the mucociliary transport produced by the sinus membrane; it continues to maintain the physiologic mobility synchronized with breathing movements during sinus elevation. This, however, depends on the quality of the mucus; if it is afflicted by infection, the increased viscosity will hinder its free movement, and it will not overcome these obstacles.

The mucus transport system has another peculiarity. Even in the presence of an accessory ostium, both natural and surgically created, the mucus is always transported toward the natural ostium avoiding these alternative drainage canals. This has rendered surgical ostia in the inferior meatus to restore normal sinus physiology obsolete. The membrane may undergo pathologic modification often due to inflammatory processes that cause a thickening observed in radiographs. A thickening of the sinus membrane is not sufficient to diagnose sinusitis. It should also be noted that sinusitis is a clinical condition, and a diagnosis cannot be made only with radiography. Although it is difficult to supply empirical data, it is advisable to request an ENT consultation when thickening of over 3–4 mm is encountered.

The success of the sinus augmentation procedure depends on the ability to maintain the integrity of the membrane and the perforation of the membrane could result in infection of the graft and implant failure. Even though the mean thickness of the Schneiderian membrane was reported to be relatively thin, only 0.3 and 0.79 mm in histologic and CBCT [22], it can be stretched more than 1.2 times its original size in an in vitro study [23]. While the thicker membranes had higher stretching ability, stronger membrane, and less perforation compared to thinner membranes, previous studies show that the membrane perforation rate was lower when the thickness was 1.5–2 mm and 1–1.5 mm for vertical and lateral sinus procedures, respectively [24, 25]. This implied that too thick membranes are also not beneficial to the sinus augmentation procedure. The thickening of the membrane more than 4 mm in CBCT scan, medical consultation is recommended as a pathological thickened membrane from sinusitis is weaker and poses a risk for sinus membrane perforation [12].

3.2   Sinus Walls: Floor, Medial-Lateral Wall Distance, Angle, Lateral Wall Thickness, Septum

The shape of the sinus walls and the presence of the septum can influence the difficulty of both vertical and lateral sinus augmentation procedures.

Sinus width [26]	The average sinus width was 8–10 mm and is ideal for lateral sinus augmentation. Wide sinus width required larger areas of membrane detachment whereas, in narrow sinus width, access for membrane manipulation is limited. However, this can be overcome with the use of the operating microscope to visualize and better manipulate the membrane
The angle between buccal and palatal alveolar walls [10]	The perforation rate was higher (62.5%) in narrow/acute angle (<30°) compared to wider angle in lateral sinus augmentation surgery. Complete osteotomy (wall-off) technique and closer outline to the sinus floor/anterior wall was recommended to facilitate access to elevate the membrane in the corners between sinus walls
Palatonasal recess [11]	Acute angle palatonasal recess (<90°) was found to be prevalent at second premolar sites and could make the membrane manipulation more challenging at the medial wall

Buccal wall thickness [12, 27]	More time is required for rotating instruments to complete antrostomy preparation in a thick buccal wall. The color contrast between thick bone and blue color of the membrane is less compared to thin buccal bone. Besides, excessive buccal bone wall thickness (>2 mm) may limit access to the instrument shank to elevate the sinus membrane and increase the risk for membrane perforation
Sinus septa (Underwood's septa) [27–32]	The sinus septa, a cortical bone plate with an average height of 8 mm, are commonly found at the first molar and premolar zone in the vestibulopalatal direction. The incidence of septa varies between 16% and 58% with an average of 30%. The presence of sinus septa has been shown to increase the risk for sinus membrane perforation for lateral sinus augmentation and was reported to have a negative relationship with the Schneiderian membrane thickness. The difficulty also increases when the septa orient in a sagittal direction with a height of more than 6 mm. Adequate identification with a computerized tomographic scan of the septa must be accomplished to avoid complications.

3.3   Residual Ridge Height and Width

Residual ridge height less than 4 mm has been reported to have a thinner Schneiderian membrane with higher perforation incidence in lateral sinus augmentation surgery [33, 34]. The possible cause of this could be a larger area of membrane elevation, thus increase the risk of perforation due to technical difficulties. In the case of vertical sinus augmentation, higher elevation in reduced residual ridge height could also result in higher force and possibly exceeds the critical perforation forces of the sinus membrane [23]. In addition, a residual ridge less than 3 mm could also jeopardize the implant survival rate for implants that were placed simultaneously in lateral sinus augmentation [35].

3.4   Vascular Supply

The vascular network in the maxilla is particularly extensive and is supplied by three arteries (Fig. 3a, b).

– Infraorbital artery
– Major palatine artery
– Alveolar antral artery originating from the internal maxillary artery

The alveolar antral artery often sprouts an intraosseous anastomosis with the infraorbital artery running inside the lateral wall of the sinus to an average distance of 19 mm from crestal bone [36]. Solar [37] showed how the anastomotic branch of the posterior superior alveolar artery is present in 100% of samples. Elian et al. [38] showed that this artery may be located in the lateral wall and visible in CT scans in 52% of sinuses. In addition, in 20% of cases, the artery is found in the projection area of the antrostomy. Previous CBCT studies demonstrated that the artery is present in

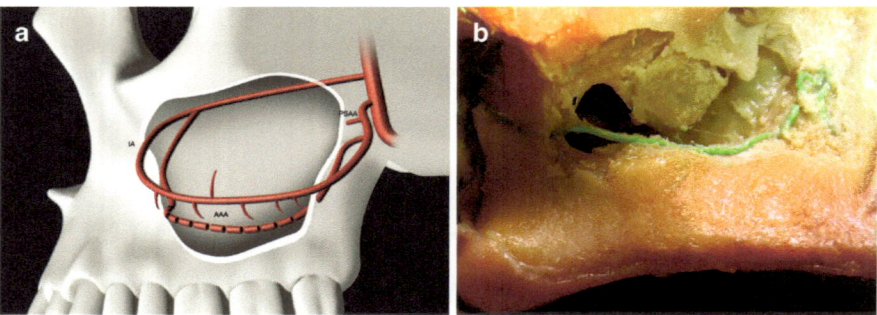

Fig. 3 (**a**) The vascular system of the vestibular wall of the maxillary sinus is supplied by three arteries: the infraorbitary artery (IA), the posterior superior alveolar artery (PSAA) and the alveolar antral artery (AAA) originating from the internal maxillary artery that could form an intraosseous (dotted line) or extra osseous anastomosis. (**b**) Macro-anatomical dissection of the sinus lateral wall: the alveolar antral artery (Green) is close to the Schneiderian membrane and no bony layer between such vessel and the membrane is visible after antrostomy. A careful pre-operative CBCT evaluation is mandatory in order to avoid intraoperative bleeding

the lateral wall; Mardinger et al. [39] reported it in 55% of cases, Temmermann et al. [40] in 49.5%, and Rosano et al. [36] in 47.5% of cases. Furthermore, the artery may run entirely externally (extraosseous, subperiosteal), run entirely internally (extraosseous maintaining contact with the membrane), or have a mixed course [36, 41]. In cases where the artery path is intraosseous, 3D imaging such as CT or CBCT reveals a circumferential radiotransparent area in the bone wall visible in the paraxial sections in particular. On the other hand, when the artery is not encased by the bony cortex, the CBCT could not be used to detect the artery in this case. This anastomosis ensures blood supply to the sinus membrane and the periosteal tissues. It is important to take note of the anastomosis preoperatively to avoid intraoperative hemorrhaging when this artery branch is sectioned during antrostomy.

It has been recommended to place the superior border of the osteotomy outline up to 15 mm from the alveolar crest in a minimal resorbed ridge to gain adequate access and avoid inadvertent penetration of the artery [39]. Massive hemorrhaging during the sinus elevation procedure is rare given that the diameter of blood vessels in the sinus is around 1 mm. Only in 5% of cases do the vessels have a diameter that exceeds 2 mm, and in these cases, if it is necessary to section the vessel because it impedes access to the sinus, proximal and distal ligation of the blood vessel is recommended [36, 42]. Venous return from the sinus is facilitated by the facial vein, sphenopalatine vein, and pterygoid plexus. It is important to note that veins can spread infection from the sinus to the surrounding tissues. The loss of maxillary teeth and advancing age cause a marked reduction in vascularization in the bones and a corresponding decrease in the number of blood vessels accompanied by a reduction in diameter rendering blood flow contorted.

Relatively small osteotomy window preparation with the adjunctive use of the microscope could potentially avoid complications as inadvertent injury to this artery during lateral sinus augmentation procedure could increase the difficulty of the membrane manipulation and subsequently cause perforation of the membrane.

3.5   Innervation

Innervation of the sinus derives directly from the maxillary nerve, the second branch of the fifth cranial nerve (trigeminal nerve). This nerve with its posterior middle and superior alveolar ramifications innervates the sinus floor in the posterior region, the ipsilateral molar, and premolar teeth. The anterior superior alveolar branch originating from the infraorbital nerve at the infraorbital foramen level reaches the anterior sinus wall and teeth in the maxilla, running below the sinus membrane. Some branches starting from infraorbital nerve branch off from the main trunk before leaving the infraorbital foramen and innervate the medial wall of the sinus. Other branches involving the sinus mucosa are those of the pterygoid palatine sphenopalatine ganglions with long and short sphenopalatine nerves. Posterior teeth on the other hand are innervated and receive blood supply from neurovascular ramifications deriving from the maxillary tuberosity forming the posterior wall of the sinus.

4   Fundamental Principles of Endoscopy as a Minimally Invasive Approach for Antral Interventions

Endoscopic sinus augmentation was first introduced in a case series as a low invasive adjunctive surgical technique in eight patients with residual bone height ranged between 4 and 8 mm [43]. Vertical sinus augmentation with simultaneous implant placement was performed with 17 titanium implants of 12–14 lengths and all subjects presented with no inflammation and displacement of the bone graft at the time of implant exposure with control sinuscopy. Recently, another case series have shown the sinus floor was lifted without perforation in 83.33% of cases using the endoscopic-assisted evaluation through lateral endoscopic approach and crestal osteotomy site [44]. The highest rate of membrane perforation in membrane thickness is less than 2 mm. Therefore, the authors recommended a blind crestal sinus augmentation approach should be used only when the sinus membrane thickness is more than 2 mm and preoperative membrane thickness evaluation by CBCT should be prescribed to evaluate the risk of membrane perforation. Minimal postoperative symptoms (e.g., inflammation, swelling, postoperative sinusitis) were observed. Furthermore, endoscopic-assisted sinus augmentation can also be used in lateral approach during the membrane elevation. Clear visualization of the endoscopic view may reduce the perforation rate, provide optimal bone graft distribution, and limit the need for huge or multiple bone windows [45]. The intraoperative continuous endoscopy allows (1) detection of sinus pathology, (2) assessment of natural ostium patency, (3) low-invasive surgical approach, (4) reduce postoperative morbidity, (5) control of graft position, (6) may reduce the risk of sinus membrane perforation, and (7) may provide proper vascularization of the graft and promote osteoregeneration.

5   Presurgical Sinus Assessment: Diagnosing Pathological Conditions of the Maxillary Sinus

Maxillary sinus elevation is a procedure that modifies the local anatomy of the sinus and may temporarily impair sinus homeostasis.

Patients in need of maxillary sinus surgery should undergo an appropriate radiological evaluation to visualize not only the upper dental arch (the maxillary sinus) but also for evaluation of the osteomeatal complex. For this reason, a proper preoperative evaluation should include not only orthopantomography but also cone-beam computed tomography (CBCT) [3, 46].

While no controlled clinical trials have been performed to assess the correlation of complications following maxillary sinus elevation and initial anatomic-physiological status of the maxillary sinus, it is reasonable to speculate that the success rate of the procedure could be partially related to the baseline condition of the maxillary sinus [47].

It can be stated that the clinician can lower the risk of postoperative complications if maxillary sinus elevation is performed starting from a healthy sinus with high compliance [47, 48]. It is therefore advisable to perform an extensive anamnestic, clinical, and radiographic assessment before sinus augmentation surgery to investigate the sinus health and subsequent sinus compliance to avoid unnecessary postsurgical complications.

It is extremely important during the first consultation to collect a complete history of potential conditions affecting the maxillary sinus, such as nasal obstructions, facial trauma, sinus infections, allergic symptoms, smell and taste dysfunction, pressure-related discomfort, chronic respiratory diseases, previous nasosinusal surgery, facial deformities, scars, and mouth breathing.

If the anamnesis is positive or there are symptoms of sinusitis, it is advisable to ask for an ENT assessment. The same assessment should be made in cases that present radiologic signs of radiopacity, previous sinus treatments, impaired nasal breathing, and chronic respiratory diseases.

Table 1 proposes a list of questions for a specific maxillary sinus anamnesis.

Table 2 summarizes the basic requirements of CT scan.

A sinus lift procedure can be impaired by preexisting odontogenic sinusitis (Table 3).

Odontogenic sinusitis has been reported to represent 10% of all cases of maxillary sinusitis [49, 50], but it is estimated that the real incidence could be between 25% and 40% [51, 52].

A survey [53] by 93 board-certified otolaryngologists and rhinologists reported that an odontogenic source is a common cause of maxillary sinusitis and reported treating an average of 2.9 patients per year with odontogenic maxillary sinusitis,

Table 1 Maxillary sinus medical history

Medical history	No	Yes	Notes
Have you ever had allergies?			
Have you ever had chronic respiratory diseases?			
Can you breathe normally using both nostrils?			
Have you ever had ENT diseases?			
Do you use nasal sprays?			
Have you ever had chronic or acute sinusitis?			
Have you ever had ENT or maxillofacial surgery?			
Can you compensate pressure through the ears, for example, when you take a plane?			
Is there ever a bitter taste at the back of your throat?			
Do you have or have you ever had any facial fillers or facelifts?[a]			

[a]This information is important during flap management. Facial fillers may cause problems in soft tissue handling

Table 2 Requirements of a basic radiologic evaluation

Radiologic evaluation	YES	NO	Notes
Does the CT allow a correct visualization of the osteo-meatal complex?			
Is the osteo-meatal complex patent?			
Are there any signs of radiopacity in the maxillary sinus?			
Final evaluation			
Ask for ENT assessment			
Patient eligible for maxillary sinus elevation			

who were initially misdiagnosed. Otolaryngologists also perceived that radiologists rarely consider dental pathology when scanning the maxillary sinus using computed tomography.

The exact pathogenesis of odontogenic sinusitis is still not fully understood although impaired Schneiderian membrane integrity due to maxillary dental infections or trauma, odontogenic disease of the maxillary bone, tooth extractions, implantology, or endodontic treatment is always present.

Microbiological sampling of sinusitis of odontogenic origin reveals a different bacterial flora than that found in rhinogenic sinusitis [54]. Usually, odontogenic sinusitis is a polymicrobial infection, and anaerobic species, from the oral cavity and upper respiratory tract, are predominant.

The development of sinusitis in patients with predisposing odontogenic disease is variable; however, a recent review suggested the possible role of the bacterial biofilm in relation to the severity and progression of odontogenic sinusitis [55].

Sinus lift procedures could be affected by many behavioral and environmental conditions affecting the normal physiology of the maxillary sinus.

Table 3 Contraindications for maxillary sinus augmentation. Modified from Mantovani M [21].

Presumably irreversible ENT contra-indications (PIEC$_S$)	Potentially reversible ENT contra-indications (PREC$_S$)
Anatomic structural alterations: – Serious deformities and posttraumatic, postsurgical, and postradiotherapy scarring on the nasal-sinus walls and/or mucosa lining	Anatomic structural alterations: Stenosis of the drainage-ventilation pathways in the maxillary sinus (sustained by one or more of the following anatomic alterations): Septal deviation, paradox curve of the middle turbinate bone, conchae bulla, hypertrophy of the agger nasi cell, presence of Haller cell), postsurgical scars or synechiae on the osteomeatal complex, oro-antral fistula. All these alterations can be resolved by surgery: The maxillary sinus appears to be well-ventilated thanks to a partial uncinectomy
Inflammatory infective processes: – Reoccurring or chronic sinusitis, with or without polyps, which cannot undergo resolution as it is associated with congenital mucociliary clearance alterations (e.g., cystic fibrosis, Kartagener's syndrome, Young's syndrome), to intolerance of acetylsalicylic acid (triad: Nasal polyps, asthma, intolerance to acetylsalicylic acid, ASA), to immunologic deficiency (e.g., AIDS, pharmacologic immunosuppression)	Inflammatory infective processes: Acute viral or bacterial rhinosinusitis, allergy-related rhinosinusitis, mycotic sinusitis (noninvasive forms), acute repeating, and chronic sinusitis sustained by one of the anatomic alterations listed above which obstruct the sinus drainage-ventilation ways, by endo-antral foreign bodies, or by nasal polyps. Functional endoscopic surgery is clearly indicated
Tumor-related: – Locally aggressive benign tumors (e.g., inverted papilloma, myxoma, ethmoidal-maxillary fibromatosis) in antrum; – Nasal-sinus malignant tumors (epithelium, neuroectodermal, bone, soft tissue, odontogenic, lymphomatosis, metastatic-originated) of the maxillary sinus and/or adjacent structures	Tumor-related: – Nonobstructive nasal-sinus benign tumors, both before and after the lifting operation could affect the sinus drainage-ventilation pathways or when removal does not affect the mucociliary transportation system (e.g., mucosa cysts, cholesterinic granuloma, antrochoanal polyp) all are easily subject to correction by functional endoscopic surgery
Nasal-sinus manifestations of a specific systemic granulomatous diseases: – Wegener's granulomatosis, "idiopathic midline granuloma," and sarcoidosis	

Modified from Mantovani M (ed.), Otorhinolaryngological implications in augmentation of the maxillary sinus. In: Testori T, Del Fabbro M, Weinstein R, Wallace S. Maxillary Sinus Surgery, Quintessence 2009 [21]

The use of cocaine, a drug usually inhaled through the nose, may have a dramatic effect on the oral mucosa [56].

In a systematic review addressing hard palate perforation in cocaine abusers, sinusitis is confirmed as one of the most common side effects [57]. From a clinical point of view, in the authors' experience, the Schneiderian membrane in these patients appears extremely thin and fragile, requiring great attention when detaching.

Smoking is a well-known risk factor for implant survival [58]. A retrospective evaluation on the survival rate of implants placed in grafted sinuses found that smoking more than 15 cigarettes per day was significantly correlated to implant failure [59].

The following recommendations could guide the implant surgeon on how to interact with an ENT specialist for the appropriate course of treatment on the radiological findings in the sinus. Any radiological findings should be interpreted along with a proper sinus history and after having evaluated any possible clinical symptoms that the patient might have.

– Mucosal thickening up to 3 mm not related to symptoms of acute rhinosinusitis does not require any further investigation if the OMC is patent. Any mucosal thickening, if related to OMC closure, needs a specific ENT evaluation.
– Mucous retention cyst does not require any further investigation if the cyst, even after the elevation of the sinus membrane, does not interfere with the OMC or if the cyst is located in a different area, i.e., distal wall of the sinus.
– Any foreign bodies (teeth, implants) should be removed before surgery. Bony wall dehiscence with soft tissue closure and healthy sinus is not a contraindication to maxillary sinus elevation.
– Missing sinus wall and bone erosion should always be regarded with great suspicion and requires specialist evaluation to exclude neoplastic conditions.

6 Pre-op Diagnosis, Planning, and Evaluation of Case Difficulty

During the diagnosis phase, an important parameter to assess is the degree of resorption in the alveolar crest. This variable must be evaluated in the apico-coronal (sinus-crestal bone floor), vestibulo-palatal, and residual crestal direction with respect to the occlusal plane (interarch distance). The "classic indication" for sinus elevation is moderate atrophy in the upper jaw without skeletal alteration. In these cases, it is possible to carry out an implant-prosthetic rehabilitation with normal-sized teeth [60]. A 3D analysis of the edentulous ridge will determine the type of surgery needed to restore vertical and/or horizontal bone volume (Fig. 4a–d). In clinical cases with an increased interarch distance and/or an alveolar ridge with a thickness of less than 6 mm in the vestibulo-palatal direction, the ideal treatment would be by reconstructive surgery [60]. The quantity of crestal bone available in the apico-coronal direction can influence the choice of the surgical approach. Many clinicians would accept 4 mm as the limit determining whether to carry out

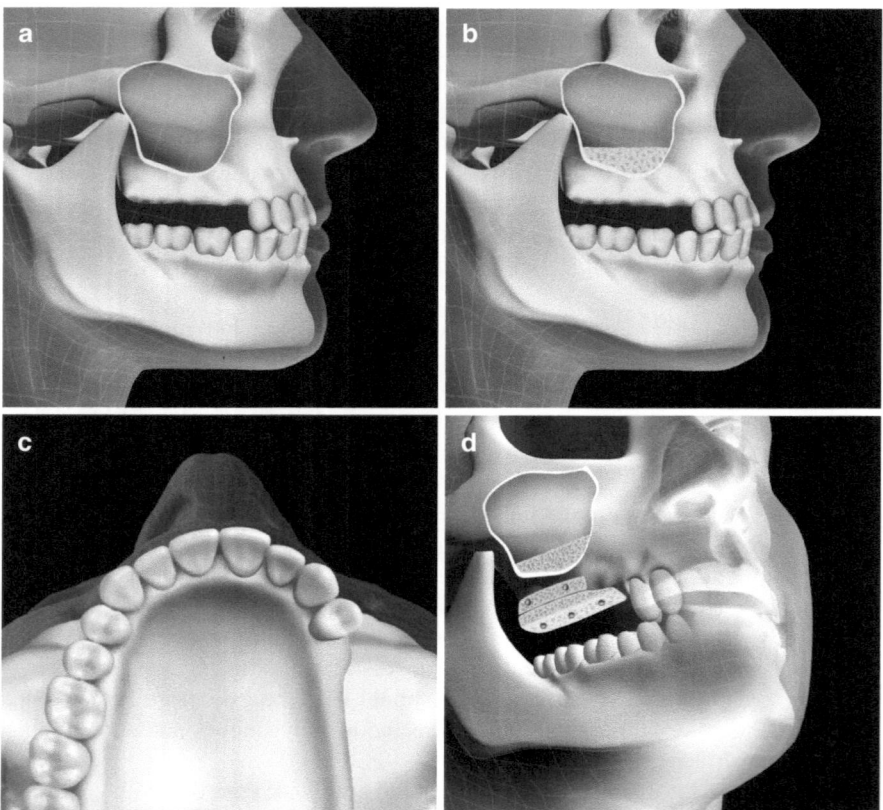

Fig. 4 (**a**) Hyper-pneumatization of the maxillary sinus with normal inter-arch distance and no horizontal atrophy is the ideal condition for maxillary sinus augmentation, (**b**) no further bone augmentation procedures are needed. (**c**) More often hyper-pneumatization of the sinus is combined with augmented inter-arch distance and/or horizontal bone atrophy. (**d**) In these clinical situations maxillary sinus augmentation alone is not enough. Adjunctive bone regenerations procedures must be carried out i.e. GBR

maxillary sinus elevation with a crestal or lateral approach. An analysis of the quality/quantity of available bone is a useful parameter to predict the primary stability of the proposed implant. Such considerations determine the choice between sinus surgery with implant placement (simultaneous protocol) and sinus surgery with implant placement at a later stage (delayed protocol).

Although it is technically possible to stabilize implants with residual crestal bone heights of 2 mm or less, the risk of early implant failure is high if implants are spontaneously exposed before graft material consolidation. In case of exposure, the physiological process establishing the biological width begins with consequent crestal bone resorption of about 2 mm. This phenomenon may result in micromotion or outright mobility of the implant due to loss of the only bone-implant contact present before graft consolidation. Premature exposure of implants is more likely to occur when thin soft tissues are present (under 1–1.5 mm), or it can be caused by compression from improperly conditioned removable prostheses. In cases with residual crestal bone of 3 mm or less, it is advisable to plan a delayed approach, after graft consolidation. The use of short implants is an appropriate therapeutic option when residual crestal height is 7 mm or more.

While studies have reported varying success, the current database is insufficient to suggest the routine clinical use of super-short implants (5 mm). On the vertical plane, to carry out a cemented prosthetic restoration, the minimum distance between the crestal bone and occlusal plane should be at least 7 mm to allow sufficient space for restorative components. In clinical practice, prosthetic crowns, in case of maxillary sinus elevation, are usually longer in the apico-coronal direction to compensate for bone resorption that has taken place (longer crowns). Future prosthetic rehabilitation must be planned in advance with a diagnostic wax-up to evaluate function, aesthetics, and maintenance with normal homecare hygiene procedures. On the transversal plane, the clinician's aim is to obtain an interarch ratio that assures a proper distribution of functional and occlusal load. On the sagittal plane, especially in the edentulous patient, intra-oral examination analyzing the state of and support available from perioral soft tissues in association with skeletal class assessment is fundamental. The vertical reduction in the lower third of the face, retraction of the upper lip, deepening of the nasolabial sulcus, and increase in nasolabial angle are clinical signs of significant atrophy. Modest atrophy of the crest can usually be treated in a manner that avoids invasive reconstruction procedures by compensating for the bone resorption with longer crowns along with adequate treatment of peri-implant tissues hence obtaining a good compromise from an aesthetic-functional point of view.

Quantity of residual crestal bone available and relative indications for the type of surgery (lateral approach, crestal, short implants).

Some clinical parameters that can be evaluated preoperatively with regard to procedures for home care include the emergence profile of prosthetic restoration, an adequate quantity of peri-implant keratinized mucosa, and sufficient arch depth. Pre-op radiological examinations recommended include a CBCT extended to the osteomeatal complex for the assessment of ostium patency and investigating the possible presence of disease in the paranasal sinuses. This examination allows for an accurate ENT diagnosis in case of sinus disease. When compared to a bi-dimensional examination (orthopantomography), CBCT allows for an accurate assessment of septal anatomy, the diameter and course of blood vessels, possible bone dehiscence, and sinus disease [46]. Using dedicated software, graft volume can be determined, and surgical guides for the antrostomy and implant positioning can be fabricated.

Once a thorough preoperative evaluation and surgical diagnosis are completed, it is possible to assess, within reason, the surgical risk and determine the level of experience/expertise that is necessary to achieve a positive outcome. The Maxillary Sinus Elevation Difficulty Score worksheet (Supplement) awards difficulty points for several clinical situations that may be encountered [10, 36, 61]. Simply add up the case score and determine if the case falls within the general guidelines of diffi-culty suggested by the authors [27]. Your own experience level should match well with the case difficulty level.

7   Microscope-Assisted Lateral Sinus Augmentation

7.1   Lateral Sinus Augmentation

7.1.1   Potential Benefits and Advantages

Flap elevation	A lateral sinus augmentation is possible in a limited space (a single tooth gap space)
	Conservative incision design and minimal flap releasing
Osteotomy site preparation	Smaller lateral window size
Sinus membrane elevation	Reduction of the incidence of the Schneiderian membrane perforation (increased visualization of irregular anatomical structures in the sinus cavity)
	Cost-effective (less bone graft is needed with less Schneiderian membrane elevation)
Implant placement	Increased visualization of the sinus cavity during simultaneous implant placement
Wound closure	Facilitate primary wound closure with high magnification and optimal illumination from the operating microscope
Healing phase	Faster bone maturation, a higher percentage of vital bone formation, and less early implant failure from the preservation of the vascularized sinus bony walls
Patient-centered outcomes	High patient satisfaction, less postoperative pain due to minimally invasive surgery

7.1.2   Incision Design and Osteotomy Preparation

After local anesthesia injection, an incision is made midcrestally of the edentulous ridge. A vertical incision is made at the line angle of the tooth adjacent to the eden-tulous area, extend 2-3 mm beyond the mucogingival junction to gain access and facilitate flap mobilization (Fig. 5). Full-thickness flap reflection is performed at approximately 3 mm just beyond the expected osteotomy border. Careful use of the elevator or retractor should be taken into consideration especially in thin lateral or crestal sinus walls as the instruments might accidentally go through the sinus wall into the sinus cavity [12]. Minnesota elevator is recommended to retract the flap altogether with lips and cheeks, which facilitate the direct vision of the operating microscope. Dimension of the osteotomy site is initially 6×6 mm in diameter at the point where the location of the future implant is previously planned (Fig. 6). A rotary diamond bur with a high-speed air-driven handpiece is used to draw the oste-otomy site outline and a piezoelectric device is subsequently utilized until the bluish-hue color is appeared (Fig. 7).

Fig. 5 Vertical incision extending beyond mucogingival junction to ensure adequate flap mobilization and access to the lateral bony wall

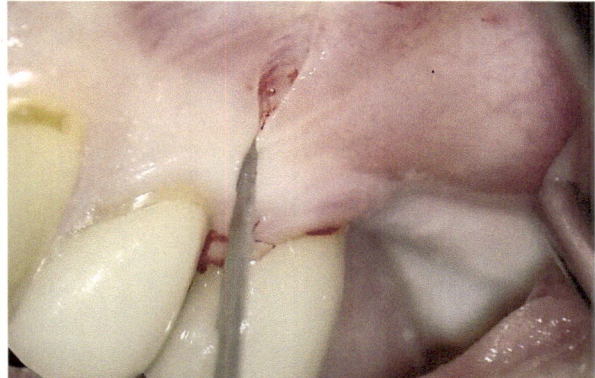

Fig. 6 Minnesota elevator is used to retract the flap altogether with lips and cheeks and reveal the location of the osteotomy site

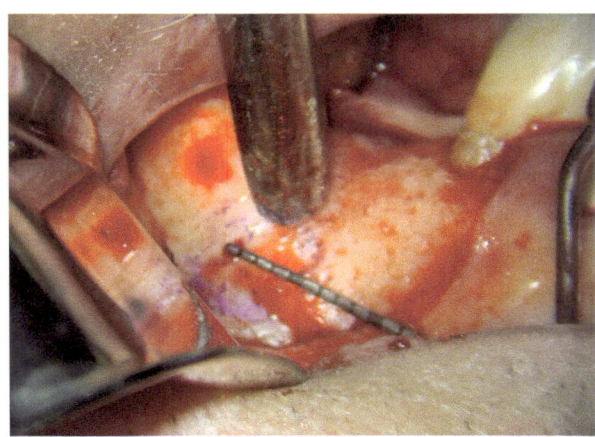

7.1.3 Schneiderian Membrane Examination and Management

The Schneiderian membrane is elevated with the use of a series of sinus elevation instruments (Fig. 8). The extent of sinus membrane elevation should be at the implant location to ensure adequate membrane release is obtained as the perforation of the sinus membrane may occur at area with the greatest amount of membrane distension [13]. The integrity of the Schneiderian membrane is assessed with the operating microscope using indirect and direct vision at an approximate magnification of 8–18× (Fig. 9). The amount of bone graft is predetermined by the amount of vertical height needed. The aim is to use the least amount of particulate bone graft as much as necessary to promote faster bone healing and save the unnecessary expense for excess particulate grafts. An absorbable human amnion-chorion membrane (BioXclude, Snoasis medical, Denver CO, USA) is used for simultaneous guided bone regeneration to augment horizontal ridge width if needed. Primary wound closure is achieved by flaps approximation, periosteal scoring at the base of the flap if necessary, and suture with 6-0 (P-3 needle) or 7-0 (P-1 needle) polypropylene sutures (AD Surgical, California, USA).

Fig. 7 Bluish hue color of the osteotomy site

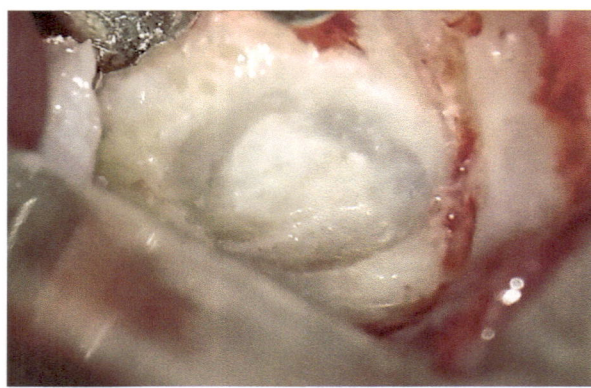

Fig. 8 The sinus membrane elevation by sinus elevation instruments (surgical curette)

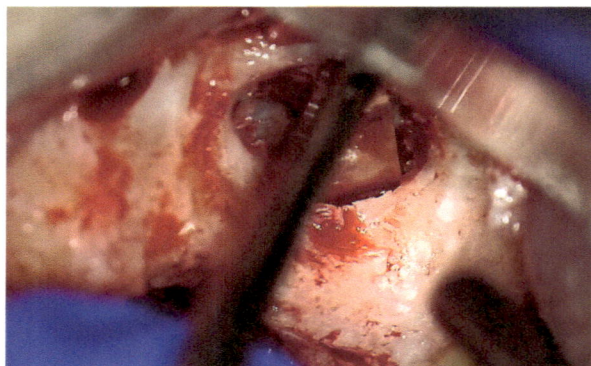

Fig. 9 The integrity of the Schneiderian membrane is assessed with the operating microscope at a magnification of 8–18×

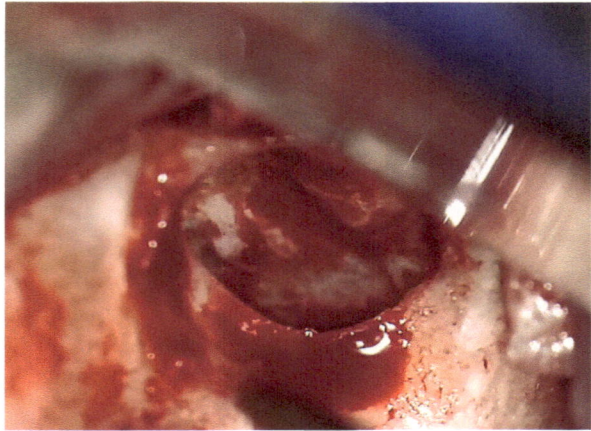

7.1.4   Management of Schneiderian Membrane Perforation

If the perforation occurs during osteotomy preparation, the window is extended until the sound sinus membrane can be accessed and elevated. The absorbable human amnion-chorion membrane is considered a membrane of choice to cover the site of perforation due to its ease of use (no membrane preparation is needed, etc.). Alternatively, an absorbable collagen membrane can be used. If the size of perforation is more than 10 mm in diameter or the location is close to the adjacent root, non-stabilized repairs (without screws or sutures) are unpredictable and the surgery should be aborted and allow approximately 4 months for the sinus membrane to heal before initiate a second attempt [12].

8   Microscope-Assisted Vertical Sinus Augmentation

8.1   Potential Benefits and Advantages

Flap elevation	Conservative incision design and minimal flap releasing
Sinus membrane	Detection of the Schneiderian membrane perforation
elevation	Predictively treat and manage membrane perforation
Wound closure	Facilitate primary wound closure with high magnification and optimal illumination from the operating microscope
Healing phase	Less incidence of postoperative sinusitis due to undetected sinus membrane perforation
Patient-centered outcomes	High patient satisfaction, less postoperative pain due to minimally invasive surgery

8.2   Osteotomy Site Preparation

After full-thickness flap elevation at the crest of the edentulous ridge, osteotomy site of vertical sinus augmentation is performed with either an osteotome approach or a set of specially designed burs (Densah® Burs, Versah, Jackson, Michigan, USA) (Fig. 10).

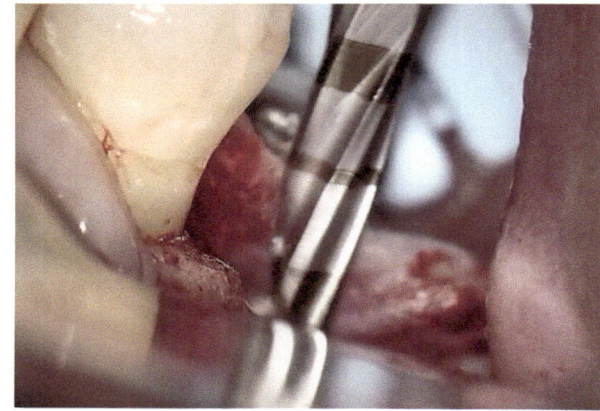

Fig. 10 The specially designed burs could be used to create an osteotomy site by simultaneously advancing the sinus floor and lifting the membrane with both allograft and compacted autograft

8.3 Detection of Schneiderian Membrane Perforation and Management

The sinus membrane is lifted and inspected for the presence of perforation if any by the use of the operating microscope at an approximate magnification of 8–18×. The illumination should be adjusted to the near maximum to facilitate the assessment of the small osteotomy site (Fig. 11a, b). The evaluation should be performed immediately after osteotomy site preparation and after sinus membrane elevation or bone graft placement. If the size of perforation is less than 2 mm, a collagen sponge or membrane could be used without bone graft. However, if the size is more than 2 mm and alternative short implant placement is not feasible, lateral sinus augmentation along with management of the perforation should be performed [15].

8.4 Bone Graft Application and Simultaneous Implant Placement

The amount of particulate allograft is tentatively calculated relative to the previously planned vertical height needed (Fig. 12a, b). Approximately, 0.1 mL of grafting material is required for 3.5 mm vertical sinus membrane elevation and 0.2 mL, 0.3 mL for 5 mm and 6 mm vertical elevation height, respectively [62].

9 Conclusions

Optimal treatment planning, accurate diagnosis, Schneiderian membrane manipulation, and detection of intrasurgical complications are prerequisites for the success of sinus augmentation procedures. Knowing the sinus anatomy and possible sinus

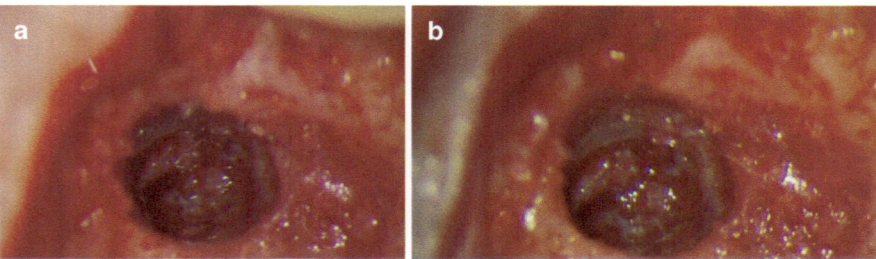

Fig. 11 (**a, b**) The integrity of the Schneiderian membrane is assessed with the operating microscope at a magnification of 8–18×

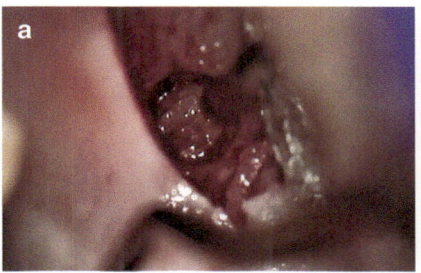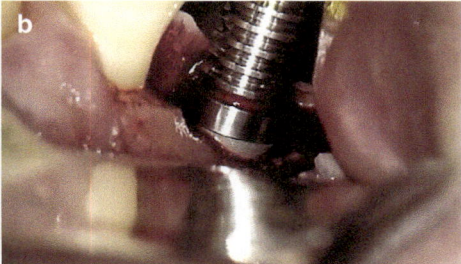

Fig. 12 (**a**) Particulate allograft is applied to the crestal osteotomy site. (**b**) Subsequently implant placement

pathology is critical. At the surgical level, minimally invasive operating microscope-assisted sinus augmentation could assist in gentler handling of soft and hard tissues, detecting intraoperative complications, promoting faster healing, resulting in less postoperative pain compared to conventional sinus augmentation procedures. Few years of clinical experiences with OM for performing lateral and vertical sinus augmentation have provided high success rate and positive patient feedback. Research is encouraged to study the benefits of using OM for enhancing sinus healing after augmentation procedures.

10   Key Points

1. The key factors to the success of sinus augmentation and reduce complications to a minimum are; (1) adequate evaluation of sinus health and identification of sinus pathology if any, and (2) understand sinus anatomy with optimal treatment planning.
2. The detection and accurate diagnosis of the size of the perforation during surgery with sufficient magnification and illumination of the operating microscope could guide clinicians to establish an optimal solution and avoid unforeseen postoperative severe complications.
3. Microscope-assisted sinus augmentation could facilitate a minimally invasive, precise hard and soft tissue manipulation and result in minimal postoperative pain with high patients' satisfaction due to smaller window size and minimal flap elevation.
4. Benefits for microscope-assisted lateral sinus augmentation are; (1) the lateral sinus augmentation surgery is possible in a limited space, (2) Smaller lateral window size, (3) possible less incidence of the Schneiderian membrane perforation, (4) Less bone graft is needed, (4) increased visualization for simultaneous implant placement, (5) faster bone maturation and primary wound closure.
5. Benefits for microscope-assisted vertical sinus augmentation are; (1) Detection of the Schneiderian membrane perforation, (2) Predictively treat and manage membrane perforation, (3) less incidence of the Schneiderian membrane perforation due to undetected sinus membrane perforation.

11   Appendix

Maxillary Sinus Elevation Difficulty Score: (MSED) Score		
A	*Extra-intraoral evaluation*	
A1	*Face type*	
	Long or normal face[a]	☐ 0 pt
	Short face[b]	☐ 2 pt
	[a]Long face usually has thin sinus wall and the zygomatic process more apically positioned (see B7)	
	[b]Short face has thicker sinus walls and zygomatic process more coronally oriented (see B7)	
A2	*Surgical access (ease to retract cheeks)*	
	Dimension of the mouth	☐ 0 pt
	Wide: 0 pt	☐ 1 pt
	Regular: 1 pt	☐ 2 pt
	Narrow: 2 pt	☐ 0 pt
	Thickness of the cheeks	☐ 1 pt
	Normal: 0 pt	☐ 2 pt
	Thick: 1 pt	☐ 0 pt
	Very thick (usually bruxers): 2 pt	☐ 1 pt
	Sinus elevation patient side	
	Left side for left-handed surgeon or right side for right-handed surgeon 0 pt	
	Left side for right-handed surgeon or right side for left-handed surgeon 1 pt	
A3	*Type of edentulism*	
	Fully edentulous	☐ 0 pt
	Partially edentulous (missing bicuspid and molars)	☐ 1 pt
	Partially edentulous (missing only molars or missing one tooth in between natural teeth)	☐ 2 pt
B	*Radiographic evaluation*	
B1	*Wall thickness*	
	Thin: ≤1 mm	☐ 0 pt
	Medium: >1, <2 mm	☐ 1 pt
	Thick: >2 mm	☐ 2 pt
B2	*Sinus membrane thickness*	
	≥1.0 to <2.5	☐ 0 pt
	≤1.0	
	>2.5	☐ 1 pt
		☐ 2 pt
B3	*Septa direction*	
	Absent	☐ 0 pt
	Bucco-nasal direction	☐ 1 pt
	Mesio-distal direction	☐ 2 pt
B4	*Septa location*	
	Middle recess	☐ 0 pt
	Posterior recess	☐ 1 pt
	Anterior recess	☐ 2 pt
B5	*Alveolar antral artery diameter[a]*	
	<1 mm	☐ 0 pt
	>1, <2 mm	☐ 1 pt
	>2 mm	☐ 2 pt
	[a]This parameter is important only if the artery interferes with the execution of the antrostomy. (if the artery is not involved, enter 0)	

Maxillary Sinus Elevation Difficulty Score: (MSED) Score		
B6	*Angle between the buccal and palatal wall*[a]	
	>30°	☐ 0 pt
	<30°	☐ 1 pt
	[a]The wider the angle the more difficult it is to perform the antrostomy	
B7	*Zygomatic process morphology*[a]	
	Apically positioned	☐ 0 pt
	Coronal positioned	☐ 1 pt
	[a]The zygomatic process of the maxilla could be apically or more coronally located with respect to the ridge. If it is apically located and there is a vertical wall, it is easier for the clinician to perform the antrostomy. If it is coronally located there is an inclined wall and it is more difficult for the surgeon to perform the antrostomy	
B8	*Osteoma/exostosis*	
	Absent	☐ 0 pt
	Present	☐ 1 pt
B9	*Bone dehiscence*	
	Absent	☐ 0 pt
	Present at the level of the buccal wall	☐ 1 pt
	Present at the level of the ridge	☐ 2 pt
	Present at the level of the nasal wall	☐ 3 pt
B10	*Palatonasal recess*	
	Absent	☐ 0 pt
	Present	☐ 1 pt

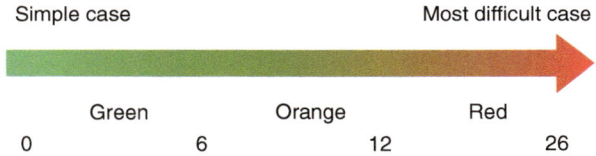

Simple case   Most difficult case

         Green   Orange   Red

0   6   12   26

References

1. Boyne PJ, James RA. Grafting of the maxillary sinus floor with autogenous marrow and bone. J Oral Surg. 1980;38:613–6.
2. Tatum H Jr. Maxillary and sinus implant reconstructions. Dent Clin N Am. 1986;30:207–29.
3. Wallace SS, Tarnow DP, Froum SJ, Cho SC, Zadeh HH, Stoupel J, et al. Maxillary sinus elevation by lateral window approach: evolution of technology and technique. J Evid Based Dent Pract. 2012;12(3 Suppl):161–71.
4. Lundgren S, Cricchio G, Hallman M, Jungner M, Rasmusson L, Sennerby L. Sinus floor elevation procedures to enable implant placement and integration: techniques, biological aspects and clinical outcomes. Periodontol 2000. 2017;73:103–20.
5. Pjetursson BE, Tan WC, Zwahlen M, Lang NP. A systematic review of the success of sinus floor elevation and survival of implants inserted in combination with sinus floor elevation. J Clin Periodontol. 2008;35(8 Suppl):216–40.
6. Tan WC, Lang NP, Zwahlen M, Pjetursson BE. A systematic review of the success of sinus floor elevation and survival of implants inserted in combination with sinus floor elevation. Part II: transalveolar technique. J Clin Periodontol. 2008;35(8 Suppl):241–54.

7. Schwarz L, Schiebel V, Hof M, Ulm C, Watzek G, Pommer B. Risk factors of membrane perforation and postoperative complications in sinus floor elevation surgery: review of 407 augmentation procedures. J Oral Maxillofac Surg. 2015;73:1275–82.
8. Vercellotti T, De Paoli S, Nevins M. The piezoelectric bony window osteotomy and sinus membrane elevation: introduction of a new technique for simplification of the sinus augmentation procedure. Int J Periodontics Restorative Dent. 2001;21:561–7.
9. Jordi C, Mukaddam K, Lambrecht JT, Kuhl S. Membrane perforation rate in lateral maxillary sinus floor augmentation using conventional rotating instruments and piezoelectric device-a meta-analysis. Int J Implant Dent. 2018;4:3.
10. Cho SC, Wallace SS, Froum SJ, Tarnow DP. Influence of anatomy on Schneiderian membrane perforations during sinus elevation surgery: three-dimensional analysis. Pract Proced Aesthet Dent. 2001;13:160–3.
11. Chan HL, Monje A, Suarez F, Benavides E, Wang HL. Palatonasal recess on medial wall of the maxillary sinus and clinical implications for sinus augmentation via lateral window approach. J Periodontol. 2013;84:1087–93.
12. Testori T, Weinstein T, Taschieri S, Wallace SS. Risk factors in lateral window sinus elevation surgery. Periodontol 2000. 2019;81:91–123.
13. Garbacea A, Lozada JL, Church CA, Al-Ardah AJ, Seiberling KA, Naylor WP, et al. The incidence of maxillary sinus membrane perforation during endoscopically assessed crestal sinus floor elevation: a pilot study. J Oral Implantol. 2012;38:345–59.
14. Gargallo-Albiol J, Sinjab KH, Barootchi S, Chan HL, Wang HL. Microscope and micro-camera assessment of Schneiderian membrane perforation via transcrestal sinus floor elevation: a randomized ex vivo study. Clin Oral Implants Res. 2019;30:682–90.
15. Tavelli L, Borgonovo AE, Saleh MH, Ravida A, Chan HL, Wang HL. Classification of sinus membrane perforations occurring during transcrestal sinus floor elevation and related treatment. Int J Periodontics Restorative Dent. 2020;40:111–8.
16. Merli M, Moscatelli M, Mariotti G, Pagliaro U, Bernardelli F, Nieri M. A minimally invasive technique for lateral maxillary sinus floor elevation: a Bayesian network study. Clin Oral Implants Res. 2016;27:273–81.
17. Sirinirund B, Chan HL, Velasquez D. Microscope-assisted maxillary sinus augmentation: a case series. Int J Periodontics Restorative Dent. 2021;41:531–7.
18. Avila-Ortiz G, Wang HL, Galindo-Moreno P, Misch CE, Rudek I, Neiva R. Influence of lateral window dimensions on vital bone formation following maxillary sinus augmentation. Int J Oral Maxillofac Implants. 2012;27:1230–8.
19. Baldini N, D'Elia C, Bianco A, Goracci C, de Sanctis M, Ferrari M. Lateral approach for sinus floor elevation: large versus small bone window - a split-mouth randomized clinical trial. Clin Oral Implants Res. 2017;28:974–81.
20. Baldini N, D'Elia C, Mirra R, Ferrari M. Minimally invasive flap compared to a trapezoidal flap in lateral approach maxillary sinus elevation procedures: four-month post-loading results from a split-mouth randomised controlled trial. Int J Oral Implantol (Berl). 2019;12:209–24.
21. M. M. Otorhinolaryngological implications in augmentation of the maxillary sinus. In: Testori T, Weinstein R, Wallace S, editors. Maxillary sinus surgery and alternatives in treatment. Chicago: Quintessence; 2009. p. 29–34.
22. Insua A, Monje A, Chan HL, Zimmo N, Shaikh L, Wang HL. Accuracy of Schneiderian membrane thickness: a cone-beam computed tomography analysis with histological validation. Clin Oral Implants Res. 2017;28:654–61.
23. Pommer B, Unger E, Suto D, Hack N, Watzek G. Mechanical properties of the Schneiderian membrane in vitro. Clin Oral Implants Res. 2009;20:633–7.
24. Wen SC, Lin YH, Yang YC, Wang HL. The influence of sinus membrane thickness upon membrane perforation during transcrestal sinus lift procedure. Clin Oral Implants Res. 2015;26:1158–64.
25. Lin YH, Yang YC, Wen SC, Wang HL. The influence of sinus membrane thickness upon membrane perforation during lateral window sinus augmentation. Clin Oral Implants Res. 2016;27:612–7.

26. Chan HL, Suarez F, Monje A, Benavides E, Wang HL. Evaluation of maxillary sinus width on cone-beam computed tomography for sinus augmentation and new sinus classification based on sinus width. Clin Oral Implants Res. 2014;25:647–52.
27. Testori T, Tavelli L, Yu SH, Scaini R, Darnahal A, Wallace SS, et al. Maxillary sinus elevation difficulty score with lateral wall technique. Int J Oral Maxillofac Implants. 2020;35:631–8.
28. Wen SC, Chan HL, Wang HL. Classification and management of antral septa for maxillary sinus augmentation. Int J Periodontics Restorative Dent. 2013;33:509–17.
29. Cakur B, Sumbullu MA, Durna D. Relationship among Schneiderian membrane, Underwood's septa, and the maxillary sinus inferior border. Clin Implant Dent Relat Res. 2013;15:83–7.
30. Velasquez-Plata D, Hovey LR, Peach CC, Alder ME. Maxillary sinus septa: a 3-dimensional computerized tomographic scan analysis. Int J Oral Maxillofac Implants. 2002;17:854–60.
31. Underwood AS. An inquiry into the anatomy and pathology of the maxillary sinus. J Anat Physiol. 1910;44(Pt 4):354–69.
32. Rosano G, Taschieri S, Gaudy JF, Lesmes D, Del Fabbro M. Maxillary sinus septa: a cadaveric study. J Oral Maxillofac Surg. 2010;68:1360–4.
33. Yilmaz HG, Tozum TF. Are gingival phenotype, residual ridge height, and membrane thickness critical for the perforation of maxillary sinus? J Periodontol. 2012;83:420–5.
34. Testori T, Yu SH, Tavelli L, Wang HL. Perforation risk assessment in maxillary sinus augmentation with lateral wall technique. Int J Periodontics Restorative Dent. 2020;40:373–80.
35. Park WB, Kang KL, Han JY. Factors influencing long-term survival rates of implants placed simultaneously with lateral maxillary sinus floor augmentation: a 6- to 20-year retrospective study. Clin Oral Implants Res. 2019;30:977–88.
36. Rosano G, Taschieri S, Gaudy JF, Weinstein T, Del Fabbro M. Maxillary sinus vascular anatomy and its relation to sinus lift surgery. Clin Oral Implants Res. 2011;22:711–5.
37. Solar P, Geyerhofer U, Traxler H, Windisch A, Ulm C, Watzek G. Blood supply to the maxillary sinus relevant to sinus floor elevation procedures. Clin Oral Implants Res. 1999;10:34–44.
38. Elian N, Wallace S, Cho SC, Jalbout ZN, Froum S. Distribution of the maxillary artery as it relates to sinus floor augmentation. Int J Oral Maxillofac Implants. 2005;20:784–7.
39. Mardinger O, Abba M, Hirshberg A, Schwartz-Arad D. Prevalence, diameter and course of the maxillary intraosseous vascular canal with relation to sinus augmentation procedure: a radiographic study. Int J Oral Maxillofac Surg. 2007;36:735–8.
40. Temmerman A, Hertele S, Teughels W, Dekeyser C, Jacobs R, Quirynen M. Are panoramic images reliable in planning sinus augmentation procedures? Clin Oral Implants Res. 2011;22:189–94.
41. Rosano G, Taschieri S, Gaudy JF, Del Fabbro M. Maxillary sinus vascularization: a cadaveric study. J Craniofac Surg. 2009;20:940–3.
42. Testori T, Rosano G, Taschieri S, Del Fabbro M. Ligation of an unusually large vessel during maxillary sinus floor augmentation. A case report. Eur. J Oral Implantol. 2010;3:255–8.
43. Engelke W, Deckwer I. Endoscopically controlled sinus floor augmentation. A preliminary report. Clin Oral Implants Res. 1997;8:527–31.
44. Elian S, Barakat K. Crestal endoscopic approach for evaluating sinus membrane elevation technique. Int J Implant Dent. 2018;4:15.
45. Giovannetti F, Raponi I, Priore P, Macciocchi A, Barbera G, Valentini V. Minimally-invasive endoscopic-assisted sinus augmentation. J Craniofac Surg. 2019;30:e359–62.
46. Harris D, Horner K, Grondahl K, Jacobs R, Helmrot E, Benic GI, et al. E.A.O. guidelines for the use of diagnostic imaging in implant dentistry 2011. A consensus workshop organized by the European Association for Osseointegration at the Medical University of Warsaw. Clin Oral Implants Res. 2012;23:1243–53.
47. Timmenga NM, Raghoebar GM, Liem RS, van Weissenbruch R, Manson WL, Vissink A. Effects of maxillary sinus floor elevation surgery on maxillary sinus physiology. Eur J Oral Sci. 2003;111:189–97.
48. Torretta S, Mantovani M, Testori T, Cappadona M, Pignataro L. Importance of ENT assessment in stratifying candidates for sinus floor elevation: a prospective clinical study. Clin Oral Implants Res. 2013;24(Suppl A100):57–62.

49. Lopatin AS, Sysolyatin SP, Sysolyatin PG, Melnikov MN. Chronic maxillary sinusitis of dental origin: is external surgical approach mandatory? Laryngoscope. 2002;112:1056–9.
50. Mehra P, Murad H. Maxillary sinus disease of odontogenic origin. Otolaryngol Clin N Am. 2004;37:347–64.
51. Melen I, Lindahl L, Andreasson L, Rundcrantz H. Chronic maxillary sinusitis. Definition, diagnosis and relation to dental infections and nasal polyposis. Acta Otolaryngol. 1986;101:320–7.
52. Albu S, Baciut M. Failures in endoscopic surgery of the maxillary sinus. Otolaryngol Head Neck Surg. 2010;142:196–201.
53. Longhini AB, Branstetter BF, Ferguson BJ. Otolaryngologists' perceptions of odontogenic maxillary sinusitis. Laryngoscope. 2012;122:1910–4.
54. Saibene AM, Vassena C, Pipolo C, Trimboli M, De Vecchi E, Felisati G, et al. Odontogenic and rhinogenic chronic sinusitis: a modern microbiological comparison. Int Forum Allergy Rhinol. 2016;6:41–5.
55. Taschieri S, Torretta S, Corbella S, Del Fabbro M, Francetti L, Lolato A, et al. Pathophysiology of sinusitis of odontogenic origin. J Investig Clin Dent. 2017;8(2)
56. Blanksma CJ, Brand HS. Cocaine abuse: orofacial manifestations and implications for dental treatment. Int Dent J. 2005;55:365–9.
57. Silvestre FJ, Perez-Herbera A, Puente-Sandoval A, Bagan JV. Hard palate perforation in cocaine abusers: a systematic review. Clin Oral Investig. 2010;14:621–8.
58. Heitz-Mayfield LJ, Huynh-Ba G. History of treated periodontitis and smoking as risks for implant therapy. Int J Oral Maxillofac Implants. 2009;24(Suppl):39–68.
59. Testori T, Weinstein RL, Taschieri S, Del Fabbro M. Risk factor analysis following maxillary sinus augmentation: a retrospective multicenter study. Int J Oral Maxillofac Implants. 2012;27:1170–6.
60. Giannì ABMR, Baj A, Carlino F, Tomic O. Maxillary atrophy: classification and surgical protocols. In: Testori TDFM, Weinstein R, Wallace S, editors. Maxillary sinus surgery and alternatives in treatment. Chicago Quintessence Publishing; 2009. p. 92–132.
61. Insua A, Monje A, Urban I, Kruger LG, Garaicoa-Pazmino C, Sugai JV, et al. The sinus membrane-maxillary lateral wall complex: histologic description and clinical implications for maxillary sinus floor elevation. Int J Periodontics Restorative Dent. 2017;37:e328–36.
62. Sonoda T, Harada T, Yamamichi N, Monje A, Wang HL. Association between bone graft volume and maxillary sinus membrane elevation height. Int J Oral Maxillofac Implants. 2017;32:735–40.

The Shanelec SMILE Technique: Immediate Microsurgical Implant and Provisional Restoration Placement in Anterior Esthetic Sites

Leonard S. Tibbetts, J. David Cross, and Bryan S. Pearson

Contents

Supplementary Information The online version contains supplementary material available at [https://doi.org/10.1007/978-3-030-96874-8_13].

L. S. Tibbetts (✉)
Private Practice, Arlington, TX, USA

J. D. Cross
Private Practice, Springfield, IL, USA

B. S. Pearson
Department of Periodontics, Louisiana State University, HSC School of Dentistry, New Orleans, LA, USA

Private Practice, Lafayette, LA, USA

Abstract

Replacement of a tooth in the anterior esthetic zone with a lifelike implant restoration can be a significant challenge. In this chapter, a microsurgical procedure for tooth extraction, implant placement, bone grafting, a connective tissue graft, and fabrication of a tissue supporting provisional crown is detailed. The SMILE Technique, developed by Dr. Dennis Shanelec, is an exacting, predictable procedure that has been used in over 1700 cases in multiple practices with a 98.58% overall success rate. The only exclusion criterion, other than ASA type IV patients, was uncontrolled diabetes and uncontrolled periodontal diseases.

Keywords

SMILE technique · Implant microsurgery · Minimally invasive extraction · 10× magnification · Socket drilling · Properly fabricated immediate provisional crown · Advancing the flap

1   Introduction

Over 22 years ago, Dr. Dennis Shanelec pioneered and changed implant dentistry with The SMILE Technique (simplified microsurgical implant lifelike esthetics), otherwise defined as immediate microsurgical implant and provisional restoration placement in anterior esthetic sites. This microscope-based procedure for immediate implant and provisional restoration placement has established an extremely predictable technique for maintaining the highest natural esthetic standards in even the most challenging clinical cases.

The loss of a tooth in the anterior esthetic zone often results in enormous distress. Dental implant placement has evolved into a successful and predictable option for the edentulous and partially edentulous patient [1–6]. Periodontists have been at the forefront in the development of this important technique in the anterior esthetic zone.

The Periodontal Practice Development Network Study Club was founded in 1984 by a small group of periodontists to share knowledge and techniques developed to stay on the cutting edge of periodontics. Dr. Dennis A. Shanelec demonstrated that microsurgical periodontal plastic surgical procedures were less traumatic and more predictable than the then currently practiced periodontal plastic surgery procedures being done without magnification (macrosurgery). The surgical microscope and the microsurgical techniques developed by Dr. Shanelec allow the surgeon to develop enhanced motor skill by using a precise hand grip and a reduction in physiologic tremor. Microsurgical procedures are less invasive, have diminished morbidity, and result in rapid healing [5, 7, 8].

Esthetics is a key marketing area in dentistry. It is understandable that patients often have a significant fear of losing a front tooth and how it is to be replaced [9]. In the past, the gold standard for replacing a missing incisor or cuspid had been a fixed partial denture. This was usually preceded by the patient wearing a removable temporary partial denture, often referred to as a "flipper," which is descriptive of its inherent limitations. Restoring the appearance of normal anatomy in the anterior esthetic zone following tooth loss is often compromised by the collapse of adjacent papillae, resorption of the buccal alveolar bone, and recession of the buccal marginal gingival. Another complication often seen with the use of a fixed partial denture for replacement of a missing tooth in the esthetic zone is that preparation of abutment teeth for use with a fixed partial denture often results in irreversible trauma to the pulp that necessitates root canal therapy.

In both medicine and dentistry, the use of microsurgery has resulted in the development of minimally invasive techniques that replaced procedures that produced more surgical trauma [7, 10–12]. By applying the principles of microsurgical techniques described in the literature, significant improvements in periodontal and implant surgical procedures are possible. As an example, the application of microsurgical principles to surgical tooth extraction can result in a significant reduction in trauma to the extraction site. The increased visual acuity made possible with the microscope allows the surgeon to increase motor movement precision and to see nuances in the direction of tooth movement during luxation. These subtle motions, which are not apparent with normal macrovision, can indicate a path of least resistance for the root during extraction. This can result in less trauma to the alveolar bone, the gingiva, and the papillae [11].

All of the phases of tooth extraction, implant osteotomy and placement, bone grafting, connective tissue grafting, and fabrication of the provisional restoration are performed using the microscope at a magnification of 10× or greater [5, 7, 13]. Because of the minimized tissue trauma resulting from microsurgical techniques for tooth extraction and implant osteotomy, patients report little or no discomfort following these procedures [7, 10, 12].

Implant osteotomy done using the microscope is a unique experience for the surgeon. Because of the enhanced illumination and visual acuity, the socket walls and apex appear large and clearly visible. In the anterior maxilla, the most favorable bone for implant placement lies to the palatal and apical aspects of the socket. The osteotomy must therefore be done at an angle to the socket wall using a lateral cutting bur. Twist drills are not designed for this purpose, as they track in the direction of least bone density and into the open socket. Without using lateral cutting burs before each incremental increase in twist drill size, the implant angulation and position will invariably move toward the buccal aspect of the extraction socket. The coaxial lighting and stereoscopic magnification provided by the microscope allows precise preparation and placement of the implant in a stable and esthetic position.

2 Immediate Implant Placement in the Maxillary Anterior Area

In most cases, implants have become the best option for restoring failed maxillary and/or mandibular anterior teeth. Several factors can influence the choice when deciding between immediate versus delayed implant placement [14]. Immediate implant placement with a provisional restoration has been shown to be a predictable procedure [9, 15–17]. The advantages of using the surgical microscope for immediate implant placement and fabrication of the provisional crown are significant and include greater precision and less trauma in tooth removal, enhanced lighting and visualization, allowing more precise osteotomy and implant placement with minimal bleeding. Using the microscope to create a provisional crown that matches the original contours of the extracted tooth allows the provisional crown to provide the correct support for the surrounding soft tissue. Such support is essential for maintaining the stability of the gingival architecture during the healing and implant osseointegration [6, 9, 13, 15, 17].

The SMILE Technique has several advantages over macrosurgical implant placement including (1) precision of the surgical procedure and enhanced motor skills; (2) minimal surgical trauma, with reduced inflammation and little to no prolonged bleeding; (3) excellent illumination of the surgical field; (4) precision of implant site preparation; (5) exactness of provisional crown design and fabrication; and (6) precise primary apposition of the connective tissue graft wound edges with an emphasis on passive primary wound closure [5].

At the present time, more than 1700 SMILE technique cases have been successfully completed and documented by Dr. Shanelec and members of Dentorati, a microsurgical study club. Of those cases, there are 18 where the implant failed to osseointegrate, and 6 cases that were lost to follow-up after implants and provisional were placed. The success of the SMILE technique is attributed to careful application of the detailed microsurgical steps described below. The goal is immediate implant and provisional implant restoration in an extraction socket with excellent esthetics and predictable dental implant osseointegration. Success is attributed to thorough, precise completion of each of the microsurgical steps associated with the technique. A level of competence through experience as a microsurgeon is required to perform the SMILE Technique.

When the implant platform is ≥5 mm below the crest of the papilla, a properly fabricated immediate provisional crown can consistently maintain the mesial and distal papillae heights. Buccal recession of approximately 1 mm will occur, however, unless a concurrent subepithelial connective tissue graft of 1.5 mm thickness is performed. Preexisting inflammation around the failing tooth has not been found to be a contraindication to treatment. However, complete debridement of the socket with the microscope at 10× magnification is required, using the protocol developed by Dr. Shanelec. Following thorough debridement of the socket it is flooded with an antibiotic (super-saturated solution of Tetracycline or Clindamycin), or sodium hypochlorite solution in order to decontaminate the site before beginning the osteotomy. A fractured or an avulsed tooth should be treated at the earliest possible time. When possible, the fractured or avulsed tooth should be retained and mimicked when the implant provisional crown is fabricated. This permits papilla regeneration by the properly supported gingiva (Table 1; Figs. 13.1, 13.2, 13.3, 13.4, 13.5, 13.6, 13.7, 13.8, 13.9, 13.10, 13.11, 13.12, 13.13, 13.14, and 13.15).

Table 1 Microscopic esthetic zone implant placement technique sequential flowchart [5]

Step	
1	All procedures performed under the microscope at magnifications 10× to 20×
2	Take a clear silicone impression of the failing tooth to light-cure composite for the provisional (Fig. 13.1a)
3	Create a flowable composite shell crown that replicates the anatomy of the failing tooth (Fig. 13.1b, c)
4	Atraumatic extraction, NO flaps (Fig. 13.3a–b, Video 1)
5	Complete microscopic socket debridement of the lateral and apical granulation tissue (Fig. 13.3a, b, Video 2)
6	Decontamination of the socket with an antibiotic or sodium hypochlorite solution for 30 s
7	Use lateral side cutting drills to align the osteotomy to the palatal wall of the socket (Fig. 13.4, Video 3)
8	The implant is placed with the implant apex positioned palatally and the implant platform approximately 2 mm toward the labial (Fig. 13.6a–b)
9	Position the implant platform approximately 5mm below the mesial and distal papillae
10	Position the palatal aspect of the platform at the palatal bony crest of the socket (Fig. 13.6a–b)
11	Use an appropriate diameter implant 12–14 mm long
12	Use a standard internal or external hex implant platform
13	Place the implant with at least 35 Ncm torque
14	Fill the buccal socket gap with osseous allograft, xenograft, or stem cell bone graft material to the level of the implant platform (Fig. 13.6c–d, Video 4)
15	Compress the surface graft material 1–2 mm to create a finely powdered bone graft seal (Fig. 13.6c, d)
16	Mold a collagen membrane free form or use Avitene (Microfibril, Collagen Hemostat, Davol, Inc., Warwick, RI, USA) over the bone autograft (Fig. 13.6e)
17	Hollow out the shell crown from step 3 (Fig. 13.1d)
18	Lute the shell crown to the opaqued abutment in the mouth (Fig. 13.7a, b)
19	Eliminate the flash and fill the subgingival contours with flowable composite
20	Create and check the emergence profile to support but not distort the buccal tissue and the papillae
21	Take an impression of the gingival half of the provisional attached to the implant analog (Fig. 13.10)
22	Highly polish and glaze the provisional (Fig. 13.7c)
23	Cure the provisional with a high intensity xenon light to eliminate free monomer
24	Harvest a connective tissue graft from the palate and place it into a buccal envelope (Fig. 13.8a, b, Videos 5 and 6)
25	Place the connective tissue graft into the tunnel
26	After freeing the papillae, advance the flap with 6-0 polypropylene suture as needed (Fig. 13.9)
27	Fill the screw space inside the implant with metronidazole gel
28	After installing the provisional crown with the proper torque (35 Ncm) place nonsterile Teflon tape above the screw head and seal the access with composite
29	Reduce the occlusion to remove all excursive movement contacts
30	Fabrication of a custom impression coping for the restorative dentist final impression of the implant restoration, with the exact same contours as the original temporary custom composite crown (Fig. 13.11a–e)
31	Perform postoperative evaluations every 4 weeks until the final restoration is done
32	Proceed to final restoration no sooner than 3 months of healing (Fig. 13.13a–b)
33	Postoperative evaluation of the ceramic crown both clinically and radiographically at 1 month post-placement and annually thereafter (Figs. 13.13c, d and 13.14a, b)

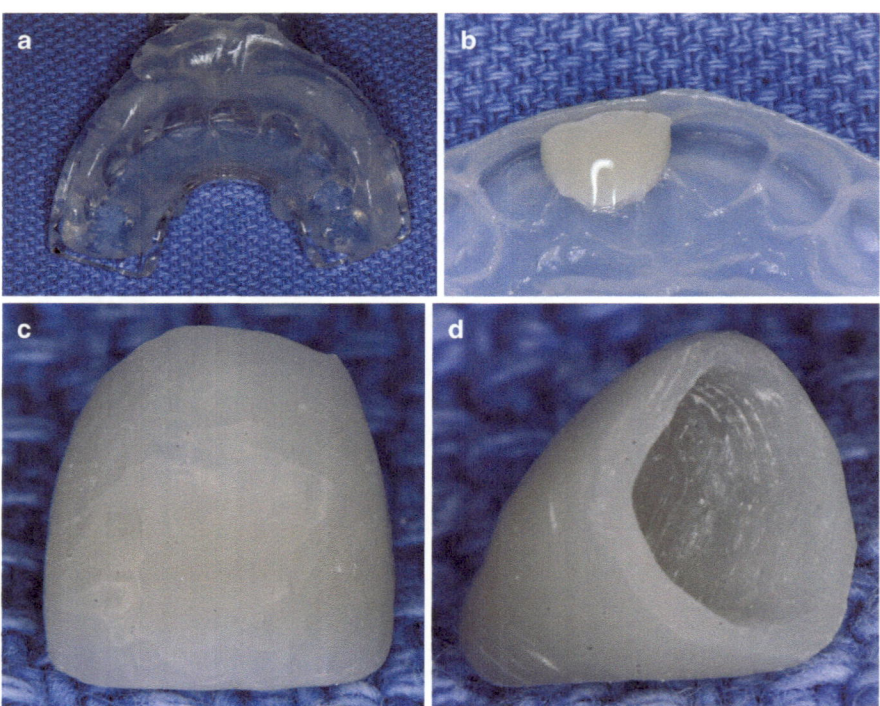

Fig. 13.1 (**a**) A clear silicone impression of the failing tooth is taken to assure duplication of the anatomy of the immediate provisional crown that is to be placed. (**b**) Impression of failing tooth is filled with flowable composite replicating the tooth anatomy and light cured. (**c**) A replicated shell crown duplicates the dento-gingival junction and the proximal contours of the extracted tooth. (**d**) Hollowed out shell crown to be joined to the opaqued impression coping attached to the implant analog

3 Case Presentation

The immediate microsurgical implant placement with implant supported provisional restorations following atraumatic extractions has been used since 2000 with a 98% success rate by clinicians competent in microsurgery.

4 Step 1: Implant Microsurgery

Cases are done using a working magnification of 10× or above for all phases of treatment. Little or no discomfort has been reported by patients following the combination of microsurgical tooth removal, precise implant placement in the socket, and seating an anatomically correct provisional restoration. The overall success rate

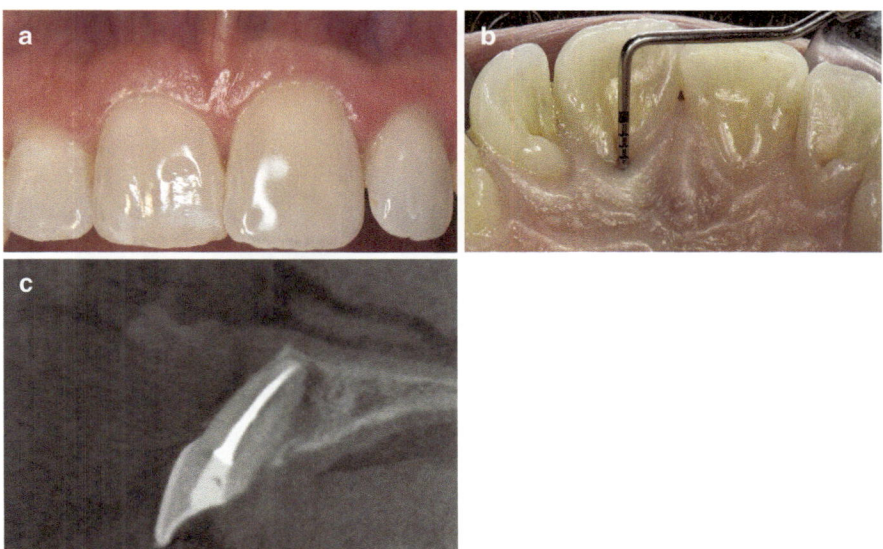

Fig. 13.2 (**a**) Failing left central incisor. (**b**) Palatal probing depth of 11 mm. (**c**) CAT scan exhibiting minimal buccal bone, with the only area of bone for implant placement apically and palatally

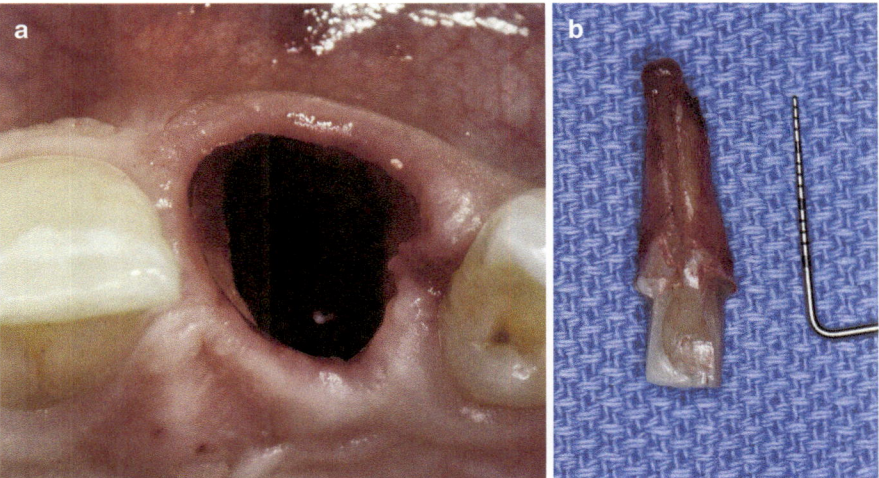

Fig. 13.3 (**a**) With enhanced visual acuity and improved surgical dexterity, the socket walls and apex appear large and clearly visible, with the gingiva and socket bone intact. (**b**) Extracted tooth with developmental root defect that contributed to probing depth

Fig. 13.4 Laterally cutting burrs for cutting into the palatal socket wall prior to using the twist drills

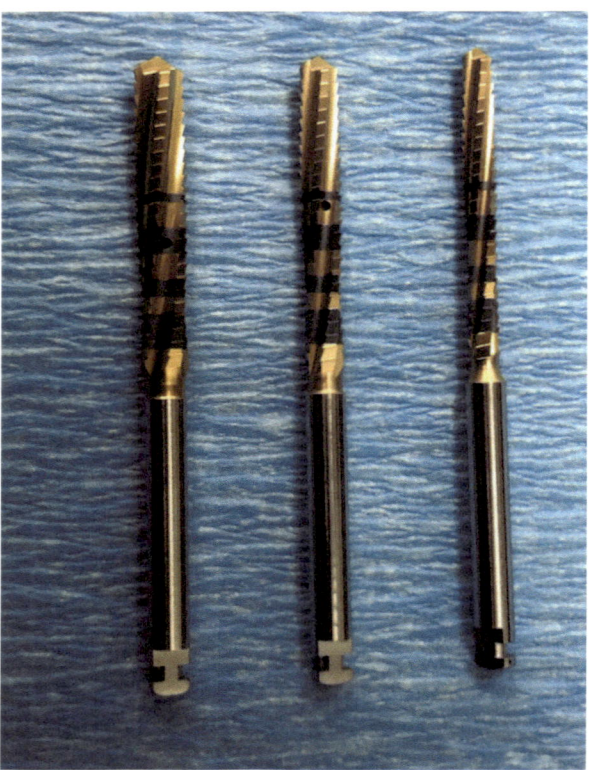

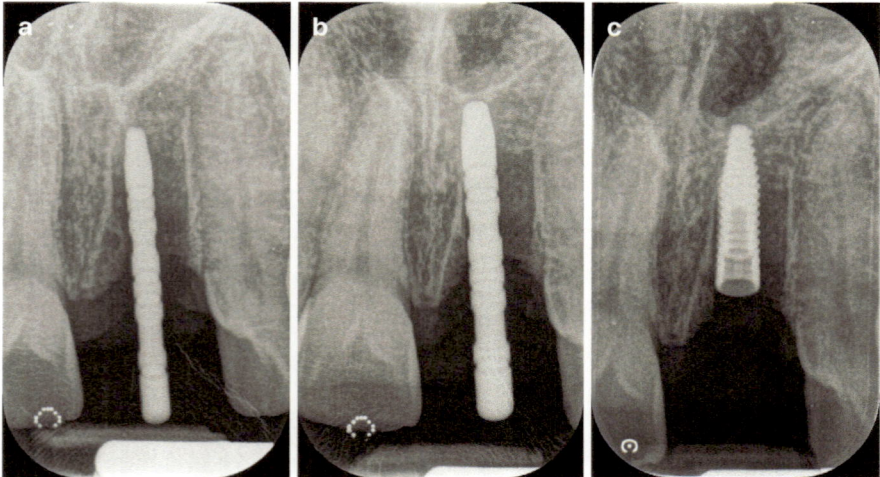

Fig. 13.5 (**a**) Palatal wall of extraction socket is drilled into with the enhanced vision to an appropriate depth, and then enlarged with twist drills. (**b**) Depth gauges are used to determine proper implant position. (**c**) Apex of tapered implant is positioned palatally, while the implant platform is positioned approximately 2mm toward the labial

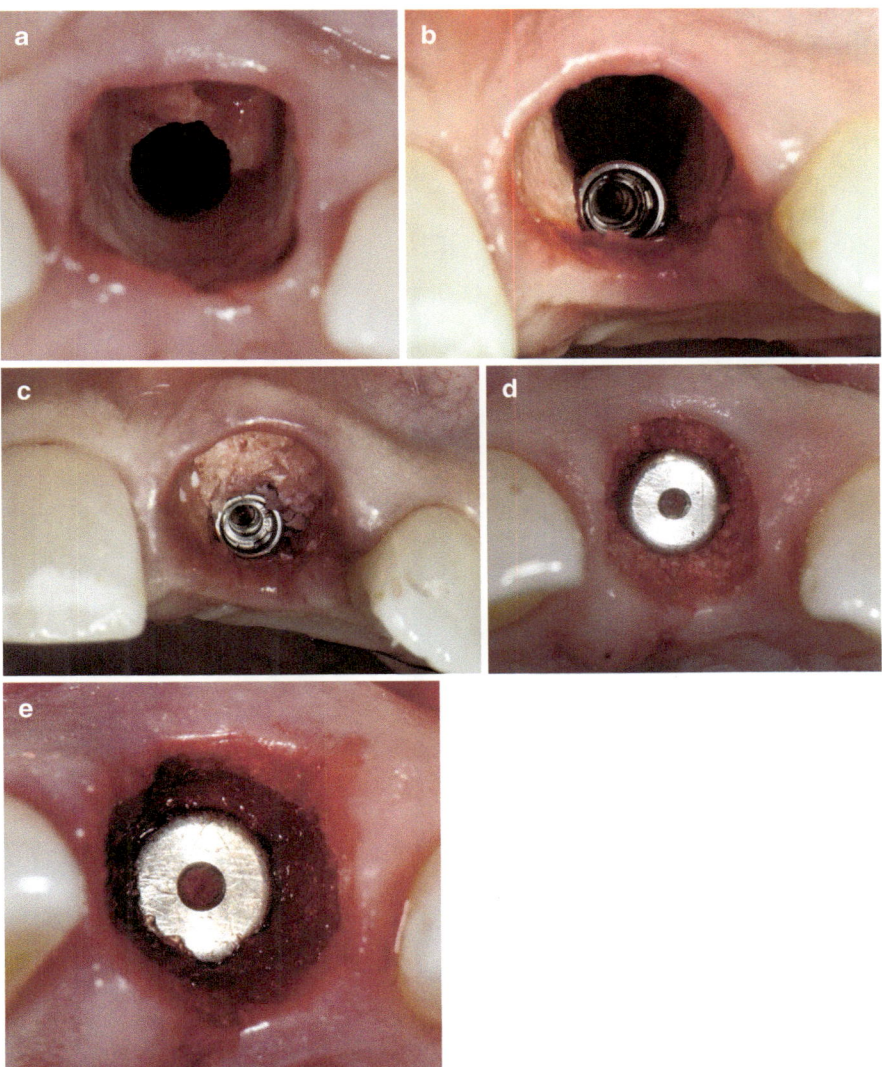

Fig. 13.6 (**a**) Osteotomy preparation for implant placement requires knowledge of both the anatomy of the maxilla and an appreciation of the cutting pattern of the drills. (**b**) Position palatal aspect of the implant platform at the palatal bony crest of the socket. (**c**) Fill the buccal socket gap with osseous allograft, xenograft, or stem cell bone graft to the level of the implant. (**d**) Compress the surface graft material 1–2 mm to create a fine powdered graft material seal. (**e**) An autograft bone graft filtered from the drilling bone dust is compressed to the platform level and covered with Avitene or a free form collagen membrane

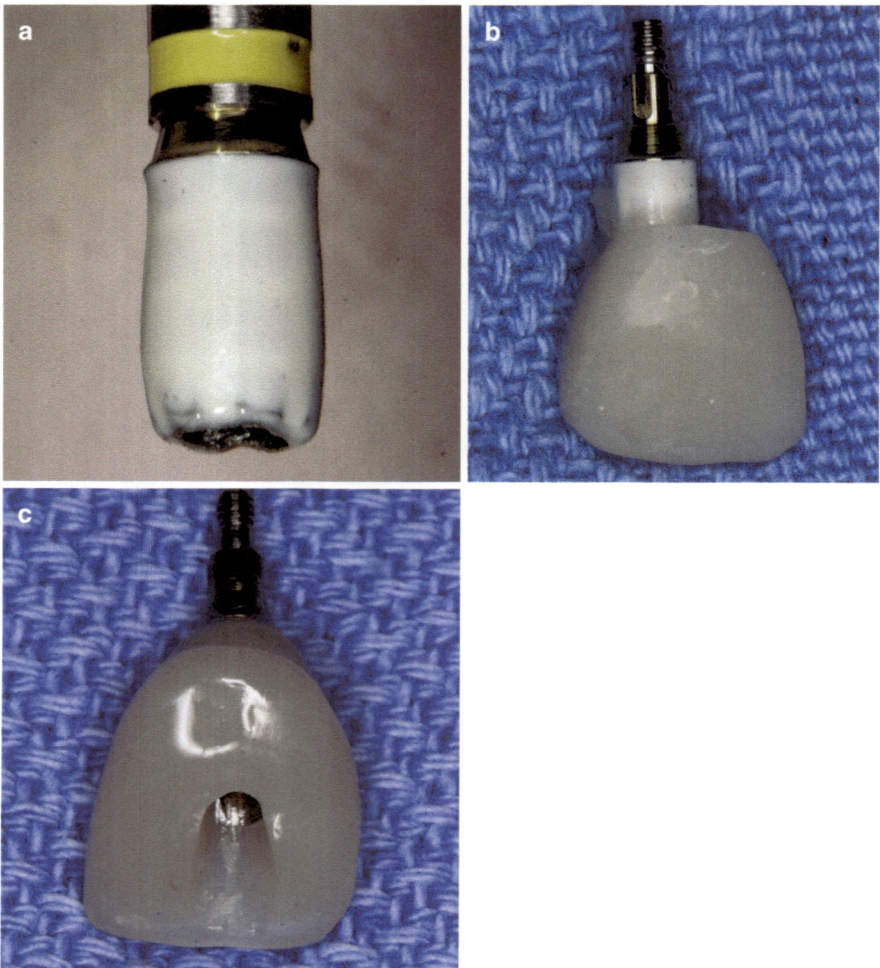

Fig. 13.7 (a) Opaqued screw retained abutment attached to an implant analog. (b) The hollowed out shell crown is luted to the opaqued screw retained abutment with light cured composite. (c) Voids and rough edges are carefully eliminated. The emergence profile is created and examined so that it supports the gingiva without distortion and is polished and glazed. The free monomer is eliminated by light curing

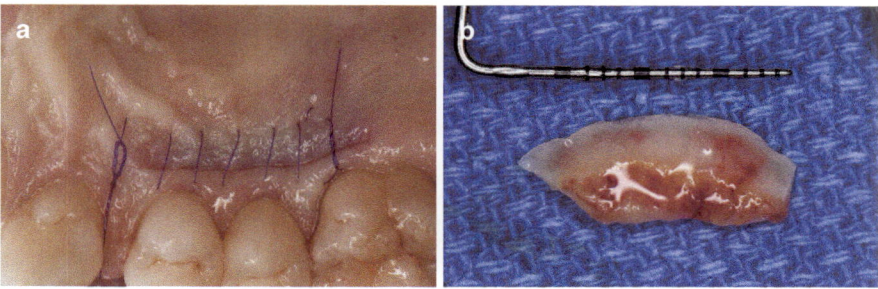

Fig. 13.8 (**a**) Sutured subepithelial connective tissue graft donor site. (**b**) A subepithelial connective tissue graft approximately 1.5 mm thick will be placed in a buccal envelope to prevent recession

Fig. 13.9 Primary passive wound closure of the connective tissue recipient site, after freeing the papillae

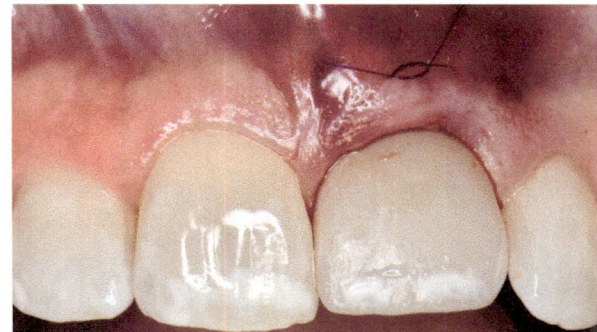

Fig. 13.10 Impression of the provisional crown used to fabricate the custom transfer coping

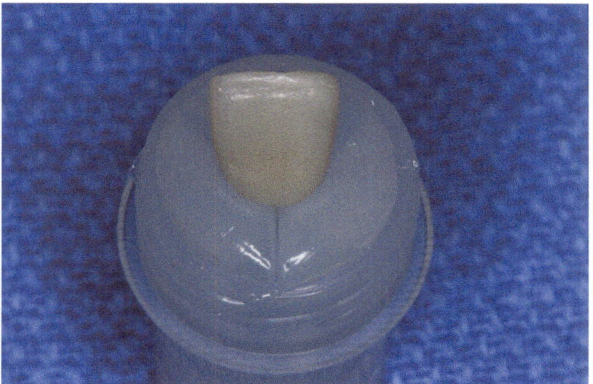

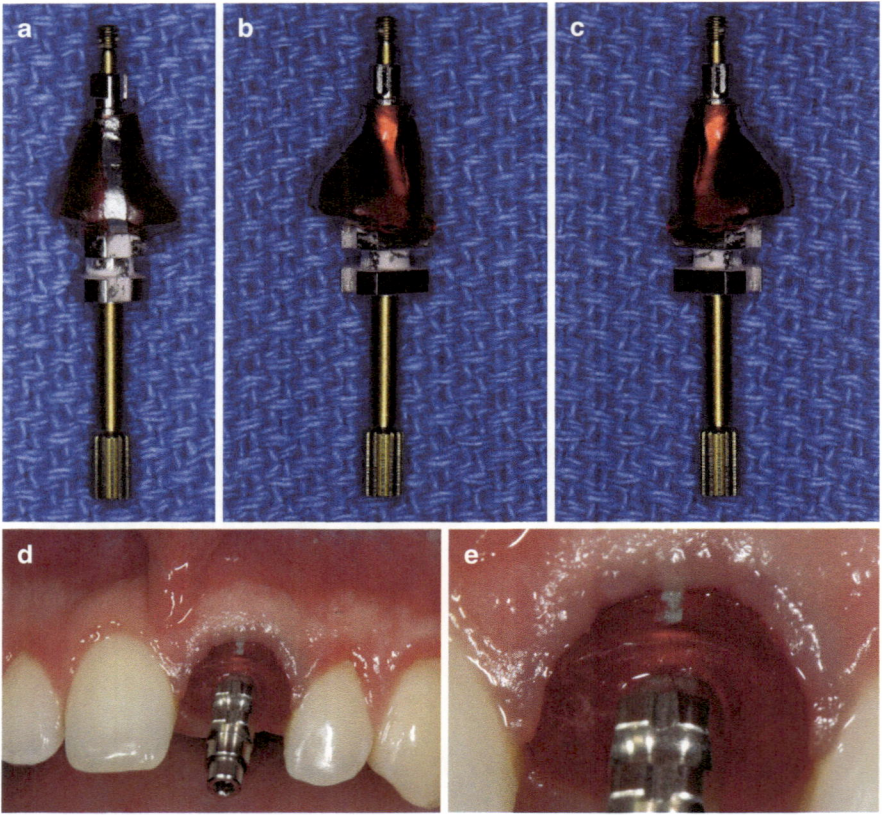

Fig. 13.11 (**a**) A custom transfer coping is made for the ceramist with a mark applied to the labial for orientation. It duplicates the natural height and contours of the gingival tissues and individually shaped to support the gingival tissue without distorting the buccal and interproximal tissues. (**b**) Distal proximal view of emergence profile. (**c**) Mesial proximal view of emergence profile. (**d**) Seated view of the custom fabricated transfer coping. (**e**) Enlarged view of transfer coping showing support of the gingiva

of the cases treated demonstrates that predictable and consistent results have been achieved with this technique for many years.

5   Steps 2, 3, 18, and 19: Preparation of Provisional Replication of the Failing Tooth

Before surgery, a clear silicone impression of the failing tooth is made to assure accurate capturing of the dento-gingival junction. A flowable light-cured composite duplication of the tooth is fabricated from the impression for the provisional fabrication, and it is trimmed to the exact location of the dento-gingival junction,

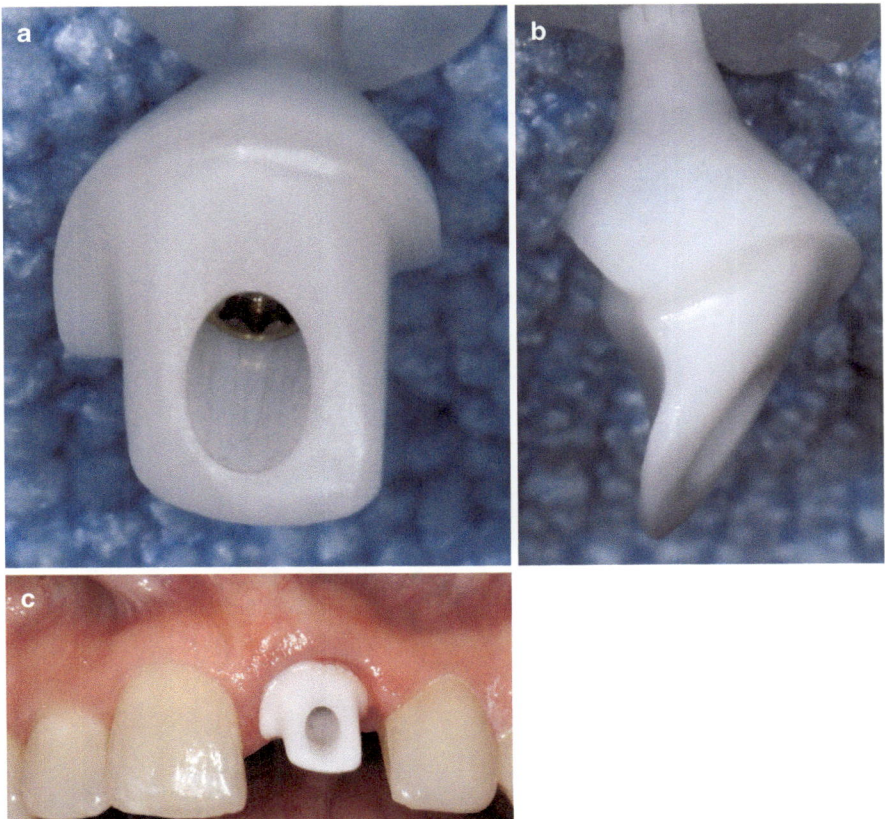

Fig. 13.12 (**a**) A zirconium abutment with the exact same contours as the impression transfer coping of the provisional emergence profile. (**b**) Mesial view of the zirconium abutment from the impression transfer coping of the provisional emergence profile. (**c**) Seated zirconium abutment with the preservation of the natural height and contour of the gingiva

establishing the emergence profile. The replicated shell crown is hollowed out to later be filled with a light-cured esthetic color-matched composite, which will be used for luting to a screw-retained temporary, opaqued titanium abutment.

6   Steps 4–6: Extraction with Minimal Trauma and Socket Debridement

With the application of enhanced visual acuity and improved surgical dexterity made possible by the microscope, gingival and osseous anatomy is preserved. Minimization of forces during the extraction protects the alveolar bone, particularly the buccal wall. Damage to the gingiva and papillae is prevented by prior atraumatic

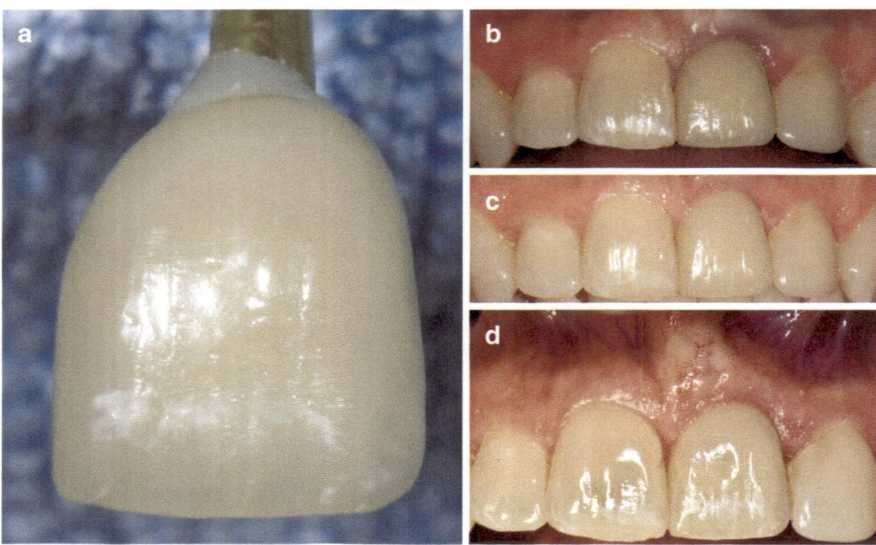

Fig. 13.13 (**a**) Final crown seated on the custom abutment. (**b**) Final restoration at the time of cementation. (**c**) Postoperative view at 24 months. (**d**) 24-month postoperative enlarged view

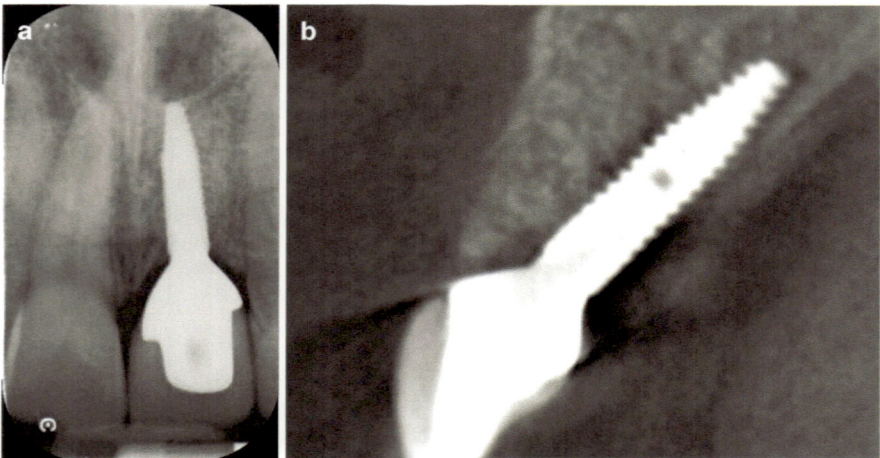

Fig. 13.14 (**a**) 24-month postoperative radiograph of implant. (**b**) 24-month CAT scan

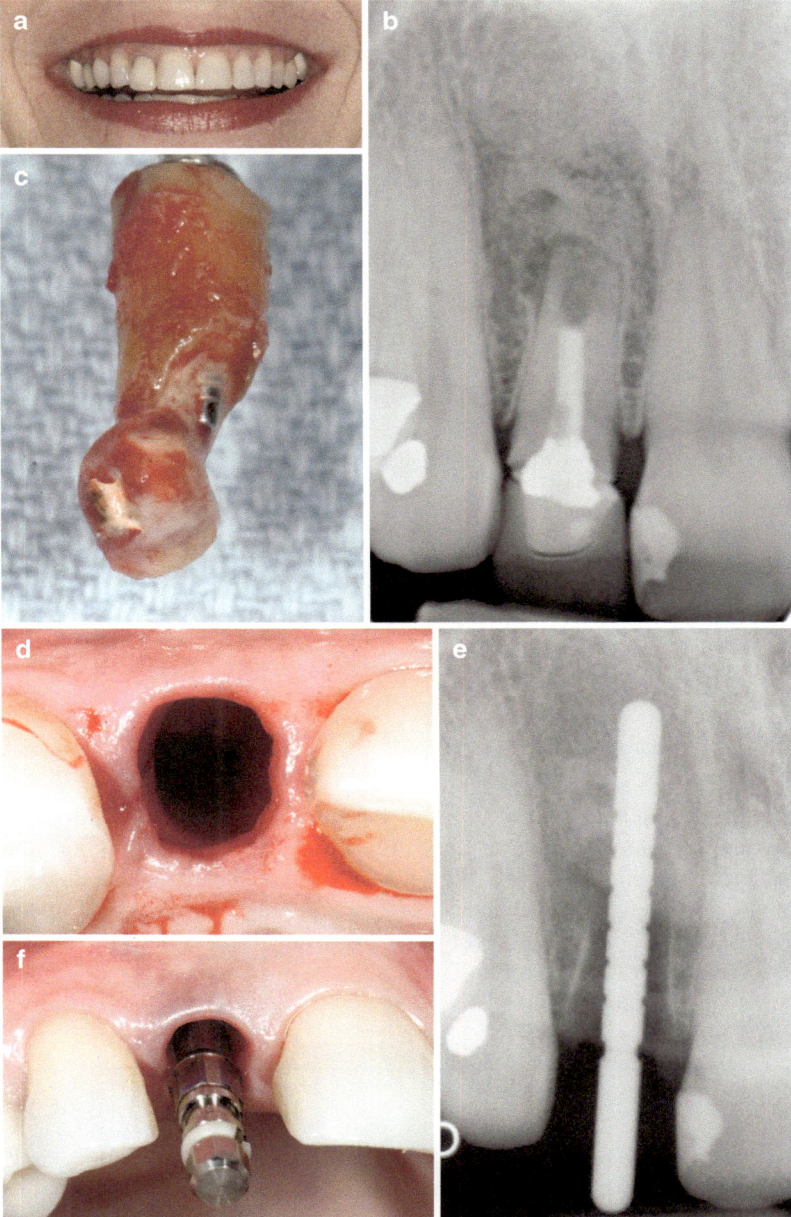

Fig. 13.15 (**a**) Preoperative view of failing maxillary right lateral incisor. (**b**) Radiograph of failing maxillary right lateral incisor. (**c**) Microsurgically assisted extracted lateral incisor. (**d**) Debrided, atraumatic extraction socket with little to no bleeding. (**e**) Depth gauge of palatally inclined implant preparation. (**f**) Implant apex positioned palatally to tip the implant platform slightly to the buccal. (**g**) Highly polished and glazed provisional crown. (**h**) Tapered implant with screw retained provisional crown prior to placement of Teflon tape and composite restoration sealing. (**i**) Final implant screw retained restoration on maxillary right lateral incisor

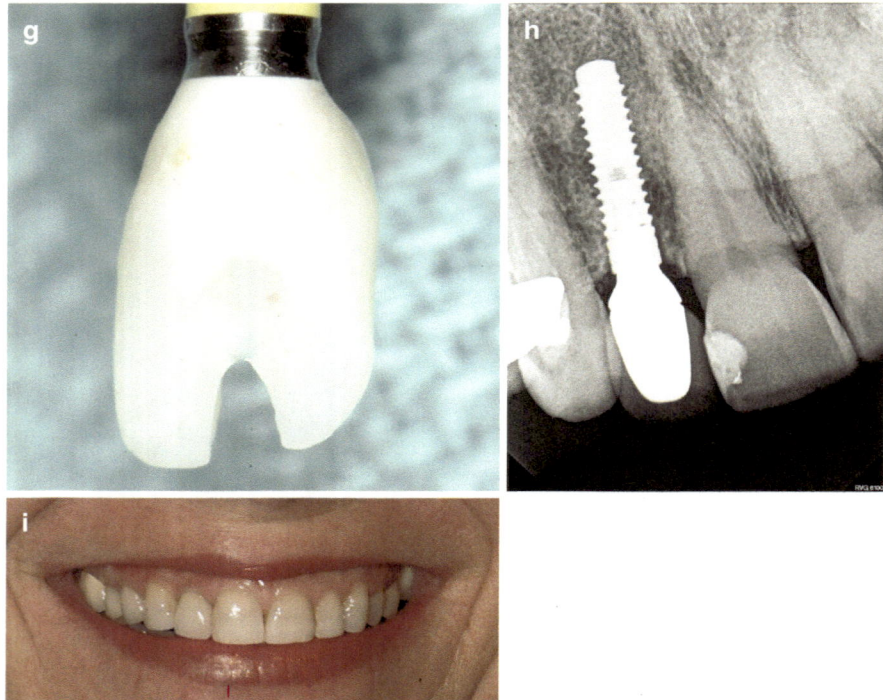

Fig. 13.15 (continued)

separation of papillae from the root of the tooth being extracted. Magnification allows surgeons to see subtle degrees in luxation direction that are not otherwise visualized. Following extraction, the sulcus is deepithelialized with a flame-shaped diamond, and microscopically the socket is thoroughly debrided of granulation tissue, irrigated and filled with one of several possible decontamination solutions for 30 s, such as super-saturated solutions of tetracycline, clindamycin, or a solution of sodium hypochlorite.

7   Step 7: Socket Drilling

The most favorable bone in the maxillary anterior is positioned both palatally and apically to the socket, requiring drilling in the extraction socket that is totally different than drilling in edentulous sites. Drilling must therefore be done at an angle to the socket wall using lateral cutting burrs or ultrasonics before each incremental increase in twist drill size. Twist drills are not designed to drill at an angle to the socket wall and tend to track in the direction of least dense bone. Attempting to use a twist drill for this step will generally result in directing the preparation toward the labial plate. With microscopic magnification and lighting, drilling on the lateral socket wall can succeed in accomplishing a stable and esthetic placement for maxillary anterior implants.

8   Steps 8–13: Implant Placement

Implants can be placed with the implant apex positioned palatally and the implant platform bucally approximately 2 mm toward the labial. Implants placed into the extraction osteotomy sites have been torqued to as much as 76 Ncm, but generally are only torqued to 35 Ncm. The thread geometry of tapered implants is felt to improve implant stability without the danger of lateral bone compression. Of the implants placed using the SMILE Technique, over half have been 12 and 14 mm in length.

9   Steps 14–16: Osseous Grafting of the Buccal Socket Gap

Both allograft and xenograft have been used to fill the labial socket gap to the level of the implant platform. The surface graft material is compressed 1–2 mm to create a fine powdered allograft or xenograft seal. A layer of microfibrillar collagen is placed over the bone before the implant provisional crown is placed. In all the cases, connective tissue was harvested from the palate and placed into a split-thickness envelope recipient site prepared on the buccal aspect of the socket. This is done to preserve and restore the gingival height that would be lost as a result of injury or inflammation.

10   Steps 17–24: Implant Provisional Crown

The implant provisional crown must support the surrounding gingiva exactly like the extracted tooth to preserve natural esthetics [18]. This involves placing an opaqued titanium screw-retained temporary abutment, creating a hollowed composite shell crown from the clear silicone impression of the failing tooth. The shell crown is luted to the opaqued abutment in the mouth and the flash is eliminated using a micro-diamond bur. The subgingival profile for each patient is individually shaped at the time of surgery, with voids and rough edges eliminated and the provisional carefully contoured to support the gingival tissue. The emergence profile is created and examined so it supports the gingiva without distorting the buccal and interproximal tissues. The provisional crown is polished and glazed as a final step. To eliminate free monomer that may be present to irritate the soft tissue or bone, a light-cured composite is used. An impression of the gingival one-half of the provisional crown attached to an implant analog is made before the crown is attached to the implant. This is used to fabricate a custom impression transfer coping. The possibility of the provisional crown loosening is reduced by the precise attachment of the machined titanium provisional abutment. Of the 1700 successful cases less than 1% of the provisional crowns have had the screw loosen.

11   Steps 25 and 27: Advancing the Flap

After placing the subepithelial connective tissue graft into the buccal envelope, the papillae are freed with a microsurgical knife, and the flap is advanced with 6-0 polypropylene suture as needed.

12   Steps 26, 28, 29, 30, 31: Provisional Restoration Seating, Adjusting Occlusion, Postoperative Care

To avoid premature loading of the screw retained provisional crown the occlusion is removed, and lateral contacts with adjacent teeth are adjusted to assure minimal, symmetrical, light proximal contacts. The screw threads are coated with metronidazole gel, and the provisional crown is positioned with the proper torque. Nonsterile Teflon tape is placed above the screw head, and the access is sealed with composite. By doing so, patients leave the office with a non-loaded esthetic provisional tooth securely anchored to the implant. Postoperative evaluations are performed at 4-week intervals.

13   Step 32: Final Restoration

Patients are never without a natural looking tooth when an immediate provisional crown with an exact emergence profile is placed at the time of the implant placement. The provisional crown ensures that the gingiva is supported during implant osseointegration. The exact emergence profile of the provisional crown is transmitted to the ceramist by using the custom impression transfer coping created from the provisional crown [19–21]. From the model made from the impression, a computer scan is used to create the permanent zirconium ceramic abutment exactly matching both the provisional emergence profile and the original tooth shape. A final restoration is fabricated and placed after 12–24 weeks [5].

14   Step 33: Postoperative CAT Scan

Creating a tooth in a natural harmony with the adjacent teeth is possible by combining the skills of a team comprised of a competent microsurgeon, a restorative dentist, and a ceramist.

15   Clinical Results and Discussion

Using the SMILE Technique for cases done in private practice settings in California, Texas, Louisiana, New York, and Illinois, over 1700 cases have been completed involving the extraction of maxillary central incisors, lateral incisors, or cuspids.

The long-term success rate over a period of 1–18 years is 98.58%. No exclusion criteria were used for the cases other than ASA type IV patients, uncontrolled diabetes and uncontrolled periodontal diseases. Patient scheduling and restorative logistics usually determined the delivery of the final restoration at about 12–24 weeks following implant placement.

Treatment success criteria included: (1) the absence of infection, mobility, pain, inflammation, or bleeding upon probing; (2) the ability to withstand rotational torque of >35 Ncm at the time of permanent abutment placement; (3) a peri-implant tissue sulcus <1 mm apical to the implant platform; (4) radiographic evidence of bone to the top most implant thread; (5) restoration of the implant that remains in function; and (6) a satisfactory objective esthetic outcome for both the patient and the provider.

Once a level of competence is achieved in microsurgical procedures, implant microsurgery offers the opportunity for implant therapy that can preserve or enhance the esthetic results.

Rapid healing, minimal discomfort, superior esthetics, and improved patient acceptance are the benefits of this technique. As use of the surgical microscope increases, the advantages of its use in many phases of dentistry will become more obvious. Use of microscopy has the potential to clinically advance dentistry in many areas. While the technique described is multifaceted requiring multiple steps for successful completion, the clinical outcome is outstanding. Successful treatment requires microscope magnification, attention to detail, and a combination of thorough microsurgical and restorative skills.

16   Key Points

1. The SMILE Technique developed by Dr. Dennis Shanelec has been shown to be a predictable, successful implant procedure with a 98.58% success rate.
2. The SMILE Technique consists of 5 microsurgical procedures including a connective tissue graft, atraumatic tooth removal, precise implant placement, bone graft, and fabrication of a screw retained custom composite temporary crown, all performed using a surgical operating microscope.
3. Due the complexity of each individual procedure, a moderate to advanced level of microsurgical experience is required.
4. The proper incorporation of each of the steps is critical to the long-term success of the procedure.
5. A highly polished, properly contoured screw retained composite temporary restoration is required to achieve ideal esthetics through precise tissue support.

References

1. Adell R, Eriksson B, Lekholm U, Branemark PI, Jemt T. Long term follow-up study of osseo-integrated implants in the treatment of totally edentulous jaws. Int J Oral Maxillofac Implants. 1990;5:347–59.

2. Widmark G, Friberg B, Johansson B, Sinder-Pedersen S, Taylor A. MK III: a third generation of the self-tapping Branemark system implant, including the new Stargrip internal grip design. A1-year prospective four-center study. Clin Implant Dent Relat Res. 2003;5:273–9.

3. Covani U, Crespi R, Cornelini R, Barone A. Immediate implants supporting single crown restoration: a 4-year prospective study. J Periodontol. 2004;75:982–8.

4. Evian CI, Emling R, Rosenberg ES, Waasdorp JA, Halpern W, Shah S, Garcia M. Retrospective analysis of implant survival and the influence of periodontal disease and immediate placement on long-term results. Int J Oral Maxillofac Implants. 2004;19:393–8.

5. Shanelec, Dennis A, Tibbetts, Leonard S. Implant microsurgery: immediate implant placement with implant-supported provisional. Clin Adv Periodont. 2011;1:161–72.

6. Buser D, Chen S, Weber HP, Belser U. Early implant placement following single-tooth extraction in the esthetic zone: biologic rationale and surgical procedures. Int J Periodontics Restorative Dent. 2008;28:441–51.

7. Burkhardt R, Lang N. Coverage of localized gingival recessions: Comparison of micro- and macrosurgical techniques. J Clin Periodontol. 2005;32:287–93.

8. Campelo LD, Dominguez Camara J. Flapless implant surgery: a 10 year clinical retrospective analysis. Int J Oral Maxillofac Implants. 2002;17:271–2.

9. Wohrle PS. Single tooth replacement in the anterior aesthetic zone with immediate provisionalization. Pract Periodont Aesth Dent. 1998;10(9):1197–14.

10. Patel C, Mehta R, Joshi S, Hiran T, Joshi C. Comparative evaluation of treatment of localized gingival recession with coronally advanced flap, using microsurgical and conventional techniques. Contemp Clin Dent. 2018;9:613–8.

11. Tibbetts LS, Shanelec DA. Periodontal microsurgery. Dent Clin N. 1998;42:339–59.

12. Tibbetts LS, Shanelec DA. A review of the principles and practice of periodontal microsurgery. Tex Dent J. 2007;124:188–04.

13. Leknius C, Geissberger M. The effect of magnification on the performance of fixed prosthodontic procedures. CDA J. 1995;23:66–70.

14. Studer S, Pietrobon N, Wohlwend A. Maxillary anterior single-tooth replacement: a comparison of three treatment modalities. Pract Periodontics Aesthet Dent. 1994;6:51–60.

15. De Rouck T, Collys K, Wyn I, Cosyn J. Instant provisionalization of immediate single-tooth implants is essential to optimize esthetic treatment outcome. Clin Oral Implants Res. 2009;20:566–70.

16. Chu SJ. A novel prosthetic device and method for guided tissue preservation of immediate postextraction socket implants. Int J Periodontics Restorative Dent. 2014;34:9–17.

17. Ross SB, Pette GA, Parker WB, Hardigan P. Gingival margin changes in maxillary anterior sites after single immediate implant placement and provisionalization: a 5-year retrospective study of 47 patients. Int J Oral Maxillofac Implants. 2014;29:127–34.

18. Croll BM. Emergence profiles in natural tooth contour. Part 1: photographic observations. J Prosthet Dent. 1989;62:4–10.

19. Hui E, Chow J, Li J, Wat P, Law H. Immediate provisional for single-tooth implant replacement with Branemark System: preliminary report. Clin Implant Dent Relat Res. 2001;3:79–86.

20. Hinds KF. Custom impression coping for an exact registration of the healed tissue in the esthetic implant restoration. Int J Periodontics Restorative Dent. 1997;17:585–91.

21. Polack MA. Simple method of fabricating an impression coping to reproduce periimplant gingiva on the master cast. J Prosthet Dent. 2002;88:221–3.

Microscope-Assisted Implant Complication Management

Ramon Gomez-Meda and Jonathan Esquivel

Contents

Abstract

Accidents and complications are unavoidable from time to time when placing implants, but the surgeon should know how to prevent and treat those complications. The use of microscope, its illumination, and magnification allow the practitioner to increase the predictability of treatment, allowing better precision in managing the tissues. In some narrow and deep spaces, the use of the OM as its

Supplementary Information The online version contains supplementary material available at [https://doi.org/10.1007/978-3-030-96874-8_14].

R. Gomez-Meda (✉) · J. Esquivel
Department of Prosthodontics, LSUHSC School of Dentistry, New Orleans, LA, USA

coaxial light facilitates a sharp field of view. The surgeon's abilities and predictability of surgical techniques increase, employing minimally invasive surgeries and solving several problems reducing treatment time, costs, and morbidity for the patient at the same time. This kind of dentistry becomes more gratifying and motivating for the practitioner and the whole team, reducing the patient's anxiety level.

Keywords

Implant complications · Accidents · Implant malposition · Periimplantitis Esthetic implant complications · Dental implants · Microscopy

1 Implant Complications

Placing implants may involve trans-surgical accidents that can affect the outcome of surgery or complications after the implant has integrated that can be categorized as early or late complications [1, 2]. With the increase in the number of implants placed, the number of complications has also increased. The clinician must be proficient, solving them to increase the chances of successful implant therapy.

Microsurgery with its increased illumination and magnification allows the practitioner to detect and manipulate the anatomical structures and soft tissues better, reducing surgical accidents and complications and, consequently, the morbidity, increasing this way the treatment success.

2 Trans-Surgical Accident

This type of accident includes implant malposition or displacement, soft tissue lesions, lesions to adjacent teeth, bleeding, dehiscence or fenestration, lack of primary stability, injury to neuro-sensorial structures, aspiration, or swallowing dental instruments, or mandibular fracture [3–8].

A thorough medical history, which includes an examination for the presence of coagulation disorders and other medical alterations that could potentially lead to complications, should be done [9].

A radiological evaluation with a cone-beam computed tomography (CBCT) is also essential to properly plan implant surgery [3]. A computer-aided design computer-aided manufacturing (CAD-CAM) generated surgical guide can avoid or reduce the chance of malpositioned implants and help to avoid dehiscence, fenestrations, or the damaging of vital structures.

Surgery in the anterior maxilla or mandible of edentulous patients with inadequate bone quality and quantity can compromise the sublingual, lingual, or submaxillary artery [6]. In these cases, the use of a microscope can help locate and identify arteries and nerves, avoiding any major bleeding or nerve damage (Figs. 1 and 2; Videos 1, 2, and 3).

Fig. 1 Dental nerve emergences can be easily detected with the help of microscope

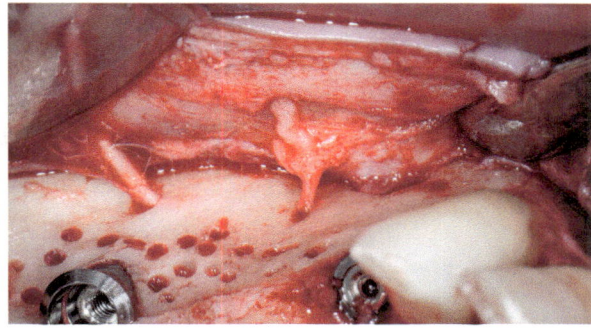

Fig. 2 Anatomical structures are isolated and visualized through the microscope preventing intraoperative accidents and early complications

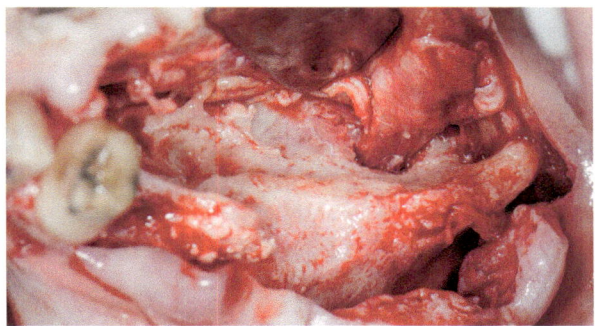

Also, the use of microscope increases the care of soft tissues with a better instrument manipulation technique, reducing other types of accidents like flap tears due to excessive traction or incorrect use of instruments (Fig. 3) [4, 10, 11]. Flap elevation can be initiated with papilla elevators to avoid tearing the margins of the gingiva (Video 4). Also, microsurgical forceps, less invasive and smaller than macro-elevators, help manipulate the flap without traumatizing it.

A microsurgical approach may reduce the incidence of bone dehiscence and fenestrations that can be unnoticed in immediate implant placement or flapless surgeries due to the lack of visibility [12]. Also, 90% of cortical plates in the anterior zone are thinner than 1 mm [13], and magnification allows for better visualization. Cortical plate integrity can be easily and quickly assessed after tooth extraction, before immediate implant placement, without the need of raising a flap. For this purpose, increasing the OM magnification above 10× and even 20× is useful (Video 5).

There is no evidence that vertical dehiscence under 2 mm needs any guided bone regeneration procedure, reducing the morbidity for the patient (Figs. 4 and 5) [14]. A dehiscence larger than 2 mm needs bone regeneration procedures with nonresorbable or resorbable membranes [15] that can nowadays be approached microsurgically, eliminating or minimizing the extent of vertical releasing incisions and covering the wound with a tension-free closure of the flaps (Fig. 6) [7]. Although many surgeons use the operative microscope every day, the techniques for suturing

Fig. 3 Small flap tear that could be avoided with a more careful approach. The reduced dimension of the lesion did not require any additional therapy

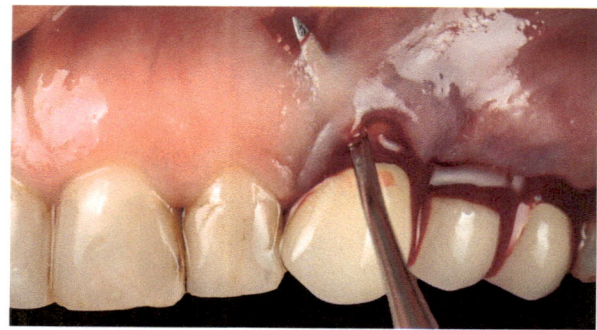

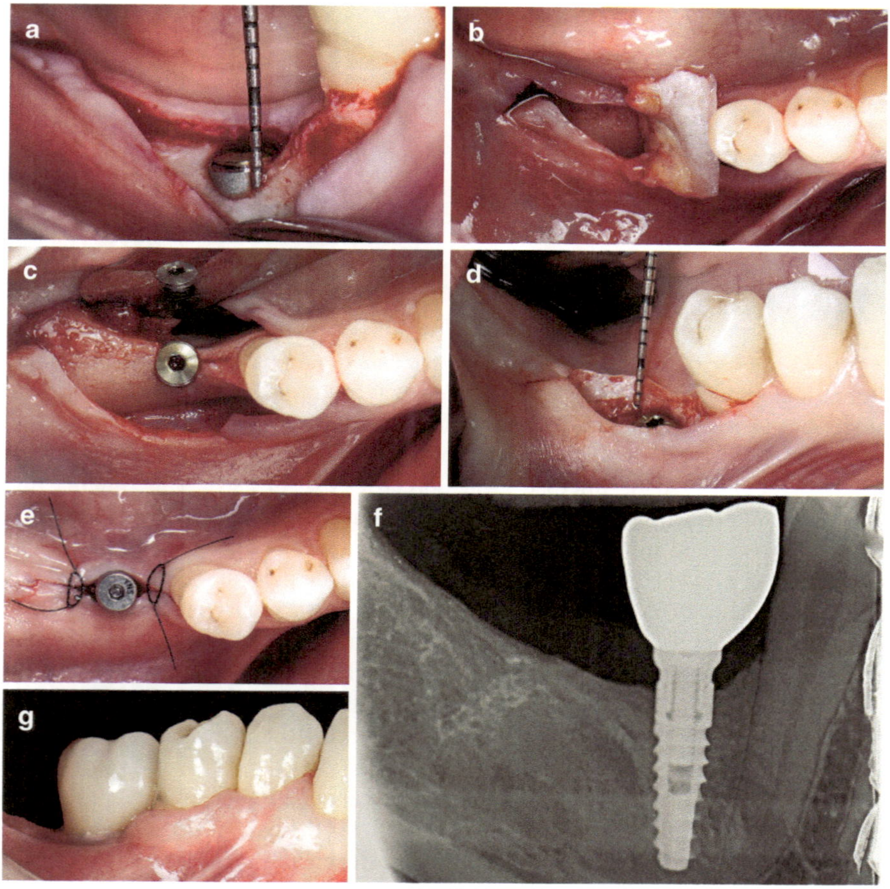

Fig. 4 (a–g) Small dehiscences under 2 mm do not need a bone regeneration procedure. Instead, the surgery can be simplified with a microsurgical approach using a CTG to increase the thickness and quality of the soft tissues around the neck of the implant reducing the bone remodeling of the crest

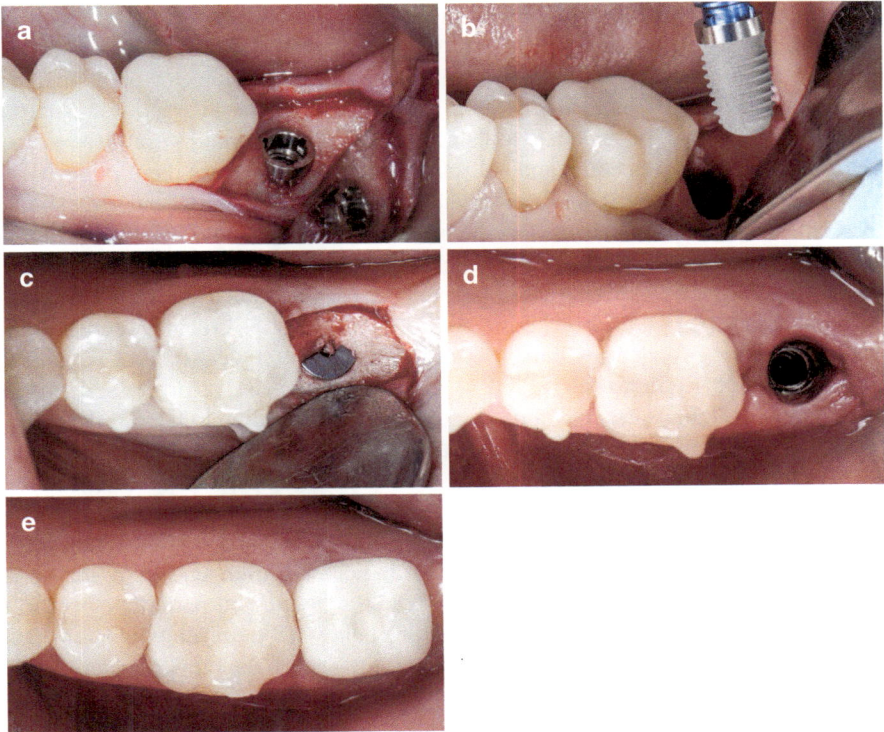

Fig. 5 (a–e) A tissue level implant is another treatment option when a small dehiscence, under 2 mm, is present due to a narrow crest. Surgery and interim restoration are shown in the pictures

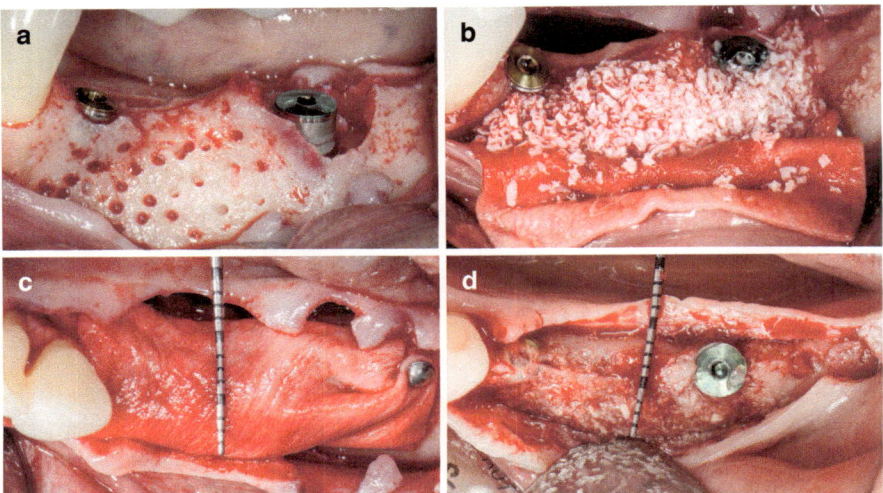

Fig. 6 (a–d) A guided bone regeneration procedure (GBR) is the treatment of choice to guarantee more than 2 mm of bone on the buccal aspect of the implant preventing a long-term dehiscence or fenestration and a possible implant failure

very small vascular and neural structures are more complex than the routinely used approach. Practicing microsurgical anastomosis techniques is beneficial for the clinician [16]. Mastering the microsurgical technique can help develop skills that can be applied to other areas of surgery [17]. To perform microvascular anastomosis, the clinician must have the adequate tools necessary. It is essential to use these instruments only for this procedure and not routine surgery to increase their longevity.

Several factors must be considered when selecting instruments. First, they should be comfortable to use; the shape of the handle affects the ability of the clinician to manipulate the instrument without losing control. The most common shapes are flat and rounded but can also have a knurled pattern. The clinician should use the handle shape and grip pattern they feel more comfortable with. It is crucial to consider the tension of spring-loaded instruments. If the tension is too weak, it will be hard to secure the tool, leading to excessive overclosure or the risk of dropping it. If the tension is too high, its use may require excessive effort leading to fatigue. The clinician should make a test for correct tension. In this test, should hold the instrument between his/her fingers and have the tips of the instrument partially closed. Then, the clinician should turn his or her hand over holding the position and check if the instrument tip rotates out of position, which would indicate a weak tension. Hand muscle fatigue after prolonged use is the best indicator of high tension in the instruments. An exercise the clinician can do is hold the instrument partially closed and measure how much time this position could be held without developing strain. The longer the instrument is held without fatigue, the longer the clinician can use the instrument in surgery.

The weight of the instrument is also important. Stainless steel instruments are heavier than titanium instruments and may have a firmer feel between the fingertips.

Finally, the length of the instrument handle determines a comfortable working distance. Regardless of the depth of the tissue, the clinician must be able to stabilize his or her hands using the fingers as support in areas close to the working surface.

3   Early Complications

Early complications can include edema, ecchymosis, hematomas, emphysema, bleeding, soft tissue dehiscence, sensitivity, and infection or implant fracture.

The microscope may reduce this kind of early complication as it allows for improved soft tissue manipulation and reducing edema and swelling.

3.1   Edema, Bleeding, Ecchymosis, and Hematoma

Swelling appears hours after a surgical procedure. It can lead to discomfort, trismus, or sensitive alterations due to compression of terminal branches of a nerve and may require corticosteroids [18]. The symptoms usually decrease with time and can quickly vanish after a few days. The extension of the surgical procedure and the general condition of the patient can induce bleeding after surgery. Minimal invasive

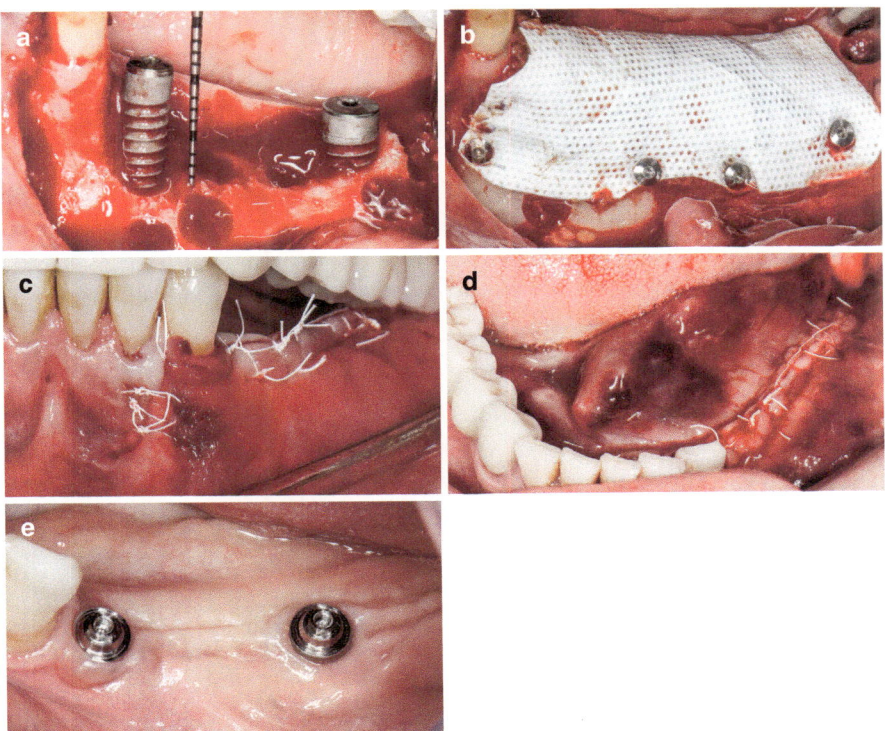

Fig. 7 (a–e) Important bleeding and swelling in the sublingual aspect of the mouth in a patient with medical problems. Even when using a careful and microsurgical approach, a previous comprehensive medical evaluation of patient condition is mandatory. Regardless of presence of an intrasurgical complication, vertical GBR procedure was eventually successful

surgeries and the identification of vital structures help avoid these kinds of complications.

Immediately placed implants and guided flapless surgery techniques have been shown to reduce the need for analgesic and anti-inflammatory drugs [19–22]. On the other hand, wider flaps like the ones necessary for guided bone regeneration of large defects are more prone to swelling, edema, and hematoma as the periosteum is cut to allow for tension-free suturing (Fig. 7). Careful management of tissues, using non-excessive tension, is paramount to reducing surgical trauma and, consequently, the edema and swelling (Fig. 8). The use of the microscope may help increase the care of the soft tissues and even allow to perform bone regeneration procedures without raising flaps, mainly at the time of implant placement (Fig. 9) [23, 24]. Traditionally, a flap was raised after detecting a cortical plate defect, and a collagen membrane plus a biomaterial or bone chips were used to regenerate the area. Nowadays, it is possible to work flapless even in the presence of large fenestrations and dehiscence, preserving the integrity of the soft tissues and avoiding the mobilization of the periosteum. Hard and soft tissues can be tunneled into the gap

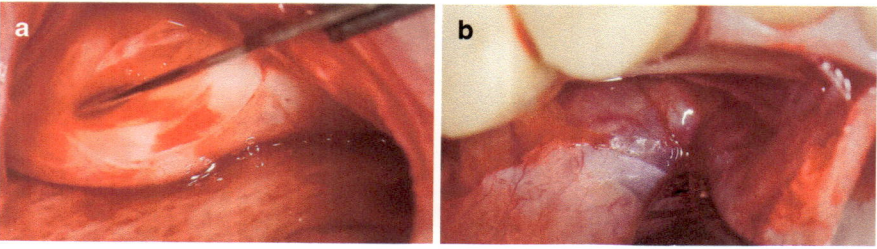

Fig. 8 (**a, b**) Magnification and good illumination are paramount when cutting periosteum to get a free-tension closure of flaps avoiding any damage to underlying tissues

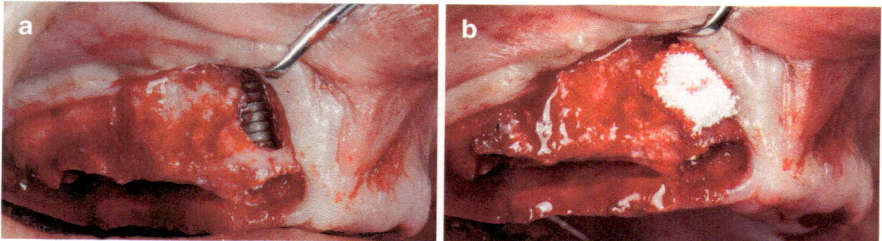

Fig. 9 (**a, b**) A microsurgical approach allows bone regeneration of a fenestration in buccal cortical plate after an immediate implant placement without fully raising a flap

between the immediately placed implant and the periosteum and therefore easily stabilized without the help of a membrane [25].

The microsurgical triad, described as the combination of magnification, illumination, and the surgical technique's increased precision, allows for the numerous advantages described above [11]. First of all, the operative microscope's (OM) magnification forces the surgeon to change protocols and ergonomics, improving his or her motor skills and surgical abilities. Better illumination makes it easier to work with tunneling techniques even in posterior areas keeping a sharp view of the surgical field and keeping the procedures minimally invasive. Finally, the possibility to use microsurgical instruments and sutures, along with the previously mentioned magnification, better illumination, and an improvement in motor skills, makes it possible to change the workflow and precision of the surgical techniques used, reducing tissue trauma and morbidity, speeding up the healing process with less swelling and pain.

3.2 Mucosal Dehiscence

The leading cause of surgical wound dehiscence is flap closure under tension [26]. In cases with thin biotype, scarring and traumatized tissues are prone to wound dehiscence, most commonly present in patients with medical problems such as diabetes, history of radiation therapy, use of corticosteroids, or heavy smoking. Connective tissue grafts are a good way to close wound dehiscence (Fig. 10), even in more complex cases where the dehiscence leads to an oroantral fistula (Fig. 10) [27].

Attention should be given to minimize flap tension [28] and preserve the flap's blood supply [29] or using tunneling techniques, when possible, to preserve the vascularization of the recipient site and the grafts (Figs. 11 and 12; Videos 6 and 7). As mentioned before, this is an advantage with the use of the dental microscope [30].

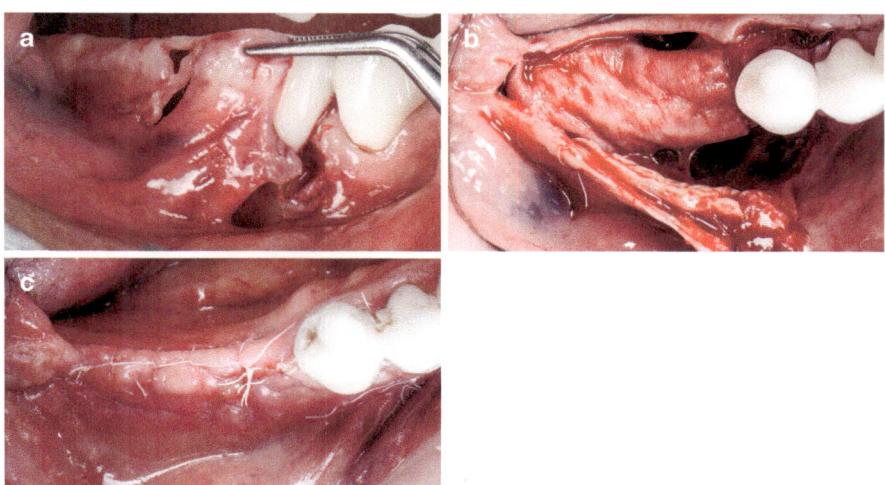

Fig. 10 (**a–c**). A more complex and bigger tear was repaired with an interpositional subepithelial connective tissue graft (sCTG) to avoid aborting bone regeneration surgery

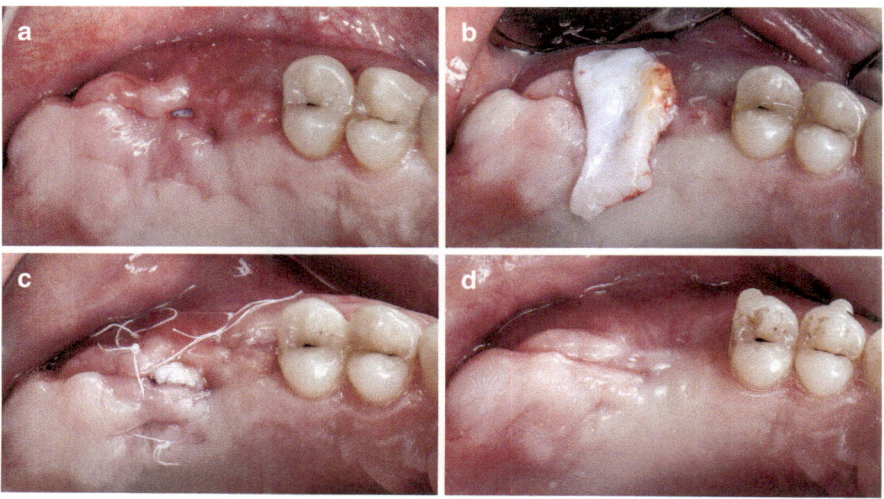

Fig. 11 (**a–d**) After a vertical GBR procedure with a non-resorbable PTFE-d titanium reinforced membrane an early small exposition was detected and solved using a sCTG tunneled through the dehiscence. Minimally invasive and microsurgical approach allowed to preserve integrity and vascularity of tissues allowing for a more predictable procedure

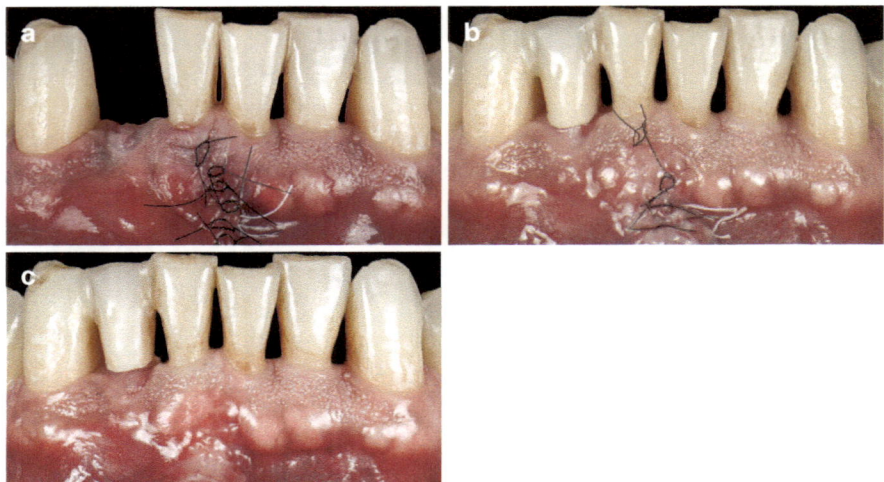

Fig. 12 (a–c). Precision of microsurgical suture after a tunneling technique to reconstruct hard tissues. After a few days healing was complete and a few weeks later no scars were visible

A well-designed flap along a microsurgical procedure reduces the chances of mucosal dehiscence. A well-designed flap is one with a minimum extension that would still allow to properly visualize the area and execute the surgical procedure without compromising its vascularization. It should have releasing incisions for tension-free closure to guarantee its integrity and avoid necrosis of the gingival margins. The use of special instruments such as smaller forceps, elevators, pliers, as well as sutures are important for success when using a microsurgical approach.

4   Late Complications

Late implant complications are classified into biological, biomechanical, and esthetic complications.

4.1   Mechanical Complications

Overload, non-axial loading, and biomechanical stress were considered for many years to compromise implant survival. Recent evidence has been published, suggesting that technical/mechanical risk factors do not affect implant survival or the surrounding bone [31].

Different mechanical complications may be present during implant therapy. The literature reports an incidence of screw loosening in 9% of the cases (Video 8), 4% for loss of prosthetic retention, and 3.5% incidence of veneering material fractures in 5 years [32].

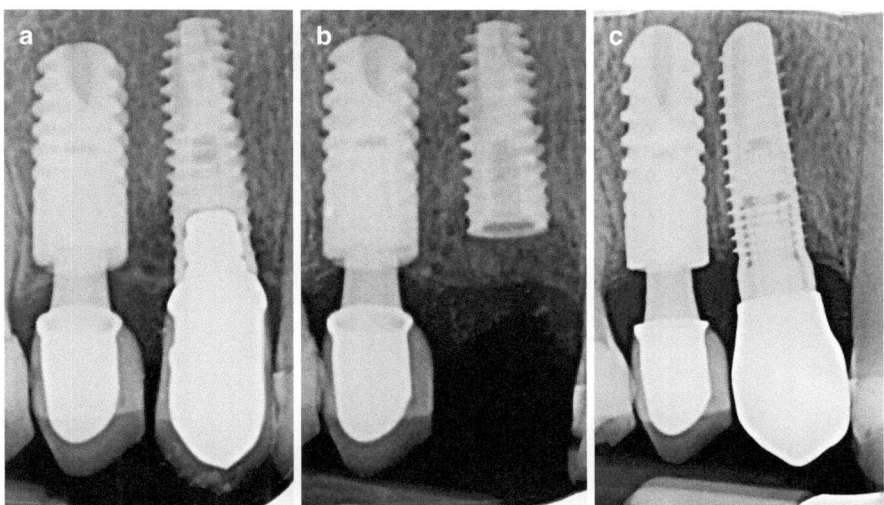

Fig. 13 (**a–c**) The microscope is extremely helpful when broken implants have to be extracted avoiding raising wider flaps and preserving most of the bone around the implant which has to be retrieved

An increase in the failure of some types of rehabilitations has been observed over 10 years. Different types of prosthetics designs exhibited varying incidence of complications: fixed dental prostheses (FDPs) with cantilever extensions on teeth (19.6%), combined tooth-implant-supported FDPs (22.3%), and resin-bonded FDPs (35.0%) [33]. These scenarios can lead to the need for multiple repairs and remakes, compromising the patient's quality of life. It has been reported that greater implant loss occurred in overdentures when compared to other prosthetic designs. Also, there is greater loss in the maxilla than mandible, and failure increases with short implants and poor bone quality [34].

Implant fracture is not frequent, among 0.2–1.5% of cases [35] and usually happens after 3–4 years of implant loading [36]. Very narrow implant design, overloading, parafunctional habits, or an ill-fitting prosthesis may lead to implant fracture (Fig. 13; Video 9) [37].

Fractures of prosthetic retaining screws are frequent due to metal fatigue [38]. The use of the microscope is advantageous when a screw has to be retrieved without damaging the implant (Video 10). In these narrow, deep, and tight spaces, it is advantageous to use the OM as its coaxial light (shadow-free) facilitates a sharp field of view, which would be otherwise almost impossible. This magnification and illumination make it easy to engage the broken screw or make a groove to retrieve it. Sometimes it is not possible to retrieve a screw because its remaining part keeps a high torque, and the engaging part gets damaged during the retrieving process (Video 11). In those cases, it is necessary to take out the implant. Magnification and

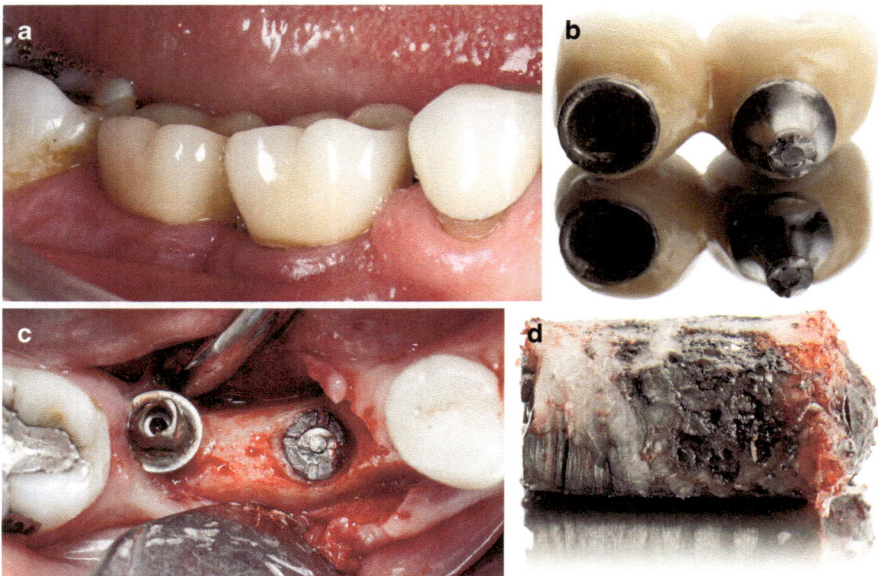

Fig. 14 (**a–d**) When the abutment inside the implant is broken it can be necessary to retrieve the implant. Good illumination and proper magnification allow a proper diagnosis and decision-taking

good visualization are helpful to retrieve the implant preserving the maximum quantity of bone around it avoiding future complex bone regeneration procedures (Fig. 14; Video 12).

4.2   Biological Complications

Biological complications include inflammation of the peri-implant tissue and implant loss [39]. Mucositis is described as an inflammation limited to the mucosa around the dental implant, whereas peri-implantitis involves losing supporting bone [40]. Biological complications and their treatment may lead to gingival recession or soft tissues collapse, compromising implant therapy's success.

Microorganisms found in peri-implantitis are very similar to those found in chronic periodontitis. Overall, the prevalence of peri-implantitis has been documented to range from 1.1% to 85.0%. The incidence has increased from 0.4% within 3 years to 43.9% in 5 years. Lack of hygiene measures, smoking, diabetes mellitus, and periodontitis were identified as risk factors of peri-implantitis [41]. Also, hard tissue resorption around the implant head can be accelerated due to an excess of cement into the peri-implant sulcus, which acts as the source of bacteria, causing inflammation and bleeding upon probing [42]. This may happen in 90% of the implant crowns inserted with cement [43].

The prevention of biological implant complications relies on careful planning, a thorough examination to assess etiological factors, and a regular maintenance recall schedule. Different treatment modalities have been suggested for the treatment of periimplantitis: non-surgical mechanical debridement, local and/or systemic antibiotics, lasers, gingivectomy with or without implantoplasty and regenerative surgery [43–46]. Mechanical and chemical decontamination techniques are still the most highly recommended [47].

The treatment option will depend on the amount of bone loss and the morphology of the peri-implant defect. Nonsurgical treatments are chosen in cases with mucositis or peri-implantitis that involve a defect smaller than 2 mm (Figs. 15 and 16). Peri-implant defects with more than 2 mm bone loss that do not respond to decontamination usually require surgical treatment: gingival resection or apically positioned flap, with or without implantoplasty or guided bone regeneration [48–50]. Although there is no consensus among previous studies, peri-implant defects, including circumferential defects within the bony housing and 2/3-wall intrabony defects, appear to have more regenerative potential (Fig. 17) than those which have lost the cortical bone plates. Conversely, resective therapy (i.e., an apically positioned flap) should be considered in defects with moderate bone loss that do not have a good regenerative potential (Fig. 18). Additionally, to reduce plaque accumulation and facilitate patient home care, implantoplasty is recommended at the time of resective surgery (Fig. 19; Video 13). Nonsurgical treatment modalities can maintain mild peri-implant disease cases [51]. Removal of the implant is the ideal treatment option if the bone loss is beyond 50% of the implant surface or if mobility is present.

With the increasing popularity of implant therapy, biological implant complications are essential issues that cannot be ignored. In addition to comprehensive examination and a thorough treatment plan understanding and preventing the risks, proper surgical technique and regular maintenance play roles in preventing implant biological complications. The microscope magnification and better illumination allow the surgeon to assess the peri-implant defect better and clean the implant's surface. The smoother soft tissue management may avoid wider flaps reducing the morbidity for the patient and increasing the predictability of the guided bone regeneration techniques due to the tension-free closure of the wound and a better clot stability.

4.3   Esthetic Implant Complications

The esthetic sector is a challenging area to treat with dental implants. Attention to detail is required to increase the chances of a successful outcome. Good visualization and lighting are crucial elements to allow for this to happen. According to Jung, the cumulative five-year esthetic complication rate is approximately 7.1% [32].

Esthetic complications in dental implant therapy include gingival recession, soft tissue collapse, grayish color around gingiva, and scaring as a consequence of previous surgeries [52–58]. These esthetic complications are mainly relevant in patients

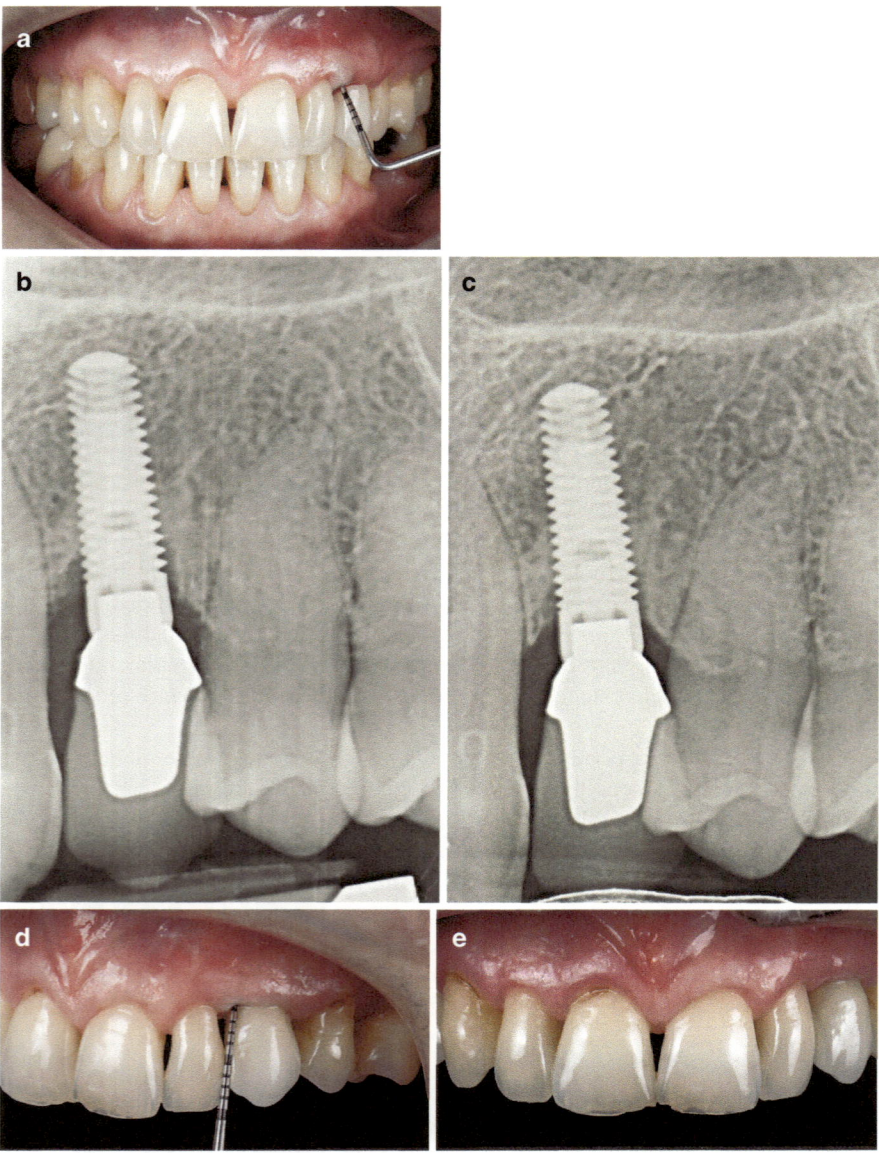

Fig. 15 (**a–e**) Mechanical debridement in a case with periimplantitis due to excess of cement

with a high gingival display, and they should be evaluated following the Pink and White esthetic scores (PES WES) [59, 60].

Several risk factors can promote esthetic implant complications: implant position and prosthesis design, hard and soft tissue condition, and the surgical technique used.

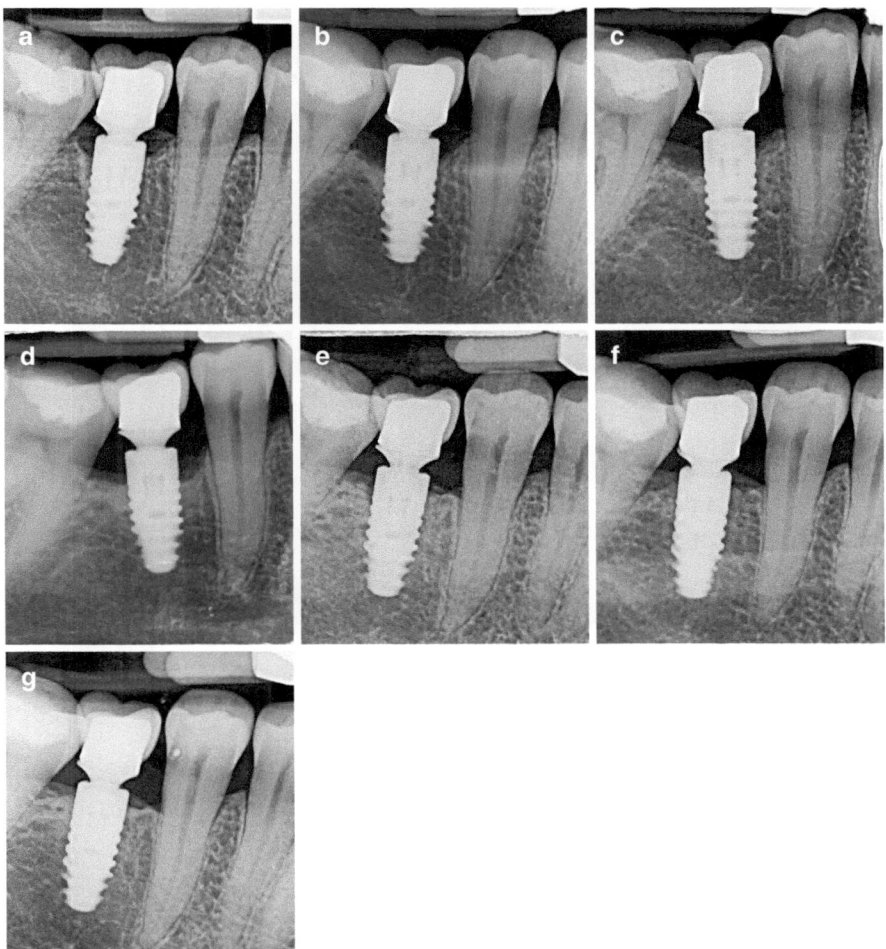

Fig. 16 (a–g) Mechanical debridement in a case with periimplantitis and very good evolution through the years without the need for a surgical procedure

4.3.1 Implant Position and Prosthesis

During the past decades, implant dentistry has evolved from a "surgically driven concept" to a "prosthetically driven concept" to avoid future esthetic, prosthodontic, and biological complications [61, 62]. When an implant is placed too facially or the implant or abutments used are too wide, a gingival recession can occur (Fig. 20).

Gingival recession is mainly present in thin phenotypes where the gingival recession can be three times larger than in a thick phenotype (1.5 vs. 0.6 mm) in only 4 years [63].

When a gingival recession is present, the implant is of adequate size and is not placed buccally, the treatment is predictable, and a partial or total cover can be

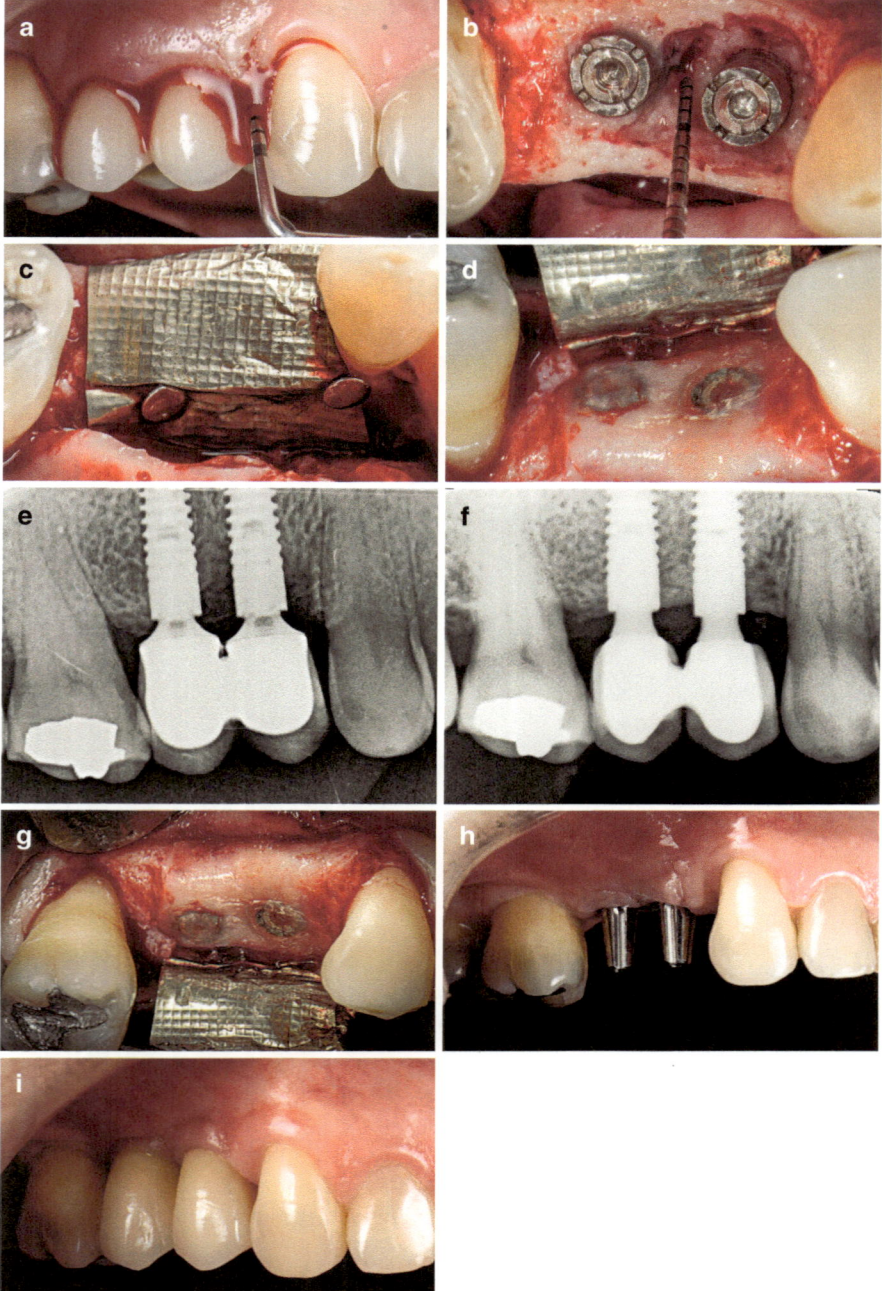

Fig. 17 (**a–i**). GBR after decontamination of the surface of the implants

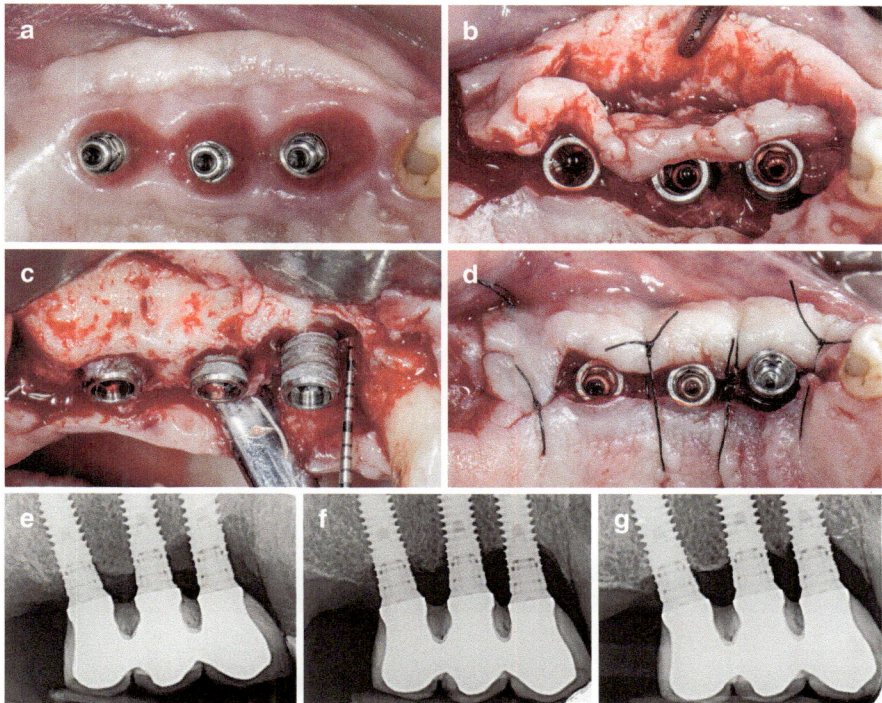

Fig. 18 (**a–g**) Gingivectomy and decontamination of the surface to treat advancing periimplantitis. As a result, a good stability of the bone crest can be observed years later. Radiographs taken in 2014, 2016, and 2020

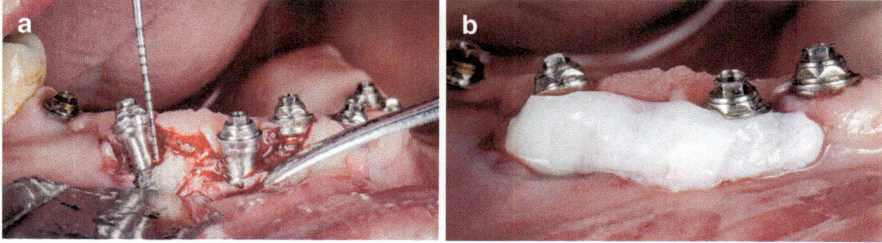

Fig. 19 (**a, b**) Implantoplasty and CTG to improve soft tissue condition on the buccal side of an implant-supported rehabilitation in a patient without gummy smile

expected [55, 64–66]. A perio-prosthodontic approach can be beneficial, combining a coronally advanced flap and a connective tissue graft with an abutment or temporary restoration with a narrower diameter [54, 64, 65]. When the abutment design is correct, a tunneling approach may be sufficient to solve the problem, and the implant crown can be replaced immediately, making the procedure simpler (Fig. 21).

Fig. 20 When the patient does not present a gummy smile implant gingival recessions do not always need to be treated if implants are healthy

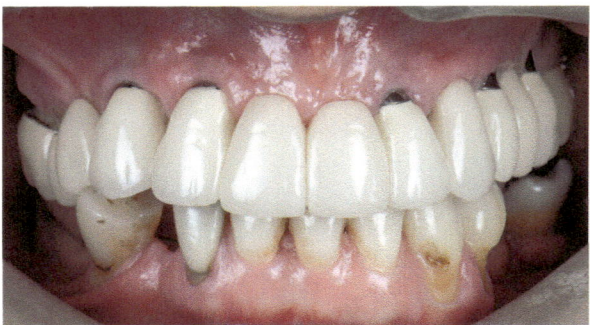

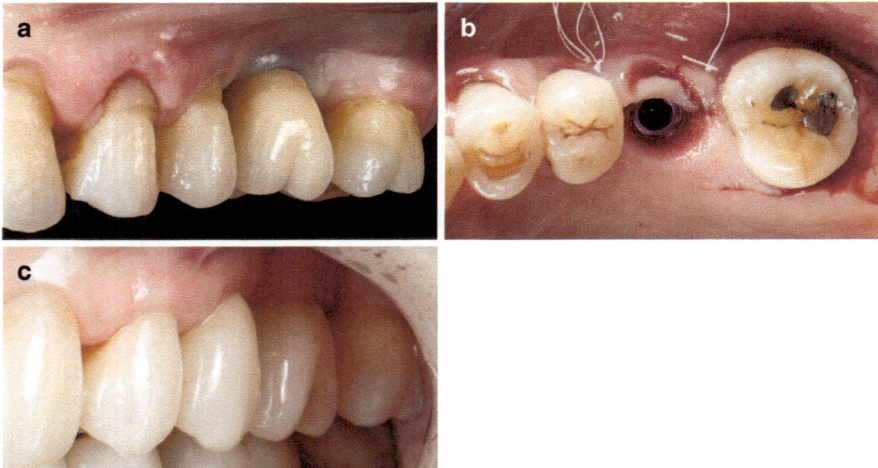

Fig. 21 (a–c) Tunneling technique is used to increase the volume of the gingiva and the band of keratinized gingiva on the buccal aspect of an implant

The implant head and the abutment contour should not surpass the line connecting the adjacent teeth cervical area. Gingival recessions can be avoided by positioning the implant neck at the cingulum of the future restoration. Filling the gap between the cortical plate and the implant body with a biomaterial reduces the socket's collapse. In thin phenotypes, connective tissue grafts tunneled on the buccal may help avoid gingival recessions [63, 67]. The abutment's emergence profile should be concave to allow space for the soft tissues (Fig. 22) [68, 69]. This space can be augmented in occasions with implantoplasty if the implant's malposition is not severe or when the esthetics implications are not relevant because the patient does not present a gummy smile (Fig. 19) [70, 71]. When implants are badly malpositioned and not restorable, the treatment should be started all over again.

If the emergence angle of the abutment is greater than 30 degrees, the space for soft tissues will be reduced and may be a significant risk indicator for peri-implantitis. A convex profile creates an additional risk for bone-level implants [72].

Fig. 22 Ideal emergence profile which includes the EBC zones, preserving the Crestal bone with a straight emergence profile emerging from the implant head, stabilizing the soft tissues with a concave Bounded buccal surface and a convex Esthetic zone

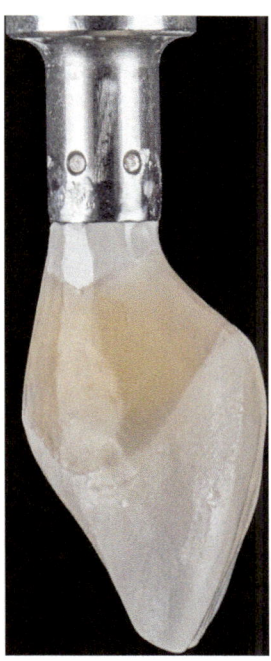

4.3.2 Phenotype

A thin buccal cortical plate and bone dehiscence's are usually related with thin phenotypes and are associated to gingival recession [73]. When the thickness of the gingiva is less than 1.5 mm, a grayish color of the abutment, or the neck of the implant can be seen through the gingiva (Fig. 23) [74].

The mucosa can be thickened to get more stable and esthetic results around implants (Fig. 24) [75–77].

The lack of keratinized tissue is still a controversy today. Some authors fail to demonstrate its relationship with inflammation and recession around implants [78]. Other authors suggest that the lack of keratinized tissue promotes bone remodeling and, consequently, gingival recession [79]. An apically positioned flap and a free gingival graft may prevent the recession, improve the patient's hygiene levels, and even prevent mucositis or periimplantitis (Fig. 25) [80, 81].

4.3.3 Surgical Technique and Morphology of the Recession

The risk of gingival recession is higher after immediate implant placement if no additional measures are taken or when many surgical procedures are executed [82, 83]. Combining a connective tissue with the immediate implant placement helps avoid many surgeries that usually compromise the proximal tissues; however, a 0.5 mm papilla contraction may still be observed [67, 84]. Papilla reconstruction procedures are unpredictable and should be prevented when possible [74, 85].

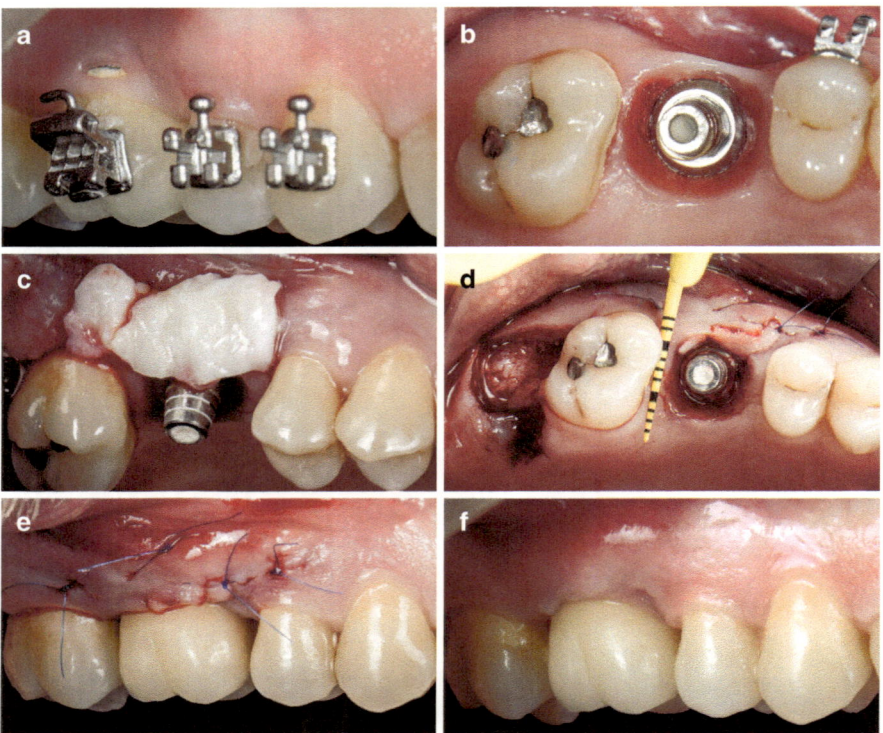

Fig. 23 (a–f). A microsurgical approach allowed to improve the quality and quantity of soft tissues after momentarily retrieving the implant-supported crown

The healing process around teeth and implants is similar, but the peri-implant soft tissues' complete maturation takes longer [86]. The stability of the blood clot between the flap and the wound bed is a key point to guarantee a healing process without complications, and suturing techniques are paramount to ensure optimal surgical outcomes [86]. With the help of microscope, the surgical results are becoming more predictable and repeatable, providing good clinical results for the patient and reducing the healing time and morbidity. Treating recessions around implants is less predictable than around teeth because of the reduced vascularization and the different orientation of the collagen fibers. For this reason, implant explantation can be a more predictable approach sometimes [87].

Before taking a final decision about preserving or explanting an implant, several points should be evaluated: the number of implants involved, size and location of the problem, design, and fit of the abutment, the quantity of bone on the buccal and proximal sides, as well as the size and condition of the gingival recession.

Coronally advanced flaps (CAF) and CTG have been used successfully to cover recessions around implants in three retrospective studies [55, 64, 71]. Only some studies show complete recession coverage, but patient satisfaction is high even

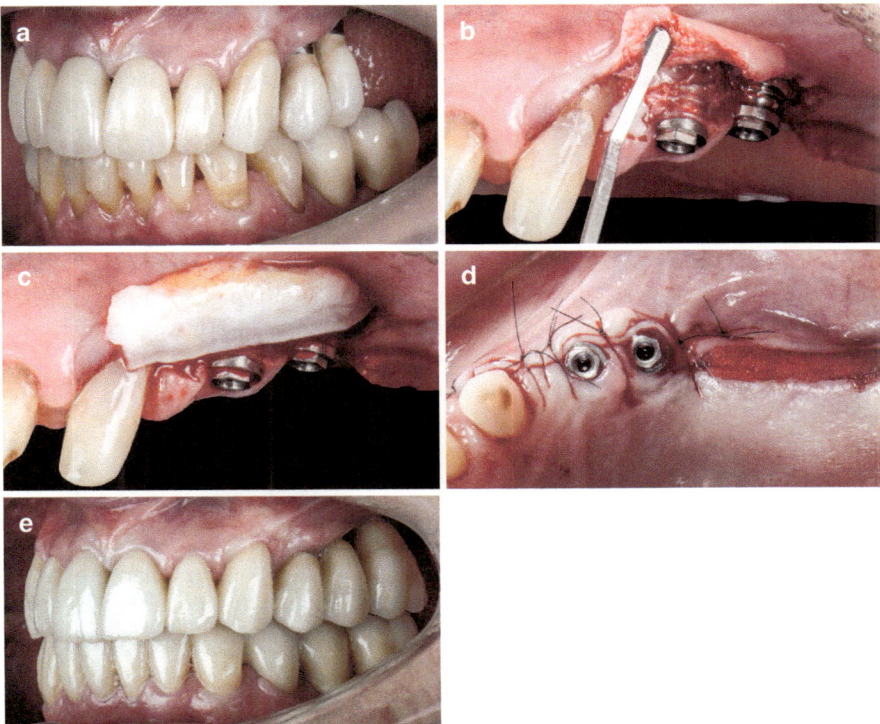

Fig. 24 (**a–e**) CAF plus a CTG is a very predictable way to treat gingival recessions on implants

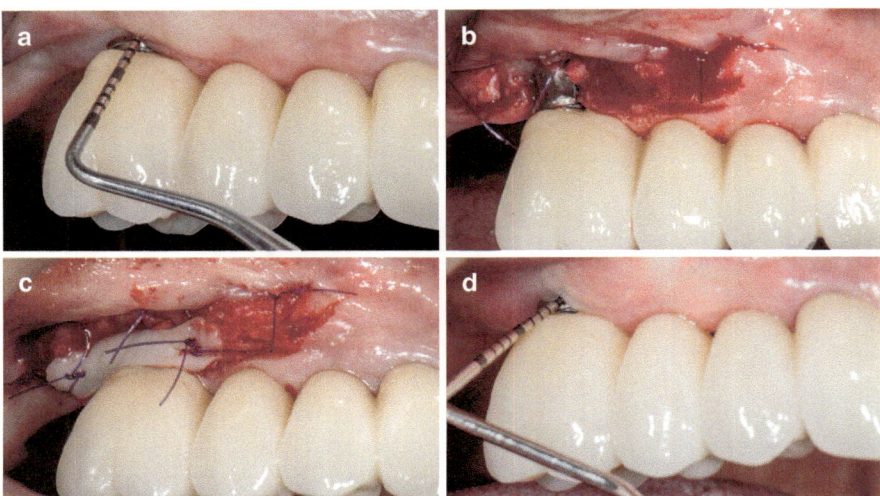

Fig. 25 (**a–d**) Apical positioned flap, implantoplasty, and FGG to increase the band of keratinized tissue and the vestibule dimensions in a patient with difficulties for hygiene

when full coverage of the recession was not achieved (Fig. 24) [71, 88, 89]. Releasing incisions to advance coronally the flap reduces the vascularization of the flap and can induce scar tissue that can be observed years later [58, 90–93]. For these reasons, a "pouch" technique is advisable for mild recessions (Fig. 23; Video 14).

Even when biomaterials have been used to cover recessions around implants such as Acellular Dermal Matrix (ADM), the connective tissue graft (CTG) seems the most predictable approach with the best results [66, 71, 94–96]. The CTG should have at least 2 mm thickness. The area or technique used to harvest the CTG may not be relevant. Single incision in the palate, de-epithelialized grafts from the palate, and tuberosity grafts have been used with similar results [97]. Connective tissue from the tuberosity is denser, and the morbidity is low, but its disadvantage is the scarce quantity and the overgrowth that may happen over time (Fig. 23) [98].

4.3.4   Papilla Reconstruction

Jemt classified the gingival papilla status into five grades: 0, lack of papilla; 1, <50% of the volume of the papilla is present; 2, between 50% and 100% of the volume of the papilla is present; 3, papilla volume is perfect; 4, overgrowth of the papilla [99]. The distance from the contact point to the bone crest can predict the filling of embrasure by the proximal soft tissue [100]. When this distance is less than 5 mm, the papilla will fill the embrasure 100% times, and this decreases as the contact point moves farther from the bone crest.

The papilla height between two implants is reduced when compared to other scenarios [101]. If a pontic site is next to the implant, the papilla height can be reconstructed to achieve even 5.5–6 mm (Fig. 26).

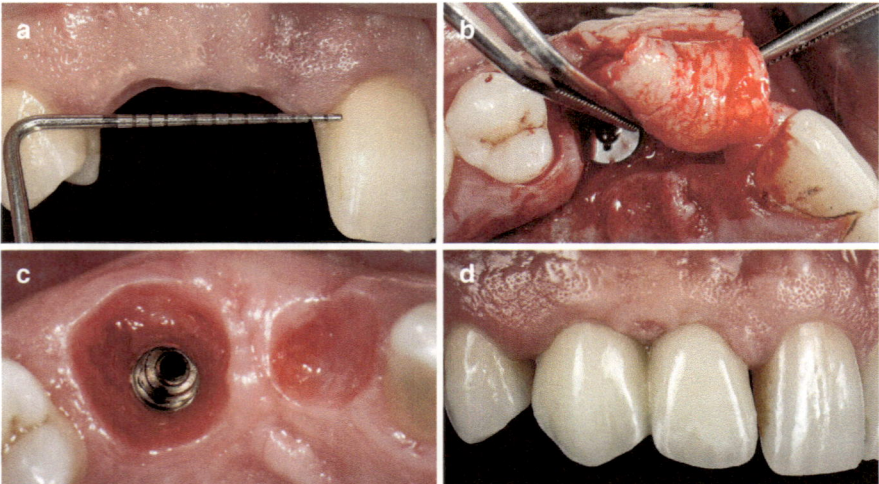

Fig. 26 (a–d) Pontic site reconstruction and papilla development using a perio-prosthodontic approach combining a pedicled palatal CTG with a long-term interim restoration

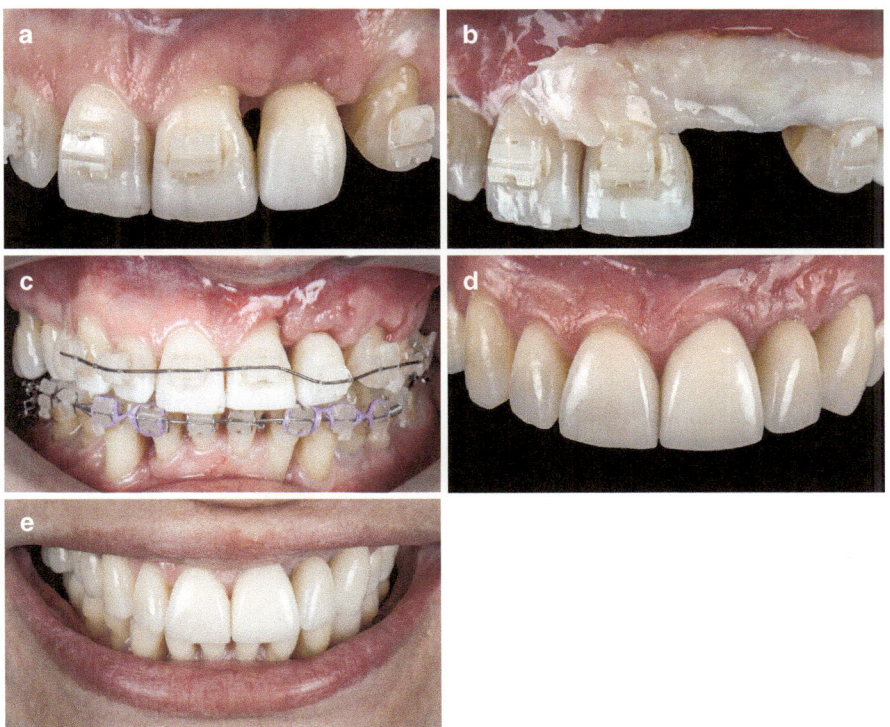

Fig. 27 (a–e) A combination of orthodontic, periodontal, prosthodontic, and restorative therapies was used in this complex case to reconstruct the soft tissues and papillae

Papilla reconstruction is unpredictable and requires microsurgical experience, but it can be done by applying several soft tissue augmentation procedures [88, 99, 102], a combination of bone regeneration and soft tissue grafting [103], orthodontic treatment plus restorative treatment (Fig. 27) [104, 105], tunneling techniques [106], or a combination of different techniques, the orthodontic extrusion being the most predictable [107–111].

Pink ceramic can also be used to resolve very severe defects, but consideration should be given to difficult hygiene maintenance and the possible esthetic non-pleasant result in patients who expose the transition area [112].

5 Conclusions

In dentistry, the expertise of the surgeon, his visual-spatial abilities, attitude, and capacity to cope with stress are determinants that affect the selection of the technique and its predictability [113–116].

Fig. 28 The microsurgical triad: the visualization is improved with a good magnification and illumination of the surgical field. This ends up improving the surgical skills of the surgeon due to the continuous challenge to his abilities

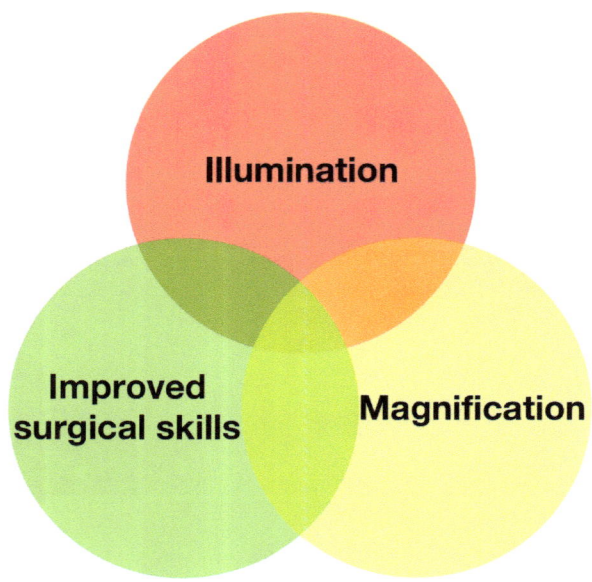

Shanelec and Tibbets introduced the use of microscopy in periodontics at the American Academy of Periodontology's Annual Meeting in 1992 [117]. Since then, many clinicians have been introducing the microscope into their practices. The combination of small microsurgical instruments and delicate surgical techniques allows for extremely fine, crisp, and accurate incisions, gentle tissue handling, and precise suturing. Other advantages are less discomfort to the back and less eye strain [118].

A better and more precise soft tissue management through magnification and a better illumination allow the surgeon to increase progressively his abilities and the predictability of his surgical techniques driving this process to a different approach employing minimally invasive surgeries and being able to solve several problems reducing treatment time, costs, and morbidity for the patient at the same time. Moreover, this kind of dentistry is more gratifying and motivating for the practitioner and the whole team, reducing the patient's anxiety level (Fig. 28).

The use of microscope has some disadvantages: need of education in the field, more time-consuming at the beginning, limited surgical field, and higher costs for the patient. So, it can only be justified if the predictability of the clinical results is increased significantly. That is the case in hard and soft tissue surgical procedures where the microsurgical handling of the anatomical structures seems to compensate for the effort of using a microscope. Of course, treating implant complications with a microsurgical approach opens a new era in dentistry, increasing the predictability of the techniques used [119].

6 Key Points

1. Implant placement may involve trans-surgical accidents that can affect the outcome of surgery or complications after the implant has integrated that can be categorized as early or late complications.
2. The microscope's use increases the care of soft tissues with a better instrument manipulation technique, reducing accidents like flap tears due to excessive traction or incorrect use of instruments.
3. The operative microscope's (OM) magnification forces the surgeon to change protocols and ergonomics, improving his/her motor skills and surgical abilities.
4. Better illumination makes it easier to work with tunneling techniques even in posterior areas, keeping a sharp view of the surgical field and minimally invasive procedures.
5. The possibility to use microsurgical instruments and sutures, along with the previously mentioned magnification, better illumination, and an improvement in motor skills, makes it possible to change the workflow and precision of the surgical techniques used, reducing tissue trauma and morbidity, speeding up the healing process with less swelling and pain.
6. OM drives the treatment to a different approach employing minimally invasive surgeries and solving several problems reducing treatment time, costs, and morbidity for the patient at the same time.
7. Moreover, this kind of dentistry is more gratifying and motivating for the practitioner and the whole team, reducing the patient's anxiety level.

References

1. Annibali S, La Monaca G, Tantardini M, Cristalli MP. The role of the template in prosthetically guided implantology. J Prosthodont. 2009;18:177–83.
2. Hanif A, Qureshi S, Sheikh Z, Rashid H. Complications in implant dentistry. Eur J Dent. 2017;11:135–40.
3. Dreiseidler T, Mischkowski RA, Neugebauer J, Ritter L, Zöller JE. Comparison of cone-beam imaging with orthopantomography and computerized tomography for assessment in presurgical implant dentistry. Int J Oral Maxillofac Implants. 2009;24:216–25.
4. Ozcelik O, Haytac MC, Akkaya M. Iatrogenic trauma to oral tissues. J Periodontol. 2005;76:1793–7.
5. Zhou W, Han C, Li D, Li Y, Song Y, Zhao Y. Endodontic treatment of teeth induces retrograde peri-implantitis. Clin Oral Implants Res. 2009;20:1326–32.
6. Mardinger O, Manor Y, Mijiritsky E, Hirshberg A. Lingual perimandibular vessels associated with life-threatening bleeding: an anatomic study. Int J Oral Maxillofac Implants. 2007;22:127–31.
7. Hur Y, Tsukiyama T, Yoon TH, Griffin T. Double flap incision design for guided bone regeneration: a novel technique and clinical considerations. J Periodontol. 2010;81:945–52.
8. Neugebauer J, Scheer M, Mischkowski RA, An SH, Karapetian VE, Toutenburg H, Zoeller JE. Comparison of torque measurements and clinical handling of various surgical motors. Int J Oral Maxillofac Implants. 2009;24:469–76.
9. Garfunkel AA, Galili D, Findler M, Lubliner J, Eldor A. Bleeding tendency: a practical approach in dentistry. Compend Contin Educ Dent. 1999;20(836–8):840–2. 844 passim.

10. Kang K, Grover D, Goel V, Kaushal S, Kaur G. Periodontal microsurgery and microsurgical instrumentation: a review. Dent J Adv Stud. 2016;4:74–80.
11. Belcher JM. A perspective on periodontal microsurgery. Int J Periodontics Restorative Dent. 2001;21:191–6.
12. Steigmann M. Aesthetic flap design for correction of buccal fenestration defects. Pract Proced Aesthet Dent. 2008;20:487–93. Quiz 494.
13. Braut V, Bornstein MM, Belser U, Buser D. Thickness of the anterior maxillary facial bone wall-a retrospective radiographic study using cone beam computed tomography. Int J Periodontics Restorative Dent. 2011;31:125–31.
14. Chiapasco M, Zaniboni M. Clinical outcomes of GBR procedures to correct peri-implant dehiscences and fenestrations: a systematic review. Clin Oral Implants Res. 2009;20:113–23.
15. Jung RE, Hälg GA, Thoma DS, Hämmerle CH. A randomized, controlled clinical trial to evaluate a new membrane for guided bone regeneration around dental implants. Clin Oral Implants Res. 2009;20:162–8.
16. MacDonald JD. Learning to perform microvascular anastomosis. Skull Base. 2005;15:229–40.
17. Derman GH, Schenck RR. Microsurgical technique—fundamentals of the microsurgical laboratory. Orthop Clin North Am. 1977;8:229–48.
18. Misch CE, Resnik R. Mandibular nerve neurosensory impairment after dental implant surgery: management and protocol. Implant Dent. 2010;19:378–86.
19. Cannizzaro G, Leone M, Esposito M. Immediate functional loading of implants placed with flapless surgery in the edentulous maxilla: 1-year follow-up of a single cohort study. Int J Oral Maxillofac Implants. 2007;22:87–95.
20. Cannizzaro G, Leone M, Consolo U, Ferri V, Esposito M. Immediate functional loading of implants placed with flapless surgery versus conventional implants in partially edentulous patients: a 3-year randomized controlled clinical trial. Int J Oral Maxillofac Implants. 2008;23:867–75.
21. Merli M, Bernardelli F, Esposito M. Computer-guided flapless placement of immediately loaded dental implants in the edentulous maxilla: a pilot prospective case series. Eur J Oral Implantol. 2008;1:61–9.
22. Arisan V, Karabuda CZ, Ozdemir T. Implant surgery using bone- and mucosa-supported stereolithographic guides in totally edentulous jaws: surgical and post-operative outcomes of computer-aided vs. standard techniques. Clin Oral Implants Res. 2010;21:980–8.
23. Elian N, Cho SC, Froum S, Smith RB, Tarnow DP. A simplified socket classification and repair technique. Pract Proced Aesthet Dent. 2007;19:99–104.
24. da Rosa JC, Rosa AC, da Rosa DM, Zardo CM. Immediate Dentoalveolar Restoration of compromised sockets: a novel technique. Eur J Esthet Dent. 2013;8:432–43.
25. Zuffía J, Blasi G, Gómez-Meda R, Blasi A. The four-layer graft technique, a hard and soft tissue graft from the tuberosity in one piece. J Esthet Restor Dent. 2019;31:304–10.
26. Lee S, Thiele C. Factors associated with free flap complications after head and neck reconstruction and the molecular basis of fibrotic tissue rearrangement in preirradiated soft tissue. J Oral Maxillofac Surg. 2010;68:2169–78.
27. Watzak G, Tepper G, Zechner W, Monov G, Busenlechner D, Watzek G. Bony press-fit closure of oro-antral fistulas: a technique for pre-sinus lift repair and secondary closure. J Oral Maxillofac Surg. 2005;63:1288–94.
28. Burkhardt R, Lang NP. Role of flap tension in primary wound closure of mucoperiosteal flaps: a prospective cohort study. Clin Oral Implants Res. 2010;21:50–4.
29. Mörmann W, Ciancio SG. Blood supply of human gingiva following periodontal surgery. A fluorescein angiographic study. J Periodontol. 1977;48:681–92.
30. Zuhr O, Rebele SF, Cheung SL, Hürzeler MB. Research Group on Oral Soft Tissue Biology and Wound Healing. Surgery without papilla incision: tunneling flap procedures in plastic periodontal and implant surgery. Periodontol 2000. 2018;77:123–49.
31. Salvi GE, Brägger U. Mechanical and technical risks in implant therapy. Int J Oral Maxillofac Implants. 2009;24:69–85.

32. Jung RE, Zembic A, Pjetursson BE, Zwahlen M, Thoma DS. Systematic review of the survival rate and the incidence of biological, technical, and aesthetic complications of single crowns on implants reported in longitudinal studies with a mean follow-up of 5 years. Clin Oral Implants Res. 2012;23:2–21.
33. Pjetursson BE, Brägger U, Lang NP, Zwahlen M. Comparison of survival and complication rates of tooth-supported fixed dental prostheses (FDPs) and implant-supported FDPs and single crowns (SCs). Clin Oral Implants Res. 2007;18:97–113.
34. Goodacre CJ, Kan JY, Rungcharassaeng K. Clinical complications of osseointegrated implants. J Prosthet Dent. 1999;81:537–52.
35. Eckert SE, Meraw SJ, Cal E, Ow RK. Analysis of incidence and associated factors with fractured implants: a retrospective study. Int J Oral Maxillofac Implants. 2000;15:662–7.
36. Kohal RJ, Wolkewitz M, Mueller C. Alumina-reinforced zirconia implants: survival rate and fracture strength in a masticatory simulation trial. Clin Oral Implants Res. 2010;21:1345–52.
37. Al Quran FA, Rashan BA, Al-Dwairi ZN. Management of dental implant fractures. A case history. J Oral Implantol. 2009;35:210–4.
38. Al Jabbari YS, Fournelle R, Ziebert G, Toth J, Iacopino AM. Mechanical behavior and failure analysis of prosthetic retaining screws after long-term use in vivo. Part 4: failure analysis of 10 fractured retaining screws retrieved from three patients. J Prosthodont. 2008;17:201–10.
39. Berglundh T, Persson L, Klinge B. A systematic review of the incidence of biological and technical complications in implant dentistry reported in prospective longitudinal studies of at least 5 years. J Clin Periodontol. 2002;29:197–212. Discussion 232–3.
40. Lindhe J, Meyle J, Group D of European Workshop on Periodontology. Peri-implant diseases: consensus report of the sixth European workshop on periodontology. J Clin Periodontol. 2008;35:282–5.
41. Dreyer H, Grischke J, Tiede C, Eberhard J, Schweitzer A, Toikkanen SE, Glöckner S, Krause G, Stiesch M. Epidemiology and risk factors of peri-implantitis: a systematic review. J Periodontal Res. 2018;53:657–81.
42. Wilson TG Jr. The positive relationship between excess cement and peri-implant disease: a prospective clinical endoscopic study. J Periodontol. 2009;80:1388–92.
43. Froum SJ, Froum SH, Rosen PS. A regenerative approach to the successful treatment of peri-implantitis: a consecutive series of 170 implants in 100 patients with 2- to 10-year follow-up. Int J Periodontics Restorative Dent. 2015;35:857–63.
44. Persson GR, Samuelsson E, Lindahl C, Renvert S. Mechanical non-surgical treatment of peri-implantitis: a single-blinded randomized longitudinal clinical study. II. Microbiological results. J Clin Periodontol. 2010;37:563–73.
45. Mombelli A, Lang NP. Antimicrobial treatment of peri-implant infections. Clin Oral Implants Res. 1992;3:162–8.
46. Deppe H, Horch HH, Henke J, Donath K. Peri-implant care of ailing implants with the carbon dioxide laser. Int J Oral Maxillofac Implants. 2001;16:659–67.
47. Subramani K, Wismeijer D. Decontamination of titanium implant surface and re-osseointegration to treat peri-implantitis: a literature review. Int J Oral Maxillofac Implants. 2012;27:1043–54.
48. Romeo E, Ghisolfi M, Murgolo N, Chiapasco M, Lops D, Vogel G. Therapy of peri-implantitis with resective surgery. A 3-year clinical trial on rough screw-shaped oral implants. Part I: clinical outcome. Clin Oral Implants Res. 2005;16:9–18.
49. Serino G, Turri A. Outcome of surgical treatment of peri-implantitis: results from a 2-year prospective clinical study in humans. Clin Oral Implants Res. 2011;22:1214–20.
50. Renvert S, Polyzois I, Claffey N. Surgical therapy for the control of peri-implantitis. Clin Oral Implants Res. 2012;23:84–94.
51. Hsu YT, Mason SA, Wang HL. Biological implant complications and their management. J Int Acad Periodontol. 2014;16:9–18.
52. Bengazi F, Wennström JL, Lekholm U. Recession of the soft tissue margin at oral implants. A 2-year longitudinal prospective study. Clin Oral Implants Res. 1996;7:303–10.

53. Oates TW, Robinson M, Gunsolley JC. Surgical therapies for the treatment of gingival recession. A systematic review. Ann Periodontol. 2003;8:303–20.
54. Shibli JA, d'Avila S, Marcantonio E Jr. Connective tissue graft to correct peri-implant soft tissue margin: a clinical report. J Prosthet Dent. 2004;91:119–22.
55. Burkhardt R, Joss A, Lang NP. Soft tissue dehiscence coverage around endosseous implants: a prospective cohort study. Clin Oral Implants Res. 2008;19:451–7.
56. Frost NA, Mealey BL, Jones AA, Huynh-Ba G. Periodontal biotype: gingival thickness as it relates to probe visibility and buccal plate thickness. J Periodontol. 2015;86:1141–9.
57. Cosgarea R, Gasparik C, Dudea D, Culic B, Dannewitz B, Sculean A. Peri-implant soft tissue colour around titanium and zirconia abutments: a prospective randomized controlled clinical study. Clin Oral Implants Res. 2015;26:537–44.
58. Wessels R, De Roose S, De Bruyckere T, Eghbali A, Jacquet W, De Rouck T, et al. The mucosal scarring index: reliability of a new composite index for assessing scarring following oral surgery. Clin Oral Investig. 2019;23:1209–15.
59. Fürhauser R, Florescu D, Benesch T, Haas R, Mailath G, Watzek G. Evaluation of soft tissue around single-tooth implant crowns: the pink esthetic score. Clin Oral Implants Res. 2005;16:639–44.
60. Belser UC, Grütter L, Vailati F, Bornstein MM, Weber HP, Buser D. Outcome evaluation of early placed maxillary anterior single-tooth implants using objective esthetic criteria: a cross-sectional, retrospective study in 45 patients with a 2- to 4-year follow-up using pink and white esthetic scores. J Periodontol. 2009;80:140–51.
61. D'haese J, Ackhurst J, Wismeijer D, De Bruyn H, Tahmaseb A. Current state of the art of computer-guided implant surgery. Periodontol 2000. 2017;73:121–33.
62. Esquivel J, Meda RG, Blatz MB. The impact of 3D implant position on emergence profile design. Int J Periodontics Restorative Dent. 2021;41:79–86.
63. Kan JY, Rungcharassaeng K, Lozada JL, Zimmerman G. Facial gingival tissue stability following immediate placement and provisionalization of maxillary anterior single implants: a 2- to 8-year follow-up. Int J Oral Maxillofac Implants. 2011;26:179–87.
64. Roccuzzo M, Gaudioso L, Bunino M, Dalmasso P. Surgical treatment of buccal soft tissue recessions around single implants: 1-year results from a prospective pilot study. Clin Oral Implants Res. 2014;25:641–6.
65. Zucchelli G, Mazzotti C, Mounssif I, Mele M, Stefanini M, Montebugnoli L. A novel surgical-prosthetic approach for soft tissue dehiscence coverage around single implant. Clin Oral Implants Res. 2013;24:957–62.
66. Anderson LE, Inglehart MR, El-Kholy K, Eber R, Wang HL. Implant associated soft tissue defects in the anterior maxilla: a randomized control trial comparing subepithelial connective tissue graft and acellular dermal matrix allograft. Implant Dent. 2014;23:416–25.
67. Frizzera F, de Freitas RM, Muñoz-Chávez OF, Cabral G, Shibli JA, Marcantonio E Jr. Impact of soft tissue grafts to reduce peri-implant alterations after immediate implant placement and provisionalization in compromised sockets. Int J Periodontics Restorative Dent. 2019;39:381–9.
68. Rompen E, Raepsaet N, Domken O, Touati B, Van Dooren E. Soft tissue stability at the facial aspect of gingivally converging abutments in the esthetic zone: a pilot clinical study. J Prosthet Dent. 2007;97:S119–25.
69. Gomez-Meda R, Esquivel J, Blatz MB. The esthetic biological contour concept for implant restoration emergence profile design. J Esthet Restor Dent. 2021;33:173–84.
70. Zucchelli G, Mazzotti C, Mounssif I, Marzadori M, Stefanini M. Esthetic treatment of peri-implant soft tissue defects: a case report of a modified surgical-prosthetic approach. Int J Periodontics Restorative Dent. 2013;33:327–35.
71. Zucchelli G, Felice P, Mazzotti C, Marzadori M, Mounssif I, Monaco C, et al. 5-year outcomes after coverage of soft tissue dehiscence around single implants: a prospective cohort study. Eur J Oral Implantol. 2018;11:215–24.
72. Katafuchi M, Weinstein BF, Leroux BG, Chen YW, Daubert DM. Restoration contour is a risk indicator for peri-implantitis: a cross-sectional radiographic analysis. J Clin Periodontol. 2018;45:225–32.

73. Wennström JL. Mucogingival considerations in orthodontic treatment. Semin Orthod. 1996;2:46–54.

74. Jung RE, Sailer I, Hämmerle CH, Attin T, Schmidlin P. In vitro color changes of soft tissues caused by restorative materials. Int J Periodontics Restorative Dent. 2007;27:251–7.

75. Speroni S, Cicciu M, Maridati P, Grossi GB, Maiorana C. Clinical investigation of mucosal thickness stability after soft tissue grafting around implants: a 3-year retrospective study. Indian J Dent Res. 2010;21:474–9.

76. Stimmelmayr M, Allen EP, Reichert TE, Iglhaut G. Use of a combination epithelized-subepithelial connective tissue graft for closure and soft tissue augmentation of an extraction site following ridge preservation or implant placement: description of a technique. Int J Periodontics Restorative Dent. 2010;30:375–81.

77. Zuhr O, Bäumer D, Hürzeler M. The addition of soft tissue replacement grafts in plastic periodontal and implant surgery: critical elements in design and execution. J Clin Periodontol. 2014;41:S123–42.

78. Wennström JL. Lack of association between width of attached gingiva and development of soft tissue recession. A 5-year longitudinal study. J Clin Periodontol. 1987;14:181–4.

79. Lin GH, Chan HL, Wang HL. The significance of keratinized mucosa on implant health: a systematic review. J Periodontol. 2013;84:1755–67.

80. Berglundh T, Armitage G, Araujo MG, Avila-Ortiz G, Blanco J, Camargo PM, et al. Peri-implant diseases and conditions: consensus report of workgroup 4 of the 2017 World Workshop on the Classification of Periodontal and Peri-Implant Diseases and Conditions. J Periodontol. 2018;89:S313–8.

81. Isler SC, Uraz A, Kaymaz O, Cetiner D. An evaluation of the relationship between peri-implant soft tissue biotype and the severity of peri-implantitis: a cross-sectional study. Int J Oral Maxillofac Implants. 2019;34:187–96.

82. Cordaro L, Torsello F, Roccuzzo M. Clinical outcome of submerged vs. non-submerged implants placed in fresh extraction sockets. Clin Oral Implants Res. 2009;20:1307–13.

83. Cooper LF, Reside G, Stanford C, Barwacz C, Feine J, Nader SA, et al. Three-year prospective randomized comparative assessment of anterior maxillary single implants with different abutment interfaces. Int J Oral Maxillofac Implants. 2019;34:150–8.

84. Ryser MR, Block MS, Mercante DE. Correlation of papilla to crestal bone levels around single tooth implants in immediate or delayed crown protocols. J Oral Maxillofac Surg. 2005;63:1184–95.

85. Froum SJ, Khouly I. Survival rates and bone and soft tissue level changes around one-piece dental implants placed with a flapless or flap protocol: 8.5-year results. Int J Periodontics Restorative Dent. 2017;37:327–37.

86. Sukekava F, Pannuti CM, Lima LA, Tormena M, Araújo MG. Dynamics of soft tissue healing at implants and teeth: a study in a dog model. Clin Oral Implants Res. 2016;27:545–52.

87. Berglundh T, Lindhe J, Ericsson I, Marinello CP, Liljenberg B, Thomsen P. The soft tissue barrier at implants and teeth. Clin Oral Implants Res. 1991;2:81–90.

88. Hidaka T, Ueno D. Mucosal dehiscence coverage for dental implant using split pouch technique: a two-stage approach [corrected]. J Periodontal Implant Sci. 2012;42(3):105–9. https://doi.org/10.5051/jpis.2012.42.3.105. Erratum in: J Periodontal Implant Sci. 2012;42:146.

89. Lai YL, Chen HL, Chang LY, Lee SY. Resubmergence technique for the management of soft tissue recession around an implant: case report. Int J Oral Maxillofac Implants. 2010;25:201–4.

90. Kleinheinz J, Büchter A, Kruse-Lösler B, Weingart D, Joos U. Incision design in implant dentistry based on vascularization of the mucosa. Clin Oral Implants Res. 2005;16:518–23.

91. Allen AL. Use of the supraperiosteal envelope in soft tissue grafting for root coverage. I. Rationale and technique. Int J Periodontics Restorative Dent. 1994;14:216–27.

92. Zabalegui I, Sicilia A, Cambra J, Gil J, Sanz M. Treatment of multiple adjacent gingival recessions with the tunnel subepithelial connective tissue graft: a clinical report. Int J Periodontics Restorative Dent. 1999;19:199–206.

93. Girbés-Ballester P, Viña-Almunia J, Peñarrocha-Oltra D, Peñarrocha-Diago M. Soft tissue response in posterior teeth adjacent to interdental single implants: a controlled randomized

clinical trial comparing intrasulcular vs trapezoidal incision. Int J Oral Maxillofac Implants. 2016;31:631–41.

94. Mareque-Bueno S. A novel surgical procedure for coronally repositioning of the buccal implant mucosa using acellular dermal matrix: a case report. J Periodontol. 2011;82:151–6.

95. Sculean A, Mihatovic I, Shirakata Y, Bosshardt DD, Schwarz F, Iglhaut G. Healing of localized gingival recessions treated with coronally advanced flap alone or combined with either a resorbable collagen matrix or subepithelial connective tissue graft. A preclinical study. Clin Oral Investig. 2015;19:903–9.

96. Thoma DS, Naenni N, Figuero E, Hämmerle CH, Schwarz F, Jung RE, et al. Effects of soft tissue augmentation procedures on peri-implant health or disease: a systematic review and meta-analysis. Clin Oral Implants Res. 2018;29:32–49.

97. Rojo E, Stroppa G, Sanz-Martin I, Gonzalez-Martín O, Alemany AS, Nart J. Soft tissue volume gain around dental implants using autogenous subepithelial connective tissue grafts harvested from the lateral palate or tuberosity area. A randomized controlled clinical study. J Clin Periodontol. 2018;45:495–503.

98. Amin PN, Bissada NF, Ricchetti PA, Silva AP, Demko CA. Tuberosity versus palatal donor sites for soft tissue grafting: a split-mouth clinical study. Quintessence Int. 2018;49:589–98.

99. Jemt T. Regeneration of gingival papillae after single-implant treatment. Int J Periodontics Restorative Dent. 1997;17:326–33.

100. Tarnow D, Elian N, Fletcher P, Froum S, Magner A, Cho SC, et al. Vertical distance from the crest of bone to the height of the interproximal papilla between adjacent implants. J Periodontol. 2003;74:1785–8.

101. Salama H, Salama MA, Garber D, Adar P. The interproximal height of bone: a guidepost to predictable aesthetic strategies and soft tissue contours in anterior tooth replacement. Pract Periodontics Aesthet Dent. 1998;10:1131–41.

102. Nemcovsky CE, Moses O, Artzi Z. Interproximal papillae reconstruction in maxillary implants. J Periodontol. 2000;71:308–14.

103. Urban IA, Klokkevold PR, Takei HH. Abutment-supported papilla: a combined surgical and prosthetic approach to papilla reformation. Int J Periodontics Restorative Dent. 2016;36:665–71.

104. Cirelli JA, Cirelli CC, Holzhausen M, Martins LP, Brandão CH. Combined periodontal, orthodontic, and restorative treatment of pathologic migration of anterior teeth: a case report. Int J Periodontics Restorative Dent. 2006;26:501–6.

105. Wittneben JG, Buser D, Belser UC, Brägger U. Peri-implant soft tissue conditioning with provisional restorations in the esthetic zone: the dynamic compression technique. Int J Periodontics Restorative Dent. 2013;33:447–55.

106. Feuillet D, Keller JF, Agossa K. Interproximal tunneling with a customized connective tissue graft: a microsurgical technique for interdental papilla reconstruction. Int J Periodontics Restorative Dent. 2018;38:833–9.

107. Geurs NC, Romanos AH, Vassilopoulos PJ, Reddy MS. Efficacy of micronized acellular dermal graft for use in interproximal papillae regeneration. Int J Periodontics Restorative Dent. 2012;32:49–58.

108. Awartani FA, Tatakis DN. Interdental papilla loss: treatment by hyaluronic acid gel injection: a case series. Clin Oral Investig. 2016;20:1775–80.

109. Bertl K, Gotfredsen K, Jensen SS, Bruckmann C, Stavropoulos A. Can hyaluronan injections augment deficient papillae at implant-supported crowns in the anterior maxilla? A randomized controlled clinical trial with 6 months follow-up. Clin Oral Implants Res. 2017;28:1054–61.

110. Korayem M, Flores-Mir C, Nassar U, Olfert K. Implant site development by orthodontic extrusion. A systematic review. Angle Orthod. 2008;78:752–60.

111. Buskin R, Castellon P, Hochstedler JL. Orthodontic extrusion and orthodontic extraction in preprosthetic treatment using implant therapy. Pract Periodontics Aesthet Dent. 2000;12:213–9.

112. Viana PC, Kovacs Z, Correia A. Purpose of esthetic risk assessment in prosthetic rehabilitations with gingiva-shade ceramics. Int J Esthet Dent. 2014;9:480–9.

113. Burkhardt R, Hämmerle CHF, Lang NP, Research Group on Oral Soft Tissue Biology & Wound Healing. How do visual-spatial and psychomotor abilities influence clinical performance in periodontal plastic surgery? J Clin Periodontol. 2019;46:72–85.
114. Wetzel CM, Black SA, Hanna GB, Athanasiou T, Kneebone RL, Nestel D, Wolfe JH, Woloshynowych M. The effects of stress and coping on surgical performance during simulations. Ann Surg. 2010;251:171–6.
115. Renouard F, Amalberti R, Renouard E. Are "human factors" the primary cause of complications in the field of implant dentistry? Int J Oral Maxillofac Implants. 2017;32:e55–61.
116. Barone A, Toti P, Marconcini S, Derchi G, Saverio M, Covani U. Esthetic outcome of implants placed in fresh extraction sockets by clinicians with or without experience: a medium-term retrospective evaluation. Int J Oral Maxillofac Implants. 2016;31:1397–406.
117. Shanelec DA, Tibbetts LS. A perspective on the future of periodontal microsurgery. Periodontol 2000. 1996;11:58–64.
118. Tibbetts LS, Shanelec D. Periodontal microsurgery. Dent Clin N Am. 1998;42:339–59.
119. Nordland WP, Sandhu HS, Perio C. Microsurgical technique for augmentation of the interdental papilla: three case reports. Int J Periodontics Restorative Dent. 2008;28:543–9.